CARDIOVASCULAR PROCEDURES
Diagnostic Techniques and
Therapeutic Procedures

CARDIOVASCULAR PROCEDURES
Diagnostic Techniques and Therapeutic Procedures

ARA G. TILKIAN, M.D., F.A.C.C.

Assistant Clinical Professor of Medicine
University of California, Los Angeles;
Codirector of Cardiology, Holy Cross Hospital
Mission Hills, California

ELAINE KIESS DAILY, R.N., B.S., R.C.V.T.

Clinical Cardiac Research Nurse
Department of Cardiology at the
University of California—San Diego Medical Center;
Consultant and Lecturer, San Diego, California

with 462 illustrations

The C. V. Mosby Company
St. Louis • Washington, D.C. • Toronto   1986

MOSBY

A TRADITION OF PUBLISHING EXCELLENCE

Editor: Don Ladig
Assistant Editor: Maureen Slaten
Project Editor: Connie Povilat
Production Coordinator: Mark Spann

Great care has been used in compiling and checking the information
in this book to ensure its accuracy. However, because of changing technology,
new discoveries, and individualization of patient care, the uses, effects,
and dosages of drugs may vary from those given here. The medications
discussed do not necessarily have specific approval by the Food and Drug
Administration for use in the diseases and dosages for which they are recommended.
Equipment design and recommendations for use may also change.
We urge that you check the manufacturer's recommendations as given in the
package insert provided with each product.

Printed in the United States of America

The C.V. Mosby Company
11830 Westline Industrial Drive, St. Louis, Missouri 63146

Library of Congress Cataloging-in-Publication Data

Tilkian, Ara G., 1944-
    Cardiovascular procedures.

    Includes bibliographies and index.
    1. Cardiovascular system—Diseases.   I. Daily,
Elaine Kiess.   [DNLM: 1. Cardiovascular Diseases—
diagnosis. 2. Cardiovascular Diseases—therapy.
WG 141 T573c]
RC667.T54   1986   616.1   86-16268
ISBN 0-8016-4965-X

C/VH/VH 9 8 7 6 5 4 3 2   17/B/606

Contributors

DAVID S. CANNOM, M.D.
Director of Cardiology, The Hospital of the Good Samaritan;
Clinical Professor of Medicine, UCLA School of Medicine
Los Angeles, California

EDWARD L. CONOVER, B.S.E.E.
Clinical Consultant on Electrical Safety;
Manager, Electronic Design Automation Department
Missile Systems Group, Hughes Aircraft,
Canoga Park, California

MARY CONOVER, R.N, B.S.
Instructor and Education Consultant
West Hills Hospital, Canoga Park, California;
Santa Teresita Hospital, Duarte, California

JACK A. PATTERSON, M.D., F.A.C.C.
Director, Department of Cardiology
Valley Presbyterian Hospital
Van Nuys, California

HARRY W. REIN, M.D.
Director, Department of Neurology
Valley Presbyterian Hospital
Van Nuys, California

ISAAC WIENER, M.D., F.A.C.C., F.A.C.P.
Associate Director, Department of Cardiology
Valley Presbyterian Hospital;
Assistant Clinical Professor of Medicine
University of California
Los Angeles, California

ROGER A. WINKLE, M.D., F.A.C.C.
Director, Center for Cardiac Surveillance Unit;
Director, Electrophysiology Laboratory, Sequoia Hospital,
Redwood City, California

Consultants

EDWIN L. ALDERMAN, M.D., F.A.C.C.
Professor of Medicine (Cardiology);
Director, Cardiac Catheterization Laboratory
Stanford University Medical Center
Stanford, California

MARGARET E. BILLINGHAM, M.B., B.S., F.A.C.C.
Associate Professor of Pathology;
Director, Department of Cardiac Pathology
Stanford University Medical Center
Stanford, California

DAVID S. CANNOM, M.D.
Director, Department of Cardiology
The Hospital of the Good Samaritan;
Clinical Professor of Medicine
UCLA School of Medicine
Los Angeles, California

J. MICHAEL CRILEY, M.D.
Chief of Cardiology
Harbor–UCLA Medical Center
Torrance, California

KEVIN K. DRAKE, M.D.
Director, Department of Radiology
Holy Cross Hospital
Mission Hills, California

DONNA EARLEY, M.S.
Director, Department of Radiation and Environmental Safety
Cedars–Sinai Medical Center,
Los Angeles, California

JAMES S. FORRESTER, M.D.
Professor of Medicine, UCLA School of Medicine;
Associate Director, Department of Cardiology
Cedars-Sinai Medical Center,
Los Angeles, California

WILLIAM J. FRENCH, M.D.
Associate Professor of Medicine, UCLA School of Medicine
Los Angeles, California;
Director, Cardiac Catheterization Laboratory
Harbor–UCLA Medical Center
Torrance, California

JULIUS H. GROLLMAN, Jr., M.D.
Clinical Professor of Radiology, UCLA School of Medicine
Los Angeles, California;
Chief, Cardiovascular Radiology
Little Company of Mary Hospital
Torrance, California

PETER M. GUZY, M.D., Ph.D., F.A.C.C.
Associate Professor of Medicine;
Director, Pacemaker Clinic
UCLA Medical Center
Los Angeles, California

E. WILLIAM HANCOCK, M.D.
Professor of Medicine
Division of Cardiology
Stanford University Medical Center
Stanford, California

STEVEN R. HIRSCHTICK, Esq.
Former Professor of Law, Loyola Law School
Los Angeles, California;
Partner in the Law Firm of Hirschtick, Chenen,
Lemon, and Curtis
Los Angeles, California

RICHARD E. KERBER, M.D.
Professor of Medicine
Cardiovascular Division
The University of Iowa
Iowa City, Iowa

JAY W. MASON, M.D.
Professor of Medicine and Chief of Cardiology
University of Utah Medical Center
Salt Lake City, Utah

JAMES T. NIEMANN, M.D.
Director of Emergency Services
Harbor–UCLA Medical Center
Torrance, California

STEPHEN OESTERLE, M.D.
Assistant Professor of Medicine;
Director, Unit for Coronary Interventions
Stanford University Medical Center,
Stanford, California

SUSAN J. QUAAL, R.N., C.V.S., M.S., C.C.R.N.
Cardiovascular Clinical Specialist
Veterans Administration Medical Center;
Adjunct Associate Clinical Professor University of Utah
Salt Lake City, Utah

STERLING SCOTT REESE, M.D.
Assistant Professor of Medicine, UCLA School of Medicine
Los Angeles, California;
Chief of Cardiology
Olive View Medical Center
Sylmar, California

JOHN B. SIMPSON, M.D., Ph.D., F.A.C.C.
Attending Physician, Sequoia Hospital
Redwood City, California

C.F. STARMER, Ph.D.
Professor of Computer Science;
Associate Professor of Medicine
Duke University Medical Center
Durham, North Carolina

DAN TICH, B.S.E.E.
Group Product Marketing Manager
Cardiac Pacemakers, Inc.
St. Paul, Minnesota

Dedicated to **Mary Conover,** Master Teacher,
without whose tireless sacrifice
this book could not have been completed.

Foreword

The rapid increase in and sophistication of invasive cardiovascular procedures and interventional cardiology during the past decade have resulted in a remarkable ability to diagnose and treat the cardiovascular patient. Older procedures such as pericardiocentesis and pacing have undergone rapid technologic changes, whereas procedures such as acute thrombolytic therapy and angioplasty for an acute myocardial infarction have been developed. During this time we have learned a great deal about the normal and pathophysiologic function of the cardiovascular system: hemodynamic and electrophysiologic monitoring are used routinely in treating seriously ill cardiovascular patients.

At the same time, our choices of access routes, catheters, and basic techniques to obtain cardiovascular information or to treat the cardiovascular patient continue to expand. *Cardiovascular Procedures* is remarkable in its scope and depth of coverage of a complicated and diverse subject. At the same time, the authors maintain a sense of organization, clarity, and brevity through liberal use of diagrams and tables.

In reading *Cardiovascular Procedures* one realizes the advantage of a one- or two-author book on cardiovascular techniques in contrast to the more common method, with each chapter written by a different author. The book is concise yet thorough in taking the reader through each procedure step by step. Different, commonly accepted approaches or techniques are presented with the advantages and disadvantages discussed.

Because of its scope this book is valuable for everyone responsible for the care of the cardiovascular patient. I strongly recommend it to the browser, the student, and the experienced cardiologist. Each will benefit in a different way, and the information is timely, accurate, and of utmost importance.

John S. Schroeder, M.D.

Professor of Medicine (Cardiology)
Stanford University Medical Center
Stanford, CA 94305

Preface

This is a book for physicians and nurses who perform cardiovascular procedures. There are areas of special interest to trainees in Cardiovascular Medicine, practicing Cardiologists, Cardiovascular Radiologists, and specialists in Critical Care, Emergency Medicine, and Cardiovascular Nursing. The text provides illustrated, in-depth coverage of commonly performed cardiovascular diagnostic and therapeutic procedures. The emphasis on procedural technique provides sufficient detail for the beginner and adequate depth for the experienced operator so that it is not only a useful text for training, but serves as a comprehensive resource in daily practice. Its use by the novice should be in conjunction with closely supervised teaching programs.

We have chosen to describe the procedures in great detail. The rationale for each procedure is fully discussed, including indications, contraindications, and risks. When more than one technique is used for a particular procedure, we describe the method with which we have had most success. When controversies or alternate methods exist, they are discussed and referenced. A very useful section of each chapter concerns how to avoid trouble or, if difficulties are encountered, how to resolve them. The personnel necessary to perform the procedure and their responsibilities are defined. Patient preparation, premedication, complications, management, and aftercare are covered in detail. Clinical interpretations and use of data obtained, or an in-depth discussion of the clinical aspects of procedures, are beyond the scope of this book. Sufficient detail is given to place the procedure in its clinical context and the reader is directed to the excellent texts on cardiovascular medicine.

The basics on the tools and techniques of vascular access, hemodynamic monitoring, and cardiac catheterization are covered in the first five chapters. This is followed by an in-depth presentation on the diagnostic techniques of pulmonary angiography, endomyocardial biopsy, and electrophysiologic studies. Commonly performed therapeutic procedures that are described step by step include pericardiocentesis, intra-aortic balloon pumping, cardioversion, and use of pacemakers. The rapidly evolving techniques of coronary angioplasty, thrombolytic therapy, and use of the implanted automatic cardioverter/defibrillator are among the procedures covered in detail. A very useful chapter deals with the retrieval of catheter fragments and resolution of intracardiac catheter knots. The chapter on emergency resuscitation is on the cutting edge of new concepts in cardiopulmonary and cerebral resuscitation. Throughout this book, the emphasis is placed on how to perform a procedure safely. Thus, we complete the text with a discussion on how to avoid or minimize the risks related to the use of contrast media, radiation, and electrical current. Medicolegal considerations are briefly discussed. We have included several appendixes of material that we have found useful in our daily practice.

The information in this book has been kept up to date through current literature and input from nationally recognized authorities who reviewed chapters in their particular field of expertise. We solicited and welcomed this critical review from our panel of consultants, but do not hold them responsible for any deficiencies in this text. This responsibility lies solely with the authors. We believe it possible that someone, somewhere, has a better way of performing a procedure. We welcome comments from our readers who would like to share their techniques with us.

Ara G. Tilkian
Elaine Kiess Daily

Acknowledgments

The names of our consultants have been listed on a separate page. They cannot be thanked enough for so generously sharing with us their vast knowledge. Their genuine interest in and critical review of the manuscript reflected their own goals of excellence in their field of expertise. For this we are most grateful.

We also wish to thank the following physicians who reviewed various sections of the manuscript: Jeffrey Aaronson, M.D., Ronald Accomozzo, M.D., John Alexander, M.D., Pat O. Daily, M.D., Walter P. Dembitsky, M.D., and Paul Sussman, M.D. We are grateful for the important contributions that they so generously and willingly made.

We are grateful to librarians Lucille Moss and Francine Kubrin for their prompt, cheerful, and thorough responses to our many requests for references and for making the library facilities available to us.

The technical help of Barbara Learned, R.N., Lana Kirkman, R.N., Tyra Solich, R.N., Erwin Schwarz, C.R.T., Bill Masters, R.T.R., C.V.T., and Eben Kermit and the photographic skills of Robert W. Williams are greatly appreciated.

Our medical illustrator was Phyllis Stookey with help from Don and Deanna Hockett.

Manufacturers of cardiovascular products were very responsive to our requests for specifications, information, and illustrations, easing our task considerably.

Special thanks are due to Brian Bates and Bruce Jingles of Cook, Inc., Karen Spivey of Oximetrix, Marsha Halfman-Franey of American Edwards Laboratories, Carl Simpson of Advanced Cardiovascular Systems, and Paul La Violette of USCI.

Elaine Daily would like to thank Dr. Kirk Peterson and the staff of the Cardiac Catheterization Laboratory at the University of California Medical Center, San Diego, for tirelessly answering questions and providing up-to-date information. In addition, she would like to thank her family, especially her daughter, Auburn, who showed understanding beyond her years and never complained when her mother had to "burn the midnight oil" to complete this text.

Ara Tilkian would like to thank his associates, Leonard P. Haber, M.D., and David Y. Naruse, M.D., who shared freely with him their vast experience in invasive cardiology, as well as Jack A. Patterson, M.D., and Isaac Wiener, M.D., who contributed to this book and carried extra burden when he was "on call" in the library. Finally, he would like to express his appreciation to his wife, Elizabeth, who shared with him the pain and the joy of completing this work.

Ara G. Tilkian
Elaine Kiess Daily

Contents

Detailed Contents

Part I

DIAGNOSTIC PROCEDURES

Chapter One

Tools for catheterization

ELAINE K. DAILY
ARA G. TILKIAN

The tools for catheterization, for either diagnostic or monitoring purposes, consist of catheters, guidewires, needles, introducers, transducers, and protective sleeve adaptors. These basic tools are available in a myriad of varieties that can be quite confusing. Some variations are dictated by function, while others are minor design alterations selected by the manufacturer. The aim of this chapter is to shed some light on the construction, design, use, and availability of commonly used catheterization equipment.

CATHETERS

Invasive diagnostic cardiology as a practice in medicine began in the 1940s with the investigative studies of Andre Cournand and Dickinson Richards.[1-3] In his Nobel lecture in 1956, Cournand stated that "the cardiac catheter was . . . the key in the lock."[4] Certainly this key has unlocked the door to expanded diagnostic capabilities and therapeutic interventions.

Material

The original cardiac catheters were rubber ureteral catheters—the only ones commercially available before World War II. After the war, numerous other inert materials that had been developed for industrial use became available. A few of these have been found suitable for medical applications. It is only within the past two decades that catheter materials have been chosen on the basis of biologic response rather than physical properties.[5] However, the perfect catheter material has not yet been developed, and compromises must continually be made when the diagnostic tool is selected. Alterations in the characteristics of the particular plastic often occur when material is incorporated to make the catheter radiopaque. Despite this, it is always desirable to utilize radiopaque catheters for any procedure.

Dacron

Catheters made of woven Dacron are very maneuverable and flexible. Most woven Dacron catheters are covered with a polyurethane coating to increase surface smoothness and reduce vascular trauma. Some Dacron angiographic catheters are reinforced with a nylon core to increase bursting pressure and thereby allow higher flow rates of contrast media for angiography. Nylon has great physical and mechanical strength and also has a reduced friction coefficient, which improves contrast media flow rates. *Examples:* USCI Cournand, "birdseye," Eppendorf, and Sones catheters.

Polyurethane

Catheters extruded from polyurethane have an excellent tensile properties memory (they recover their original shape well at body temperature). This is a particularly desirable feature for superselective preformed catheters whose tip design may be altered during insertion and manipulation. Polyurethane catheters are also somewhat softer than those made of polyethylene or Teflon, which reduces the risk of vascular trauma or perforation. This feature often permits easier, smoother passage of the catheter in a tortuous vascular system. While polyurethane may be associated with increased thrombogenicity, this can be countered with systemic administration of heparin, which can be reversed at the end of the procedure. Polyurethane can be reshaped if immersed in boiling water or exposed to steam for varying periods of time, depending on wall thickness. *Examples:* Cordis Corp. pigtail angiographic catheters and the original Judkins coronary catheters.

Polyethylene

Polyethylene is utilized in both preformed and custom-made catheters. Its degree of stiffness lies somewhere between the stiffness of polyurethane and that of Teflon. Because polyethylene does not soften much at body temperature, it also maintains its shape and thus is very popular for selective catheterization. This material can also be easily reshaped by means of the method described later in this chapter. This is a desirable feature when the patient's size or anatomy requires a change in the catheter's preformed shape. Recent data suggest that polyethylene catheters tend to be more thrombogenic than catheters made of polyvinylchloride (PVC), polyurethane, or silicone rubber.[6] Therefore, systemic administration of heparin is recommended. Some preformed polyethylene angiographic catheters (Torcon) also have an inner stainless steel mesh braid, which improves the rotational control of the catheter and increases the catheter's bursting point so that greater injection pressures can be used. *Examples:* Cook pigtail angiographic catheters, Judkins catheters, National Institutes of Health (NIH) catheters, and Cournand catheters.

Teflon

Teflon catheters are the stiffest vascular catheters. The advantage of Teflon is its extremely low friction coefficient, which reduces vascular trauma, increases ease of insertion and passage, and improves flow rates of contrast media. A low friction coefficient is also an important characteristic whenever anything will be passed through the catheter or sheath. Teflon has poor curve memory and is therefore more appropriate for nonselective catheterization and angiography where placement does not depend on specific catheter curve. If necessary, Teflon catheters can be reshaped, but the use of a heat gun is required to reach a temperature of 750° F. Unfortunately, Teflon's poor memory does not promote retention of the new shape. *Examples:* Brockenbrough catheters (Cook, Inc.), transducer-tip catheters, and introducer sheaths.

Polyvinylchloride

PVC catheters are softer than catheters of the aforementioned materials. This characteristic makes the material quite supple and flexible and therefore ideal for flow-directed catheters. PVC has a high friction coefficient, which may reduce ease of catheter passage and increase the incidence of venous spasm. PVC catheters are also associated with increased thrombogenicity,

have very poor tensile properties (memory), and cannot be reformed.

Of all the commonly used catheter materials, PVC is the most hydrophilic, with a high rate of moisture absorption (Table 1-1). Of particular importance is the absorption of certain drugs by the PVC material of the catheter. Drugs reported to be absorbed include nitroglycerin, isosorbide, insulin, diazepam, thiopental, and chlordiazepoxide.[7,8] The loss of drugs to the catheter material occurs rapidly during the initial administration. Concentration eventually returns to normal after binding sites in the plastic become saturated (approximately 20 to 30 minutes). This delay in drug delivery should be considered when these drugs are administered through PVC catheters and intravenous (IV) tubing. The clinical importance of this observation has not been fully validated and may not be of concern when drugs are titrated according to symptomatic response, such as with nitroglycerin. *Examples:* Balloon-tip, flow-directed catheters and triple-lumen right atrial catheters.

Design

The ideal cardiac catheter is one that provides the most accurate information (hemodynamic pressures and angiographic opacification) with no risk to the patient. Unfortunately, such a catheter is not available, and compromises must often be made between the two ideals, with the patient's safety receiving first consideration.

Some basic design features that are important for successful catheterization include material used, curve shape, flexibility, memory, catheter tip, end and side holes, and catheter hub.

Material

The types of materials used in construction of cardiac catheters have already been discussed. Selection of a particular material should be dictated by the purpose and need for its application. However, at times there are no options with regard to material, as the catheter

Table 1-1. Characteristics of catheter materials

Characteristic	Teflon	Polyethylene	Polyurethane	PVC
Friction coefficient (f = F/W)	0.04	0.21	1.35	2.0
Stiffness	+4	+3	+2	+1
Memory (curve retention)	Good with very high heat	Excellent	Excellent	Fair
Moisture absorption (%/24 hours)	0	0.015	0.9	0.75

f, Friction coefficient; *F,* force required to move a 5 lb. weight over a nonlubricated polished surface; *W,* 5 lbs.

of a desired shape may be available in only one type of material (e.g., the Brockenbrough or balloon flotation catheter). Catheter surfaces should be smooth with low friction coefficients to reduce trauma at the puncture site as well as along the endothelia. Catheter stiffness has been implicated as an important factor in thrombus formation of central venous catheters.[9,10] Virtually all intravascular catheters are thrombogenic (some more so than others).[6] For this reason, systemic administration of heparin is necessary to reduce thrombus formation during catheterization.

Certain catheter materials are hydrophilic, resulting in the absorption of water or moisture over time. This absorption leads to softening and weakening of the catheter. In addition, certain drugs are absorbed into plastic, resulting in inaccurate drug delivery (see p. 4). Teflon is the only catheter material that absorbs no water or moisture. (See Table 1-1.)

Curve shape

The curve shape of the catheter tip is an important consideration in catheters used for selective angiographic studies. Preformed catheters are available in an array of primary and secondary curvatures to facilitate selective placement and positional stability of the catheter. In addition, polyethylene and polyurethane tubing can be custom shaped to any particular curve shape required (see p. 18). A nonspecific, gentle curve in preformed catheters is adequate for many purposes, including pressure measurements and nonselective catheter placement.

Flexibility

The construction of the catheter determines its flexibility and the safety and ease with which it can be manipulated. The ability to finely control the rotation or torque of the catheter's tip by manipulation of the catheter's hub is an essential feature for successful selective catheterization. Catheters with an inner stainless steel wire braid provide the greatest amount of torque transmission. However, the tip of these catheters remains flexible (without braiding) to allow safe, atraumatic selective vascular entry (e.g., Sones coronary catheter and Schoonmaker-King multipurpose catheter). Catheters with a flexible tip and a stiffer shaft may also be useful in tortuous vessels.

Memory

Memory is the ability of the catheter to resume or keep its original preformed shape and is a function of the material used in catheter construction. Catheters with preformed curves often must be straightened with a guidewire to permit passage through the vascular system. It is important that upon removal of the guidewire, the catheter resumes its original preformed curve. It is also important that at body temperature the catheter does not soften sufficiently to lose its preformed curve. Both polyurethane and (to a lesser extent) polyethylene have good curve memory. Some Dacron and polyethylene catheters (e.g., Sones and Schoonmaker-King catheters) can be shaped or reshaped intravascularly with brief, transient curve retention. This technique requires experience and a thorough knowledge of intravascular anatomy. Neither PVC nor Teflon retains shape well.

Tip

The catheter tip should be neither blunt nor too sharp and should be soft and flexible. Catheters with a slightly tapered ("bullet-nose") tip produce the least amount of trauma during insertion and reduce the risk of vascular dissection, which can occur with the passage of blunt-tip catheters. However, too sharp a taper, producing a pointed tip, can increase the risk of catheter tip penetration and should be avoided. The soft and flexible catheter tip helps to avoid damage to the endothelium or subendocardium.

End and side holes

Most multipurpose cardiac catheters have an end hole at the tip of the catheter, permitting percutaneous introduction over a guidewire. (Before the widespread use of catheter introducer sheaths, all catheters inserted percutaneously required an end hole for insertion over a guidewire. This is no longer a requirement for percutaneous catheterization.) Although the presence of an end hole at the tip of the angiographic catheter allows more complete flushing of the catheter, thus reducing the risk of thrombus formation at the tip, the absence of an end hole (with only side holes) reduces the risk of intramural injection of contrast medium and catheter recoil during angiography.

Staggered side holes near the distal portion of the catheter are advantageous in angiographic catheters because they permit rapid delivery of large boluses of contrast medium. However, the risk of clot formation is increased with multihole catheters, necessitating more vigorous aspiration and manual flushing.

Although the pigtail catheter does possess an end hole, its coiled tip places the end hole back inside the curve, away from the endocardium; staggered placement of 4 to 12 side holes allows ejection of most of the contrast material via the side holes rather than the end hole, thereby reducing catheter recoil and the risk of intramural injection. These features have made the pigtail angiographic catheter the most widely used catheter for ventricular or aortic angiography.

Hub

Whether the catheter hub is made of plastic or metal, it should not be significantly smaller than the lumen of the catheter. Such narrowing could markedly affect the rate of injection of contrast medium. If metal catheter hubs are used, Teflon guidewires should be inserted through them with caution, lest the Teflon coating be abraded. Tapered hubs permit easier insertion of a guidewire.

Sizes
Diameter

The outside diameter of cardiac catheters continues to be measured in French (Fr) gauge (1 Fr = 0.335 mm or 0.013 inches), which was the standard measurement of the ureteral catheters originally used in cardiac catheterization. Some manufacturers have color coded their catheters to facilitate size identification. Actual measurement of the inside and outside diameters of the catheter (in millimeters) provides a more accurate assessment of size as well as essential information for ap-

propriate selection of corresponding components (i.e., guidewires and sheaths). The outside diameter (in millimeters) of a catheter can quickly be determined by dividing the French gauge by 3. The inside diameter of the catheter will vary depending on the thickness of the catheter wall. Table 1-2 lists the French gauges and diameters of cardiovascular catheters.

Size selection

Catheter size selection represents a compromise between use of the largest size possible for more accurate pressures and faster delivery of large boluses of dye and use of the smallest size possible to reduce the risk of vascular trauma, thrombus formation, or bleeding.

Accurate waveforms can best be obtained with an 8 Fr or larger catheter and a minimal amount of plumbing equipment (tubing, stopcocks, etc.). The decreased lumen size of a 6 or 7 Fr catheter results in resonance that artifactually accentuates the pressure waveform, with early systolic overshoot and diastolic dips. Some cardiac catheters are available in a thin-wall version, which provides an increased inside diameter with the same outside diameter. This not only improves hemodynamic pressure measurement and blood sampling and flushing abilities but also decreases the risk of thrombus formation. However, thin-wall catheters possess less torque control and are less suitable for high-pressure injection of contrast media.

A 7 or 8 Fr catheter is suitable for cardiac catheterization and angiography in most adults. Smaller catheters (5 Fr) are popular for outpatient angiographic procedures in adults.

Length

Catheter length selection is determined by the insertion site and the desired eventual location of the catheter tip. In general, the catheter should be no longer than necessary to reach the intended location. Long catheters reduce operator control of the catheter tip, require a higher pressure injection for rapid delivery of contrast material, and alter the pressure waveform. Increased length and size of catheters, as well as prolonged catheterization times, predispose to thrombus formation. Right heart catheters for adults are generally 100 to 125 cm long, with a shorter catheter suitable for internal jugular vein insertion. Left heart catheters are generally 100 to 110 cm long; this is usually sufficient for placement of the catheter tip in the left ventricle (LV) via the femoral artery approach. Occasionally, in the case of a very tall person, this length does not allow proper placement. In this case a longer (125 cm) catheter will usually suffice.

Table 1-2. Size specifications for cardiovascular catheters

	Inside diameter		Outside diameter	
Size (Fr)	Inch	mm	Inch	mm
Standard wall				
4	0.018	0.46	0.052	1.33
5	0.026	0.66	0.065	1.67
6	0.036	0.91	0.078	2.00
7	0.046	1.17	0.091	2.33
8	0.056	1.42	0.104	2.67
9	0.064	1.63	0.118	3.00
10	0.072	1.83	0.131	3.33
11	0.083	2.11	0.144	3.67
12	0.094	2.39	0.157	4.00
14	0.144	2.90	0.183	4.67
Thin wall				
4	0.023	0.58	0.052	1.33
5	0.034	0.86	0.065	1.67
6	0.046	1.17	0.078	2.00
7	0.058	1.47	0.091	2.33
8	0.068	1.73	0.104	2.67
9	0.078	1.98	0.118	3.00
10	0.088	2.24	0.131	3.33
11	0.098	2.49	0.144	3.67
12	0.108	2.74	0.157	4.00
14	0.128	3.25	0.183	4.67

General-purpose right heart catheters
Cournand catheter (Fig. 1-1)

Originally designed by Andre Cournand in 1939, the Cournand catheter was the first catheter specifically made for use in the heart.

CONSTRUCTION: The Cournand catheter is a standard-wall, end-hole radiopaque woven Dacron catheter with an outer coating of polyurethane. It has a very gradual distal curve, which lends itself well to passage through the right side of the heart. It is reusable.

USE: This is an all-purpose right heart catheter used in the cardiac catheterization laboratory for pressure measurements, including wedge pressure and blood sampling.

SIZES: The Cournand catheter is available in sizes 5 through 8 Fr, with 100 and 125 cm lengths.

Lehman catheter (Fig. 1-2)

CONSTRUCTION: The Lehman catheter is a thin-wall variation of the Cournand catheter with a slightly shorter distal curve. Its thinner wall increases the inside diameter of the catheter and decreases its stiffness. It is reusable. (*Note:* This catheter should not be confused with the Lehman ventriculography catheter.)

USE: Use of the Lehman catheter is the same as that of the Cournand catheter.

SIZES: It is available in sizes 4 through 9 Fr, with 50, 80, 100, and 125 cm lengths.

Goodale-Lubin catheter (Fig. 1-3)

CONSTRUCTION: The Goodale-Lubin catheter is constructed of woven Dacron coated wtih polyurethane. Unique characteristics are the two laterally opposed side holes near the distal open end (sometimes referred to as a "birdseye" because of these oval side holes near the tip). It is reusable.

USE: The Goodale-Lubin catheter is a standard catheter used in the cardiac catheterization laboratory for routine right heart pressure measurements and blood sampling.

SIZES: It is available in sizes 4 through 8 Fr, with 80, 100, and 125 cm lengths.

VARIATIONS: There are standard-wall and thin-wall versions of this catheter. The curve of the standard-wall variation resembles the curve of the Cournand catheter, while the curve of the thin-wall type resembles that of the Lehman catheter.

DISADVANTAGES: Although the inside diameter of the thin-wall catheter is somewhat larger than that of the standard-wall variety, the thin-wall catheter is less radiopaque and its reduced stiffness may inhibit passage through the heart. This catheter is also not suited for obtaining an accurate pulmonary artery wedge pressure (PAWP).

Balloon flotation catheters (Fig. 1-4)

CONSTRUCTION: Balloon flotation catheters are PVC, multilumened, right heart catheters wtih a balloon at the tip, which, when inflated with air, carries the catheter along with the blood flow through the right side of the heart and into the pulmonary artery (PA), allowing measurement of PA pressure (PAP) and PAWP.

USE: These catheters are employed for diagnostic purposes in the cardiac catheterization laboratory or for continuous bedside hemodynamic monitoring. They can be used for either short- or long-term measurement of right heart pressures (including PAWP), and allow

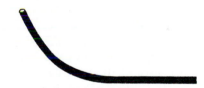

Fig. 1-1. Cournand catheter.

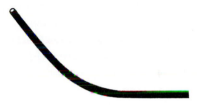

Fig. 1-2. Lehman catheter.

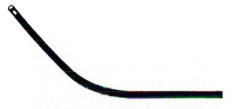

Fig. 1-3. Goodale-Lubin catheter.

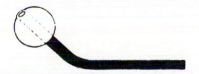

Fig. 1-4. Balloon flotation catheter.

blood sampling and cardiac output measurement via the thermodilution method. PAWP can be obtained through the distal port by inflation of the balloon of the catheter, which carries the catheter tip forward and occludes the lumen of the vessel proximal to the tip.

The balloon flotation catheter is particularly useful for catheterization in children, in whom exact anatomy is not always predictable. However, its greatest use is for continuous bedside monitoring of the critically ill patient.

SIZES: Standard adult sizes are 5, 7, and 7.5 Fr, 110 cm long. Pediatric sizes are 4 and 5 Fr, 60 cm long. The balloon capacity of the different sizes varies and is marked on the hub of the catheter (Table 1-3).

ADVANTAGES: The ease and accuracy of obtaining PAWP have been markedly improved with the use of the balloon flotation catheter. Its flotation feature permits passage without the use of fluoroscopy, thereby allowing bedside insertion and positioning of the catheter. When used in the cardiac catheterization laboratory, it markedly reduces the time and use of fluoroscopy for right heart catheterization. Because the inflated balloon protrudes slightly beyond the tip of the catheter, trauma to the endocardium is prevented, the incidence of arrhythmias during catheter manipulation is reduced, and the complication of cardiac perforation is essentially eliminated.

DISADVANTAGES: The soft, flexible nature of the PVC balloon flotation catheter may present difficulties in passage, with looping of the catheter in the right atrium (RA) or right ventricle (RV) and predisposing to catheter knotting, particularly when these chambers are enlarged and cardiac output is low. Prolonged catheter insertion time further softens the catheter and prevents

Table 1-3. Balloon capacity of flotation catheters

Catheter	Size (Fr)	Balloon capacity (cc)
Berman angiographic	4	0.5
	5	0.75
	6	1.0
	7	1.25
	8	1.25
Bynum-Wilson	7	1.5
	8	1.5
Swan-Ganz	4	0.5
	5	0.75
	7	1.5
	7.5	1.5

successful passage out to the PA. Injection of sterile, iced saline solution into the catheter may stiffen it temporarily. The adult-size catheter (7 or 7.5 Fr) allows insertion of an 0.025-inch (0.6 mm) guidewire into the distal port if further stiffening is required. An 0.018-inch (0.46 mm) and an 0.014-inch (0.36 mm) guidewire can be inserted through the 6 and 5 Fr catheters, respectively.

VARIATIONS: Balloon flotation catheters are available with two to five lumens, a distal thermistor for thermodilution measurement of cardiac output, and a ventricular pacing wire.

The two-lumen catheter has a distal port for PAP and PAWP monitoring and one lumen for the balloon. The three-lumen catheter has the distal port for PAP and PAWP monitoring and a proximal port for RAP monitoring. The four-lumen catheter has all of these features plus a thermistor and computer connecting cable for thermodilution cardiac output measurements (Fig. 1-5). The five-lumen catheter has an additional RA port for infusion of fluid or drugs without interruption during cardiac output measurements.

A four-lumen Swan-Ganz thermodilution catheter is also available with a lumen that terminates near the thermistor. This lumen has no distal port and is intended only for the insertion of an 0.025- or 0.028-inch guidewire. It is intended for use in patients in whom insertion is anticipated to be difficult or prolonged (patients with large RA or RV, tricuspid regurgitation, or pulmonary hypertension), where increased catheter stiffness may be needed to avoid catheter coiling and encourage forward flow.

A recent innovation in the conventional balloon flotation PA catheter involves fiberoptics for continuous monitoring of the oxygen saturation of mixed venous blood (Svo_2) when the catheter is attached to a bedside microprocessor. This feature allows physiologic integration and is particularly desirable for monitoring critically ill patients. Increases in the number of lumens within the catheter may increase its functional capabilities, but they also increase the likelihood of dampened pressure waveforms and the risk of clotting.

Balloon flotation catheters without recessed balloons require use of a sheath that is one-half to one French size larger than the catheter to accommodate the balloon.

Angiographic catheters
Gensini catheter (Fig. 1-6)

CONSTRUCTION: The Gensini catheter is made of woven Dacron with a polyurethane coating and three pairs (six) of laterally opposed oval side holes within

1.5 cm of its open tip. The tip is tapered to provide a close fit over the appropriate-size guidewire.

USE: The catheter is intended specifically for percutaneous insertion into the right or left side of the heart for purposes of retrograde aortic and ventricular as well as pulmonary and vena caval angiographic studies.

SIZES: The Gensini catheter is available in sizes 5 through 8 Fr, with 80, 100, and 125 cm lengths. The tapered tips of the 5 and 6 Fr catheters fit an 0.025-inch (0.6 mm) guidewire; the 7 and 8 Fr catheters fit on 0.035-inch (0.9 mm) or 0.045-inch (1.1 mm) guidewires.

DISADVANTAGES: The straight tip of this catheter is more arrhythmogenic than the tip of a pigtail catheter and often recoils during injection of contrast medium, particularly at high flow rates. The risk of intramyocardial injection and myocardial perforation is also increased with this straight-tip end-hole catheter.

National Institutes of Health catheter (Fig. 1-7)

CONSTRUCTION AND VARIATIONS: The National Institutes of Health (NIH) catheter is a closed-end, side-hole catheter with a gentle curve. It is available in two versions, made by USCI and Cook, Inc. The USCI version has six side holes near its flexible tip. It is a thin-wall catheter constructed of woven Dacron reinforced with a nylon core, which permits injections at very high flow rates.

The Cook catheter has either four or six side holes near its tip and is constructed of polyethylene with an inner stainless steel braid (Torcon Blue), which imparts rotational control to the catheter shaft (improved torque) and allows higher injection pressures. However, the flow rates achievable with this NIH catheter are lower than those possible with the USCI version.

USE: The NIH catheter is used for angiographic visualization of either the RV or LV, the arterial or pulmonary vasculature, and the great veins. It was originally designed for insertion via an arteriotomy. However, the use of vascular sheaths now permits percutaneous insertion of this closed-end catheter.

SIZES: The USCI NIH catheter is available in sizes 5 through 8 Fr and lengths of 50, 80, 100, and 125 cm. The Cook NIH catheter is available in sizes 6.5, 7.3, and 8.2 Fr, all 100 cm long.

DISADVANTAGES: The NIH catheter is stiff and may recoil and cause extrasystoles. The risk of cardiac perforation is considerable in inexperienced hands.

Eppendorf catheter (USCI) (Fig. 1-8)

CONSTRUCTION: The Eppendorf catheter is a thin-wall catheter of woven Dacron with polyurethane coating. Its distinguishing feature, however, is that only the area 20 cm proximal to the hub of the catheter is reinforced with nylon fibers, thus making this catheter less stiff than the NIH catheter while permitting torque control and the ability to withstand high-pressure injections. The design of the Eppendorf catheter is similar to that of the NIH catheter, with a closed end and six laterally opposed side holes.

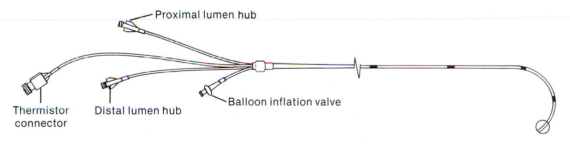

Fig. 1-5. Four-lumen thermodilution balloon flotation catheter.

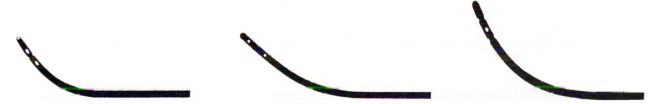

Fig. 1-6. Gensini angiographic catheter.

Fig. 1-7. NIH catheter.

Fig. 1-8. Eppendorf catheter.

USE: Uses of the Eppendorf catheter are the same as those of the NIH catheter.

SIZES: The catheter is available in sizes 7 and 8 Fr, either 100 or 125 cm long.

Lehman ventriculography catheter

CONSTRUCTION: The Lehman ventriculography catheter is a thin-wall, closed-end, woven Dacron catheter with polyurethane coating. The unique feature of this catheter is its slightly curved tip, tapered to 5 Fr, with four side holes beginning 2.5 cm from the tip.

USE: This catheter is usually fairly stable in the LV and is designed primarily for left ventriculography.

SIZES: It is available in sizes 5 through 8 Fr, with 80, 100, and 125 cm lengths.

ADVANTAGES: The tapered tip makes this catheter useful for traversing a tortuous subclavian system or for crossing a tight aortic valve. In addition, the location of its side holes allows one to calculate a left ventricular/aortic pressure gradient by means of a pull-back technique without removing the tip of the catheter from the LV.

DISADVANTAGES: If the LV chamber is very small, it is possible for the curved tip of the Lehman ventriculography catheter to come in contact with the wall of the ventricle before the side holes are within the ventricular chamber.[11]

Pigtail angiographic catheters (Fig. 1-9)

CONSTRUCTION: A pigtail angiographic catheter is made of polyurethane or polyethylene with a tapered tip, the terminal 5 cm of which is coiled back onto itself in a tight loop ("pigtail"). The catheter is available with an open or closed end with 4 to 12 non–laterally opposed side holes located in the terminal 5 cm of the catheter.

While pigtail catheters with 12 side holes are commonly used, there is evidence to indicate that a catheter with four to six side holes performs as well in terms of catheter recoil, reduced ventricular irritability, and absence of intramyocardial injection during angiography.[12,13]

USE: This is the most commonly used catheter for left ventricular and aortic angiography and is also successfully used for pulmonary angiography.[14]

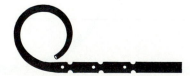

Fig. 1-9. Pigtail angiographic catheter.

Pigtail catheters were designed in the 1960s to allow safer passage across cardiac valves and safer injection of contrast medium into the ventricles and great vessels. An end-hole pigtail catheter may be useful in evaluation of hypertrophic heart disease because it provides a single port for pressure monitoring and the ability to fluoroscopically verify that the end hole is free within the ventricle.

ADVANTAGES: The coiled tip reduces the incidence of ventricular arrhythmias, catheter recoil, intramyocardial injection, and cardiac perforation. This type of catheter is the least traumatic with the exception of the balloon flotation catheter. The pigtail coil easily crosses the normal aortic valve, but usually the tip must be straightened with a slightly protruding guidewire to cross a stenotic aortic valve.

DISADVANTAGES: The risk of thrombus formation is increased with all pigtail catheters because of the inability to adequately flush the terminal portion of the coiled tip (beyond the side holes). It is therefore recommended that the catheter be forcibly aspirated and manually flushed every 3 to 5 minutes in the heparinized patient. A reduction in the number of side holes should permit more effective manual flushing and therefore reduce the incidence of thrombus formation. In addition, it is recommended that multihole pigtail catheters be utilized primarily for injection of contrast media and not for prolonged hemodynamic data collection.

Torcon Blue or Green pigtail catheter (Cook, Inc.)

CONSTRUCTION: Torcon Blue and Green catheters are of polyethylene with an inner stainless steel braid for better torque control and the ability to withstand high injection pressures.

USE: They are intended for angiographic studies of the LV, aorta, and vena cava.

SIZES: These catheters are available in sizes 6.5, 7.3, and 8.2 Fr, with 65, 80, 100, and 110 cm lengths and the option of 4, 6, 8, or 12 spiraled side holes.

Positrol II pigtail catheter (USCI)

CONSTRUCTION: The Positrol II catheter is made of polyurethane with an inner stainless steel braid. It is available with a standard-coil pigtail as well as a tighter coiled, smaller radius pigtail.

USE: This catheter is employed for angiographic studies of the LV and aorta.

SIZES: It is available in sizes 7 and 8 Fr, 110 cm long, with eight non–laterally opposed side holes, which minimize the weakening of the catheter at the side holes.

Nycore high-flow pigtail catheter (USCI)

CONSTRUCTION: The Nycore catheter has a permanently bonded jacket of polyurethane over a thin nylon

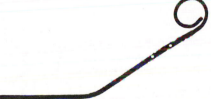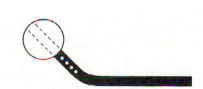

core. The unique feature of the nycore pigtail catheter is its larger inside diameter. Therefore, this catheter is capable of injecting contrast media at higher flow rates. The flow rates are equal to one French size larger than designated.

USE: It is employed for angiographic studies of the LV and aorta.

SIZES: The Nycore catheter is available in sizes 7 and 8 Fr, with 65, 80, and 110 cm lengths, an open end, and eight side holes.

Ducor high-flow femoral-ventricular pigtail catheter (Cordis Corp.)

CONSTRUCTION: Polyurethane encapsulates a stainless steel wire braid (except in the tip), which provides torque control and allows high-pressure injections (up to 1000 psi). (*Note:* The thin-wall version of this catheter has no wire braid reinforcement and therefore is only able to withstand injection pressures of 500 psi or less. However, the thin-wall catheters can deliver a higher flow rate at a lower pressure than standard catheters.)

USE: The Ducor catheter is also used for angiographic studies of the LV and aorta.

SIZES: This catheter is available in sizes 5, 7, and 8 Fr, in 65, 90, and 110 cm lengths, with 12 side holes.

VARIATIONS: A new, super-flow Ducor end-hole pigtail catheter with eight side holes is available and is suitable for aortic angiographic studies in which lower injection pressures are used to prevent extravasation. This catheter can be used at higher flow rates with lower pressures and can withstand a maximal pressure of 800 psi.

Grollman pigtail catheter (Cook, Inc.) (Fig. 1-10)

CONSTRUCTION: This end-hole pigtail catheter is made of soft polyethylene material and contains four spiraled side ports near its terminal end.

USE: Because of its shape and softer material, this catheter is suitable for angiographic studies of the RV and PA, where there is greater danger of cardiac perforation (see Chapter 7 for a detailed discussion of this catheter).

VARIATIONS: This catheter is available in two curves. The standard Grollman catheter has a 60° bend. A Grollman catheter with a 60° bend and a reverse curve is also available.

Van Tassel angled pigtail catheter (USCI) (Fig. 1-11)

CONSTRUCTION: The Van Tassel catheter is similar to the Nycore high-flow pigtail catheter, with polyurethane over a thin nylon core. The unique feature of this end-hole catheter is a 145° or 155° angle 7 cm from the tip.

USE: The catheter is employed for angiographic studies of the LV and aorta in patients with normal or stenosed aortic valves. This design is particularly helpful for crossing a stenotic aortic valve, because it permits better alignment of the catheter as it approaches the aortic valve orifice. The curved pigtail can be straightened with a straight guidewire to direct the catheter tip across the aortic valve. Once the tip of the catheter is inside the ventricle, the angle lifts the tip away from the posterior wall of the ventricle and thus reduces myocardial irritability and the risk of intramyocardial injection during angiography.

SIZES: It is available in sizes 7 and 8 Fr, 110 cm long, with eight side holes.

Ducor angled pigtail catheter (Cordis Corp.)

CONSTRUCTION: The Ducor angled pigtail catheter is made of polyurethane with an inner stainless steel wire braid, which permits an ejection pressure of 1000 psi. This open-end catheter has 12 (rather than 8) elliptical side holes, which allow maximal flow rate.

USE AND SIZES: Uses and availability of this catheter are identical to those of the Van Tassel angled pigtail catheter.

Flow-directed angiographic catheters

Berman angiographic catheter (Fig. 1-12)

CONSTRUCTION: The Berman angiographic catheter is a double-lumen PVC catheter with side holes near the balloon tip.

USE: The catheter is intended for selective pulmonary angiography in adults or for right and left heart cathe-

Fig. 1-10. Grollman pigtail catheter.

Fig. 1-11. Van Tassel angled pigtail catheter (USCI).

Fig. 1-12. Berman angiographic catheter.

terization and angiography in infants and small children. It allows use of a single catheter for hemodynamic pressure monitoring and angiography. It is not suitable for PAWP recording, as the side holes are *proximal* to the balloon. During contrast injection the inflated balloon keeps the catheter away from the wall of the heart or vessel, reducing the risk of arrhythmia and penetration. The tapered tip permits the catheter to maintain its outside diameter when the balloon is deflated. A sheath one-half or one French size larger is recommended for percutaneous insertion.

Bynum-Wilson angiographic catheter (special order, American Edwards Laboratories) (Fig. 1-13)

CONSTRUCTION: The Bynum-Wilson catheter is a double-lumen PVC catheter with side holes near the tip *distal* to the balloon, which is 1 cm from the tip.

USE: It is employed for superselective balloon occlusion PA angiography in adults. With the catheter tip positioned in a branch of the PA, the balloon is inflated, blood flow to the vessel is stopped, and 2 to 5 ml of contrast medium is slowly injected by hand into the vessel while filming is done. This catheter is also suitable for standard-power angiography, with the balloon deflated. It can be used to measure PAWP. (See Chapter 5 for details.)

The tip of this catheter is not tapered, therefore the deflated balloon increases the diameter of the 7 Fr to 8.5 or 9.0 Fr and the diameter of the 8 Fr to 9 or 10 Fr. Thus, the 7 Fr catheter requires a 9 Fr sheath for percutaneous insertion. The fit of the sheath and catheter should be checked before insertion. Venous cutdown is recommended for insertion of the 8 Fr catheter.

SIZES: The catheter is available in sizes 7 Fr (yellow) and 8 Fr (tan), 110 cm long.

Preformed coronary catheters*
Judkins coronary catheter (Fig. 1-14)

CONSTRUCTION: All major catheter manufacturers produce Judkins-type left and right coronary artery catheters—end-hole catheters with no side holes. The primary differences concern the material with which the catheter is composed, affecting torque control and flow rate characteristics. The original Judkins catheter is constructed of polyurethane.

USE: Dr. Melvin Judkins designed the catheter for selective catheterization of the left and right coronary arteries by means of the percutaneous transfemoral approach. The uniquely preformed 90° curved tip of both the left and right coronary catheters facilitates placement in each coronary artery with relatively little ma-

nipulation. The secondary arm of the curved tip (a 30° curve in the right coronary catheter and a 180° curve in the left coronary catheter) is available in three lengths to accommodate variations in size of the ascending aorta. While the 7 or 8 Fr, 4 cm long Judkins left or right coronary catheter is the standard for normal-size aortas, the longer ones may be necessary for aortic dilatation, elongation, or tortuosity (see p. 136).

SIZES: Both right and left coronary catheters are available in 4.5, 5, 7, 7.3, 8, or 8.2 Fr with the tip tapering to 5 Fr or less. All are 100 cm long and are available with secondary curves of 3.5, 4, 5, or 6 cm.

ADVANTAGES: The new 5 Fr Judkins coronary catheters facilitate outpatient coronary artery catheterization and angiography.

Amplatz coronary catheters (Fig. 1-15)

CONSTRUCTION: All major catheter manufacturers produce Amplatz-type left and right coronary catheters—end-hole catheters constructed of either polyurethane or polyethylene.

USE: Dr. Kurt Amplatz designed the catheter for selective catheterization of the left or right coronary artery from the percutaneous femoral approach. The uniquely designed tip and curve of this catheter are shaped to fit the anatomy of the sinus of Valsalva. This reduces the dangers of occlusion of the coronary ostium as well as spontaneous dislodgment or advancement of the catheter.

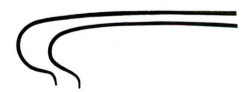

Fig. 1-13. Bynum-Wilson angiographic catheter.

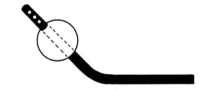

Fig. 1-14. Judkins coronary catheters.

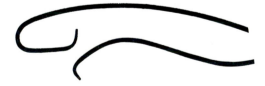

Fig. 1-15. Amplatz coronary catheters.

*See also Chapter 5.

SIZES: It is available in sizes 7, 7.3, 8, and 8.2 Fr, all 100 cm long.

VARIATIONS: The catheter is available with several broad secondary curve sizes (L1 to L4) to accommodate variations in aortic root size. The L1 and L2 are suitable for left coronary arteriography in patients with normal aortic roots; the L3 is used for dilated aortic roots or in very large men; and the L4 is used for marked aortic dilatation or for patients with high branching of the left coronary artery.

The Amplatz right coronary catheter is available in only three secondary curve sizes (R1 to R3). The R1 is used for coronary arteriography in patients with normal aortic roots, while the R2 and R3 are useful for abnormal position of the right coronary artery as well as for bypass graft visualization.

ADVANTAGES: Because of the marked difference between the configurations of the Amplatz and Judkins coronary catheters, the Amplatz catheter can usually be selectively placed in the right or left coronary artery if placement of the Judkins catheter is unsuccessful. If the percutaneous transfemoral approach is used, it is wise to have both Amplatz and Judkins catheters available. Although the Amplatz catheter was intended for and is most commonly used with the percutaneous femoral artery technique, it has also been successfully used from the brachial artery, particularly if there is difficulty in placement of the Sones catheter.

Schoonmaker multipurpose catheter (Fig. 1-16)

CONSTRUCTION: The Schoonmaker catheter is an open-end polyurethane catheter with an inner wire braid and two side holes.

USE: Dr. Fred W. Schoonmaker designed the multipurpose angiographic catheter for opacification of the

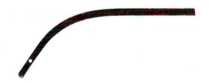

Fig. 1-16. Schoonmaker multipurpose catheters.

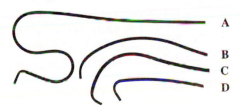

Fig. 1-17. Coronary bypass catheter(s).

left and right coronary arteries as well as the LV using a single catheter.

SIZES: The catheter is available in sizes 7 and 8 Fr, 100 cm long.

DISADVANTAGES: Although eliminating the need for multiple catheter exchanges would permit more rapid visualization of the coronary arteries and LV, successful selective placement in the left coronary artery can sometimes be difficult with this catheter. Increased ventricular irritability during left ventriculography makes this catheter suboptimal for LV angiograms.

Coronary bypass catheters (Fig. 1-17)

CONSTRUCTION: Coronary bypass catheters are made of polyurethane, with an open end and no side holes.

USE: It is specifically designed and curved for postoperative opacification of right and left coronary bypass grafts from the femoral percutaneous approach.

SIZES: Coronary bypass catheters come in sizes 7 and 8 Fr, 100 cm long.

Left coronary bypass catheter (Fig. 1-17, *C*). Dr. Melvin Judkins designed this catheter for visualization of a left coronary bypass graft affixed to the left anterior descending or circumflex artery. The tip has a 90° bend with a secondary curve of approximately 70°.

Right coronary bypass catheter (Fig. 1-17, *B*). This catheter is the same as the left, except for a 110° to 120° bend of the catheter tip. It is used for visualization of either right or left coronary bypass grafts.

Coronary bypass catheter II (Fig. 1-17, *A*). Designed by Drs. B.H. Greenberg and C.J. Trahm, this is employed for visualization of right coronary bypass grafts located superiorly on the aorta. It has two oppositely directed circular bends with a small, 90° curved tip.

Internal mammary bypass catheter (Fig. 1-17, *D*). Designed for opacification of both right and left internal mammary artery bypass grafts, this is similar to the Judkins right coronary catheter with a shallower primary curve (80° to 85°) and a 1.5 to 2 cm tip.

Catheters for brachial artery cutdown

Sones coronary catheter (Fig. 1-18)

CONSTRUCTION: The Sones coronary catheter is constructed of polyurethane or woven Dacron with an end hole and four side holes. USCI makes a Sones catheter with an inner nylon core and/or stainless steel mesh braid for increased torque control and strength.

USE: Dr. F. Mason Sones designed this catheter for selective catheterization of either the right or left coronary artery from the brachial artery cutdown approach. The tip of the Sones catheter is tapered and is available with curve lengths of 2.5, 4, or 7.6 cm. While the long,

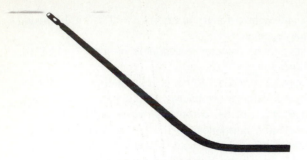

Fig. 1-18. Sones coronary catheter.

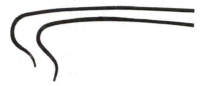

Fig. 1-19. Castillo coronary catheter.

Fig. 1-20. Softip coronary catheter.

tapered tip is very suitable for shaping in the aortic root and for selective coronary artery catheterization and injections, it is not ideal for rapid delivery of contrast media (i.e., ventriculography or aortography). However, this catheter can provide diagnostic-quality ventriculograms and is useful at times for crossing stenotic aortic valves.

SIZES: The catheter is available in sizes 7, 7.5, and 8 Fr, 80 and 100 cm lengths. The Dacron Sones catheter is available in three different curve types (A, B, and C curves).

VARIATIONS: Several variations of the Sones catheter offer different tip curves, curve lengths, and lengths of taper from the distal tip. Type I Sones catheters have a longer taper (1½ inches) than type II (1 inch). Catheter curve A has a long tip (7.5 cm); catheter curve B has shorter curve (3.8 to 4 cm); and catheter curve C has a rounder and even shorter curve (2.5 cm).

Castillo coronary catheter (Fig. 1-19)

CONSTRUCTION: The Castillo coronary catheter is a polyurethane, open-end catheter with no side holes.

USE: This end-hole catheter was designed by Dr. C.A. Castillo for selective catheterization of the right and left coronary arteries from the brachial artery cut-

down approach. The tip of the Castillo coronary catheter is curved (similar to the Amplatz) to permit selective placement in patients with a tortuous subclavian artery, a dilated aortic root, or high branchoff of the left coronary artery. Often the Castillo coronary catheter can be successfully placed when placement of the Sones catheter fails.

SIZES: Type I (small), type II (normal), and type III (large) catheters correspond to variations in the size of the aortic root. The catheter is available in sizes 7 and 8 Fr, 80 and 100 cm lengths.

Softip coronary catheter (Angiomedics, Inc.)
(Fig. 1-20)

CONSTRUCTION: This new soft-tip catheter is constructed of a special blend of polyurethane with a wire braid body for effective torque control and maneuverability. Its distinguishing feature is its soft, deformable tip, which has a thinner wall than the body of the catheter, with a slight bulblike design (see Fig. 1-20). This catheter is available in the Judkins, Amplatz, and multipurpose configurations for coronary arteriography as well as the pigtail design for ventriculography.

USE: This catheter was developed to considerably reduce intimal trauma, plaque dislodgment, and vessel dissection during coronary angiography. There has been limited clinical documentation of the use of the Softip catheter.

SIZES: It is available in sizes 7 and 8 Fr, 100 cm long.

ADVANTAGES: In vitro studies demonstrate that the Softip catheter has a lower frictional coefficient than some other diagnostic catheters and a marked reduction in tip penetration.[15] The softness and bulblike shape of the tip, with its ability to hinge inward, allow the tip to deform upon vessel wall contact, absorbing wall forces. This deformation does not interfere with pressure measurements or rapid injection of contrast medium.

Specialized catheters
Shirey transvascular catheter (Fig. 1-21)

CONSTRUCTION: The Shirey transvascular catheter is made of woven Dacron with a polyurethane coating. It is available in three different types, all having six laterally opposed side holes: type I has a closed end and a 5 Fr tapered tip; type II has an open end and a 6 Fr tapered tip; type III has a closed end and a 6 Fr tapered tip.

USE: Drs. Shirey and Sones designed this catheter specifically for retrograde catheterization and angiography of the left atrium (LA). The catheter has an aortic curve (7.5 cm) similar to that of the Sones catheter. It can be maneuvered into the LV, loop first, with its tip facing the aortic and mitral valves. Slow withdrawal of the extra loop will usually guide the tip of the catheter into the LA. Types I and III, which have a closed end, are also suitable for ventriculography or aortography. The type II Shirey catheter, which has an open end, is used for carotid arteriography and, on occasion, coronary arteriography.[16]

SIZES: The catheter comes in sizes 7 and 8 Fr, 110 cm long (the 8 Fr catheter is reinforced with nylon core, making it much stiffer).

Brockenbrough transseptal catheter (Fig. 1-22)

CONSTRUCTION: This is a Teflon-coated end-hole catheter with four specially arranged side holes and a tapered tip of varying curvature.

USE: The Brockenbrough transseptal catheter was specially designed to be inserted over the Brockenbrough transseptal needle into the LA. Its curve facilitates advancement into the LV for ventriculography.

SIZES: It is available in sizes 8 and 8.5 Fr in lengths of 55, 69, and 70 cm, with tip curvatures of 2.0, 2.5, 3.0, or 3.5 cm.

Double-lumen catheter (Fig. 1-23)

CONSTRUCTION: The double-lumen catheter is constructed of woven Dacron with a polyurethane coating. It has two lumens of equal size—one at the tip and the other 12 cm from the tip. From the proximal lumen to the distal lumen, the tip of the catheter tapers approximately two French sizes.

USE: This catheter is very useful for simultaneous measurement of pressures to determine a gradient between the RA and the RV or between the RV and the PA. The double-lumen catheter is used in hemodynamic evaluation for cases of suspected tricuspid stenosis or pericardial constriction. However, in the 7 Fr size, the lumen diameters are so small as to yield damped pressure tracings. For accurate evaluation of tricuspid or pulmonic stenosis, dual identical catheter/transducer systems are useful.

SIZES: The double-lumen catheter comes in sizes 7, 8, and 9 Fr, 125 cm long.

Multilumen catheter (Fig. 1-24)

CONSTRUCTION: The multilumen catheter is made of radiopaque polyurethane with three separate lumens whose distal exit ports are 2.2 cm apart. The corresponding lumen hubs are marked and color coded (white—proximal; blue—middle; and brown—distal). The distal lumen is the largest (16 gauge), while the middle and proximal lumens are both 18 gauge.

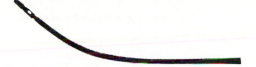

Fig. 1-21. Shirey transvascular catheter.

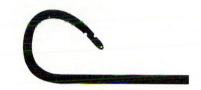

Fig. 1-22. Brockenbrough transseptal catheter.

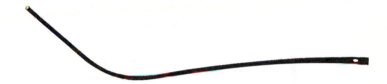

Fig. 1-23. Double-lumen catheter.

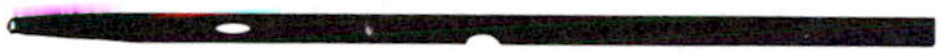

Fig. 1-24. Multilumen catheter.

USE: This catheter was designed for central venous pressure (CVP) monitoring; continuous or intermittent drug infusions; hyperalimentation; administration of blood, blood products, or viscous or high-volume fluids; and venous blood sampling.

This catheter can be inserted directly into the subclavian or jugular vein over a guidewire or through a catheter sheath. When it is inserted through a sheath with a side port, a fourth infusion lumen becomes available. The multilumen catheter provides multiple infusion lines through a single venipuncture. Because each lumen is completely separate, simultaneous IV administration of incompatible drugs is possible. This catheter is very useful in critical care medicine, as it permits IV hyperalimentation, chemotherapy, antibiotic therapy, and venous blood sampling, all carried out through a single catheter.

SIZES: The catheter is size 7 Fr, 30 cm long.

Fogarty catheter (Fig. 1-25)

CONSTRUCTION: The Fogarty catheter is a small vinyl catheter with a balloon near its tip.

USE: It is used to perform peripheral vascular embolectomy through a surgical cutdown. The catheter is packaged in stiff cylindric tubes with a sized stylet in-

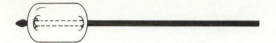

Fig. 1-25. Fogarty catheter.

side the catheter. Insertion can be made with or without the stylet, depending on the degree of stiffness desired. The balloon is inflated with sterile liquid after the stylet is removed. The volume of fluid required for balloon inflation is marked on its end and varies from 0.2 to 2.5 ml. Half the maximal liquid capacity is usually sufficient for clot removal.

SIZES: The Fogarty catheter is available in sizes 2 through 7 Fr, with 40, 60, 80, and 100 cm lengths.

Transducer-tip catheters

Millar catheter
CONSTRUCTION: The Millar catheter has an ultraminiature semiconductor strain gauge pressure transducer located at the tip.

USE: It is employed for high-fidelity diagnostic hemodynamic pressure acquisition. It is particularly helpful when first and second derivatives of the pressure waveforms are to be computed. Newer variations of the transducer-tipped catheter also permit blood sampling and high-speed injection of contrast medium for angiography.

SIZES: The Millar catheter comes in 3, 4, 5, 6, 7, and 8 Fr, with 75, 110, 120 and 140 cm lengths.

VARIATIONS: There are no-lumen catheters with one or two distal pressure sensors (3 to 6 cm apart); catheters with one lumen opening on the side approximately 4 mm proximal to the single pressure sensor at the tip; and catheters with one lumen and two pressure sensors. They are available in a straight or pigtail configuration.

ADVANTAGE: High-fidelity diagnostic pressure determination is possible.

DISADVANTAGES: The catheters are stiff and difficult to manipulate; zeroing the transducer after insertion is impossible; drift is a common problem; the catheters are expensive.

Camino Laboratories catheters
CONSTRUCTION: These are Teflon or PVC catheters with fiberoptics and a miniaturized pressure transducer at the tip. Pressure changes sensed by the transducer are transmitted via a fiberoptics system to a microprocessor for analysis and conversion into digital and analog pressure signals.

USE: The Camino Laboratories catheters are used for high-fidelity diagnostic hemodynamic pressure acquisi-

tion of both the right and left sides of the heart as well as long-term hemodynamic monitoring of RAP, PAP, PAWP, LAP, or arterial pressure.

SIZES: The 4 Fr catheter has no lumen. There is an 8 Fr thermodilution PA catheter.

VARIATIONS: Variations include a no-lumen 4 Fr catheter and a four-lumen thermodilution flotation PA catheter.

ADVANTAGES: These catheters permit high-fidelity diagnostic pressure acquisition. They are stable, convenient to set up and maintain, and relatively inexpensive. ˙

DISADVANTAGES: The stiffness of the catheters requires a guiding catheter for passage of 4 Fr; zeroing the transducer after insertion is impossible.

Angioscopic catheters
CONSTRUCTION: These multilumened, reusable fiberoptic catheters are constructed of polyurethane (Tremedyne, Inc.), shrinkable fluoride-based polymer jacket (American Edwards Laboratories), or PVC (Olympus Corp.). Each of the endoscopes contains fibers for light transmission (illumination) as well as an optical bundle of fibers for imaging. In addition, the Olympus endoscope contains a small (1.2 mm) lumen for flushing. The Tremedyne endoscope contains a lumen for flushing and inflation of a 2.5 or 4.6 cc balloon, positioned 2 to 4 mm from the tip. Inflation of the balloon prevents forward blood flow to improve visualization.

The proximal end of endoscopic catheters can be attached to video or camera equipment for photography or viewing with a monitor.

USE: The catheters are used for intraluminal examination of blood vessels to detect the presence and exact location of atherosclerotic plaque, thrombi, or suture lines (after operation). These catheters are currently employed primarily for investigation.

SIZES: Angioscopic catheters are available in sizes 4.5 Fr (1.5 mm), 7.5 Fr (2.5 mm), and 11 Fr (3.7 mm), 150 cm long.

Pacing catheters

Temporary emergency or elective transvenous pacing can be accomplished with a variety of pacemaker catheters depending on the patient's needs. Pacing catheters, despite other variations, are either unipolar or bipolar. Unipolar catheters have one wire terminating in a distal electrode (cathode), which comes in direct contact with the myocardium. The indifferent electrode (anode) is located outside the heart, either within the subcutaneous tissue or within the pulse generator itself. The unipolar pacing catheter is infrequently used for temporary pacing. Bipolar pacemaker catheters have two wires terminating in two electrodes located 1 to 2 cm apart at the tip of the catheter. The distal stimulating electrode is negative and the proximal electrode is positive. At the terminal end of the catheter the electrode wires bifurcate into positive and negative poles for connection to the pulse generator. The bipolar pacing catheter can be used for both temporary and permanent pacing. Multielectrode catheters (tripolar, quadrapolar, and hexapolar) are also available for use in electrophysiologic studies (see Chapter 9).

The types of bipolar pacing catheters commonly used are the semifloating 4 Fr pacing electrode, the heavier 5 and 6 Fr pacing electrodes, and the 3 Fr floating balloon electrode.

Many pacing electrodes and catheters are available with heparin bonded to the surface to reduce thrombogenicity.

Standard pacing electrodes (Fig. 1-26)

CONSTRUCTION: These are no-lumen catheters with two platinum electrodes located 1 or 2.5 cm apart at the tip of the catheter and two electrode connectors at the base.

USE: They are employed for temporary atrial or ventricular pacing.

SIZES: Standard pacing electrodes come in sizes 3, 4, 5, 6, and 7 Fr, 110 cm long.

VARIATION: A J-shaped curve (13 mm radius) of the catheter tip is available for atrial pacing or sensing. This curve aids in achieving a stable position in the atria. A J-curve atrial lead with a proximal-orienting wing aids in directional orientation of the catheter when fluoroscopy is not used. A flotation bipolar pacing electrode is available with a balloon located between the distal and proximal electrodes. With inflation of the balloon (1.3 cc of air or less), the electrode is flow directed into the appropriate position.

Specialized pacing catheters

Balloon flotation monitoring and pacing catheter

CONSTRUCTION: This is a PVC, bipolar pacing catheter with a balloon lumen and an infusion or pressure lumen ending 12 cm from the tip.

USE: The balloon flotation monitoring and pacing catheter is employed for temporary transvenous right ventricular pacing during central venous drug or fluid administration, blood sampling, and CVP measurements.

SIZES: It is available in sizes 5 and 7 Fr, 110 cm long. The 5 Fr size has a 1.3 cc maximal balloon capacity.

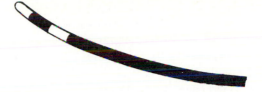

Fig. 1-26. Standard bipolar pacing electrodes.

VARIATION: There is a balloon pacing catheter with a distal lumen for PA pressure monitoring with positioning of the electrodes 14 and 15 cm from the balloon tip for right ventricular pacing.

Thermodilution pacing catheters

CONSTRUCTION: This is a standard PVC thermodilution catheter with an additional lumen terminating 19 cm from the tip for insertion of a temporary pacemaker probe into the RV.

USE: It is used for hemodynamic pressure monitoring of patients at high risk for developing complete heart block.

SIZES: Thermodilution pacing catheters come in sizes 5 and 7 Fr, 110 cm long.

VARIATION: One type has bipolar electrodes mounted 14 to 15 cm from tip. It is 7 Fr, 110 cm long and is used for hemodynamic monitoring and ventricular pacing.

DISADVANTAGES: It is difficult to obtain consistent capture in the RV when the catheter is manipulated for PAWP measurements. Also, it is difficult to position the RV port correctly in patients with enlarged or small hearts.

Zucker pacing catheter

CONSTRUCTION: The Zucker pacing catheter is a single-lumen, Dacron catheter with an end hole and two electrodes spaced 1.5 cm apart.

USE: It is used for right heart catheterization, including pressure measurements, blood sampling, and atrial or ventricular pacing. It is most commonly used to catheterize patients at high risk of developing heart block.

SIZES: It comes in sizes 6 and 7 Fr, with 100 and 125 cm lengths.

DISADVANTAGE: The catheter is relatively stiff for manipulation in the right side of the heart.

Custom-made catheters

The appropriate shape and the size of the catheter are primary determinants of successful selective angiography. Most angiographers today use commercially available preformed catheters and are encouraged to do so by catheter manufacturers, who are more than willing to custom make any shape catheter desired. Despite this, it is not uncommon to have to at least modify preformed catheters for successful catheter placement. However, because of the material used, not all catheters can be reshaped.

PVC is not suitable for shaping or reshaping because of the radiopaque material (bismuth salts), which alters the characteristics of the catheter. Teflon can be reshaped if a heat gun is used to reach a temperature of 750° F. Although polyethylene also loses its shape at high temperatures, it changes the least when made radiopaque, and therefore it is the most suitable for catheter shaping or reshaping.

Reshaping polyethylene or polyurethane catheters

1. Insert either the stiff end of a guidewire or a catheter-shaping, malleable piece of wire into the catheter segment to be reshaped.
2. Hold the catheter in the desired shape over a steam jet or under sterile conditions in a bowl of boiling water for several seconds to heat the polyethylene (to 200° F). Polyurethane requires a longer exposure to heat (up to 5 minutes for nontapered proximal portions) for reshaping.
3. Quickly immerse the whole assembly in cold, sterile fluid to allow the catheter to retain its new shape.
4. Remove the shaping wire or guidewire.

Forming catheters from polyethylene tubing

Polyethylene catheter material is available in numerous color-coded French sizes in 10- to 20-foot rolls of tubing. The following steps are involved in making a radiopaque catheter from polyethylene tubing.

1. Tapering the catheter tip (Fig. 1-27, *A* and *B*)
   a. Insert a guidewire whose size matches the inside diameter of the polyethylene tubing being used (see Table 1-1).
   b. With the guidewire inside the polyethylene tubing, evenly rotate the tubing over an alcohol lamp until it becomes soft and the heated segment can be pulled apart to form an evenly tapered segment.
   c. Cut the tapered end (with the guidewire still in

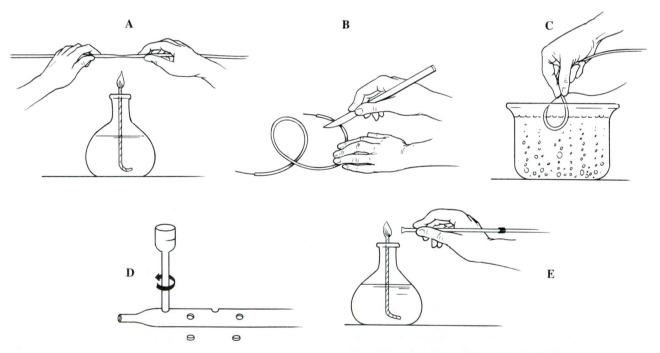

Fig. 1-27. Formation of a catheter using polyethylene tubing. **A,** With a guidewire inside the polyethylene tubing, rotate the tubing evenly over an alcohol lamp until the tubing softens and can be stretched apart. **B,** Cut the tapered end (with the wire still in place) with a sharp scalpel. **C,** With the wire still in place, bend the catheter to the desired shape and heat the tubing in hot water. **D,** Punch the desired holes in the catheter by rotating the punching instrument against the catheter until its wall is punctured. **E,** Flange the proximal end of the catheter by holding it near the underside of an alcohol flame.

place) to a desired length by rolling it on a flat surface while exerting slight pressure with a sharp razor or scalpel.
2. Shaping the catheter (Fig. 1-27, *C*)
   a. With the stiff end of the guidewire or shaping wire in place, bend the catheter tubing into the desired shape.
   b. Immerse the catheter tubing and guidewire into hot water (>160° F) to heat and soften the tubing. (Do not immerse the thin, tapered tip into the hot water.)
   c. Maintaining the curve, immerse the catheter tubing and guidewire into cold water to retain its shape.
   d. Remove the guidewire. If necessary, smooth the edges of the tip by rubbing with 4-0 emory polishing paper.
3. Punching side holes (Fig. 1-27, *D*)
   a. Lay the catheter on a hard, flat surface.
   b. Using a special punching tool, press the cannula against the wall of the tubing near its tip. (Do not place holes in either the tapered or curved portion of the catheter, where they would weaken the catheter.)
   c. Rotate the cannula to remove a plug from the catheter. (Make sure all small plugs are accounted for and removed, to prevent their inadvertent injection during angiography.)
4. Flanging the end (Fig. 1-27, *E*)
   a. Cut the catheter tubing to the desired length.
   b. Attach an appropriate-size Luer fitting onto the catheter.
   c. Hold the proximal end of the catheter near the underside of an alcohol flame in a horizontal fashion.
   d. Rotate the proximal end of the catheter until an even flange is obtained.

Cleansing, sterilization, and storage

Most catheters used today are intended for one-time use only. The burden of risk involved when single-use items are reused falls on the hospital and physician, not on the manufacturer or distributor. In response to intense pressure to reduce costs some hospitals reuse catheters on a limited basis, but only if health standards and patient safety can be maintained. Multilumen balloon-tip catheters should not be reused, as balloon integrity would be compromised. Catheters suitable for reuse should be cleansed in the following way:
1. Immediately after use, flush the catheter manually with 20 to 40 ml of tap water and rinse the outer surface with tap water.
2. Connect the catheter to a pressure flush system and flush with water for 30 to 45 minutes.
3. Cleanse the catheter by soaking in Detergicide solution for 30 minutes or by ultrasonic cleansing in Detergicide solution for 15 minutes.
4. Flush the catheter with 1000 ml of Detergicide solution with either a pressure flush system or a gravity drip setup.
5. Rinse the catheter with 1000 ml of distilled water using a pressure flush system or a gravity drip setup.
6. Dry the catheter.

Sterilization is best achieved with ethylene oxide followed by an appropriate aeration period. Other methods of sterilization (autoclaving or cold sterilization with glutaraldehyde) subject the catheter to temperatures or chemicals that could damage it. Care must be exercised when clean catheters are packaged for sterilization to prevent coiling of the catheter more than 8 inches in diameter. This not only would shape the catheter in a way that could impede manipulation, but also could introduce stress points and increase the risk of catheter damage. Radiation sterilization may degrade certain plastics depending on the polymer and the radiation dose and duration.[5]

Single- or multiple-use catheters are best stored in a vertical hanging position, which prevents any damage that could occur from added weight or folding. With age, catheters can become brittle and break, therefore it is important that all stock be inventoried and the expiration date carefully noted (3 years for Cordis polyurethane and USCI polyurethane catheters).[17] The oldest equipment should be used first, if it is not outdated.

GUIDEWIRES

Guidewires (originally steel guitar strings) are very delicate devices used in cardiac catheterization to straighten a catheter curve, traverse vessels, and permit percutaneous insertion of an introducer or catheter.

Guidewires are constructed of finely coiled stainless steel over a straight wire core (Fig. 1-28). This tapered core can be either fixed, terminating 3 cm from the tip, or movable, in which a portion of the guidewire separates allowing movement of the core. This feature allows the operator to vary the length of "floppiness" at the tip by adjusting the position of the rigid core.

All guidewires (except some early guidewires used in coronary angioplasty) have an inner safety wire, which is bonded or welded at both ends to prevent separation in the event of guidewire breakage and to contain the coils of the spring wire during manipulation. The wire

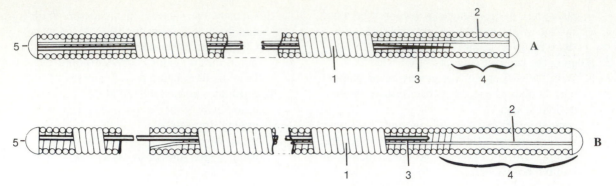

Fig. 1-28. Guidewire construction. **A,** Fixed-core guidewire. **B,** Movable-core guidewire. Parts of the guidewire include the *(1)* spring coils, *(2)* inner safety wire, *(3)* mandrel core, *(4)* flexible tip, and *(5)* proximal end. Note that the proximal end of the movable-core guidewire separates from the remaining guidewire to permit alterations in the length of core within the wire.

tips are welded and polished for strength and smoothness to minimize vessel trauma.

Guidewire measurement is somewhat confusing. In North America the diameter of the wire is measured in thousandths of an inch (Table 1-4), while the length is measured in centimeters. Much confusion could be avoided if all guidewire diameters were expressed in millimeters. For the sake of tradition and clarity we will refer to guidewire diameters in both inches and millimeters.

Material

Guidewires are constructed of fine stainless steel. Some guidewires are also coated with a thin film of Teflon to reduce the friction coefficient of the guidewire within the catheter. Care must be exercised when a Tef-

lon guidewire is passed through a metal needle or catheter hub, as the Teflon coating can become abraded and flake off. Most important, a Teflon guidewire should never be abruptly withdrawn from a metal needle.

Types

Guidewires basically are of two shapes, straight and J curve, and may have either a fixed or movable core.

Straight guidewires

The straight guidewire has a flexible tip (generally 3 cm) and is appropriate for passage through vessels of linear configuration. Since both the proximal (stiff) and the distal (flexible) ends of the straight guidewire appear the same, it is imperative to check the ends before insertion to ensure that the *flexible* end is inserted.

Table 1-4. Standard guidewire measurements and usage

Outside diameter		Minimal thin-wall needle size	Common usage
Inch	*mm*		
0.006	0.15	—	PTCA
0.010	0.25	—	PTCA
0.012	0.30	—	PTCA
0.014	0.36	—	PTCA
0.016	0.41	—	PTCA
0.018	0.46	21 gauge	PTCA & small vessel puncture
0.025	0.6	19 & 20 gauge	Percutaneous arterial cannulation; adding stiffness to 7 Fr balloon flotation catheters
0.032	0.8	18 gauge	Monitoring catheters
0.035	0.9	18 gauge	Standard diagnostic catheters
0.038	1.0	17 gauge	Standard diagnostic catheters
0.045	1.14	16 gauge	Brockenbrough catheter
0.063	1.6	14 gauge	PTCA guiding catheters

PTCA, Percutaneous transluminal coronary angioplasty.

Some straight guidewires are constructed such that both ends are flexible, to prevent inadvertent insertion of a stiff end into a vessel.

J-Curve guidewires

The J-curve guidewire generally has a 1.5, 3, or 6 mm curved radius at its tip (Fig. 1-29). It is particularly useful for passage through tortuous vessels. Use of the J-curve guidewire for negotiating the external jugular vein has been associated with a higher incidence of successful passage than the use of a standard straight wire.[18]

Many percutaneous catheter introducer sets now supply a 3 mm curve radius J-curve guidewire with their kit. This size curve, initially intended for pediatric use, has become commonly used for catheterization in adults. The larger J-curve (6 mm radius) guidewire is often appropriate for negotiating a tortous femoral vein. An even larger J-curve (15 mm radius) guidewire is available for cases of extreme vessel tortuosity.

A multipurpose, double-end guidewire offers a long (10 cm), flexible, straight tip at one end with a small (1.5 mm) J curve on the other end. This two-in-one combination potentially reduces the number of guidewires used for a single procedure.

J-curve guidewires are packaged with a small plastic sleeve that, when advanced over the tip of the guidewire, straightens the wire and permits it to be introduced into the hub of a needle or catheter (Fig. 1-30).

Fixed-core guidewires

Fixed-core guidewires (Fig. 1-28) have a straight inner core wire (mandrel) that is fixed at one end and terminates usually 3 cm from the tip. The core provides necessary stiffness to the body of the coiled wire, while allowing flexibility at the tip. Variations in the tapered length (10 or 15 cm) of the mandrel alter the degree of tip flexibility and improve the transition from flexible distal coil to supported mandrel. This is an important feature in PTCA guidewires. Both straight and J-curve guidewires are available with a fixed core.

Movable-core guidewires

Guidewires that have the straight core attached only at the distal end are designed to allow movement of the tip of the core for the purpose of increasing or decreasing the length of the flexible tip (Fig. 1-28). This is accomplished by not welding the proximal end of the mandrel core to the end of the guidewire, but instead securing the inner mandrel to a 5 cm handle that is attached to the distal end of the wire. Variations in the tapered length of the core (5, 10, or 15 cm) alter the

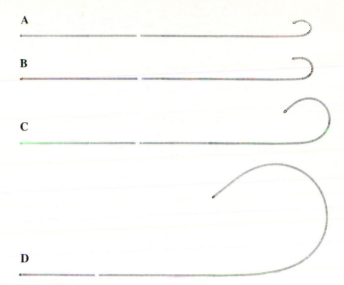

Fig. 1-29. Various-size curves of the J-curve guidewire. **A,** Small (1.5 mm) curve; **B,** 3 mm curve; **C,** 6 mm curve; **D,** large (15 mm) curve.

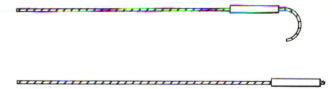

Fig. 1-30. The curve of the J-curve guidewire is straightened out before vascular entry by sliding the accompanying plastic sleeve over the distal wire tip.

degree of tip flexibility or, in the case of J-curve wires, vary the radius of the floppy wire. This ability to increase or decrease the length of the wire's flexible tip is often desirable for traversing local areas of tortuosity. While the movable-core guidewire requires some experience and skill of operation, it has become the guidewire of choice for many angiographers. On occasion, readvancement of the inner mandrel may be difficult. This is usually due to bending or kinking of the unsupported flexible tip. In general, the inner mandrel should never be forced if resistance is met. If this occurs, the entire guidewire should be removed.

Core-flex guidewires

CONSTRUCTION: Core-flex guidewires have a solid stainless steel mandrel with a safety wire constructed of spring coil soldered to the end (Fig. 1-31). Although the outside diameter of this guidewire is only 0.018 inch (0.46 mm), the guidewire offers the same support

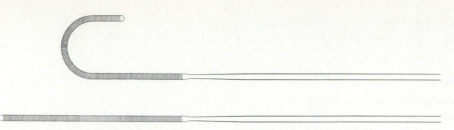

Fig. 1-31. Core-flex guidewire has a solid wire body with spring coils only at its distal tip.

and rigidity as an 0.035-inch (0.9 mm) guidewire because of its solid steel mandrel.

USE: The rigidity of this guidewire permits percutaneous cannulation with a smaller 22-gauge needle, rather than the standard 18-gauge needle.

SIZES: It is available straight or with a J curve in appropriate lengths for percutaneous insertion.

Exchange guidewires

The exchange guidewire is a straight wire unique only in its length of 260 or 300 cm. It is used exclusively for catheter exchange purposes as it is long enough to allow the removal and insertion of a catheter while the tip remains in the selected chamber. This is often desirable for exchanging catheters in the LV if difficulty was encountered in crossing the aortic valve. Exchange guidewires are also used in coronary angioplasty.

Open-end guidewire/catheter

CONSTRUCTION: This new Teflon guidewire has an open end and a removable inner mandrel. In this way it can function both as a guidewire and, with the mandrel removed, as a catheter.

USE: This guidewire is of greatest use in traversing tortuous or stenotic arteries during peripheral angioplasty.[19] Pressures can be monitored during this procedure through the lumen of the guidewire. Clinical use is limited at this time.

SIZES: The outside diameters are 0.035 and 0.038 inch (0.9 and 1.0 mm), and the respective inside diameters are 0.018 and 0.02 inch (0.46 and 0.6 mm), with either a straight or J-curved tip.

Sizes

Most guidewires are available in sizes ranging from 0.018 to 0.038 inch (0.4 to 1.0 mm). In general, the smaller sizes (0.4, 0.5, and 0.6 mm) are used in children. The exception is the 0.025-inch (0.6 mm) guidewire, which can be inserted into the distal lumen of the Swan-Ganz catheter to increase its stiffness. For spe-

cialized procedures (coronary angioplasty), guidewires as small as 0.010 inch (0.25 mm) and 0.012 inch (0.30 mm) may be used for the dilatation catheters, and those as large as 0.063 inch (1.6 mm) for the guiding catheters. Table 1-4 lists standard guidewire measurements and common usages.

The guidewire most commonly used for percutaneous catheterization of adults is the 0.035-inch (0.9 mm) guidewire, as it will pass through sizes 6, 7, and 8 Fr catheters (see Table 1-1). Ideally, the catheter tip should fit closely over the guidewire, with no excess space between the wire and the catheter. This promotes smooth insertion of the catheter into the vessel.

Guidewires are available in lengths varying from 50 to 300 cm. The guidewire's length is dictated by the length of the specific catheter to be used. The guidewire should be at least 20 cm longer than the catheter to allow insertion of the catheter over the guidewire with some wire always exposed at the hub for manipulation and retention. In the cardiac catheterization laboratory, a 145 cm long guidewire is most commonly used, as the majority of vascular catheters are 110 to 125 cm long. In the critical care area, a 50 cm long guidewire is sufficient for percutaneous insertion of a catheter sheath.

Desired features

Important considerations in guidewire selection include stiffness, flexibility, and smoothness. These features are important for both patient safety and improved operation.

Stiffness

The stiffness of the guidewire is a function of both the core and the diameter of the wire. The wire must be sufficiently stiff to be pushed forward without collapsing back on itself or coiling within the vasculature. Increased stiffness can be obtained by use of a larger guidewire, if possible, or (more practically) use of a guidewire with a heavy-duty larger mandrel. This increase in stiffness may be most helpful in arterial catheterization of an obese patient to prevent buckling of the catheter prior to entry into the artery.[20]

Flexibility

The degree of flexibility of the guidewire is related to the core as well as to the single helix of stainless steel wire around it. It is essential that the guidewire be flexible enough to be bent sharply without kinking or breaking and that the proximal tip of the wire be soft and flexible (to minimize vascular trauma).

Smoothness

The smoothness of the wire is a result of its surface. Certainly, the Teflon-coated wires are smoother and produce less friction when passed through catheters. However, certain precautions must be exercised when Teflon-coated guidewires are used, as the Teflon coating may not always be evenly applied and can result in an increase of the guidewire's diameter. It is essential to check that the wire will pass through the selected cannula and catheter *prior* to its use. At times it may be necessary to use a slightly smaller diameter Teflon guidewire.

Some Teflon guidewires are treated with benzalkonium heparin to reduce thrombogenicity. However, one radioimmunoassay study of these wires showed a release of fibrinopeptide shortly after insertion.[21] Since most guidewires are in place only for a brief period, this initial increase in thrombogenicity may be of clinical importance. Thus, for most vascular procedures we recommend use of either a noncoated stainless steel or a Teflon guidewire in conjunction with systemic administration of heparin, rather than a benzalkonium heparin–treated wire.

Special precautions and complications

In general, all guidewires should be regarded as fragile devices susceptible to bending and breaking. This risk increases with repeated manipulations, which place stress on weak areas of the wire and predispose to wire damage.

Despite the presence of a safety wire, the guidewire can separate and embolization of a portion of the wire can occur.[22] Other reported complications include knotting of the guidewire tip, separation of the wire with protrusion of the core, and displacement of the rounded tip of a J-curve guidewire.[23] To decrease these risks, the operator should take the following precautions:

1. Carefully inspect the guidewire before use.
2. Immediately remove and inspect the guidewire when resistance is encountered.
3. Wipe off and inspect the wire after each removal.
4. Minimize the number of guidewire manipulations.
5. Minimize the time guidewires are in the vessel.
6. Do not resterilize guidewires.

Cleansing and sterilization

Because of the guidewire's construction, complete cleansing is impossible even with an ultrasonic cleaner. When placed in hydrogen peroxide, an apparently clean wire will frequently bubble, indicating the presence of blood. Under high-power magnification, used stainless steel guidewires cleansed in Detergicide, ultrasonic cleaner, and hydrogen peroxide revealed dehydrated blood particulate between the coils.[24] Used, cleaned Teflon wires showed breaking of the Teflon with detachment of Teflon particles. For this reason, as well as to reduce the hazards that accompany frequent manipulation and use, it is recommended that all guidewires be discarded after one use. If contamination has occurred prior to intravascular use, guidewires in their holders can be gas sterilized.

NEEDLES

Percutaneous vascular access into either the artery or the vein is gained via introduction of a needle. Basically, any needle can be used to puncture the vessel. Hypodermic needles are useful for entering a blood vessel to withdraw blood. However, their long bevel makes them less suitable for cannulation of a vessel, in which the entire needle lumen must be within the vessel to allow insertion of a guidewire. Virtually all vascular entry needles have thin walls; this permits passage of a guidewire without increasing the outside diameter and, therefore, the size of the puncture hole. This is not true of hypodermic needles.

Vascular needles also differ from hypodermic needles at the hub. It would be very difficult to insert a guidewire into the nontapered flat hub of a hypodermic needle. For this reason, the inside of the hub of vascular needles is gently tapered.

Percutaneous cannulation needles are frequently referred to as Seldinger needles, after Dr. Sven-Ivar Seldinger, who first described the percutaneous catheterization technique.[25]

The choice of the type of needle depends on its intended use.

Design

Vascular needles are constructed of rigid stainless steel with a beveled tip possessing two sharp cutting edges (Fig. 1-32). This type of point aids in puncturing the vessel and smoothly sliding through it. Vascular

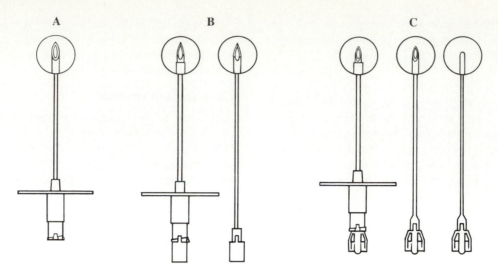

Fig. 1-32. Three types of percutaneous vascular entry needles. **A,** One-part needle. **B,** Two-part needle consisting of an inner beveled stylet and an outer cannula of metal or plastic. **C,** Three-part needle consisting of an inner beveled stylet, an outer cannula, and a rounded obturator (note the two cutting edges of the needle tip).

needles have a relatively short bevel to ensure full entry into the lumen with the appearance of blood. Needle puncture is usually performed with the bevel directed upward so that the sharp point of the needle penetrates the vessel. Percutaneous entry needles can be categorized according to the number of parts. Many companies produce the one-, two-, and three-part vascular needles discussed below with slight modifications in design. Most can be used for both venous and arterial access.

Most vascular needles possess a metal or plastic grip shield to facilitate controlled advancement and slow withdrawal of the needle. During insertion the thumb is usually placed behind the hub of the inner stylet with the index and middle fingers resting in front of the shield.

One-part needle (Fig. 1-32, A)

The one-part needle is currently the most commonly used needle for percutaneous vascular entry. This needle is *intended for single-wall puncture* of either an artery or a vein. For venous puncture, a syringe is usually attached to its hub for the purpose of aspiration during entry. A guidewire or a catheter can be inserted through the needle into the vessel. This is the method of choice for percutaneous cannulation of the subclavian and internal and external jugular veins, in which a double-wall venous puncture could result in serious damage to nearby vessels and produce bleeding. A single-wall arterial puncture is recommended for puncture of a small

artery, such as the radial artery, as well as patients who are on anticoagulants or who may receive thrombolytic therapy in the immediate future. This type of needle can also be used for single-wall arterial graft puncture, thus reducing hematoma formation.

Two-part needle (Fig. 1-32, B)

The two-part needle consists of a sharp, solid inner needle (stylet) with a blunt or slightly tapered metal or Teflon outer cannula that fits snugly over the stylet and terminates just proximal to the bevel of the needle. This needle is used for transfixation of the vessel in which both the anterior and posterior walls are punctured. For arterial puncture, the inner needle is then removed and the cannula slowly withdrawn into the lumen of the vessel. For venous puncture, a syringe is attached to the cannula for aspiration during withdrawal. This is not necessary for arterial puncture, as the higher pressure causes blood to pulsate from the cannula when it enters the lumen of the artery.

Three-part needle (Fig. 1-32, C)

The three-part needle consists of an inner needle and an outer cannula plus a round-end obturator that fits inside the cannula after the inner needle is withdrawn. The purpose of the obturator is to provide a round, nontraumatic end to the cannula for safe advancement into the vessel once the cannula is within the lumen. This needle formerly was used in the cardiac catheterization

Table 1-5. Thin-wall needle sizes

| | Inside diameter | | Outside diameter | |
Gauge	Inch	mm	Inch	mm
12	0.091	2.3	0.104	2.6
13	0.077	1.9	0.092	2.3
14	0.071	1.8	0.080	2.0
15	0.059	1.5	0.072	1.8
16	0.052	1.3	0.064	1.6
17	0.046	1.1	0.056	1.4
18	0.042	1.0	0.048	1.2
19	0.031	0.8	0.040	1.0
20	0.025	0.6	0.036	0.9
21	0.022	0.6	0.032	0.8
22	0.018	0.5	0.028	0.7
23	0.015	0.4	0.024	0.6
24	0.014	0.4	0.022	0.6
25	0.012	0.3	0.020	0.5
26	0.012	0.3	0.018	0.5
27	0.010	0.3	0.016	0.4

laboratory when an intra-arterial needle was used for pressure measurements and blood sampling. The obturator was inserted so that the cannula could be fully advanced and stabilized in the vessel. The three-part needle is rarely used today.

Sizes

The size of a needle is measured in needle gauge, which refers to its outside diameter. However, for appropriate guidewire matching it is essential to know the inside diameter of the needle (see Tables 1-4 and 1-5). For the same needle gauge, the inside diameter can vary depending on whether the needle is a standard- or thin-wall type.

Needle size selection depends primarily on the size of the patient and the target vessel. An 18-gauge needle is suitable for venous and femoral artery puncture in most adults, while a 20-gauge needle/catheter is usually inserted into radial and brachial arteries. A general rule for vascular invasion is to use the smallest diameter device that provides optimal information. Table 1-5 lists the inside and outside diameters of various needle sizes.

Types

Reusable stainless steel needles, such as the Cournand, Riley, and Potts-Cournand needles, have been traditionally used in the cardiac catheterization laboratory for percutaneous cannulation of the femoral or brachial artery or vein. Today, disposable needles are almost universally used for the same purpose. A percutaneous entry needle is used for subclavian or internal jugular vein puncture for insertion of central venous or PA catheters for hemodynamic pressure monitoring purposes. The peel-away needle is used most commonly for transvenous pacemaker insertion into the subclavian vein.

Cournand needle

CONSTRUCTION: The Cournand needle consists of at least two stainless steel parts: an outer cannula with a very short beveled tip that fits closely over an inner cannula, and an inner cannula whose sharp pointed tip protrudes beyond the tip of the outer cannula. An available third portion of this needle is a blunt, rounded obturator used only to occlude the lumen of the outer cannula when intermittent blood sampling is desired.

USE: The 18-gauge thin-wall Cournand needle is frequently used in the cardiac catheterization laboratory for both arterial and venous access for percutaneous catheter insertion. It is reusable with proper care and maintenance.

SIZES: The Cournand needle is available in 15 through 20 gauge, with regular or thin walls. All Cournand needles are 5.5 cm long.

Riley needle

CONSTRUCTION: The construction of the Riley needle is the same as that of the Cournand needle.

USE: The Riley needle is used for brachial artery puncture in small individuals, including small women and some adolescents.

SIZE: This is a 20-gauge, shorter (4 cm) version of the Cournand needle.

Potts-Cournand needle

CONSTRUCTION: The Potts-Cournand needle is identical to the thin-wall Cournand needle with the exception of the Luer-Lok hub, shield, and stylet handle, which are made of plastic.

USE: It is intended for both arterial and venous puncture (Seldinger technique). It is reusable with proper care and maintenance.

SIZES: The Potts-Cournand needle is available in 16 through 20 gauge, with thin walls; it is 5.5 cm long.

Percutaneous entry needle

CONSTRUCTION: The percutaneous entry needle is a one-part thin-wall multipurpose needle constructed of stainless steel with a plastic Luer-Lok hub, available with or without the grip shield.

USE: The needle is employed for central venous, single-wall puncture cannulation of the internal and external jugular and subclavian veins in which a syringe is attached for aspiration during puncture. It may also be used for brachial and femoral artery puncture as well as pericardiocentesis. It is disposable.

SIZES: It is available with an 18-, 19-, or 20-gauge outer cannula in lengths of 2.5, 4, 5, and 7 cm.

Arterial catheter/needle combinations

CONSTRUCTION: This set usually consists of a thin-wall short (2½-inch) Teflon tube, a sharp stainless steel needle, and a fitted inner stylet.

USE: Long-term arterial access for continuous monitoring or blood sampling is obtained through the use of a catheter/needle combination. The 18-gauge catheter is commonly used for femoral artery catheterization, while the 20-gauge catheter is used for radial artery catheterization.

SIZES: The catheter is available in sizes 15, 16, 18, and 20 gauge with inner needle sizes of 17, 18, 19, and 23 gauge, respectively.

Peel-away needle

CONSTRUCTION: The peel-away or break-away needle is a completely disposable metal needle that consists of two halves tightly placed together to function as a single 14-gauge needle. Once the needle is placed in the vessel, the catheter can be directly inserted through it without the use of a guidewire. The needle is then pulled back and peeled away from the catheter. This reduces the risk of damage to the catheter from the needle.

USE: This needle has been successfully used for percutaneous subclavian vein catheterization.[26]

Brockenbrough needle

CONSTRUCTION: The needle set consists of two parts—a long (70 or 71 cm), 18-gauge, standard-wall needle and an inner stylet. The needle has a gentle 4 cm curve at the tip to facilitate passage across the atrial septum. An indicator at the hub of the needle shows the direction of the tip of the needle. This needle is made of stainless steel, and with proper care and maintenance it can be reused.

USE: The Brockenbrough needle was designed specifically for transseptal left heart catheterization via the Brockenbrough catheter.

Desired features

Desired features of needles include a *sharp needle point,* a *smooth beveled end* of the outer cannula or catheter, and *appropriate size.*

Successful vessel puncture and reduced risk of vascular trauma requires an extremely sharp needle tip with a smooth cutting edge. Since this is the greatest problem with reusable needles, the needle tips should be

inspected frequently and sharpened if necessary. If the needle is sharpened, it is necessary to include the outer cannula so that its length and shape can be matched with the inner needle. Prior to use, the reusable needle's tip should be carefully wiped with a gauze sponge to check for irregularities that may not be visually noticeable. Any snags indicate rough areas and the needle should not be used.

The beveled end of the outer cannula or catheter should snugly fit the inner needle and should have a smooth, tapered end to minimize vascular trauma. Disposable catheters made of Teflon have a low friction coefficient, therefore trauma is reduced and blood flow is not inhibited.

As mentioned previously, an inner stylet is desirable for transfixing the anterior and posterior vessel walls (classic Seldinger technique), such as in puncture of the femoral artery or vein.

Cleansing and sterilization

Most needles used today are of the disposable, one-use type. Reusable Cournand, Riley, or Potts needles can be carefully cleaned and sterilized for reuse in the following way:

1. Upon removal, rinse all needle parts and manually flush them with water.
2. Place needle parts in Hemasol or in an ultrasonic cleaner for further cleansing.
3. Check for thorough cleaning by placing the needle in a hydrogen peroxide solution. The formation of any bubbles indicates the presence of blood, and further cleaning is required.
4. After cleaning, rinse the needles thoroughly and dry them.
5. Carefully protect the tip and package the needle components in an unassembled fashion.
6. Sterilize the set by gas or autoclaving.

CATHETER INTRODUCERS

Catheter introducers have become an integral part of the Seldinger technique. Their purpose is to facilitate the passage and exchange of catheters through a closely fitting sheath. With the exception of balloon catheters, catheters of the same French size as the sheath could be inserted. Introducers allow multiple catheter exchanges without use of, or with reduced use of, guidewires and with much less patient discomfort, as manual compression of the vessel is not required during catheter exchanges.

Design

Introducer sets originally consisted of a tapered dilator within a slightly shorter sheath. Advances in catheter introducer design have resulted in the addition of a gasket seal (hemostasis valve) on the hub of the sheath and a side port tubing with a stopcock attached directly to the hub of the sheath. These improvements eliminate blood loss during catheter exchange, decrease thrombolytic complications, and reduce the risk of air embolism in central venous catheterization. The side port tubing conveniently affords the options of fluid or drug administration as well as pressure monitoring. During coronary angiography peripheral artery pressure can be monitored through the side port of the sheath in addition to the aortic pressure to determine dampening of the catheter tip pressure. However, substantial dampening of the peripheral arterial pressure may occur depending on the size of the catheter within the sheath. In general, adequate arterial pressures can be obtained if the difference between the sheath and the catheter is at least one French size. Simultaneous arterial pressure measurements can also be made to determine gradients within the aorta or across the aortic valve.

Use of a sheath during cardiac catheterization permits exchange and passage of all types of catheters, including those without an end hole such as the NIH, Lehman, Eppendorf, or pacing catheters. Insertion of endhole catheters through a sheath allows the use of a J-curve guidewire to straighten the tip of the catheter and permit safe passage to the abdominal aorta.[27] Ideally, removal of such catheters should also be done with the use of a guidewire to reduce the risk of vessel trauma. In clinical practice, however, most catheters are removed without the help of a guidewire. Use of a guidewire in removing a pigtail catheter is recommended.

Longer introducer sets (23, 45, or 60 cm) are sometimes very helpful for passing catheters through a tortous femoral-iliac system. Once in place, multiple catheters can be exchanged without difficulty and with no vascular injury. Catheter rotation and torque transmission are also facilitated. However, the poor radiopacity of sheaths makes fluoroscopic visualization of the advancement and location of this long sheath difficult. Filling the sheath with contrast medium may help.

Catheter introducer sets with a side port are useful in arterial and venous percutaneous catheter insertion, for either short- or long-term catheterization. They are used widely for percutaneous venous catheterization when fluid or drug administration through the side port presents a distinct advantage, such as in large-volume fluid resuscitation. When a Y–type blood/solution administration set is attached to an 8 Fr, 5-inch, UMI catheter introducer, flow rates up to 184 ml/minute can be achieved.[28] Because of differences in side port inside diameter among the various types of catheter introdu-

cers, there are marked variations in flow rates (Table 1-6). Certainly high flow rates will decrease when a catheter lies within the sheath. Nonetheless, Benumof, Wyte, and Rogers[29] have reported flow rates through the side port of an 8.5 Fr Arrow introducer with a 7.0 or 7.5 Fr PA catheter in place to be equivalent to flow rates through a 16- to 19-gauge IV catheter (see Table 1-6).

The use of catheter introducers has permitted catheterization of arterial grafts for angiographic studies. The sheath allows nontraumatic insertion of multiple catheters.[30]

Types

Several manufacturers produce catheter introducers of similar basic design with minor variations.

CONSTRUCTION: Catheter introducers are assembled as a three-piece set containing a 17 to 20 cm Teflon or polyethylene, tapered-tip dilator, a 10 to 13 cm blunt Teflon or polyethylene sheath, and a short (45 cm) J-curve guidewire of corresponding diameter. The sheath possesses a gasket seal at its proximal end with an attached side port tube.

SIZES: Catheter introducers are available in sizes 5 through 9 Fr.

VARIATIONS: Longer versions (30 to 98 cm) of catheter introducers are also available for use in transluminal coronary angioplasty, ventricular biopsy, and Brockenbrough transseptal needle insertion (Mullins transseptal catheter introducer set). One catheter introducer has an adjustable Tuohy-Borst adaptor on the proximal end of the sheath instead of the check-flow valve to prevent blood reflux. If this port should remain open for any reason (during accidental or deliberate removal of the catheter), a large volume of air could enter the venous circulation.[31] The operator must take special

Table 1-6. Crystalloid flow rates of catheter introducers[28,29]

Introducer (manufacturer)	Flow rate (ml/minute)
Cordis 8 Fr, 11 cm, with side arm	50*
UMI 8 Fr 12½ cm, without side arm	184*
Arrow 8.5 Fr	
without 7 Fr PA catheter	300†
with 7 Fr PA catheter	175†
Cook, 8.5 Fr with side arm	
without 7 Fr catheter	450†
with 7 Fr catheter	250†

*Using regular IV tubing.
†At infusion pressure of 300 mm Hg.

care to inspect this valve and to make sure it has been closed tightly.

Desired features

General features to consider when selecting a catheter introducer set include smoothness and ease of insertion, a self-sealing hemopneumatic valve to prevent blood loss and air intake, and a side port with a large enough bore to deliver fluids unimpeded.

A balance must be reached between a degree of sheath stiffness to minimize vascular trauma and thrombus formation and the maintenance of sheath shape to prevent kinking or bending with the patient's movement. It is imperative that the hub of the sheath be securely bonded to prevent shearing at this junction during long-term use. If large-volume fluid administration is intended, it is best to use one of the sheaths with a very large bore side port.

Because of manufacturer variations in catheter introducer sets, it is imperative to insert the intended catheter through the sheath prior to use to ensure appropriate sizing. Ideally there should be some space between the catheter and the sheath to allow free movement as well as fluid administration.

Cleansing and sterilization

Catheter introducer sets are disposable and intended for one-time use only. If contamination should occur before actual use, the set can be gas sterilized.

PROTECTIVE SLEEVE ADAPTORS

Manipulation of the PA catheter or pacing wire is sometimes necessary, particularly during the first 24 hours after catheter insertion. Although withdrawal is the usual intervention for the PA catheter, advancement of the catheter or pacemaker may occasionally be nec-

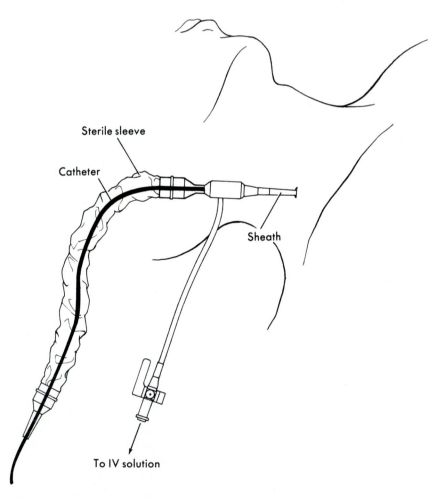

Fig. 1-33. Sterile plastic sleeve placed over a balloon flotation catheter permitting advancement of the catheter, if necessary. (From Daily, E.K., and Schroeder, J.S.: Techniques in bedside hemodynamic monitoring, ed. 3, St. Louis, 1985, The C.V. Mosby Co.)

essary. This maneuver can be performed without risk of contamination if a sterile plastic sleeve adaptor has been placed on the catheter at the time of its introduction and attached to the hub of the sheath (Fig. 1-33). This collapsible sleeve protects and maintains sterility to approximately 20 cm of catheter length. The catheter is passed through the sleeve before insertion. After the catheter has been properly positioned and sterile field and technique have been maintained, the sleeve is advanced over the catheter to the sheath, where it is securely attached to the hub of the sheath. Unless this sterile sleeve adaptor is in place, readvancement of the catheter cannot safely be performed.

TRANSDUCERS

All invasive pressure monitoring requires the transmission of a physiologic pressure to a pressure-sensitive transducer for conversion to an electric signal. The most commonly used transducers today are located outside the body, utilizing a fluid-filled system (catheter and tubing) for the transmission of physiologic pressures. Most external transducers are strain gauge transducers wired to form a Wheatstone bridge beneath its diaphragm and are a direct adaptation of strain gauges used in industry. When pressure is applied to the diaphragm of the transducer, the wires physically distort (increasing in length and decreasing in diameter), which changes the resistance to the flow of current through the wires.

The actual change in resistance can be accomplished in two ways depending on the construction of the strain gauge. If the strain gauge is *unbonded,* the connected resistor filaments or wires are suspended on a frame within the transducer, which is activated when the diaphragm moves. The *bonded* strain gauge has wire grids bonded to a thin silicone or quartz plate within the transducer. When the plate bends in response to pressure on the diaphragm, the wires are stretched and a resistance change occurs. Because the wires are very thin, strong signals can be obtained from a very small movement of the diaphragm. If voltage is applied to the resistance, the resulting current changes with the resistance variations according to Ohm's law (voltage = current × resistance). Because the transducer is connected to an instrument that amplifies, filters, and balances, the resultant electric signal can be amplified, displayed, measured, and, if calibrated, is proportional to the pressure change.

The unbonded strain gauge transducers are usually noted for their accuracy, whereas the bonded strain gauges are noted for their durability and dependability.

Technical advances have resulted in the manufacture of the *disposable pressure transducer,* consisting of an etched silicone diaphragm with a single transverse voltage piezo resistor diffused into it. Although much smaller (⅛-inch square semiconductor chip), these transducers work on the same general principle as the bonded and unbonded strain gauge transducers. This feature, along with reduced risk of infection and increased ease of use, has popularized the use of disposable transducers. The high sensitivity of the semiconductor chips has improved the frequency response of disposable transducers.

The most recent technologic advance in transducers is the placement of a miniaturized pressure-sensing device and fiberoptics within a disposable intravascular catheter. Pressure changes result in alterations in light flow, which are converted into digital and analog pressure signals. These transducer-tip catheters yield high-fidelity diagnostic pressures without the use of a fluid-filled system (see p. 16 for a complete description).

Desired features
Accuracy

The basic requirement of all transducers is accurate measurement of an applied pressure. Static pressure readings by the transducer alone should be accurate within 3% or 1 mm Hg, whichever is greater. When combined with other components that contribute errors in measurement (the monitor and the plumbing system), total system measurement error should not exceed 5%. Disposable transducers alone are as accurate as reusable ones.

Linearity

Linearity refers to the accuracy of measurements over a wide range of pressure (-30 to $+300$ mm Hg). Transducers that are not linear may be accurate at specific pressures but inaccurate at other pressures. Transducer calibration checks should be performed over a wide range of pressures (e.g., 20 to 200 mm Hg).

Temperature stability

Changes in temperature (environmental changes or flush solution) may cause zero drift and changes in the sensitivity of the transducer, resulting in erroneous pressure measurements. Transducers should accurately measure pressures within 3% or 2.5 mm Hg (whichever is greater) over a temperature range of 15° to 40° C. Disposable transducers are more sensitive to temperature than nondisposable transducers, causing zero drift beyond the criterion of 3% or 1 mm Hg.[32] This can be offset by always rezeroing before obtaining pressure readings.

Ruggedness

A transducer should be able to withstand some abuse (e.g., accidental dropping) and still remain accurate within 3% of 1 mm Hg.

Electric isolation

Electric isolation of the transducer is necessary to protect the electrically sensitive patient from even very small amounts of electric current leakage to the heart (see Chapter 22). Such currents could result in ventricular fibrillation. Electric isolation also protects the transducer during instances of defibrillation. All modern transducers (reusable and disposable) have adequate electric isolation.

Ease of use

The design of all transducers should facilitate detection and removal of air bubbles from the dome and tubing. It should be possible to assemble the transducer and monitoring equipment with ease and without jeopardizing the equipment's sterility. Transducers should easily be positioned in a mounting bracket or (preferably) attached to or near the patient. Table 1-7 lists some of the advantages and disadvantages of disposable transducers.

Care and maintenance

General guidelines for the use and handling of reusable transducers are as follows:

1. Handle reusable transducers carefully to maintain accuracy and improve longevity.
2. After use, clean and disinfect reusable transducers with an effective chemical disinfectant (e.g., glutaraldehyde) or sterilize them with ethylene oxide.
3. Store the transducers in such a manner as to prevent contamination or physical damage.
4. Before use on a patient, check the calibration of reusable transducers against a known pressure (ei-

ther with mercury or water). Do this carefully with a sterile dome to prevent transducer contamination. A new sterile dome is then needed for use on a patient.

5. Change disposable transducers every 48 to 72 hours according to hospital policy; they should not be sterilized and reused.

Table 1-7. Advantages and disadvantages of disposable transducers

Advantages	Disadvantages
Increased ease and reduced time for setup	Cost efficiency (?)
Increased stock can meet increased monitoring demands	Increased possibility of supply problems (from manufacturer or vendor)
Less risk of cross-contamination	Not compatible with every monitor
	Assumes accuracy of factory calibration without recheck

REFERENCES

1. Cournand, A.F., and Ranges, H.S.: Catheterization of the right auricle in man, Proc. Soc. Exp. Biol. Med. **46:**462, 1941.
2. Richards, D.W. Jr.: Cardiac output by the catheterization technique in various clinical conditions, Fed. Proc. **4:**215, 1945.
3. Cournand, A.F.: Measurement of cardiac output in man using the technique of catheterization of the right auricle or ventricle, J. Clin. Invest. **24:**106, 1945.
4. Cournand, A.F.: Nobel lecture, Dec. 11, 1956. In Nobel Lectures, Physiology and Medicine 1942-1962, Amsterdam, 1964, Elsevier Publishing Co., p. 529.
5. Boretos, J.W., and Eden, M.: Contemporary biomaterials, material and host response, clinical applications, new technology, and legal aspects, Park Ridge, N.J., 1984, Noyes Publications.
6. Hecker, J.F., and Scandrett, L.A.: Roughness and thrombogenicity of the outer surfaces of intravascular catheters, J. Biomed. Res. **19:**381, 1985.
7. D'Arcy, P.F.: Drug interactions and reactions update, Drug Intell. Clin. Pharm. **17:**726, 1983.
8. Jacobi J., et al.: Loss of nitroglycerin to central venous pressure catheter, Drug Intell. Clin. Pharm. **16:**331, 1982.
9. Stenqvist, O., Curelaru, I., Linder, L.E. and Gustavsson, B.: Stiffness of central venous catheters, Acta Anaesthesiol. Scand. **27:**153, 1983.
10. Curelaru, I., et al.: Material thrombogenicity in central venous catheterization. II. A comparison between plain silicone elastomer and plain polyethylene long antebrachial catheters, Acta Anaesthesiol. Scand. **27:**158, 1983.
11. Grossman, W.: Cardiac catheterization and angiography, ed. 3, Philadelphia, 1986, Lea & Febiger.
12. Schwartz, L., and Vaughan-Neil, E.: Comparison of the performance of pigtail catheters with different numbers of sideholes, Cathet. Cardiovasc. Diagn. **3:**421, 1977.
13. Judkins, M.P., and Judkins, E.: Coronary arteriography and left ventriculography: Judkins technique. In King, S.B., and Douglas, J.S.: Coronary arteriography and angioplasty, New York, 1985, McGraw-Hill Book Co.
14. Grollman, J.H.: Pigtail catheters in pulmonary angiography (Editorial). Cathet. and Cardiovasc. Diagn. **10:**389, 1984.
15. VanTassel, R.A., et al.: A less traumatic catheter for coronary angiography, Cathet. Cardiovasc. Diagn. **11:**187, 1985.
16. Heupler, F. Jr.: Coronary arteriography and left ventriculography: Sones technique. In King, S.B., and Douglas, J.S.: Coronary arteriography and angioplasty, New York, 1985, McGraw-Hill Book Co.
17. Schneider, R.M., et al.: Fracture of a polyurethane cardiac catheter in the aortic arch: a complication related to polymer aging, Cathet. Cardiovasc. Diagn. **9:**197, 1983.
18. Blitt, C.D., Carlson, G.L., Wright, W.A., and Otto, C.W.: J-wire versus straight wire for central venous system cannulation via the external jugular vein, Anesth. Analg. **61:**530, 1982.
19. Sos, T.A., et al.: A new open-ended guidewire/catheter, Radiology **154:**817, 1985.

20. Gerlock, A.J., and Mirfakhraee, M.: Essentials of interventional angiographic techniques, Philadelphia, 1985, W.B. Saunders Co.

21. Casarella, W.J., and Wilner, G.D.: Guide wire thrombogenicity measured by fibrinopeptide A radioimmunoassay, AJR **128:**363, 1977.

22. Cope, C.: Intravascular breakage of Seldinger spring guide wires, JAMA **180:**161, 1962.

23. Schwartz, A.J., Horrow, J.C., Jobes, D.R., and Ellison, N.: Guide wires—a caution, Crit. Care Med. **9:**347, 1981.

24. Anderson, J.H., Gianturco, C., Wallace, S., and Dodd, G.D.: A scanning electron microscopic study of angiographic catheters and guidewires, Radiology **111:**567, 1974.

25. Seldinger, S.-I.: Catheter replacement of the needle in percutaneous arteriography: a new technique, Acta Radiol. [Diagn.] **39:**368, 1953.

26. Crowley, W.C., and Klein, M.D.: New break-away needle for subclavian vein cannulation, Am. J. Surg. **147:**817, 1984.

27. Hillis, L.D.: Percutaneous left heart catheterization and coronary arteriography using a femoral sheath, Cathet. Cardiovasc. Diagn. **5:**393, 1979.

28. Haynes, B.E.: Catheter introducers for rapid fluid resuscitation, Ann. Emerg. Med. **12:**606, 1983.

29. Benumof, J.L., Wyte, S.R., and Rogers, S.N.: A large catheter sheath with an increased side-port functional gauge, Crit. Care Med. **11:**660, 1983.

30. Schatzki, S.C.: Catheter angiography through prosthetic vascular grafts using a Teflon sheath, Radiology **148:**565, 1983.

31. Doblar, D.D., Hinkle, J.C., Fay, M.L., and Concon, B.F.: Air embolism associated with pulmonary artery catheter introducer kit, Anesthesiology **56:**307, 1982.

32. Disposable pressure transducers, Health Devices **13:**267, 1984.

Chapter Two

Venous access

ELAINE K. DAILY
ARA G. TILKIAN

Rapid, successful, access into the venous and arterial systems is a necessary skill in caring for critically ill patients and in performing certain cardiovascular procedures. Entry into either system ranges from a simple needle puncture to obtain a blood sample to more complex cannulation methods with exchange of multiple catheters. This chapter discusses placement of catheters into the central venous system via the percutaneous and surgical approaches. (Arterial access is discussed in Chapter 3.) Variations in techniques will occur dependent on the specific goal of cannulation (short- or long-term catheterization). Where pertinent, specific variations are included. Basic steps and equipment used in performing the Seldinger technique and the surgical cutdown technique are presented initially, whereas details relevant to particular sites are presented later in discussion of that site.

Chapter 1 details the type of equipment utilized in either venous or arterial cannulation. Because of user preference, an effort has been made to make equipment recommendations general in nature.

GENERAL GUIDELINES FOR CANNULATION PROCEDURES

Certain aspects of vascular access are common to both the cutdown and percutaneous approaches of arterial and venous cannulation. These include use of aseptic technique, local anesthesia, adequate personnel, and patient and equipment preparation. Recommendations for all elective percutaneous insertions of central venous or cardiac catheters and for cutdown catheter insertion are presented below and will not be repeated for each technique.

Aseptic technique

Insertion of catheters into the central venous or arterial system should be performed by means of aseptic technique. If it becomes necessary in an emergency situation to insert a catheter without regard to sterile tech-

nique, the catheter should be replaced at the earliest opportunity.

1. Wash your hands with an antiseptic agent and wear sterile gown and gloves; wear a cap and mask for cutdown catheter insertion.
2. Vigorously scrub the intended entry site and surrounding area with an antiseptic agent (e.g., povidone-iodine [Betadine] or chlorhexidine [Hibiclens]) for 1 minute. (Begin the scrub at the puncture site and gradually extend peripherally 4 to 6 inches in a concentric fashion.)
3. Cover the surrounding area with sterile drapes, leaving a small opening at the puncture site. (Plastic adhesive–backed drapes with a small central hole work very well for this.)

Local anesthesia

For all conscious patients, administration of a local anesthetic should precede cutdown or percutaneous cannulation of an artery or a vein. Although local anesthetic agents block sensory impulse in selective nerve endings within seconds of injection, the duration of action depends on the particular agent used (Table 2-1), the concentration of the drug, and the presence or absence of epinephrine. Epinephrine causes vasoconstriction, resulting in decreased absorption and a marked increase in the duration of action. Nonetheless, administration of an anesthetic containing epinephrine is discouraged for patients with cardiac disease.

While actual allergic reactions to local anesthetic agents are quite rare,[1] systemic toxic reactions may occur as a result of rapid absorption of high doses of anesthetic or increased patient sensitivity. Systemic toxic reactions also tend to occur more frequently in elderly patients. Signs of local anesthetic reaction appear within seconds and should be recognized and treated promptly. Early signs include apprehension and somnolence, whereas later signs are circulatory and respiratory collapse with hypotension, pallor, cool clammy

32

Table 2-1. Concentration, suggested maximal dosage, and duration of action of local anesthetic agents

Drug	Concentration (%)	Maximal dose (without epinephrine) (mg/kg)	Duration of action	
			Without epinephrine	*With epinephrine*
Lidocaine (Xylocaine)	0.5	4	1¼ hr	3½ hr
	1.0-1.5	4	2 hr	6½ hr
Procaine (Novocain)	0.5	1	20 min	1 hr
Mepivacaine (Carbocaine)	0.5	4	1½ hr	4 hr
Bupivacaine (Marcaine)	0.5	2	5 hr	9 hr

skin, and respiratory irregularity, including periods of apnea. Twitching and generalized convulsions may occur later if appropriate therapy is not administered. Management of local anesthetic reaction consists of vasopressor therapy, if necessary, to maintain blood pressure; administration of oxygen and ventilation of the lungs, if necessary; and administration of barbiturate if convulsions occur. Full resuscitation equipment should be immediately available whenever local anesthetics are given. See Chapter 19 for more details.

Lidocaine dosage

Because of its rapid onset of action, lidocaine is the most commonly used local anesthetic. The dosage is 5 to 30 ml of 1% solution, with a maximal dose of 300 mg without epinephrine or 500 mg with epinephrine.[2]

Technique of lidocaine injection

1. Puncture the skin with a 25-gauge needle, bevel side down, and inject enough lidocaine (approximately 0.5 ml) to raise a small wheal on the skin.
2. Advance the needle through the subcutaneous layers along the intended path of cannulation or incision, slowly injecting more lidocaine. Precede all deep injections of lidocaine by aspiration to make sure that the injection will not be into the vessel.
3. In order to inject lidocaine in several directions, free the needle from the subcutaneous tissue by withdrawing it and then readvancing it. Do not turn or bend the hub of the needle while its tip is within the subcutaneous tissue; this will not change the direction of the needle and could cause it to break at the hub.

Use of the needle to locate the vein. The small anesthetic infiltrating needle is frequently used as a "locator" needle in "blind" venous cannulation (e.g., internal jugular or subclavian vein). If at the time of infiltration one locates the vein by aspirating venous blood into the syringe, one can mark this location by leaving a small drop of blood at the puncture site upon

removal of the infiltrating needle, or by removing the syringe and leaving the infiltrating needle in place (placing a thumb over its open hub). The larger cannulating needle is then inserted along this identified track. Location of the vein with the small-diameter needle reduces the risk of inadvertent puncture of an artery with the large cannulating needle; if puncture should occur with the small-diameter needle, bleeding and hematoma formation are considerably reduced.

Personnel

Personnel required for all vascular access procedures include both a physician experienced in the particular technique of vascular access and a nurse to assist the physician as well as to monitor and comfort the patient.

Patient preparation

For all vascular access procedures, preparation of the patient consists of the following steps:
1. Explain the procedure to the patient, if appropriate, and to the patient's family, if possible.
2. Obtain informed consent.
3. Place the patient in a supine position and in such a way as to provide maximal exposure of the intended insertion site.

Basic percutaneous catheterization equipment

The basic tools of the Seldinger technique of catheterization consist of an introducing needle, a guidewire, and a catheter. While any type of needle could be used for the Seldinger technique, thin-wall needles are preferred, as the lumen can accommodate a guidewire without substantially increasing the outside diameter. Consequently, virtually all percutaneous puncture needles today have thin walls. Needles used in the Seldinger technique are available with one, two, or three parts (see Fig. 1-32).

One-part needle

The one-part needle, with a plastic grip shield, is used for *single-wall puncture of an artery or vein.* For venous cannulation of the external jugular, internal jugular, and subclavian veins, a fluid-containing syringe is attached to the needle's hub and negative pressure maintained in the syringe during needle insertion to verify venous location.

Two-part needle

The two-part vascular needle consists of an outer cannula with an inner solid stylet or needle. This needle is used for transfixation of the artery or vein in which *both* walls of the vessel are punctured. It is most commonly used for cannulation of the radial, brachial, or femoral artery or femoral vein. For femoral vein cannulation, the needle is inserted through the vessel; a syringe containing a small amount of heparin or lidocaine is then attached to the hub of the needle and the needle slowly withdrawn while negative pressure is maintained within the syringe.

Three-part needle

The three-part vascular needle consists of an outer cannula, an inner stylet, and an obturator. This needle is used only rarely for arterial cannulation for purposes of intermittent blood sampling or pressure measurements in the cardiac catheterization laboratory. After successful insertion of the needle and cannula into the artery, the needle is removed and the round-tip obturator inserted into the cannula. The cannula can then be safely advanced slightly. Pressure measurements and blood sampling can be obtained by temporary removal of the inner obturator.

Additional equipment

Additional equipment that facilitates percutaneous catheterization and reduces some of its risks includes the catheter introducer set containing a guidewire, dilator and sheath, and sterile plastic sleeves. The dilator component of this unit tunnels through the subcutaneous tissue, preparing a track for insertion of the catheter. This prevents damage to the catheter tip and promotes successful catheter passage. The sheath of the unit remains in place, providing a conduit for catheter insertion and exchange, if necessary. Sheaths with a pneumatic seal at the hub and a side extension port reduce bleeding from the sheath hub, prevent air intake through the hub, and allow fluid or drug administration as well as pressure monitoring through the side port. This type of sheath is recommended for all internal jugular and subclavian vein catheterizations to prevent air embolism.

Generally, catheter introducer sheaths will accept catheters of the same French size. The exceptions to this are some of the balloon-tip catheters that require a sheath one size larger than the catheter because of the addition of the balloon. However, this is not true of all balloon catheters, as some have a tapered tip, which maintains an equal diameter. For this reason, it is necessary to know the manufacturer's recommendations and check the compatibility of the equipment before insertion. Precautions required in the use of catheter introducers are discussed on p. 42.

Sterile plastic sleeves should be placed over all long-term venous monitoring catheters that may require further manipulation (see Fig. 1-33). The sleeve covers the outside of the catheter from the hub of the sheath to the proximal end of the catheter, maintaining its sterility for up to 12 hours should future catheter advancement be necessary. The sleeve should be slipped over the catheter prior to insertion. After the catheter has been positioned, the sleeve is slid forward and attached to the hub of the sheath. Care must be taken to avoid sealing the sleeve to the sheath too tightly, which could compress the lumen of the catheter.

Many companies manufacture a disposable, sterile percutaneous cannulation package containing all the equipment necessary for percutaneous catheterization at the bedside. However, in the cardiac catheterization laboratory, trays are usually assembled containing the equipment listed below. IV heparin solution, transducer tubing, and monitoring equipment are also necessary for hemodynamic pressure measurements.

Fluoroscopy is ideally available for all central venous catheterizations, but it is essential for elective placement of any pacing catheters as well as for right heart catheterization via the femoral vein. The balloon flotation PA catheter, introduced via an antecubital, subcla-

---

BASIC PERCUTANEOUS CATHETERIZATION EQUIPMENT

Antiseptic solution
Drapes, towels, and towel clips
Bowl of sterile saline with heparin
4 × 4-inch gauze pads
Lidocaine 1% without epinephrine
25- and 21-gauge needles, 1½ and 2 inches long
3, 5, and 10 ml syringes
#11 scalpel
18-gauge, thin-wall, one- or two-part percutaneous entry needle, 2½ inches long
Catheter introducer set containing 0.035-inch (0.9 mm) J-curve guidewire, a dilator, and a catheter sheath
3-0 silk suture on a cutting needle
Needle holder
Catheter of choice

vian, or internal jugular vein, can be positioned in the PA without the aid of fluoroscopy by monitoring of hemodynamic waveforms. X-ray confirmation of catheter position is necessary if fluoroscopy is not used.

Emergency resuscitation equipment, including a defibrillator, should be available for all percutaneous and surgical insertions of central venous catheters.

Care of vascular catheters

Complications associated with catheters can be prevented by assiduous care and maintenance of catheter patency as well as sterility. The following steps should be taken:

1. Promote catheter patency through use of a continuous flush and periodic gentle manual flushing with heparinized saline solution.
2. Aspirate all vascular catheters prior to manual flushing.
3. Flush the arterial catheter gently with fresh sterile heparinized saline (excluding any of the aspirated fluid).
4. Never flush the catheter if aspiration is difficult or unsuccessful.
5. Carefully remove air from all flushing equipment.
6. Inspect the insertion site and change the dressing daily (with use of an iodophor ointment). All long-term monitoring catheters and tubing (including transducer domes) should be changed every 48 to 72 hours.

THE SELDINGER TECHNIQUE

In 1953 Dr. Sven-Ivar Seldinger,[3] a Stockholm radiologist, described the procedure for percutaneous arterial insertion of a catheter using a guidewire. This simple but revolutionary technique has stood the test of time and now is the preferred method of catheter insertion into either an artery or a vein. It is ideal for femoral artery cannulation and introduction of angiographic catheters as well as venous cannulation for insertion of CVP, PA, or pacing catheters.

Basic procedure

1. Make a small (2 to 3 mm) skin incision with a #11 scalpel to facilitate catheter or dilator passage (this can alternatively be done after the insertion of the guidewire into the vessel).
2. Bluntly dissect the subcutaneous tissue along the direction of the vessel using a straight or curved Kelly forceps.
3. Puncture the vessel with an 18-gauge thin-wall needle with a stylet positioned at a relatively shallow angle (30° to 40°) (Fig. 2-1, *A*).
4. Remove the stylet and slowly withdraw the needle

until blood flows freely from the needle (or spurts with arterial cannulation) (Fig. 2-1, *B*).

5. When free flow of blood is obtained, reduce the angle of the needle and advance it slightly into the vessel, making sure it remains in the vessel as indicated by continued free blood flow.
6. Insert the soft flexible tip of an appropriate-size guidewire through and a short distance beyond the needle into the vessel (approximately 15 to 20 cm) (Fig. 2-1, *C*).
7. Remove the needle with one hand while firmly holding the guidewire in place between the thumb and index finger of the other hand (Fig. 2-1, *D*). Place the remaining three fingers of the hand holding the guidewire over the insertion site, applying light pressure for puncture of a vein and firm pressure for an artery.
8. Wipe the guidewire with a sterile, moist gauze pad.
9. Thread the appropriate-size catheter over the guidewire. Approximately 10 cm of guidewire should protrude from the catheter hub before the catheter is inserted into the skin.
10. Hold the catheter and wire together firmly near the skin and insert the tip of the catheter through the skin into the vessel using a slight rotating motion (Fig. 2-1, *E*).
11. Advance the catheter and guidewire well into the vessel, making sure at all times that the guidewire protrudes from the hub of the sheath.
12. Remove the guidewire, aspirate and discard the aspirate, flush the catheter, and connect it to a manifold or other flush system. Aspiration of freely flowing blood confirms intravascular location and clears the system of any clots or air bubbles.
13. Direct the catheter to the position desired and suture it to the skin if long-term indwelling use is planned.
14. Obtain a chest radiograph for centrally positioned catheters if fluoroscopy is not used.

Variations

A small skin incision is usually made at the puncture site before needle insertion to facilitate skin entry and to avoid skin plugs in the needle lumen. However, some physicians prefer to make this incision after inserting the guidewire in preparation for dilator, sheath, and catheter insertion through the skin.

Use of a catheter introducer sheath

1. Follow steps 1 through 8 of the basic Seldinger technique.
2. Thread the appropriate-size sheath with its tapered dilator over the guidewire until approximately 6 to 10

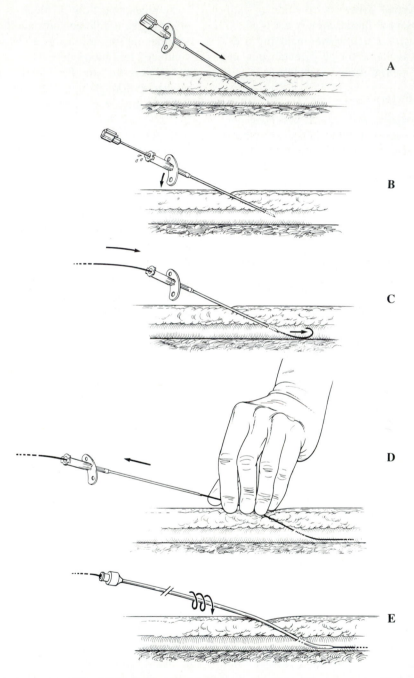

Fig. 2-1. Basic procedure for the Seldinger technique. **A,** The vessel is punctured with the needle at a 30° to 40° angle. **B,** The stylet is removed and free blood flow is observed; the angle of the needle is then reduced. **C,** The flexible tip of the guidewire is passed through the needle into the vessel. **D,** The needle is removed over the wire while firm pressure is applied at the site. **E,** The tip of the catheter is passed over the wire and advanced into the vessel with a rotating motion.

cm of guidewire protrudes from the hub of the sheath (Fig. 2-2, *A*).

3. Firmly hold the wire and dilator tip near the skin and insert the unit through the skin into the vessel using a rotating motion. Make certain that the tapered dilator precedes the sheath during insertion (Fig. 2-2, *B*). Adequate blunt dissection preceding the introduction of the guidewire will ensure easy cannulation; otherwise the dilator sheath edges may wrinkle or fray, preventing easy entry into the vessel.

4. Fully advance the unit into the vessel, making sure at all times that the guidewire protrudes from the hub of the sheath.

5. Remove the guidewire and dilator together, leaving the sheath in the vessel (Fig. 2-2, *C*).

6. Aspirate and flush the sheath with sterile saline (through the hub of a standard sheath or through the side arm, if available).

7. Insert the appropriate-size catheter through the hub of the sheath and direct it to the desired position.

8. Attach the side arm of the sheath, if available, to a heparinized flush system.

This system can be used for multiple catheter exchanges, insertion of end-hole cardiac catheters during catheterization, insertion of catheters without end holes, and long-term monitoring or fluid administration.

Insertion of multiple catheters through a single vein

Insertion of multiple catheters through a single venipuncture without significant complications has been described by several authors.[4-6] While use of a single multilumen catheter (p. 15) could at times suffice, this technique does seem advantageous in select instances, such as electrophysiologic studies, where simultaneous placement of multiple catheters is necessary. Use of

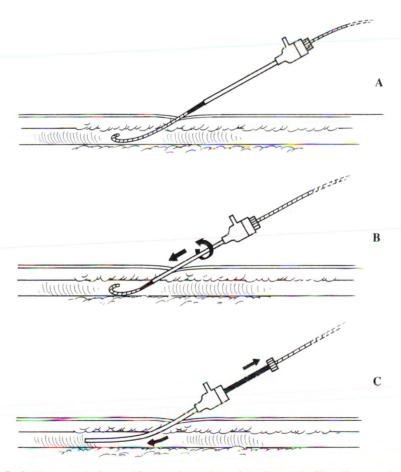

Fig. 2-2. Seldinger technique with use of a catheter introducer. **A,** The dilator and sheath are advanced over the guidewire until 6 to 10 cm of wire protrudes from the hub. **B,** The dilator and sheath are advanced through the skin into the vessel using a rotating motion. **C,** The guidewire and dilator are removed as a unit, leaving the sheath in place within the vessel.

this procedure should be limited to central veins or a large peripheral vein such as the femoral vein.

1. Follow steps 1 through 8 of the basic Seldinger technique.

2. Follow steps 2 through 5 of the technique described for use of a catheter introducer.

3. Insert two flexible guidewires through the sheath and into the vein (Fig. 2-3, *A*).

4. Remove the sheath, leaving only the two guidewires in the vein.

5. Insert a second catheter introducer set (dilator and sheath) into the vein over one of the guidewires, making certain that the other guidewire does not advance further into the vein during this manipulation (Fig. 2-3, *B*).

6. Remove the dilator and guidewire, leaving the second sheath in the vein (Fig. 2-3, *C*).

7. Aspirate and flush the sheath with sterile saline.

8. Insert a pacing electrode or catheter through the second sheath and position it correctly in the heart (Fig. 2-3, *D*).

9. Withdraw the second sheath back over the pacing catheter to make room for another catheter introducer.

10. Insert a third catheter introducer set (dilator and sheath) into the vein over the remaining guidewire and adjacent to the pacing catheter (Fig. 2-3, *E*).

11. Remove only the dilator from the third introducer, leaving the sheath and guidewire in place.

12. Introduce a second guidewire through the sheath into the vein (Fig. 2-3, *F*).

13. Remove the sheath, leaving two guidewires (and the pacing catheter) in the vein.

14. Insert a fourth catheter introducer set (dilator and sheath) into the vein over one of the guidewires, making sure that the catheter and other guidewire do not advance into the vein during this manipulation.

15. Remove the dilator and guidewire from the sheath, leaving the sheath, adjacent guidewire, and pacing catheter in the vein.

16. Aspirate and flush the sheath with sterile saline.

17. Insert a catheter or pacing electrode through the sheath and position it in the desired location.

18. Withdraw the sheath back over the catheter to make room for another catheter introducer.

19. Insert a fifth catheter introducer set (dilator and sheath) into the vein over the remaining guidewire, making sure that the other catheters do not advance.

20. Remove the dilator and guidewire from the sheath, leaving the sheath and two catheters in the vein.

21. Aspirate and flush the sheath with sterile saline.

22. Insert a catheter or pacing electrode through the sheath and position it correctly in the heart. This last sheath can remain within the vessel (Fig. 2-3, *G*).

23. If fluoroscopy is not used, obtain a chest radiograph to confirm the position of the catheter(s).

The catheter introducer sets may be reused several times during this procedure if close inspection reveals no evidence of damage (i.e., kinks, bends, or frayed edges). The dilator and sheath must be rinsed and flushed with sterile saline prior to each reuse.

While the sizes of the catheter introducer sets used will vary depending on the size of the catheters or electrodes to be inserted, the placement of multiple catheters requires a large vessel and is usually performed via the femoral vein, although the subclavian vein could also be used. The femoral vein can usually accommodate a total diameter of 14 to 18 French sizes (e.g., three catheters, each 5 to 6 Fr). The sheath must be one French size larger than the intended catheter. IV administration of 5000 units of heparin is recommended at the initiation of the procedure for short-term catheterization; use of heparin anticoagulation should be continued for prolonged catheterization.

Special precautions with the Seldinger technique and related vascular access methods
Procedure for guidewire passage if resistance is met

Never pass a guidewire if any resistance is met. First, remove and inspect the guidewire for damage. Aspirate the needle to confirm intravascular location. Use a small- or large-curve J wire for tortuous vessels. If resistance is still met, inject a small amount (2 to 3 ml) of contrast medium through the needle and observe by means of fluoroscopy. This aids in determining true intravascular access as well as the location and extent of vessel tortuosity.

Correct guidewire insertion

Never insert the stiff end of the guidewire. Check the guidewire tip before each insertion.

Verification of catheter position

For catheters inserted into central veins without the aid of fluoroscopy, obtain a chest radiograph film immediately after catheter positioning to confirm correct location. Do not infuse fluids or medications until intravascular location of the catheter is confirmed.

Compression of puncture site

After removing the catheters, manually compress the puncture site (3 to 5 minutes of gentle pressure for venous puncture; 10 minutes of firm pressure for arterial puncture).

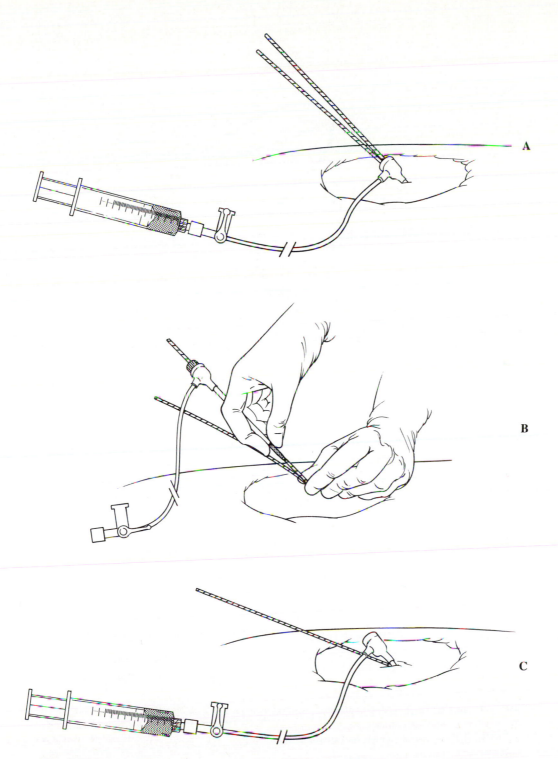

Fig. 2-3. Percutaneous insertion of multiple catheters through a single vessel. **A,** The flexible ends of two guidewires are inserted through the sheath into the vessel. **B,** After the sheath is removed, a second dilator/sheath set is inserted over one of the guidewires. **C,** The guidewire and dilator are removed leaving one sheath and guidewire in place in the vessel.

Continued.

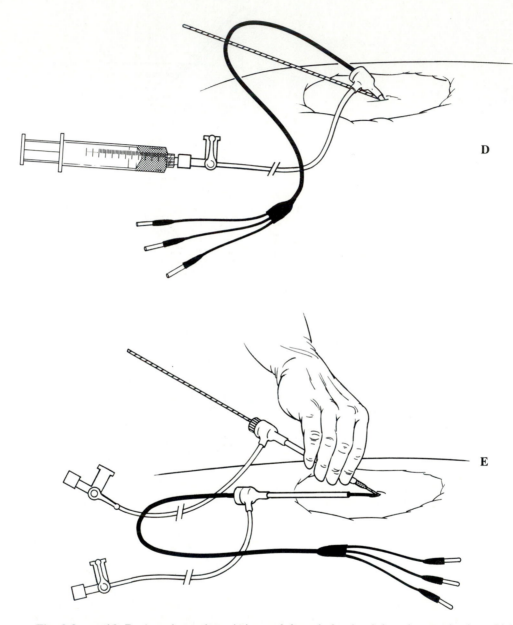

Fig. 2-3, cont'd. D, A pacing catheter is inserted through the sheath into the vessel, after which the second sheath is withdrawn. **E,** A third dilator/sheath set is inserted over the remaining guidewire into the vein, after which the dilator is removed, leaving the sheath and guidewire in the vessel.

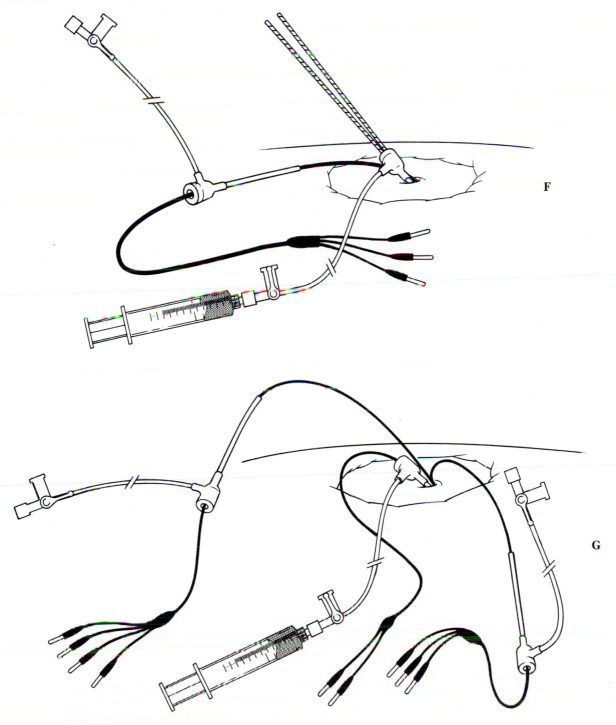

Fig. 2-3, cont'd. F, A second guidewire is inserted through the sheath into the vein, and the sheath is removed, leaving both guidewires in the vessel. Steps **B** through **E** are then repeated until three pacing catheters are inserted **(G).**

Use of a catheter introducer sheath

1. To insert the dilator/sheath system into the skin and vessel, hold the unit at the junction of the sheath and dilator to prevent buckling, kinking, or fraying. If you encounter difficulty advancing the dilator/sheath through the subcutaneous tissue into the vein, *do not forcefully advance the unit*. Remove the dilator/sheath unit leaving the guidewire in the vein, and reinsert only the dilator over the wire to dilate the tissues sufficiently for passage of the sheath. Carefully inspect the edges of the used sheath. If there are any kinks, rough or frayed edges, or buckling, use a new sheath. Remove the dilator from the vein, reassemble inside the sheath, and insert the unit over the guidewire through the redilated passage.

2. After removing the guidewire and dilator, hold the sheath firmly in place in the vessel. The unsupported sheath can easily bend or kink during this time, causing difficulty in subsequent guidewire or catheter passage. If you note resistance to guidewire passage, slowly withdraw the sheath while advancing the guidewire. This usually removes the obstruction. Forceful advance-

ment of a catheter or guidewire through a bent sheath may cause it to puncture through the wall of the sheath.

3. Catheters should be inserted and advanced through the sheath with a short piece of flexible guidewire protruding from its proximal tip, to reduce vascular trauma. This maneuver is essential for insertion of a pigtail catheter into a sheath to straighten out its tip (Fig. 2-4).

4. If you are using a sheath without a gasket or pneumatic seal, place a thumb over the hub after removing the dilator and wire to control bleeding and prevent air intake (see p. 60).

5. Continuously infuse or intermittently flush the side arms of the sheath to prevent thrombus formation and possible embolization.

Flushing the catheter

Manual flushing of vascular catheters is routinely performed to prevent clot formation. For venous catheters, aspirate and then flush the catheter (or sheath). For arterial catheters, aspirate the catheter (or sheath), discard the aspirated fluid, and flush the line with a fresh

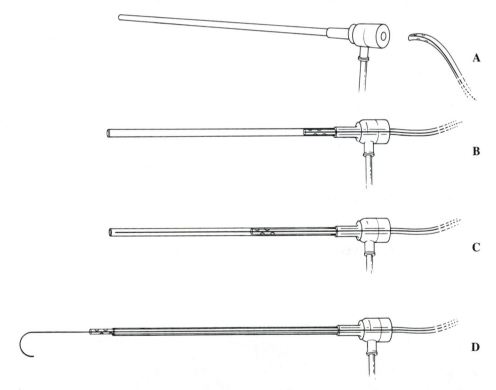

Fig. 2-4. Insertion of a pigtail catheter through a sheath with use of a guidewire. **A,** The catheter is advanced over the guidewire until the flexible tip of the wire is just at the tip of the catheter. **B,** The catheter with the guidewire is inserted through the sheath. **C,** When well into the sheath, the wire is advanced beyond the tip of the catheter. **D,** The catheter and guidewire are then advanced with the guidewire exiting the sheath first, followed by the catheter.

solution of heparinized sterile saline. Arterial flushing should be done gently (particularly in the radial artery) and should never be performed against resistance.

Correct withdrawal

If you introduce a catheter directly through the needle (either a standard needle or a peel-away one) into the vein and you encounter difficulty in advancement, *never withdraw the catheter through the needle*. To prevent shearing and embolization of the catheter, you must withdraw the needle and catheter *together*.

SURGICAL CUTDOWN TECHNIQUE

Although percutaneous catheterization provides more rapid access into the vascular system, surgical cutdown may be necessary in some emergency situations. This procedure was first described in 1940 as an alternate access procedure in patients in shock with collapsed veins, or in patients with very small veins.[7] This technique continues to be useful in hypovolemic patients and children.

The basic equipment necessary for arterial or venous cutdown is listed on this page. Additional equipment includes sterile heparinized IV solution for maintenance of catheter patency and appropriate transducer components for hemodynamic pressure monitoring.

Basic procedure

1. Make a transverse incision through the skin and superficial fascia directly over the selected vessel with a #15 blade. The incision should be wide enough to permit adequate exposure of the vessel.

2. Separate the tissues by gentle, blunt, longitudinal dissection with a curved forceps (Fig. 2-5, *A*).

3. Identify the selected vessel and bring it to the surface by placing the forceps tips underneath it (Fig. 2-5, *B*).

4. Tag the vessel both proximally and distally using 3-0 or 4-0 silk (6 to 10 cm long) for the vein and umbilical or silicone rubber (Silastic) tape for the artery (Fig. 2-5, *C*). For arterial cutdown, the Silastic tapes are usually double-wrapped around the proximal and distal portions of the vessel. The ends of each tape are then secured with a small straight forceps.

5. Occlude blood flow through the vessel. (Retract the upper tie around the artery or tie the lower tie in the vein.)

6. While pinching the top portion of the vessel with a forceps, make a small incision (approximately one-third the diameter) into the vessel using a #11 blade (sharp side up) (Fig. 2-5, *C* and *D*). Some vascular sur-

geons prefer to use a #15 blade to avoid the risk of penetrating the posterior wall of the artery with the sharp point of the #11 blade.

7. Insert the selected catheter into the vessel. A small vein introducer hook may facilitate venous entry (Fig. 2-5, *E*).

8. Temporarily release tension on the upper umbilical tape of the artery and advance the catheter to the desired position. If necessary, apply tension to proximal and distal umbilical or Silastic ties to control any bleeding.

9. For long-term indwelling catheters in a vein, tie and cut off the upper tie around the catheter and vein, taking care not to occlude the catheter. For long-term use of catheters in an artery, remove the proximal and distal ties and compress the artery for several minutes.

10. Irrigate the wound with sterile saline and carefully observe for any bleeding.

11. Close the skin with three or four interrupted sutures of 4-0 silk.

12. Suture the catheter to the skin at the insertion site.

13. Clean the incision with sterile saline, and apply povidone-iodine ointment and a sterile dressing.

BASIC EQUIPMENT FOR VASCULAR CUTDOWN

Antiseptic solution
Drapes, towels, and towel clips
Bowl of sterile saline with heparin
4 × 4-inch gauze pads
Lidocaine 1% without epinephrine
25- and 21-gauge needles, 1½ and 2 inches long
   5 and 10 ml syringes
#11 and #15 scalpels
Curved mosquito forceps
Plain forceps
Self-retracting retractors
Small rakes
Fine-toothed forceps (for arterial cutdown)
Two pieces of umbilical tape and/or Silastic tape (for arterial cutdown)
4-0 Silk suture
6-0 Monofilament suture
Iris scissors
Small plastic introducer
Needle holder
Heparin
Catheter of choice

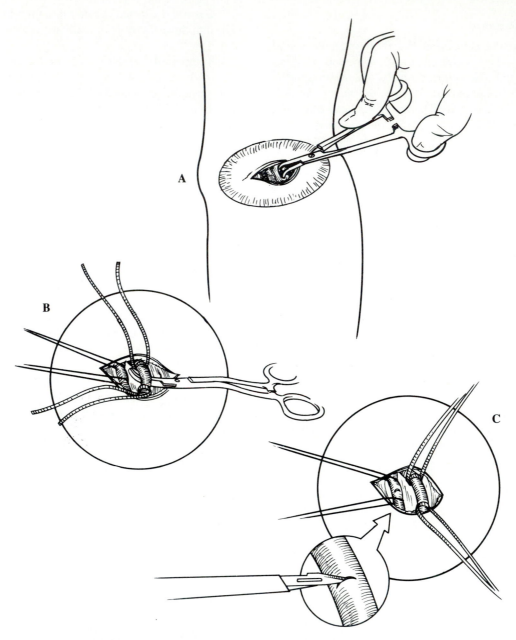

Fig. 2-5. Arterial and venous cutdown technique. **A,** Through a transverse skin incision, the subcutaneous tissues are longitudinally dissected. **B,** The selected vessel is brought to the surface with use of a forceps and the proximal and distal segments of the vessel are tagged. A small incision is made into the vein (**C**) or into the artery (**D**) with the sharp point of a #11 scalpel. **E,** Venous catheter insertion is facilitated with use of a small vein dilator. **F,** Arterial and venous catheter insertion.

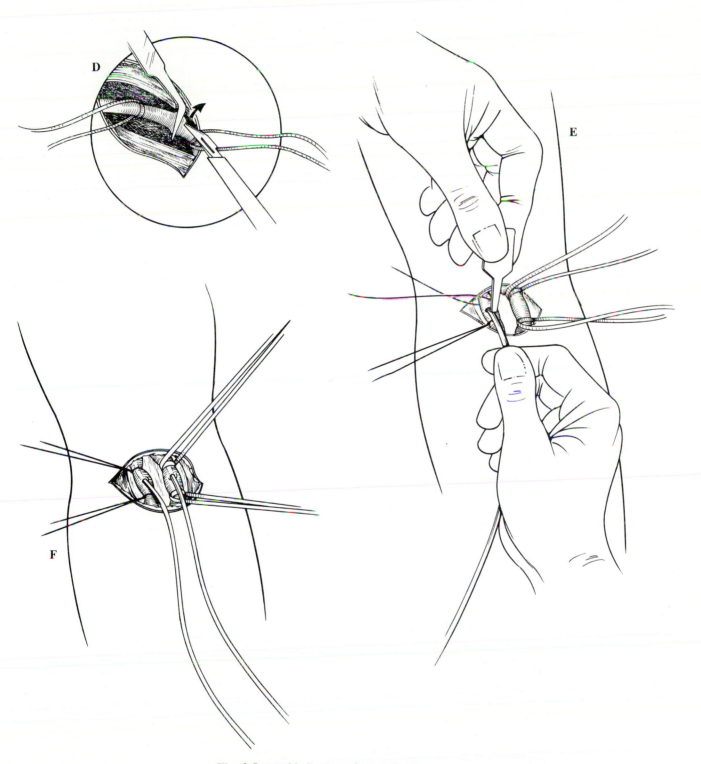

Fig. 2-5, cont'd. For legend see opposite page.

Special precautions
Discrimination between veins and arteries

Palpate vessels frequently before any dissection and take great care to differentiate the vein from the artery. The vein is a pulseless, thin-wall vessel with a slightly bluish color in contrast to the lighter gray pulsatile artery. Avoid nerves; if in doubt, aspirate with a small (25-gauge) needle to ensure vascularity.

Avoiding vessel spasm

Vessel spasm of either the vein or artery can prevent catheter advancement. Withdrawal of the catheter 20 to 30 cm followed by brisk back-and-forth movements may terminate the spasm. Injection of small amounts of lidocaine through the catheter into the vessel may also help. In addition, you may try removing the catheter and saturating the outside of the catheter with lidocaine before reinserting it. Nitroglycerin (300 to 400 μg) sublingually or directly infused into the vessel and/or papaverine (30 to 40 mg) infused intravascularly over 1 to 2 minutes may also be used. If these maneuvers fail, you must remove the catheter and insert a smaller catheter. Additional sedation of the patient may be required to prevent further spasm.

CENTRAL VENOUS ACCESS

Placement of a central venous catheter is the most commonly used invasive monitoring method for short- and long-term management of critically ill patients. In addition, many cardiovascular procedures require access to the right side of the heart, via either a peripheral vein or a central vein.

Indications

Central venous access is indicated for the administration of fluids and drugs, procurement of central venous blood samples, and insertion of catheters into the central circulation for many purposes, including hemodynamic pressure monitoring, cardiac output measurement, right cardiac and pulmonary angiography, endomyocardial biopsy, pacing or electrophysiologic evaluation and treatment, and total parenteral nutrition (TPN).

Contraindications

Although there are no absolute contraindications to venipuncture, special precautions should be exercised in patients with known bleeding disorders. In this subgroup of patients central venous catheterization should be carefully executed with a minimal number of needle punctures into sites at which bleeding can be readily observed and controlled with compression (i.e., arm or leg veins). In these instances direct puncture of incompressible central veins is best avoided, although successful cannulation of the internal jugular vein in patients with coagulopathies has been reported[8] with an overall complication rate of 7% (carotid artery puncture), which is comparable to that observed in patients without bleeding disorders. Puncture of a central, incompressible vessel is contraindicated for patients re-

Table 2-2. Venous cannulation sites: Indications and relative contraindications

Site	Indications	Relative contraindications
Basilic or median cephalic vein	Administration of drugs and moderate volume of fluids Preferred route during CPR	Not ideal for long-term monitoring or pacing catheters Arm injury Local infection
Femoral vein	Administration of large volumes of fluid during emergency resuscitation	Severe obesity Local infection
Internal jugular vein	Placement of a central catheter(s) or temporary pacemaker Administration of large volumes of fluid Administration of irritating medications or hypertonic solutions	Neck injury Local infection Coagulopathies (thrombolytic treatment) CPR Severe agitation
Subclavian vein	Placement of a central catheter(s) or temporary pacemaker Administration of large volumes of fluid Administration of irritating medications or hypertonic solutions TPN	Severe scoliosis Chest trauma or deformity Severe agitation Coagulopathies Positive-pressure ventilation Emphysematous patient

CPR, Cardiopulmonary resuscitation; *TPN*, total parenteral nutrition.

ceiving thrombolytic therapy. Table 2-2 lists the indications and relative contraindications for each insertion site.

Complications

Complications common to all venous cannulation techniques include hematoma, thrombosis, phlebitis, sepsis, cellulitis, and air embolism. Other complications are specific to the site of insertion and are presented in Table 2-3, along with rates of successful insertion, central venous catheter malposition, and overall complications. Experience and meticulous attention to technique are the best safeguards against these complications. Even then, life-threatening complications may occur.

Venous air embolism

Venous air embolism is a rare but catastrophic complication of central venous catheter placement, with a mortality of approximately 50%. Lethal air embolism occurs with central injection of 200 to 300 cc of air at a rate of 70 to 150 cc/second, although as little as 20 cc of air may cause harm to a critically ill patient.[9] The rate of air entry depends on both the inside diameter and the length of the tubing inserted. Air can enter a vein, particularly a large vein such as the internal jugular or subclavian, by one of three methods: (1) through a disconnection of or leak in the catheter, the infusion tubing, or the connecting sites; (2) through the needle or sheath at the time of insertion into the vein; or (3)

Table 2-3. Insertion success rate, central venous catheter malposition, overall complication rate, and specific complications associated with various venous insertion sites*

Site	Insertion success rate (%)	Catheter malposition rate (%) (without fluoroscopy)	Complication rate (%)	Specific complications and rate (%)
Basilic	58-98†	25-52	3-5	Thrombophlebitis (3-5) Thrombosis (<1-5) Phlebitis/cellulitis (1-20)
Internal jugular	80-94‡	0-6 (Right) 0-20 (Left)	<1-13	Carotid artery puncture (1-15) Myocardial perforation of pacing catheter (1-10) Pneumothorax (<1) Hemothorax (<1) Air embolism (<1) Catheter embolism (<1) Nerve damage (rare) Thrombosis (rare) Horner's syndrome (rare)
Subclavian vein	85-98‡	20-33	<1-17	Pneumothorax (<1-10) Subclavian artery puncture (1-20) Sepsis (<1-2) Hemothorax (1) Hydrothorax (1) Air embolism (<1) Thrombophlebitis (<1) Thrombosis (rare) Catheter embolism (rare) Brachial plexus injury (rare) Phrenic nerve injury (rare) Sternoclavicular osteomyelitis (rare)
Femoral vein	89-95†	—	4-20	Evidence of thrombus (15-20) Infection (3-20) Femoral artery puncture (4-10)
External jugular vein	61-99†	6	0-4	Hematoma (<5) Air embolism (rare) Thrombosis (rare)

*References 9, 11 to 16, 28, 29, and 32.
†Easier for people with minimal training and experience.
‡In trained hands.

along the formed track of a removed catheter that had been in place for a prolonged period, especially in a thin person with little subcutaneous tissue. This complication is more likely to occur when the patient is in an upright position, takes a deep breath, or is in a state of hypovolemia with low central venous pressure.

Massive air embolism can cause obstruction of the right ventricular outflow tract and interfere with gas exchange, presenting with manifestations that are similar to that of pulmonary thromboembolism. The diagnosis of venous air embolism is primarily clinical; the condition should be suspected whenever sudden cardiovascular collapse occurs in patients with a central venous catheter in place. Two-dimensional echocardiography has been shown to be of value in the diagnosis of venous air embolism.[10] High-resolution computerized tomographic (CT) scanning and magnetic resonance imaging (MRI) are helpful in the diagnosis of arterial air emboli of the central nervous system.[12] The clinical manifestations and methods of prevention and treatment of venous air embolism are listed on this page.

Special precautions
Avoiding puncture of the artery

When performing "blind" venous cannulation, use a small needle for exploration to avoid inadvertently puncturing the adjacent artery with a large-diameter cannula. The attached syringe should contain only a scant amount of lidocaine or saline so as not to significantly dilute the aspirated blood and prevent accurate discernment of oxygen saturation (venous or arterial). If there is any doubt, draw a blood sample for oxygen saturation analysis. This is especially helpful for avoiding arterial puncture in hypotensive patients, particularly if the venous pressure is elevated.

Verification of catheter position

Verify that the position of the catheter tip is correct by means of chest x-ray examination immediately after catheter placement. The tip of the CVP catheter should lie in the upper part of the superior vena cava. Placement of the catheter in the lower superior vena cava, RA, or even RV could result in perforation leading to pericardial hemorrhage and cardiac tamponade. The tip of the PA catheter should lie in the right or left main PA. Do not begin large-volume fluid administration until the correct position of the catheter has been radiographically verified.

Venous access sites

Venous access sites include peripheral arm veins (basilic, cephalic, median, cubital, axillary), peripheral leg veins (femoral, saphenous), the peripheral neck vein (external jugular), the central neck vein (internal jugular), and the central chest vein (subclavian). Selection of a particular site depends on the patient's needs, individual anatomic considerations, and the operator's experience. Most clinicians have experience with cannulation of the arm veins; however, this site is less suitable for pacing or long-term monitoring purposes. Nonetheless, in an emergency setting the first choice is any site that is available for rapid cannulation with the least amount of harm. Successful cannulation has been shown to closely correlate with the amount of operator experience.[13,14] Table 2-4 lists some of the advantages and disadvantages for each venous insertion site.

MANIFESTATIONS, PREVENTION, AND TREATMENT OF AIR EMBOLISM

Manifestations
- Acute respiratory distress, apnea, occasional wheezing
- Sudden hypotension and syncope
- Profound hypoxia, cyanosis
- Audible machinery ("mill wheel") murmur
- Elevated CVP (or JVP)
- Neurologic deficits (hemiplegia, aphasia) in presence of right-to-left shunt
- Cardiac arrest with asystole or VF

Prevention
- Use meticulous technique, occluding needle and catheter hub as necessary
- Elevate venous pressure (Trendelenburg position; volume expansion, if venous pressure is low)
- Use sheaths with pneumatic valve and check competency of valve prior to use
- Use Luer-Lok connections
- Securely seal all central catheters and connections
- Restrain uncooperative, agitated, or confused patients
- Do not allow containers of IV solutions to completely empty

Treatment
- Immediately place patient in left lateral Trendelenburg position
- Have the patient perform the Valsalva maneuver, if possible
- Administer 100% oxygen and ventilatory support
- Aspirate air via CVP or PA catheter
- Hyperbaric oxygen treatment (DAN)
- CPR if necessary

CVP, Central venous pressure; *JVP*, jugular venous pressure; *VF*, ventricular fibrillation; *PA*, pulmonary artery; *DAN*, Diving Accident Network telephone #919-684-8111 to locate nearest hyperbaric chamber, *CPR*, cardiopulmonary resuscitation.

Methods of percutaneous venous cannulation

Percutaneous insertion of central venous catheters has become widely accepted, not only because of speed of placement, but also because of the reduced risk of infection. In addition, percutaneous venous catheterization often preserves the integrity of the vessel, thus permitting future access. Catheters may be placed into the central venous system via percutaneous cannulation of either peripheral veins or the larger, deeper, and more central veins.

Arm vein

Cannulation of a vein in the antecubital fossa has long been the most popular technique for inserting central venous catheters and has the lowest major complication rate. In some institutions it still remains the first choice, although catheterization of the central veins directly has become more common since the advent of balloon flotation PA catheters. When fluoroscopy is not used, improper positioning of central venous catheters from an arm vein occurs much more frequently than

Table 2-4. Advantages and disadvantages of venous insertion sites

Site	Advantages	Disadvantages
Internal jugular vein	Less risk of pleural puncture and pneumothorax Easier insertion with constant landmarks If hematoma occurs, it is visible and can usually be compressed Malposition of central venous catheter is rare with direct path to right heart from right internal jugular vein Best approach for emergency transvenous pacing during chest and abdominal surgery (most accessible direct route to right heart)	Difficult to cannulate in hypovolemic patients "Blind" puncture Restriction of patient's neck mobility Increased risk of catheter movement or kinking with head movements Trendelenburg position for catheter insertion may not be possible for some patients Risk of carotid artery puncture
Subclavian vein	Remains open even in profound circulatory collapse Catheter fixation more secure Less restricting for patient Direct route to right heart	Pleural space easily entered "Blind" puncture Risk of subclavian artery puncture Difficult to apply compression if the subclavian artery is inadvertently punctured Higher incidence of catheter malposition
Femoral vein	Easy to cannulate Fewer major complications Accessible during CPR, but may not be best route (see Chapter 18)	Increased risk of infection Increased risk of thrombosis and pulmonary embolism "Blind" puncture Less mobility for the patient Risk of femoral artery puncture Malposition of the central venous catheter unless fluoroscopy is used
External jugular vein	Fewer major complications "Nonblind" puncture Accessible during operation	Increased difficulty negotiating catheter for central venous placement Increased risk of central venous catheter malposition Vein not always visible
Basilic and median cubital veins	Easy to cannulate when visible or palpable Safe Preferred route during CPR	Vein not always visible or palpable Difficult to cannulate in hypovolemic patients High rate of malposition if fluoroscopy is not used for central catheter placement Not optimal for rapid fluid infusion or emergency transvenous pacing
Cephalic vein	Same as for basilic and median cubital veins	Same as for basilic and median cubital veins Sharp angle at shoulder may preclude entry into central vein without use of a guidewire

clinically suspected, with reported incidences of from 36% to 52%.[15,16] In addition, arm movement can cause catheter tip movement of several centimeters, increasing the risk of phlebitis. For pacemakers, this movement may result in electrode dislodgment or RV perforation.

A central venous line can usually be inserted through the median vein or the basilic vein distal to the antecubital fossa. The cephalic vein is an equally large vein, but its sharp angle at the shoulder makes it more difficult to navigate.

Anatomy. Venous blood from the arm drains through two main intercommunicating veins—the basilic and the cephalic veins. The basilic vein is deeper and ascends along the ulnar surface of the forearm (Fig. 2-6). It is joined by the median cubital vein in front of the elbow and continues up along the medial side of the brachial artery to the lower border of the teres major, where it becomes the axillary vein. The cephalic vein ascends on the radial aspect of the forearm. It communicates with the basilic vein through the median cubital vein just in front of the elbow and ascends laterally until it curves sharply as it pierces the clavipectoral fascia, crosses the axillary artery, and passes beneath the clavicle to join the axillary vein, or occasionally the external jugular vein. Because of this anatomy, the cephalic

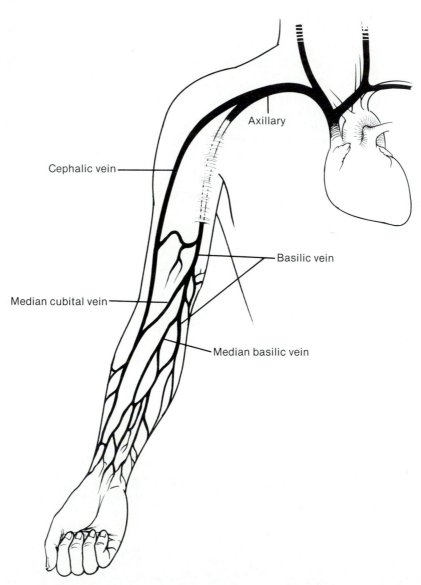

Fig. 2-6. Anatomic locations of the arm veins.

vein is more difficult to catheterize, making the basilic vein preferable.

Equipment. The basic equipment for venous cannulation consists of the basic percutaneous catheterization tray, a needle, and a catheter (central venous or PA) that is sufficiently long to reach the central vein. A small catheter can be inserted through a needle into the superior vena cava for CVP monitoring. However, it is more common today to insert PA catheters to monitor both CVP and PAP or PAWP. The PA catheter is inserted over a guidewire or through a catheter sheath by means of the Seldinger technique (p. 35).

Patient preparation. The patient is first prepared as described on pp. 32 to 33. Additional specific preparation is conducted as follows:

1. Locate the vein. This may be easier if you temporarily apply a tourniquet above the antecubital fossa and the patient makes a fist to distend the veins.

2. Abduct the selected arm 30° to 45° from the body and secure it on a flat, padded arm board.

3. For placement of a central venous catheter without fluoroscopy, estimate the length of catheter needed by extending the packaged catheter from the insertion site to the approximate position of the superior vena cava.

Procedure. This discussion will be limited to insertion of a PA catheter into an antecubital vein via the Seldinger technique.

1. Apply a venous tourniquet to the upper arm.

2. While retaining traction on the skin distal to the insertion with one hand, puncture the vein with the needle held bevel side upward at a 15° to 20° angle.

3. With the appearance of the backflow of blood in the needle, insert the guidewire into the vein approximately 2 to 4 cm beyond the tip of the needle.

4. Release the tourniquet and slowly continue to advance the guidewire several centimeters.

5. Withdraw the needle from the vein while firmly holding the guidewire in place in the vessel.

6. Wipe the guidewire with a sterile moist gauze pad.

7. Insert the catheter of choice or a catheter introducer sheath over the guidewire into the vein.

8. Remove the guidewire. If a catheter introducer set is used, remove the inner dilator along with the guidewire, flush the sheath's side arm, and temporarily close the stopcock. Insert the catheter of choice into the sheath.

9. Aspirate and flush the catheter and connect both the catheter and side arm of the sheath to a heparinized flushing solution.

10. Position the catheter in the proper location.

11. Suture the catheter to the skin with 3-0 silk. (If a

catheter sheath is used, suture the sheath and catheter separately to the skin.)

12. Apply an iodophor ointment and a sterile dressing to the insertion site and tape securely.

13. Immobolize the arm with an arm board.

14. Perform chest x-ray examination to verify the position of the catheter (if fluoroscopy is not used).

Special precautions

• *Meeting resistance:* Do not force the catheter to advance. Withdraw the catheter 2 to 3 cm, rotate it slightly, and readvance it. Other maneuvers that may facilitate catheter passage include further abduction of the arm, having the patient move his or her shoulder anteriorly or posteriorly, having the patient inspire deeply, having the patient turn his or her head to the side of the venipuncture to prevent the catheter from entering the internal jugular vein, and partial inflation of the balloon of the catheter, if available.

• *Ensuring visibility:* Do not attempt placement of a central venous catheter into a vein that cannot be made visible or palpable by means of a tourniquet, warm compresses, or placement of the arm in a dependent position with opening and closing of the hand. Choose another site in such a case.

Femoral vein

Percutaneous cannulation of the femoral vein is appropriate for relatively short-term venous catheterization. In the cardiac catheterization laboratory the femoral vein is commonly used for right heart catheterization, while the femoral artery is used for left heart catheterization.

In emergency settings the femoral vein may be very useful for many purposes, including rapid fluid resuscitation in critically ill patients through short, large-bore catheters.[17] The risk of deep venous thrombophlebitis and pulmonary embolism is increased with prolonged catheterization of this vein.

Anatomy. The femoral vein lies medially adjacent to the femoral artery in the upper thigh. Located in the femoral triangle just beneath the inguinal ligament are the femoral nerve, artery, vein, and lymph channel (NAVL) (Fig. 2-7). It is important to remember the relationship of these structures for successful femoral vein cannulation. The inguinal ligament, which lies just over the femoral artery and vein, runs between the anterior superior iliac spine and the pubic tubercle. The inguinal crease usually lies just caudal to the inguinal ligament. Location of the femoral artery by palpation identifies the location of the femoral vein, which is approximately 1 cm medial and parallel to the artery. The femoral vein possesses several valves, which may be encountered during catheter passage.

Equipment. The equipment required for this procedure includes the basic percutaneous catheterization tray, the selected catheter or pacemaker, and a fluoroscope, if the catheter is to be advanced to the right side of the heart or manipulated into the PA.

Patient preparation. The patient is prepared as described on pp. 32 to 33. The procedure then is as follows:

1. Place the patient in a supine position. Slightly abduct and externally rotate the thigh by having the patient extend his or her knee.

2. Shave the groin of the side to be catheterized.

Procedure. Either femoral vein may be used, although the right femoral vein is preferred because of the lesser degree of angulation at the junction with the inferior vena cava. The right-handed operator may also find cannulation of the right femoral vein more comfortable.

1. Palpate the femoral artery and locate the femoral

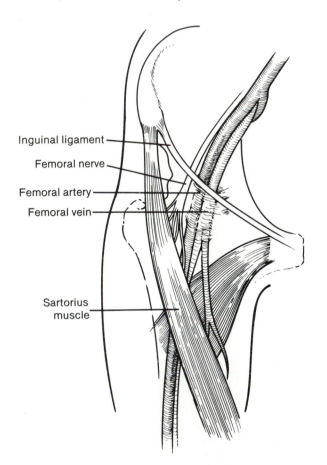

Inguinal ligament

Femoral nerve

Femoral artery

Femoral vein

Sartorius muscle

Fig. 2-7. Anatomy of the femoral triangle showing the relationship of the femoral nerve, artery, and vein.

vein approximately 1 cm medial to the artery and 3 to 4 cm below the inguinal ligament.

2. With a #11 scalpel make a small (3 mm), shallow skin incision at the proposed insertion site. Form a small insertion tunnel by gentle blunt dissection with a Kelly forceps.

3. Insert the percutaneous vascular needle and stylet beveled side upward through the skin incision at a 30° to 45° angle aiming medially toward the umbilicus (Fig. 2-8).

4. Gently advance the needle through the femoral triangle until the needle touches the periosteum of the ileum.

5. Remove the stylet and attach a 5 or 10 ml syringe with 3 to 5 ml of 1% lidocaine to the needle.

6. While applying gentle negative pressure, slowly withdraw the needle until the femoral vein is entered as indicated by the appearance of venous blood in the syringe. (Occasional flushing of the needle tip with lidocaine will ensure needle patency and adequate anesthesia.)

7. Remove the syringe with one hand while securely holding the needle in place with the other hand. Place a thumb over the needle hub to control the bleeding and prevent air aspiration.

8. Insert the soft flexible tip of the guidewire into the needle and advance it into the femoral vein approximately 20 cm.

9. Remove the needle while firmly holding the guidewire in the vessel with your thumb and index finger. Wipe the guidewire with a sterile, moist gauze pad.

10. Insert the catheter introducer set (dilator and sheath) over the guidewire, making sure approximately 5 to 10 cm of wire extends beyond the hub of the sheath.

11. While holding the dilator between the thumb and index finger just at the skin insertion site, start to advance the unit into the vessel using a rotating motion. (Keeping the dilator sheath at a very shallow angle will aid in advancement.)

12. After the sheath is entirely situated in the vessel, remove the guidewire and the dilator together from the sheath.

13. Aspirate and flush the side arm of the sheath. Close the side arm stopcock temporarily, or connect it to an IV infusion.

14. Insert the catheter of choice through the sheath and advance it to the correct position in the heart under fluoroscopic guidance.

15. Aspirate and flush the catheter, sheath, and side arm. Connect the IV infusion or pressure tubing to the catheter hub and an IV infusion to the sheath side arm.

16. Suture both the sheath and side arm to the skin.

17. Apply an iodophor ointment and carefully dress the area.

Special precautions

• *Inadvertent femoral artery puncture:* If the femoral artery is inadvertently punctured and is not intended to be cannulated later, the needle should be removed and firm compression applied over the puncture site for 5 minutes. If femoral artery cannulation is intended, it is best to proceed at this time.

• *Locating the femoral vein:* If difficulty is encountered in locating the femoral vein, having the patient perform the Valsalva maneuver will distend the vein and facilitate successful entry.

• *Long-term femoral vein catheterization:* Management of femoral vein catheters on a long-term basis (24 hours or longer) requires meticulous care and attention to prevent infection. Subcutaneous tunneling of the catheter to move the catheter skin exit site away from the perineal area may reduce the risk of infection. Systemic heparinization is recommended for prolonged femoral vein catheterization, unless it is contraindicated.

External jugular vein

The external jugular vein is less frequently used for central venous catheter insertion than either the internal jugular or subclavian vein. This is primarily due to

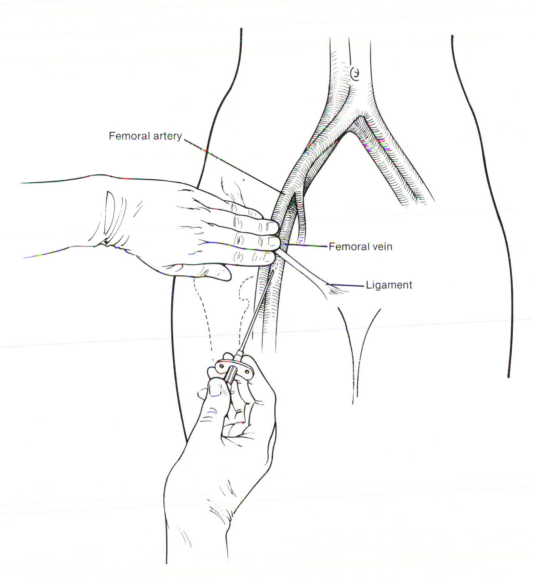

Fig. 2-8. Femoral vein puncture with the needle at a 30° to 45° angle aiming medially toward the umbilicus.

technical difficulties encountered in catheter passage. However, use of a J-tip guidewire has aided in the success of central venous and PA catheter placement.[18,19] The superficial location of the external jugular vein permits visualization of the vein during cannulation, thus reducing the traumatic complications involved with "blind" venipuncture techniques. Use of the external jugular vein for cannulation is recommended only as an alternative to arm veins and when expertise in internal jugular or subclavian vein cannulation is lacking. This vein should only be cannulated if it is clearly visible or palpable.

Anatomy. The external jugular vein is formed by a union of the posterior auricular vein and the posterior division of the retromandibular vein. It extends from the angle of the mandible, crosses the sternocleidomastoid muscle obliquely, and terminates behind the middle of the clavicle, where it joins the subclavian vein (see Figs. 2-9 and 2-10). The vein varies in size and possesses valves approximately 4 cm above the clavicle, just before its junction with the subclavian vein. These valves may be encountered during catheter passage.

Equipment. Equipment required for external jugular vein catheterization includes the basic percutaneous catheterization tray (p. 34) plus the selected catheter (central venous, PA, or pacing).

Patient preparation. First prepare the patient as described on pp. 32 to 33. Additional patient preparation consists of the following:

1. If possible, have the patient practice the Valsalva maneuver.

2. If the patient is obese or very muscular with a short neck, place a small pillow or rolled towel under the shoulder to extend the neck.

3. Turn the patient's head to the contralateral side.

4. Place the patient in a 15° to 25° Trendelenburg position to distend the vein and prevent air embolism.

Procedure. The basic procedure for catheterization of the external jugular vein is as follows:

1. Identify the external jugular vein (distending the vein by lightly pressing just above the midclavicular area or having the patient briefly perform the Valsalva maneuver will aid in identification and puncture).

2. Attach an 18- or 16-gauge needle to a 3 or 5 ml syringe containing several milliliters of sterile saline.

3. Align the needle cannula parallel to the axis of the vein with the bevel facing upward.

4. With the vein distended, puncture the external jugular vein at a point midway between the angle of the jaw and the midclavicular line (Fig. 2-9) while maintaining negative pressure within the syringe.

5. When you notice a free flow of venous blood in the syringe, ask the patient to hum while you quickly remove the syringe and insert a J-tip guidewire through the needle approximately 10 cm.

6. Withdraw the needle with one hand while carefully holding the guidewire in place with the other hand.

7. Instruct the patient to stop humming and resume breathing.

8. Wipe the guidewire with a sterile, moist gauze pad.

9. Insert the catheter introducer set over the guidewire, making sure the wire extends 10 cm beyond the hub of the sheath.

10. Advance the dilator and sheath through the skin into the vein using a rotating motion.

11. Ask the patient to hum again and quickly remove the dilator and guidewire together from the sheath.

12. Aspirate and flush the side arm of the sheath and close the stopcock or connect it to heparinized saline IV infusion system.

13. Insert the selected catheter through the sheath, instruct the patient to resume breathing, and position the catheter as desired.

14. Aspirate and flush the catheter (and sheath side arm) with saline and connect them to an IV infusion or pressure tubing as needed.

15. Suture the sheath and the catheter separately to the skin near the insertion site.

16. Apply an iodophor ointment and a sterile dressing to the site and tape it securely.

17. If fluoroscopy is not used, obtain a chest x-ray film to confirm catheter position.

Special precautions

• *Use of a J-tip guidewire to ease catheter passage:* Because of the direction of the external jugular vein and the presence of venous valves, difficulty may be encountered during catheter passage. Use of the J-tip guidewire for the Seldinger technique usually alleviates this problem. A J-tip guidewire can also be inserted through the 16-gauge Teflon catheter to facilitate catheter advancement if resistance is encountered during its passage.

• *Passage of the catheter during inspiration:* The valves within the vein are open during inspiration, so it might help to advance the catheter at this time.

Internal jugular vein

Catheterization of the internal jugular vein in the adult was first described by Hemosura in 1966.[20] Since that time the internal jugular vein has been commonly used for percutaneous insertion of central venous, PA, and pacing catheters because its anatomic location provides a straight path to the right side of the heart, its landmarks are more definite and constant, and the complication rate is lower than with the subclavian approach.

Anatomy. The internal jugular vein emerges from the base of the skull to enter the carotid sheath, which also contains the carotid artery and the vagus nerve. Initially, the internal jugular vein is posterior and lateral to the more superficial carotid artery. However, near the terminal portion of the vein, above its juncture with the subclavian vein, the internal jugular vein becomes lateral and slightly anterior to the carotid artery.

The lower portion of the internal jugular vein lies within the triangle formed by the sternal and clavicular heads of the sternocleidomastoid muscle (Fig. 2-10). It is within this triangle that the internal jugular vein is best cannulated. Behind the sternal end of the clavicle, the internal jugular vein unites with the subclavian vein to form the innominate vein.

Equipment. The basic percutaneous equipment tray (p. 34) is required, as well as the catheter of choice (central venous, PA, or pacing).

Patient preparation. The patient should first be prepared as described on pp. 32 to 33. Additional specific patient preparation consists of the following:

1. If the patient is obese or muscular with a short neck, place a small pillow or rolled towel under the shoulders to extend the neck.

2. Locate the carotid artery by palpation.

3. Identify the internal jugular vein and mark it if necessary.

4. Turn the patient's head to the contralateral side.

5. Place the patient in a 15° to 25° Trendelenburg position to distend the veins and prevent air embolism.

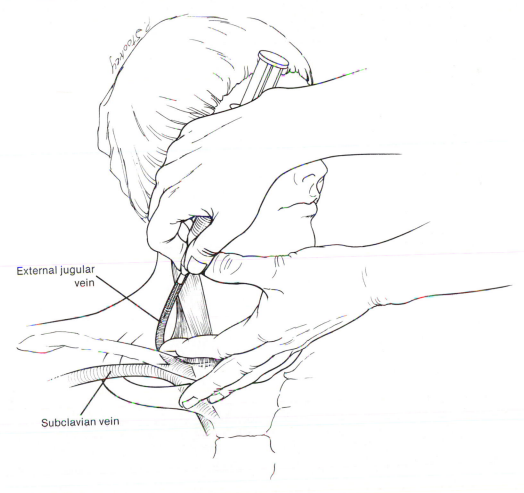

External jugular vein

Subclavian vein

Fig. 2-9. External jugular vein puncture at the midpoint between the angle of the jaw and the midclavicle.

Procedure. The literature describes at least 13 different variations of two basic approaches to percutaneous internal jugular vein cannulation. A high entry can be approached via a posterior (or lateral) route,[21] an anterior (or medial) route,[22] or a central route.[23] Likewise, a low internal jugular puncture can be approached from a lateral[24] or central route.[25-27] Fig. 2-11 illustrates the entry sites for the various approaches. In addition, either the right or left internal jugular vein can be cannulated. Most physicians prefer the right internal jugular vein because it is larger, forms a straight line to the superior vena cava and RA, the dome of the right lung and pleura lies lower than on the left side, and the large thoracic duct is not endangered. However, when right internal jugular vein cannulation fails and there is no hematoma, successful cannulation can usually be carried out on the left side.

Discussion here will be limited to three approaches to cannulation of the internal jugular vein—the central approach described by Daily et al.,[26] the posterior (or

lateral) approach described by Jernigan and Gardner,[24] and the anterior (or medial) approach described by Mostert et al.[22] The studies cited in the references at the end of the chapter describe other approaches.

Central approach[26]

1. Identify the internal jugular vein by drawing a triangle from marks placed on the medial aspect of the clavicle, the medial aspect of the sternal head, and the lateral aspect of the clavicular head of the sternocleidomastoid muscle (Fig. 2-12). The center of the triangle is directly over the center of the internal jugular vein. (Having the awake patient lift his or her head slightly off the bed makes this triangle more visible and palpable.)

2. With a #11 blade, make a small (2 to 3 mm) stab wound at the insertion site (or do this after guidewire insertion).

3. Administer a local anesthetic and locate the internal jugular vein via a small (22- or 25-gauge) needle 3 to 4 cm above the medial aspect of the clavicle and 1

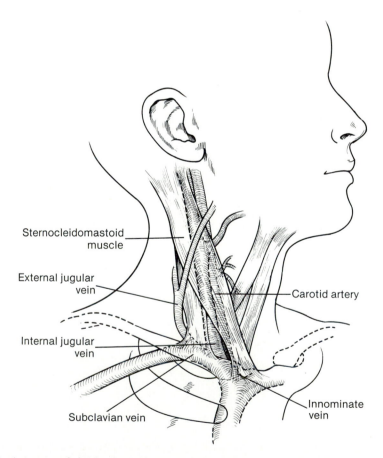

Fig. 2-10. Anatomy of the internal jugular vein showing its lower location within the triangle formed by the sternocleidomastoid muscle and the clavicle.

to 2 cm within the lateral border of the sternocleido-mastoid muscle.

4. Attach a 3 or 5 ml syringe containing 2 or 3 ml of sterile saline or 1% lidocaine to the 18-gauge vascular needle. (The smaller syringe is easier to handle.)

5. Align the needle with the syringe (Fig. 2-12) parallel to the medial border of the clavicular head of the sternocleidomastoid muscle. Direct the needle caudally at a 30° angle to the frontal plane directly over the internal jugular vein and aiming toward the ipsilateral nipple. (If the needle is positioned with its bevel side directed medially, the bevel aids in directing the guidewire medially into the central circulation.)

6. Puncture the skin and advance the needle while maintaining a slight negative pressure in the syringe until free flow of blood is obtained.

7. If the internal jugular vein is not entered initially, withdraw the needle while maintaining suction with the syringe and then redirect it 5° to 10° more laterally. If the vein has still not been entered, direct the needle more in line with the sagittal plane. Do not direct the needle medially across the sagittal plane lest the carotid artery be punctured. If possible, having the patient perform the Valsalva maneuver will distend the vein and improve the chance of successful cannulation.

8. After you observe free flow of venous blood in the syringe, instruct the patient to hold his or her breath and hum. During this time, quickly remove the syringe from the needle, place a thumb over the needle hub, and insert the soft, flexible tip of the appropriate guidewire through the needle approximately 10 to 15 cm. Remove the needle and wipe the guidewire with a sterile, moist gauze pad. Instruct the patient to resume normal breathing.

9. Insert the catheter introducer set over the guidewire until 10 to 15 cm of wire extends beyond the hub of the sheath. Advance the dilator and sheath through the skin and subcutaneous tissue into the vein. If the introducer has a side arm, this should be closed to the patient.

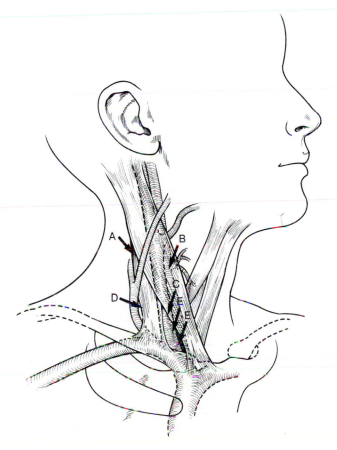

Fig. 2-11. Various puncture sites of the internal jugular vein. *A,* High posterior entry. *B,* High anterior (medial) entry. *C,* High central entry. *D,* Low lateral entry. *E,* Low central entry.

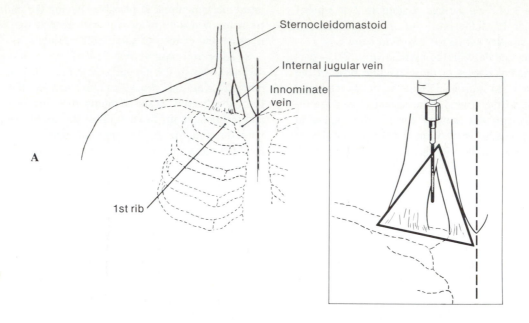

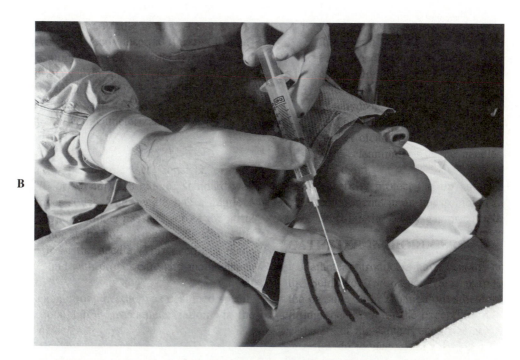

Fig. 2-12. A, Relationship of external anatomic landmarks to underlying internal jugular vein. Triangle drawn over clavicle and sternal and clavicular portions of sternocleidomastoid muscle is centered over internal jugular vein (*inset*). (From Daily, P.O., Griepp, R.B., and Shumway, N.E.: Percutaneous internal jugular vein cannulation, Arch. Surg. **101:**534-536, 1970. Copyright 1970, American Medical Association.) **B,** Alignment of the needle in the central portion of the triangle formed by the sternal and clavicular sections of the sternocleidomastoid muscle.

10. Remove the dilator and the guidewire together from the sheath.

11. Aspirate and flush the sheath side arm with saline and temporarily close the stopcock toward the patient or connect it to a heparin IV infusion.

12. Insert the catheter of choice through the sheath and position it in the heart.

13. Aspirate and flush the catheter and sheath side arm and connect them to a heparinized IV infusion or pressure tubing.

14. Suture the sheath and catheter to the skin.

15. Apply an iodophor ointment and sterile dressing to the insertion site and tape it securely.

16. Return the patient to a flat position and remove the pillow or roll from the shoulders.

17. Perform chest x-ray examination to verify catheter position (if fluoroscopy was not used).

Posterolateral approach[24]

1. Identify the sternal and clavicular heads of the sternocleidomastoid muscle as directed in step 1 of the central approach.

2. Administer a local anesthetic and locate the vein via a small (21- to 25-gauge) needle inserted under the lateral border of the sternocleidomastoid muscle, approximately 5 cm above the clavicle, just above the point where the external jugular vein crosses the sternocleidomastoid muscle (Fig. 2-13).

3. Direct the needle caudally at a 15° angle to the frontal plane, aiming medially toward the suprasternal notch (Fig. 2-13). Maintain gentle, negative pressure on the barrel of the syringe while advancing the needle.

Entry into the vein should occur within 5 to 7 cm of insertion. If the vein is not entered with the first attempt, slowly withdraw the needle while maintaining slight negative pressure within the syringe. Often the vein will be entered upon needle withdrawal. If entry is still unsuccessful, remove the needle and reinsert it at a slightly more shallow angle (approximately 10° to the frontal plane).

4. Follow steps 8 through 16 of the central approach.

Anterior (medial) approach[22]

1. Separate the carotid artery from the anterior border of the sternocleidomastoid muscle with the index and middle fingers of the left hand (Fig. 2-14). (Arterial pulsations should be palpable.)

2. Administer a local anesthetic and locate the vein via a small (21- or 25-gauge) needle inserted at the midpoint of the anterior border of the sternocleidomastoid muscle, approximately 5 cm above the clavicle and 5 cm below the angle of the mandible (Fig. 2-14).

3. Attach a saline- or lidocaine-filled 5 or 10 ml syringe to the 18-gauge cannulating needle and insert it in the same location as the locator needle.

4. Direct the needle caudally at a 30° to 45° angle to

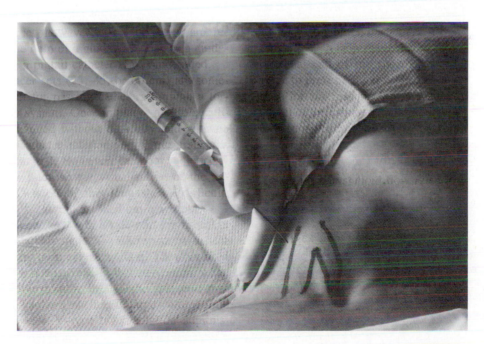

Fig. 2-13. Posterolateral puncture of the internal jugular vein with the needle inserted under the lateral border of the sternocleidomastoid muscle approximately 5 cm above the clavicle.

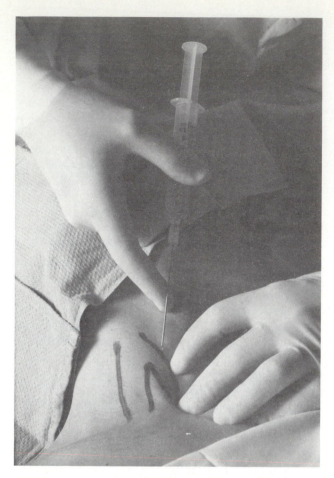

Fig. 2-14. Anterior or medial puncture of the internal jugular vein showing manual separation of the carotid artery with the needle inserted at the midpoint of anterior border of the sternocleidomastoid muscle approximately 5 cm above the clavicle.

the frontal plane, aiming toward the ipsilateral nipple or toward the junction of the medial and middle thirds of the clavicle.

5. Advance the needle while maintaining slight negative pressure within the syringe.

6. Entry into the vein should occur within 2 to 4 cm of insertion. If the vein is not entered with the first attempt, slowly withdraw the needle while maintaining slight negative pressure within the syringe. The vein may have been transfixed and the lumen will be entered during withdrawal.

Special precautions

• *Prevention of aspiration of air into the venous system:* Remove the syringe from the needle while the patient holds his or her breath or hums (or during expira-

tion with the uncooperative patient) and immediately place the thumb or index finger over the hub of the needle. Likewise, the guidewire and catheter sheath should be inserted during withheld breath or expiration. Catheter sheaths with pneumatic seals should be used. All connections must be tightly secured. Hyperinflation of the lung (either mechanical or spontaneous) during entry into the internal jugular vein should be avoided to reduce the risk of pneumothorax.

• *Procedure for inadvertent puncture of the carotid artery:* If the carotid artery is inadvertently punctured, immediately remove the needle and apply moderate compression for 5 to 10 minutes to control bleeding. Puncture of the contralateral internal jugular vein is not advised lest the same complication occur on the other side, compromising the patient's airway. Most punctures of the carotid artery are quite innocuous and require no treatment, although rare fatalities have been reported.[28]

• *Procedure for inadvertent placement of the catheter introducer set into the carotid artery:* In hypotensive, hypoxic patients, it may not be easy to distinguish between the internal jugular vein and the internal carotid artery, and the artery may be cannulated inadvertently. Such an event is documented by the appearance of an arterial waveform when a transducer system is connected to the sheath. Should this occur, the catheter or sheath should be left in place, all connections secured to prevent air embolism, and an anesthesiologist and a vascular surgeon notified to prepare for possible endotracheal intubation and exploratory operation. To prevent this serious complication, some authors recommend that the pressure waveform be assessed through the 21-gauge needle used for local anesthetic infiltration before insertion of the larger needle and catheter introducer if there is any doubt regarding venous entry.[29] An alternate method would be to withdraw a blood sample from the vessel and analyze it for oxygen saturation to confirm venous or arterial location.

• *Consideration of alternate puncture sites in elderly patients:* Since even mild compression of the carotid artery in elderly patients with atherosclerosis can result in neurologic damage, other venipuncture sites may be preferred in this subgroup.

• *Doppler technique:* Use of the Doppler technique to locate the internal jugular vein has been reported in a small series of patients with an increased success rate.[30] Using this technique, only one needle puncture was required to successfully cannulate the internal jugular vein in the majority of patients. Theoretically, this would result in a reduced complication rate. We have no clinical experience with this technique.

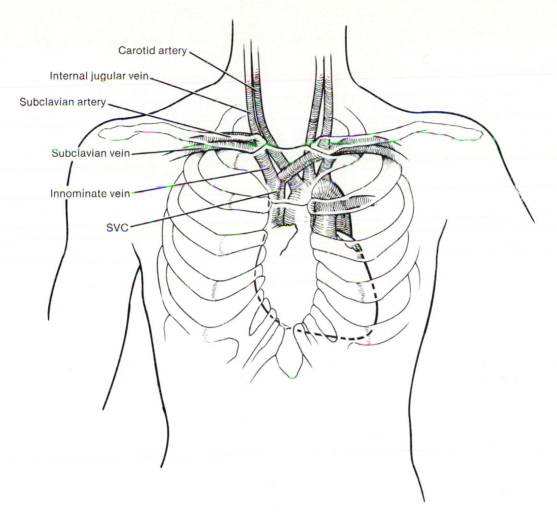

Carotid artery

Internal jugular vein

Subclavian artery

Subclavian vein

Innominate vein

SVC

Fig. 2-15. Anatomic location of the subclavian vein and surrounding structures. The subclavian vein joins the internal jugular vein to become the innominate vein at about the manubrioclavicular junction. The innominate vein becomes the superior vena cava *(SVC)* at about the level of the midmanubrium.

Subclavian vein

Cannulation of the subclavian vein for venous catheterization has grown in popularity since 1962, when Wilson et al.[31] described their successful experience with subclavian insertion of central venous catheters. Percutaneous catheterization of the subclavian vein has become a common approach to insertion of central venous, PA, and pacing catheters. This approach has been very popular for long-term placement of TPN catheters because it is easier to secure the catheter and there is less interference with the patient's mobility. The subclavian vein is also the easiest vein to cannulate in patients with profound circulatory collapse.

Anatomy. The subclavian vein begins at the lateral border of the first rib as the continuation of the axillary vein, and it ends at the medial border of the anterior scalene muscle. It joins the internal jugular vein behind the sternoclavicular joint to form the innominate vein (Fig. 2-15). The vein is separated from its artery by the anterior scalene muscle, which is approximately 10 to 15 mm thick. The vein crosses the first rib and lies anteroinferior to the artery (posterior to the middle third of the clavicle). The apical pleura lies approximately 5 mm posterior to the junction of the jugular and subclavian veins (Fig. 2-16). The subclavian vein is a large vein with an inside diameter of 1.5 to 2.0 cm or more.

Equipment. The equipment required is the same as that for the internal jugular vein approach (p. 34).

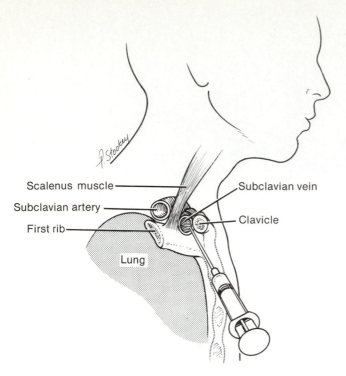

Fig. 2-16. Sagittal view showing the close relationship of the subclavian vein and artery as well as the apical pleura necessitating accurate and careful direction of the needle insertion.

Patient preparation. The patient should first be prepared as described on pp. 32 to 33. Additional preparation consists of the following:

1. Place a rolled towel under the patient's back between the scapulae.

2. Turn the patient's head to the contralateral side.

3. Place the patient in a 15° to 25° Trendelenburg position.

Procedure. The subclavian vein can be approached from either the superior or inferior direction. Overall success and complication rates of both methods are very similar. However, the supraclavicular approach offers several practical advantages: there is a shorter distance between the vein and the skin (0.5 to 4 cm); it is a more direct path to the superior vena cava; it is more easily performed during CPR with minimal or no interruption of chest compression; and the rate of correct catheter tip location is greater than with the infraclavicular approach.[32]

Practical advantages not withstanding, the infraclavicular approach to percutaneous subclavian catheterization remains the most popular method, and discussion here will be limited to this technique. Either the right or left subclavian vein may be cannulated, although the left subclavian vein may be preferred for catheter insertion because it gently curves into the innominate vein and no sharp bends of the catheter are required. However, the pleural dome is not as high on the right side as on the left side.

1. Identify the junction of the middle and medial thirds of the clavicle where the first rib proceeds beneath the clavicle. Needle insertion should be approximately 1 or 2 cm lateral and inferior to this location. A frequent error is use of a more lateral insertion site at the midclavicle area. Another means of identification is to palpate the inferior surface of the clavicle and locate a tubercle on the clavicle approximately one-third to one-half the length of the clavicle from the sternoclavicular joint. This tubercle marks the site of needle entry.[33]

2. Make a small (3 mm) skin nick at the insertion site using a #11 blade, sharp side upward (or do this after guidewire insertion).

3. Depress the area 1 to 2 cm beneath the junction of the distal and middle thirds of the clavicle with the thumb of the nondominant hand and place the index finger of the same hand approximately 2 cm above the sternal notch.

4. Administer a local anesthetic and locate the vein via a small (21- or 25-gauge) needle directed toward the index finger above the notch and at a 20° to 30° angle with the thorax. (Direct the bevel of the needle inferiomedially to encourage guidewire passage into the innominate vein.)

5. Insert the needle under the clavicle at the point identified in step 1 (Fig. 2-17).

6. Advance the needle, "walking" it down until it slips beneath the clavicle while maintaining gentle negative pressure within the syringe.

7. When the vein is entered, remove the smaller needle and attach the 18-gauge needle to a syringe containing 5 or 10 ml of heparin or lidocaine and repeat steps 3 to 6 while maintaining negative pressure in the syringe.

8. When the vein is entered with the cannulating needle, ask the patient to hold his or her breath or hum, while you quickly remove the syringe from the 18-gauge needle and immediately cap the needle hub with your thumb or index finger.

9. Insert the flexible tip of the guidewire 10 to 15 cm through the needle and remove the needle, maintaining gentle pressure on the puncture site. Instruct the patient to resume breathing.

10. With the sheath's side arm closed to the patient,

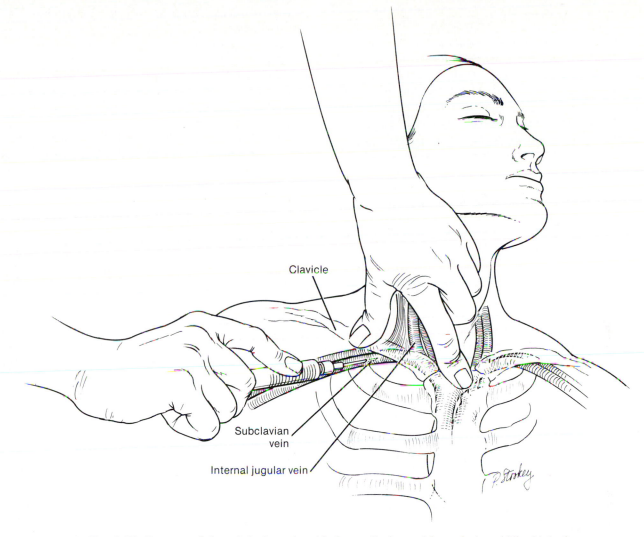

Clavicle

Subclavian
vein

Internal jugular vein

P. Stokey

Fig. 2-17. Puncture of the subclavian vein with the needle inserted beneath the middle third of the clavicle at a 20° to 30° angle aiming medially.

advance the catheter introducer set (dilator and sheath) over the guidewire into the vein, using a slight twisting motion (the side arm is closed to the patient).

11. Remove the guidewire and dilator together from the sheath.

12. Aspirate and flush the side arm of the sheath and close its stopcock to the patient.

13. Insert the catheter of choice. Having the patient bring his or her ear to the shoulder on the side of the insertion site creates a sharp angle between the jugular and subclavian veins and helps prevent misdirection of the catheter into the internal jugular vein during advancement.[34]

14. Advance and position the catheter in the heart.

15. Aspirate and flush the catheter and the side arm of the sheath and connect the side arm of the sheath and the hub of the catheter to a heparin IV infusion and pressure tubing.

16. Suture the sheath and catheter to the skin near the insertion site.

17. Apply an iodophor ointment and sterile dressing to the insertion site and tape it securely.

18. Return the patient to a flat position and remove the roll from his or her back.

19. Obtain a chest x-ray film to verify catheter position if fluoroscopy is not used.

Special precautions
• *Prevention of aspiration of air into the venous sys-*

tem: Aspiration of air should be prevented as for internal jugular vein cannulation (see p. 60).

• *Prevention of guidewire misdirection into the jugular vein:* If guidewire passage is not entirely smooth, the wire may have entered the jugular vein. The patient may complain of an unpleasant sensation in the area of the ipsilateral ear. The guidewire location should be confirmed with fluoroscopy and the wire repositioned before the catheter is advanced over it. A caudal direction of the bevel of the needle and having the patient bring his or her ear down to the shoulder on the insertion side during guidewire passage are steps that may prevent guidewire misdirection into the jugular vein.

• *Passage of the needle under the clavicle:* If it proves difficult to depress the needle sufficiently to pass under the clavicle into the vein, the needle may be bent smoothly over its entire length to form a gentle arc.[35] The needle should then be inserted at a 45° angle under the clavicle, and following its 30° arc, it will usually enter the vein.

• *Reducing the risk of pneumothorax:* The operator can reduce the risk of pneumothorax by avoiding too lateral or too deep a needle insertion. Multiple attempts at cannulation should be avoided. Generally, if three attempts prove unsuccessful, another site should be chosen.[14] Patients with chronic obstructive pulmonary disease with overinflated stiff lungs, especially those receiving ventilatory support, are at a higher risk for pulmonary complications resulting from attempted subclavian cannulation. Thus, subclavian vein cannulation is best avoided in these patients. If cannulation is attempted but unsuccessful, a chest radiograph should be obtained to rule out pneumothorax before contralateral insertion.[36]

• *Correct aim of the needle in the elderly:* In elderly patients the subclavian vein may be more inferior, requiring aiming of the needle toward the inferior margin of the sternal notch.[37] These patients may also have a bony prominence beneath the medial portion of the clavicle, making cannulation difficult.

• *Prevention of puncture of the subclavian artery:* The operator can avoid puncture of the subclavian artery by keeping the puncture site away from the most lateral course of the vein and not angulating the needle too far posteriorly (Fig. 2-16). If the subclavian artery is punctured, the needle should be removed and firm pressure applied over the puncture site for 10 minutes.

Brachial or basilic vein cutdown

The basic cutdown procedure is described on p. 43. Venous cutdown for placement of a central venous catheter is usually performed on the median basilic or brachial vein.

Anatomy. See the discussion of percutaneous cannulation (p. 50).

Equipment. The equipment required includes the basic tray for the cutdown technique plus a central venous, PA, or pacing catheter or other right heart catheter.

Patient preparation. The patient should first be prepared as described on pp. 32 to 33. The selected arm should then be abducted 30° to 40° and placed on a padded board or table.

Procedure

1. Palpate the brachial artery above the antecubital fold.

2. With a #15 blade make a 1.5 to 2.5 cm transverse incision through the skin and superficial fascia 3 to 4 cm above the antecubital fold medial to the brachial artery pulsation.

3. Follow the steps for basic venous cutdown (pp. 43 to 46).

Catheter removal

1. Release the proximal tie around the vein and catheter and remove the catheter.

2. Double tie the proximal tie to ligate the vein, or, if the vein is quite large, repair it with 6-0 monofilament suture.

3. Flush the incision with sterile heparinized saline solution.

4. Close the skin with three or four 4-0 interrupted mattress sutures.

5. Cleanse the skin with sterile water, apply an iodophor ointment and sterile dressings, and secure the dressing with tape.

An alternate method of venous catheter insertion involves a modified cutdown in which the vein is located and exposed through a surgical incision and the vein then directly punctured with a needle. The venous catheter is then inserted via the Seldinger technique over a guidewire. This direct approach is helpful in patients with very small or inaccessible veins and eliminates the necessity to ligate the vein.

Special precautions. Precautions to be used are the same as those described on pp. 46 and 51.

REFERENCES

1. de Jong, R.H.: Local anesthetics, ed. 2, Springfield, Ill., 1977, Charles C Thomas, Publisher.
2. Snow, J.C.: Manual of anesthesia, ed. 2, Boston, 1982, Little, Brown & Co.
3. Seldinger, S.-I.: Catheter replacement of the needle in percutaneous arteriography: a new technique, Acta Radiol. Diagn. **39:**368, 1953.

4. Cooper, M.W.: A simple method for insertion of multiple catheters through a single venipuncture site. Cathet. Cardiovasc. Diagn. **8:**305, 1982.

5. Skowronski, G.A., and Pearson, I.Y.: A technique for insertion of two intravascular catheters via a single puncture, Crit. Care Med. **10:**404, 1982.

6. Jacob, A.S., and Schweiger, M.J.: A method for inserting two catheters, pulmonary arterial and temporary pacing, through a single puncture into a subclavian vein, Cathet. Cardiovasc. Diagn. **9:**611, 1983.

7. Keeley, J.L.: Intravenous injections and infusions, Am. J. Surg. **50:**485, 1940.

8. Goldfarb, G., and Lebrec, D.: Percutaneous cannulation of the internal jugular vein in patients with coagulopathies: an experience based on 1000 attempts, Anesthesiology **56:**321, 1982.

9. Kashuk, J.L., and Penn, I.: Air embolism after central venous catheterization, Surg. Gynecol. Obstet. **159:**249, 1984.

10. Gottdiener, J.S., et al.: Detection of venous air embolism by 2D echocardiography: evidence for entry of air into intracardiac shunt. Circulation **72**(suppl. III):III-352, 1985.

11. Feliciano, D.V., et al.: Major complications of percutaneous subclavian vein catheters, Am. J. Surg. **138:**869, 1979.

12. Kearns, P.J., Haulk, A.A., and McDonald, T.W.: Homonymous hemianopia due to cerebral air embolism from central venous catheters, West. J. Med. **140:**615, 1984.

13. Bernard, R.W., and Stahl, W.M.: Subclavian vein catheterizations: a prospective study. I. Non-infectious complications, Ann. Surg. **173:**184, 1971.

14. Sznajder, J.I., et al.: Central vein catheterization: failure and complication rates by three percutaneous approaches, Arch. Intern. Med. **146:**259-261, 1986.

15. Johnston, A.O.B., and Clark, R.G.: Malpositioning of central venous catheters, Lancet **2:**1395, 1972.

16. Langston, C.S.: The aberrant central venous catheter and its complications, Diagn. Radiol. **100:**55, 1971.

17. Swanson, R.S., Uhlig, P.N., Gross, P.L., and McCabe, C.J.: Emergency intravenous access through the femoral vein, Ann. Emerg. Med. **13:**244, 1983.

18. Schwartz, A.J., Jobes, D.R., and Levy, W.J.: Intrathoracic vascular catheterization via the external jugular vein, Anesthesiology **56:**400, 1982.

19. Blitt, C.D., Wright, W.A., Petty, W.C., and Webster, T.A.: Central venous catheterization via the external jugular vein: a technique employing the J-wire, JAMA **229:**817, 1974.

20. Hemosura, B.: Measurement of pressure during intravenous therapy, JAMA **195:**181, 1966.

21. Brinkman, A.J., and Costley, D.O.: Internal jugular venipuncture, JAMA **223:**182, 1973.

22. Mostert, J.W., Kenny, G.M., and Murphy, G.P.: Safe placement of central venous catheter into internal jugular vein, Arch. Surg. **101:**431, 1970.

23. Civetta, J.M., Gabel, J.C., and Gemer, M.: Internal-jugular-vein puncture with a margin of safety, Anesthesiology **36:**622, 1972.

24. Jernigan, W.R., and Gardner, W.C.: Use of the internal jugular vein for placement of central venous catheter, Surg. Gynecol. Obstet. **130:**520, 1970.

25. Rao, T.L.K., Wong, A.Y., and Salem, M.R.: A new approach to percutaneous catheterization of the internal jugular vein, Anesthesiology **46:**362, 1977.

26. Daily, P.O., Griepp, R.B., and Shumway, N.E.: Percutaneous internal jugular vein cannulation, Arch. Surg. **101:**534, 1970.

27. English, I.C.W., Frew, R.M., and Pigott, J.F.G.: Percutaneous cannulation of the internal jugular vein, Thorax **24:**496, 1969.

28. Schwartz, A.J., Jobes, D.R., and Gruchow, E.: Carotid artery puncture with internal jugular cannulation using the Seldinger technique: incidence, recognition, treatment, and prevention, Anesthesiology **51:**S160, 1979.

29. Lipton, J.S., Trooskin, S.Z., and Rosenberg, N.: Carotid artery injury during attempted jugular vein catheterization, Heart Lung **13:**416, 1984.

30. Legler, D., and Nugent, M.: Doppler localization of the internal jugular vein facilitates its cannulation (abstract), Anesthesiology, 1983, p. A179.

31. Wilson, J.N., Grow, J.B., and Demong, C.: Central venous pressure in optimal blood volume maintenance, Arch. Surg. **85:**563, 1962.

32. Dronen, S., Thompson, B., Nowak, R., and Tomlanovich, M.: Subclavian vein catheterization during cardiopulmonary resuscitation: a prospective comparison of supraclavicular and infraclavicular percutaneous approaches, JAMA **247:**3227, 1984.

33. Simon, R.R., and Brenner, B.E.: Procedures and techniques in emergency medicine, Baltimore, 1984, Williams & Wilkins Co.

34. Linos, D.A., Mucha, P., and Van Heerden, J.A.: Subclavian vein, a golden route, Mayo Clin. Proc. **55:**315, 1980.

35. Asimacopoulos, P.J., Bagley, F.H., and McDermott, W.F.: A modified technique for subclavian puncture, Surg. Gynecol. Obstet. **150:**241, 1980.

36. Kaiser, C.W., et al.: Choice of route for central venous cannulation: subclavian or internal jugular vein: a prospective randomized study, J. Surg. Oncol. **17:**345, 1981.

37. O'Reilly, M.V.: The technique of subclavian vein cannulation, Can. Med. Assoc. J. **108:**63, 1973.

Chapter Three

Arterial access

ELAINE K. DAILY
ARA G. TILKIAN

The first documented arterial cannulation occurred in 1733 when Rev. Stephen Hales inserted a brass rod into the surgically exposed artery of a horse and measured the pressure via a manometer.[1] Since that time, access to the arterial system has become essential in the care and management of critically ill patients. Arterial punctures for the determination of blood gases are still performed today but have largely given way to the placement of arterial catheters, particularly if frequent blood gas determinations are anticipated or continuous monitoring of the arterial blood pressure is required. This discussion is directed to cannulation of the arterial system with short or long catheters.

GENERAL GUIDELINES

Aseptic technique, personnel, patient preparation, equipment preparation, and care of vascular lines are the same as for venous access (Chapter 2), as is local anesthesia, except that care must be taken to avoid administering excessive lidocaine, particularly around the radial artery, because it may cause pulsations to disappear. If the radial artery pulse is faint to begin with, administration of lidocaine may be omitted.

BASIC ARTERIAL CATHETERIZATION EQUIPMENT

The basic equipment needed for arterial catheterization is as follows:
- Basic percutaneous or cutdown tray (pp. 34 and 43)
- 6, 7, or 8 Fr catheter introducer set (J-curve guidewire/dilator/sheath with pneumatic seal and side arm) for use in cardiac catheterization laboratory
- Catheter of choice for the brachial, femoral, and axillary arteries and arterial grafts
- Additional specific equipment includes a 20-gauge Teflon catheter-over-needle with a small (0.018 inch or 0.46 mm) guidewire for percutaneous cannulation of the radial artery, and additional Teflon dilators (sizes 5, 6, 7 and 8 Fr) for cannulation of arterial grafts (p. 77)

INDICATIONS

Catheterization of the arterial system is indicated for pressure measurements, angiography, cardiac output determination, and counterpulsation. In addition, continuous intra-arterial pressure monitoring and multiple arterial blood sampling are frequently necessary in patients with unstable ischemic heart disease (with or without myocardial infarction), adult respiratory distress syndrome, severe arterial hypertension undergoing afterload-reducing therapy, hypotension or shock, and in patients who have undergone cardiac surgery.

CONTRAINDICATIONS

Arterial catheterization is relatively contraindicated in patients with severe atherosclerosis with diminished blood flow at or distal to the insertion site. In patients with bleeding disorders or those receiving thrombolytic therapy, bleeding disorders may occur.

COMPLICATIONS

Complications common to all intra-arterial techniques include:
- Bleeding (hematoma)
- Distal ischemia or necrosis
- Thrombosis
- Infection
- Embolism
- Vasculitis
- Arterial dissection

ARTERIAL CANNULATION SITES

The arterial system can be cannulated either percutaneously or via a cutdown at several sites. If necessary

Table 3-1. Advantages and disadvantages associated with percutaneous cannulation of specific arterial sites

Site	Advantages	Disadvantages
Radial artery	Readily accessible Good collateral circulation Superficial location Collateral circulation can be assessed before the procedure	High risk of occlusion because of small size High rate of catheter malfunction In shock states with low blood pressure and peripheral vasoconstriction this site may not reflect central aortic pressure
Brachial artery	Accessible in most patients with peripheral vascular disease	Higher complication rate Deeper location makes control of bleeding more difficult Closely surrounded by major tendons, veins, and nerves
Axillary artery	Arm position permits biplane angiography and oblique views Less patient immobilization Left axillary artery insertion associated with successful selective catheter placement Decreased risk of occlusion because of large size Extensive collateral circulation	Increased risk of nerve damage Risk of hematoma or pseudoaneurysm
Femoral artery	Large vessel easy to cannulate with decreased risk of occlusion Easier to cannulate in presence of vasoconstriction or hypotension Accurate central pressures even in shock states Long catheter life Easy to compress after catheter removal	Reduced patient mobility Insertion site not as easily located in obese patients Risk of hematoma in very obese patients in whom direct compression may be difficult

the arterial system can also be entered via cannulation of arterial grafts. To reduce complications and obtain the most accurate hemodynamic data, catheters are preferably placed in the large-diameter arteries. In order of size this would be the femoral, axillary, brachial, and radial arteries. However, in clinical practice, cannulation of the axillary artery is infrequently used. Femoral and brachial arteries have traditionally been cannulated primarily in the cardiac catheterization laboratory on a short-term basis for pressure measurements and arteriography. This practice may be changing as more clinicians become aware of the benefits and familiar with the skills of femoral artery cannulation.[2,3] Because of the poor collateral supply, cannulation of the brachial artery for long-term pressure monitoring is discouraged.

Table 3-1 lists some advantages and disadvantages of each arterial insertion site. Table 3-2 lists the insertion success rate, the overall complication rate, and specific complication rates for each arterial insertion site.

PERCUTANEOUS CANNULATION

Percutaneous insertion of arterial catheters is the preferred method of cannulation because of its ease and speed of insertion, reduced infection rate, and fewer equipment requirements.

Radial artery

Percutaneous cannulation of the radial artery is traditionally the most common means of arterial access in the critical care or emergency setting.

Anatomy

The radial artery is a small, superficially located terminal branch of the brachial artery (Fig. 3-1). It arises in the antecubital fossa and passes downward to the wrist along the radial side of the forearm. Its pulsations can be readily palpated at the wrist before the flexor carpi radialis tendon of the lateral anterior border of the radius.

The radial artery anastamoses with the ulnar artery in the hand, forming the deep palmar arch, the dorsal arch, and the superficial palmar arch.

Patient preparation

Modified Allen test. Before cannulation of the radial artery it is imperative to assess the adequacy of collateral blood flow to the hand. This can be done via a

Table 3-2. Insertion success rate and specific complications associated with percutaneous cannulation of arterial insertion sites

Site	Insertion success rate (%)	Specific complications and reported rates (%)*
Radial artery	85	Thrombosis 2.5-60
		Hematoma 0-30
		Emboli 0-23
		Infection 0-14
		Diminished pulse 1-15
		Distal ischemia 1-7
		Sepsis 0-5
		Bleeding 1
		Distal necrosis <1
		Pseudoaneurysm <1
Femoral artery	99	Hematoma 1-5
		Thrombosis 1-4
		Distal ischemia 3
		Emboli <2
		Sepsis 0-4
Brachial artery	Varied data	Diminished pulse 0-45
		Ischemia 0-1.5
Axillary artery	70-90	Brachial plexus injury <1-9
		Hematoma 1-6
		Neuropathy 0-3
		Pseudoaneurysm <1
		Sepsis <1

*References 2, 3, 6 to 10, 15, 25 to 27.

Doppler flow probe, a finger pulse monitor, or performance of the Allen test. A modified Allen test is performed in the manner described below.

1. Elevate the patient's arm well above the heart level.

2. Clench the fist of the elevated arm, either passively or actively.

3. Place the thumb of one hand over the ulnar artery and the thumb of the other hand over the radial artery and firmly compress both arteries for approximately 5 seconds.

4. While maintaining arterial compression, lower the arm and relax the hand, which will be very white.

5. Release the pressure only on the ulnar side of the artery.

6. Observe and time the appearance of a pink flush over the palm, including the thumb and fingers. The entire hand should regain color in less than 15 seconds; if so, the test is negative. Ulnar filling is deemed slow if flushing does not occur before 7 to 15 seconds and suggests that part of the hand depends on radial circulation for perfusion. This would be a positive Allen test and and is an absolute contraindication for placement of

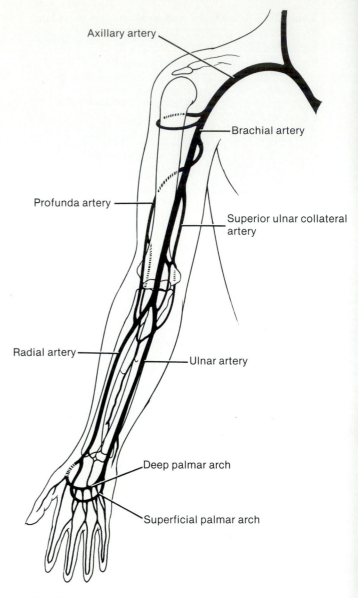

Fig. 3-1. Anatomic locations of the arteries of the arm.

a cannula in the radial artery; such placement would seriously compromise perfusion to the hand. The Allen test should be repeated, releasing compression on the radial artery only to evaluate radial adequacy. If either artery demonstrates a delay in color return, the radial artery should not be cannulated.

The Allen test may be difficult to perform in dark-skinned persons or in uncooperative patients. Under these circumstances the use of a Doppler flow probe, and more particularly the finger-pulse transducer, provides accurate assessment of the adequacy of ulnar collateral blood flow to the hand.[4]

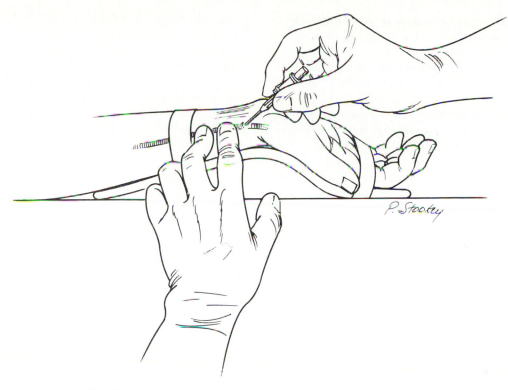

Fig. 3-2. Puncture of the radial artery with the needle at a 30° angle.

7. General patient preparation as described on pp. 32 to 33.

8. Immobilize the patient's nondominant hand (if possible) palm side up on a padded arm board, providing approximately 60 ° extension of the wrist.

9. Secure a peripheral IV line or heparin lock.

Procedure

1. Palpate the radial artery to determine its exact location and direction.

2. Make a shallow 1 to 2 mm skin incision over the radial artery with a #11 scalpel.

3. Align a 20-gauge needle with stylet at a 20° angle over the radial artery approximately 3 to 4 cm proximal to the styloid process of the radius.

4. While palpating the pulse with one hand, insert the needle into and through the radial artery (Fig. 3-2).

5. Remove the inner stylet and slowly withdraw the needle until it is located in the artery; proper location is indicated by bright red blood pulsating from the needle hub.

6. Insert the soft flexible tip of an 0.018-inch (0.46 mm) guidewire 10 to 15 cm into the artery. While securely holding the wire in place, remove the needle. Wipe the guidewire with a moistened gauze pad. Insert a short (5 cm) 3 Fr catheter over the guidewire into the artery; remove the guidewire. Alternately, and more commonly, a catheter-over-needle is inserted into the radial artery for long-term monitoring. If a catheter-over-needle is being used, remove the stylet and slowly withdraw the catheter and needle until bright red blood pulsates from the needle hub. Advance the Teflon catheter into the artery while simultaneously withdrawing the needle.

7. Aspirate, discard the aspirate, and gently flush the catheter. Attach the heparinized IV solution and stopcock to the catheter.

8. Suture the hub of the catheter to the skin with 3-0 silk.

9. Cleanse the area and apply an iodophor ointment and a sterile dressing secured with tape.

Special precautions

Diminished radial pulse. Occasionally the radial artery pulse will diminish or disappear after infiltration with lidocaine. This is usually temporary. However, return of the pulse can sometimes be hastened by gentle massage of the surrounding tissues.

Pulsatile blood cessation. If cessation of pulsatile blood occurs at any time during catheter advancement, slowly withdraw the catheter until blood flow resumes. Withdraw the catheter 1 to 2 mm more, then readvance the catheter. If no blood flow reappears during the second catheter withdrawal, remove the catheter entirely and apply compression for 5 minutes before repuncturing the artery. If there never was evidence of blood flow, the artery was probably never punctured; in this case compression is not necessary before repuncturing the artery.

Methods of cannulation (Fig. 3-3). Cannulation can be sucessfully performed by either direct threading or fixation, as described in step 5. Transfixation of the vessel by deliberate puncture of both the anterior and posterior wall of the artery is a commonly used

method in the smaller arteries. Reports indicate no significant difference in the complication rates of these methods.[5,6]

Determinants of radial artery thrombosis. The most significant determinants of radial artery thrombosis seem to be catheter size, shape, and composition and the length of time the catheter is left in the artery. For these reasons it is strongly recommended that the radial artery be cannulated with a nontapered Teflon catheter no larger than 20 gauge and that the catheter be removed as soon as clinically possible. Short-term cannulation for less than 4 hours can be safely performed with little risk of thrombosis.[7] The risk of arterial occlusion is also higher if the artery is punctured more than

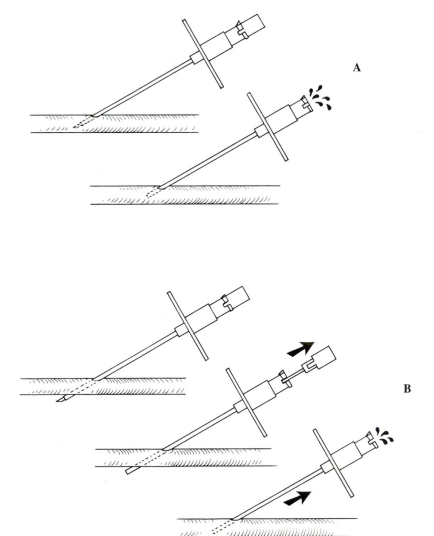

Fig. 3-3. Methods of arterial cannulation via (**A**) direct puncture or (**B**) transfixation in which both walls are punctured, after which the inner stylet is removed and the cannula is slowly withdrawn until blood flow appears at the hub.

once during attempted cannulation. Despite the high rate of thrombotic complications with radial artery catheters, permanent damage occurs infrequently, with resolution of symptoms usually within 48 hours to 7 days of catheter removal.[8] Therapeutic maneuvers that may improve distal blood flow include heparin infusion, administration of lidocaine, performance of a sympathetic nerve block, or thrombectomy via a Fogarty catheter (see p. 81). Careful attention to technique, use of a small, preferably nontapered Teflon catheter for short periods of time, and meticulous nursing care can markedly reduce the risk of serious complications.

Circulatory assessment of the hand. Circulation in the hand should be assessed every 4 hours and the catheter removed immediately upon any signs of circulatory compromise.

Prevention of bleeding. Bleeding from the puncture site can be prevented by applying firm pressure for 5 to 10 minutes after catheter removal. The puncture site should then be observed for several minutes to assure the adequacy of hemostasis. This should be followed by application of a light pressure dressing and frequent evaluations of the radial pulse and blood flow to the hand.

A loose connection from the arterial line can quickly cause hemorrhage. For this reason, only Luer-Lok connections should be used. All connections should be secured tightly and all connectors should be readily visible so that leaks can be immediately detected.

Femoral artery

The femoral artery has long been the artery of choice for percutaneous insertion of catheters retrogradely into the arterial system and left ventricle and is being used with increasing frequency by cardiologists with experience in femoral artery cannulation for long-term monitoring in the critical care setting. Other intensive care specialists are discovering the advantages of using such a large artery. The large size of the femoral artery decreases the risk of occlusive complications, facilitates successful cannulation, and permits a more accurate measurement of central arterial pressure.

Concerns about the alleged high incidence of infection or thrombotic complications associated with this approach have not materialized. Several studies have revealed similar complication rates (including infection) between femoral and radial artery cannulation.[8,9]

Anatomy

The femoral artery continues from the external iliac artery and begins just beneath the inguinal ligament in the upper thigh. If a line is drawn from the symphysis pubis to the anterior superior iliac spine, the femoral artery passes through the midpoint of that line at the inguinal ligament (see Fig. 2-7). The femoral nerve lies on the lateral side of the femoral artery, and the femoral vein on the medial side within the femoral triangle (NAVL relationship—lateral to medial direction).

The femoral pulse can be palpated in the femoral triangle approximately 2 to 3 cm below the inguinal ligament. Firm pressure is required to palpate the femoral artery because it is located deep beneath the fascia.

Patient preparation

Patient preparation for femoral artery cannulation is the same as that for cannulation of the femoral vein (p. 52).

Procedure

1. Palpate and locate the direction of the femoral artery above, below, and as it crosses the inguinal ligament, using three fingers of the left (or nondominant) hand.

2. With a #11 scalpel, make a 2 to 3 mm incision in the skin at the proposed insertion site. Bluntly dissect along the anticipated path of the catheter with a curved Kelly forceps.

3. While holding a vascular needle between the middle and index fingers of the right (dominant) hand, with the thumb resting on the hub, align the needle at a 45° angle inclined 10° to 20° medially over the femoral artery 3 to 4 cm below the inguinal ligament. Continue to palpate the femoral pulse with the left hand (Fig. 3-4).

4. Fully advance the needle with its stylet into (and through, if desired) the femoral artery until the periosteum is felt. A slight popping sensation may be felt as the needle enters the artery.

5. If the femoral artery is perforated, the needle may bounce with each pulsation. Remove the stylet and slowly withdraw the needle until the tip rests within the lumen of the artery (indicated by a pulsating jet of blood).

6. Place a thumb over the hub to control bleeding.

7. Gently depress the hub of the needle to better align the needle with the artery and insert the flexible end of the guidewire through it and into the vessel approximately 15 to 20 cm.

8. Remove the needle from the vessel while securely holding the guidewire in place and firmly compressing the insertion site with the nondominant hand to control bleeding.

9. Wipe the guidewire with a moist gauze pad.

Steps 10 through 17 (cardiac catheterization) are followed by steps 10 through 14 (long-term hemodynamic monitoring).

For cardiac catheterization:

10. Advance the dilator/sheath system over the guidewire, making sure the guidewire protrudes 10 to 15 cm from the hub of the sheath before entering the skin.

11. While applying pressure at the insertion site with the nondominant hand, hold the dilator tip between the thumb and index finger of the other hand. Advance it through the skin and into the artery with a clockwise motion.

12. Once the sheath is fully inserted in the artery,

remove the dilator and guidewire from the sheath, leaving the sheath in place.

13. Aspirate, discard the aspirate, and flush the side-arm of the sheath. Connect the sheath to heparinized and pressurized IV solution. Suture the sheath to the skin.

14. Administer heparin (5000 U) through the arterial sheath or IV line.

15. Insert the catheter of choice, with its guidewire leading through the sheath and into the vessel (see Fig. 2-4). Advance the guidewire and catheter into the ascending aorta and aortic arch, using fluoroscopic guidance.

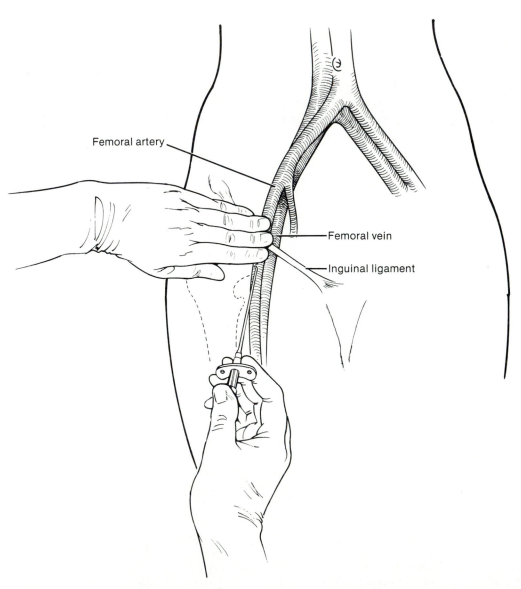

Fig. 3-4. Puncture of the femoral artery 2 to 4 cm below the inguinal ligament with the needle inclined 10° to 20° medially.

16. Remove the guidewire, aspirate, discard the aspirate, flush the catheter, and connect it to the fluid or contrast-filled manifold.

17. Advance the catheter to the desired position, using fluoroscopy (see Chapter 5).

For long-term hemodynamic monitoring:

10. Advance the monitoring catheter of choice over the guidewire until 10 to 15 cm of the wire extends beyond the hub of the catheter.

11. While continuing to apply pressure at the insertion site with one hand, firmly grasp the tip of the catheter between the index finger and thumb of the other hand. Advance the catheter through the skin and into the artery using a clockwise motion.

12. Once the catheter is fully inserted in the artery, remove the guidewire.

13. Aspirate, discard the aspirate, and gently flush the catheter. Connect it to pressurized and heparinized flush solution with a three-way stopcock.

14. Suture the catheter to the skin near the insertion site. Apply an iodophor ointment and a sterile dressing and tape securely.

Femoral artery catheter removal

To remove a long-term hemodynamic monitoring catheter or a sheath, proceed as follows.

1. Attach a 20 ml syringe to its hub.

2. Place the middle and index fingers of the nondominant hand just above the puncture site and the thumb just below the puncture site. Firmly grasp the catheter (and sheath, if used) with the other hand.

3. With an assistant applying negative pressure via the plunger of the syringe, quickly withdraw the catheter (or sheath) from the femoral artery while occlusive pressure is applied below the puncture site to prevent any thrombi moving distally.

4. Allow the puncture site to bleed for a few seconds; then apply compression just above the puncture site for 10 minutes.

5. Check femoral and dorsalis pedis pulses frequently during compression to make certain manual compression does not obliterate the pulses. If pulses are weak or absent, reduce the intensity (not the time!) of compression.

6. If bleeding from the puncture site is still apparent after 10 minutes, manual compression must be continued, uninterrupted, for an additional 10 minutes. (Check for use of heparin, aspirin, or coagulopathy.) Sandbags or compression devices should not be used until adequate hemostasis is established.

7. After hemostasis is obtained, observe the site for several minutes before applying iodophor ointment, a sterile dressing, and an elastic bandage to the site.

8. A 5 to 10 lb sandbag may be applied to the site, although it may be preferable to have an unobstructed view of the puncture site while the patient is kept on 4 to 6 hours of complete bedrest. Any bleeding occurring after this will require prolonged compression.

9. Check distal circulation (color, movement, and sensation) frequently after catheter removal. A Doppler flow probe is also useful to evaluate distal blood flow.

Special precautions

Resistance. If *any* resistance is met during passage of the guidewire through the vessel, carefully withdraw the guidewire and make certain the wire is truly intravascular by observing pulsatile blood flow through the needle. Diminished or "trickling" blood flow indicates the needle tip is not freely positioned in the lumen of the artery and requires repositioning of the needle until brisk blood flow is again observed. If good blood flow is observed, insert a J-curve guidewire instead of a straight guidewire. If the artery is extremely tortuous, a J-curve wire with a movable inner core may facilitate wire and catheter passage. A small amount of contrast media injected through the arterial needle during fluoroscopic observation may reveal the anatomy and extent of tortuosity. *Under no circumstances should a guidewire or catheter be advanced against resistance.*

Level of puncture. If the arterial needle is inserted too low, cannulation of the superficial femoral artery, rather than the common femoral artery, may result. If the superficial femoral artery is small, this could result in occlusion of the vessel. In addition, pseudoaneurysm more commonly develops after puncture of the superficial femoral artery, where there is no femoral sheath to control bleeding nor any bony structure against which to adequately compress the artery[10] (Fig. 3-5). Consequently, hemostasis is difficult to achieve if the puncture site is distal to the common femoral artery. Puncture of the common femoral artery should be approximately 3 to 4 cm below the inguinal ligament.

Brachial artery

Although the brachial artery is usually cannulated via a cutdown, it may at times be desirable to perform percutaneous entry of the brachial artery for hemodynamic monitoring or catheterization and angiography of the left heart. Patients with peripheral vascular disease of the lower extremities, large, muscular arms, or a previous cutdown that would involve an extensive and lengthy arteriotomy may be candidates for percutaneous brachial artery cannulation. However, experience with this technique is not as widespread as that of femoral artery and radial artery cannulation.

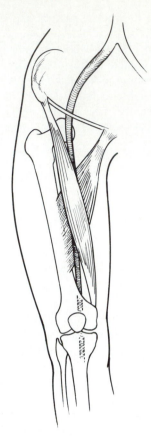

Fig. 3-5. Drawing of the femoral artery showing its relationship to the head of the femur just below the inguinal ligament. Puncture of the artery over this location provides better compression.

Anatomy

The brachial artery continues from the axillary artery in the upper arm just under the medial edge of the biceps muscle and lies medial to the biceps tendon and lateral to the median nerve at the antecubital fossa (Fig. 3-1). Below the antecubital fossa the brachial artery divides into the ulnar and radial arteries. Its course through the upper arm is superficial and palpable and is represented by a line connected between the midpoint of the clavicle with the midpoint of the antecubital fossa.

Patient preparation

1. Prepare the patient as described on pp. 32 to 33.
2. Locate the brachial artery by palpation approximately 5 cm above the antecubital fossa.
3. Evaluate the brachial artery in both arms to determine equality of pulses or the presence of a bruit.

4. Check the blood pressure in both arms. If the systolic pressure difference between the two arms is greater than 20 mm Hg, use the arm with the higher pressure because of the possibility of subclavian artery stenosis.
5. Leave the sphygmomanometer cuff under the selected arm (not around it at this time).
6. Abduct the selected arm 30° to 45° from the body and secure it on an arm board.

Procedure

The method described here utilizes a catheter sheath as described by Pepine et al.,[11] which is suitable for cardiac catheterization procedures. For insertion of a single catheter (usually a 4 Fr catheter) for long-term hemodynamic monitoring purposes, follow steps 1 through 7 below. Thereafter, follow steps 7 to 9 as described for radial artery catheterization on p. 69.

1. After local infiltration (p. 33), fix the brachial artery by pressing the index and middle finger of one hand above and below the anticipated puncture site just 5 cm above the antecubital fossa, directly over the brachial artery.
2. Insert an 18-gauge needle, with its stylet, at a 20° to 30° angle, through the skin into the artery. Take care not to puncture the posterior wall of the artery.
3. Remove the stylet and, with the appearance of pulsatile blood flow through the needle, insert the flexible end of the short J-curve guidewire through the needle and approximately 10 to 15 cm into the artery.
4. Withdraw the needle with one hand while compressing both above and below the puncture site and firmly holding onto the guidewire with the other hand.
5. Wipe the guidewire with a sterile moist gauze pad.
6. With a #11 scalpel, make a 2 to 3 mm nick in the skin at the insertion site to facilitate catheter passage.
7. Insert the 6 Fr or 7 Fr sheath/dilator unit over the guidewire, making sure the guidewire protrudes 5 to 10 cm from the hub of the sheath before inserting it into the skin. While holding the dilator between the thumb and index finger, advance it into the artery with a slight twisting motion. For hemodynamic monitoring, insert a 4 Fr Teflon catheter (rather than the sheath/dilator) over the guidewire.
8. After the sheath is fully inserted into the artery, remove the dilator and guidewire together, leaving the sheath in place.
9. Aspirate, discard the aspirate, and flush the side arm of the sheath.
10. Inject heparin (5000 units) into the side arm of the sheath and close the stopcock.

11. Secure the sheath to the skin very near the insertion site with a 3-0 suture.

12. Insert the catheter of choice with its guidewire through the sheath into the artery and position it in the usual manner, using fluoroscopy.

Catheter removal. On completion of the study (hemodynamic measurements and angiography) removal is performed as follows.

1. Remove the catheter from the sheath with the help of a guidewire.

2. Remove the securing sutures from the sheath.

3. Tightly roll several 4 × 4-inch gauze pads and place them longitudinally on the skin over the body of the sheath. Secure them with an elastic bandage.

4. Wrap a sphygmomanometer cuff around the upper arm, incorporating the rolled gauze.

5. Administer 30 to 40 mg of protamine intravenously to partially reverse the heparinization (see p. 147).

6. Attach a 10 ml syringe to the side arm of the sheath.

7. Inflate the blood pressure cuff to approximately 10 mm Hg *above* the patient's systolic pressure.

8. While aspirating through the side arm of the sheath, quickly remove the sheath from the artery.

9. Reduce cuff blood pressure to 10 mm Hg *below* the patient's systolic pressure and maintain that pressure for 10 minutes. Check frequently to make sure this does not obliterate the patient's radial pulse. If so, slightly release the pressure in the cuff.

10. After 10 minutes, slowly deflate the blood pressure cuff approximately 10 mm Hg per minute until a pressure of 50 mm Hg is reached. At this time release and remove the cuff.

11. Check the radial pulse; if it is strong, apply an elastic bandage firmly over the dressing already in place.

12. Loosen and check the dressing every 4 hours; remove it after 24 hours.

The hemodynamic monitoring catheter (4 Fr) may be removed from the brachial artery in the same manner as from the femoral artery (p. 73). Hemostasis is accomplished by manual compression.

Percutaneous brachial artery catheterization for the purpose of coronary arteriography has been performed, with minor modifications, in over 400 patients and has been found to be both a safe and successful alternate method of arterial access.[12,13]

Special precautions

Reducing vessel trauma. Use of a twisting motion during insertion of the sheath is recommended to reduce trauma to the vessel and the risk of thrombosis.

Hemostasis during catheter manipulation. Using a sheath with a pneumatic seal is highly recommended for this technique to control blood loss during catheter manipulation. However, the presence of such a seal may make it difficult to manipulate selective preformed catheters. If marked impairment of catheter movement occurs, a regular sheath (without the pneumatic seal) can be used. Hemostasis during catheter exchange is achieved by inflation of the blood pressure cuff above the patient's systolic blood pressure.[14]

Axillary artery

Percutaneous cannulation of the axillary artery may occasionally be used in the cardiac catheterization laboratory for left heart studies in those patients with peripheral vascular disease of the lower limbs. Although the brachial artery is more commonly employed in these cases, the axillary approach can also be used. The axillary approach may also facilitate performance of biplane angiograms because of the patient's arm position. In addition, percutaneous cannulation of the axillary artery for long-term hemodynamic monitoring is preferred by some physicians because of the reduced incidence of major ischemic complications with this large artery.[15]

Anatomy

The axillary artery is a large artery that continues from the subclavian artery as it enters the axilla. It ends at the axilla at the inferior border of the teres major muscle and enters the arm as the brachial artery. The axillary artery is divided in three parts by the pectoralis minor muscle, which crosses it in front. The first part traverses a fatty space extending from the lateral border of the first rib to the upper border of the pectoralis minor; the second part lies close behind the pectoralis minor, a finger's breadth from the tip of the coracoid process; the third and longest part crosses the three posterior axillary muscles near their insertions and extends to the lower border of the teres major muscle (Fig. 3-6). The axillary artery and vein and the brachial plexus form a neurovascular bundle within the axillary sheath.

Patient preparation

1. Begin patient preparation by following the steps described on pp. 32 to 33.

2. Hyperabduct and externally rotate the selected arm by placing the patient's hand under his or her head.

3. Shave the patient's underarm area.

4. Locate the axillary artery in the axillary fossa at the posterolateral border of the pectoralis muscle (Fig. 3-7).

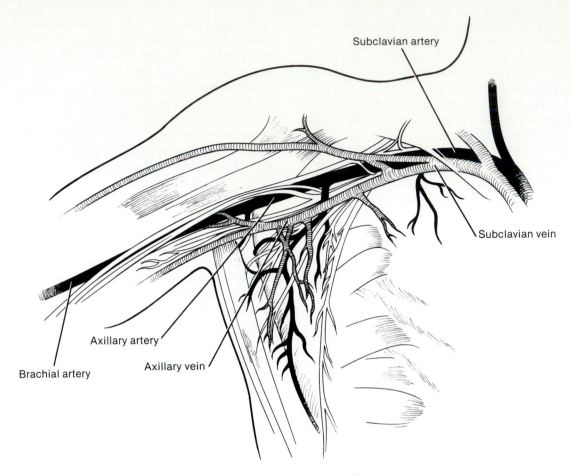

Fig. 3-6. Anatomic location of the axillary artery.

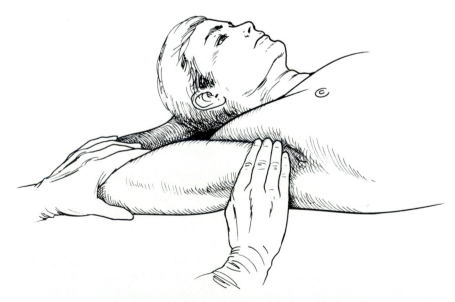

Fig. 3-7. Location of the axillary artery by palpation of the axillary fossa.

Procedure

1. Palpate and locate the direction of the axillary artery and, after local infiltration, fix it by pressing the index and middle fingers of one hand below and above the anticipated puncture site 3 to 4 cm proximal to the pectoralis muscle or the deltopectoral groove. (The puncture should be at the highest point at which the artery is palpable.)

2. With the other hand, insert an 18-gauge needle into the axillary artery.

3. When pulsatile blood flow appears in the needle hub, insert a J-tip guidewire through the needle into the vessel approximately 10 to 15 cm.

4. Follow the usual steps in percutaneous arterial cannulation. Securing the sheath in place with 3-0 silk aids in catheter manipulation and exchange without risk of sheath removal.

5. On completion of the procedure, remove the sheath and apply manual compression to the puncture site for 10 minutes. If bleeding has ceased at the end of this time, apply an iodophor ointment and a compression bandage to the site.

6. Advise the patient not to use the punctured arm for 24 hours to avoid possible bleeding from the site.

Special precautions

Infiltration of local anesthetic into the axillary area must be performed with care because the area is richly innervated.

Left versus right axillary artery. Valeix et al.[16] suggest cannulation of the left rather than the right axillary artery because of reduced patient limitations (most patients are right-handed), reduced risk of catheter malposition into the right carotid via the innominate trunk, easier insertion of preformed catheters into the coronary ostia, and easier catheterization of aortocoronary bypass grafts from the left side. Their described use of a catheter sheath for catheter insertions into the axillary artery markedly reduces the overall complication rate.

Emboli. Meticulous technique must be observed in flushing the catheters in the axillary artery because air, clot, or particulate matter could embolize to the brain via the carotid artery. This risk may be less with catheter insertions into the left axillary artery.

Arterial grafts

Patients with aortofemoral, femoral-popliteal, or femoral-tibial grafts frequently require angiographic studies for evaluation. Insertion of arterial angiographic catheters in these patients is often approached from a percutaneous brachial, axillary, or translumbar aortic puncture, or via a cutdown of the brachial artery. These routes are preferred by some physicians because of the potential hazards of graft cannulation, including uncontrollable bleeding, disruption of graft suture line with false aneurysm formation, disruption of the neointima of the graft, thrombosis, and infection.[17] Other vascular radiologists consider cannulation of the axillary artery technically more difficult to perform, with less successful selective catheterization of the aortic branches. For these reasons, and because of ease of cannulation, some physicians consider percutaneous cannulation of the arterial graft the procedure of choice for evaluation of graft patency.[18, 19]

Use of a catheter introducer sheath has improved this technique by permitting multiple catheter exchanges with much less trauma to the neointima, better control of bleeding, and improved catheter torque control. This technique has also been successfully applied to percutaneous transluminal angioplasty in patients with recurrent disease after bypass surgery.[20]

Anatomy

Most grafts are anatomically positioned, either tunneled deeply from a more superficial origin or tunneled into subcutaneous tissue.

Patient preparation

Prepare the patient as described on pp. 32 to 33.

Procedure

1. Palpate and locate the direction of the graft.

2. After local infiltration, make a small nick (2 to 3 mm) in the skin at the intended puncture site using a #11 scalpel.

3. Insert an 18-gauge, one or two-part needle at a 20° angle into the graft, *taking care not to puncture the posterior wall of the graft.*

4. With the appearance of pulsatile blood flow through the needle hub, insert the flexible end of the J-curve guidewire through the needle 15 to 20 cm into the graft.

5. Remove the needle with one hand while applying compression above and below the puncture site and firmly holding the guidewire in place with the other hand.

6. Wipe the guidewire with a sterile moist gauze pad.

7. Insert the 5 Fr dilator over the guidewire into the graft, using a slight twisting motion to enter the skin.

8. Remove the dilator, wipe the guidewire, and continue to progressively dilate the insertion site up to one half to one French size larger than the largest size catheter to be inserted.[21]

9. Remove the last dilator and insert the catheter in-

troducer (dilator and sheath) over the guidewire into the graft.

10. Remove both the dilator and guidewire from the sheath.

11. Aspirate, discard the aspirate, and flush the side port of the sheath.

12. Administer 5000 units of heparin through the side port and connect the side port to a heparinized and pressurized flush system.

13. Insert the selected catheters through the sheath and position properly for angiography.

Catheter removal. On completion of the procedure, the catheter is removed in the manner described below.

1. Follow the steps for the removal of the femoral artery catheter (p. 43).

2. Apply manual pressure to the puncture site for 15 minutes to control bleeding (check distal pulses frequently to make certain compression does not obliterate pulsations).

3. When bleeding is stopped, observe the puncture site for several minutes, then apply an iodophor ointment and a compression dressing.

Special precautions

Vascular entry needle. Because of the necessity of performing a clean, nontraumatic puncture of the graft, a reusable vascular needle should not be used for graft cannulation. A disposable or new needle should be used. Multiple punctures should be avoided in this higher risk population.

Safe use of tapered dilators. Tapered dilators should not have their full length inserted into the graft. Their sharply tapered tips could damage the posterior wall of the graft. It is only necessary to insert the dilator through the skin and just inside the graft wall. A twisting motion during the insertion is less traumatic to the graft.

Catheter sheath. Catheterization of an arterial graft without the use of a catheter sheath causes increased damage to the vessel and the catheter. The tight fit of the catheter at the puncture site increases resistance, requiring greater rotational force to insert and advance the catheter. This has resulted in weakening and subsequent separation of the catheter on withdrawal.[22, 23] This serious complication can be diminished with the use of a Teflon catheter introducer sheath, which reduces the stresses imposed on the catheter during insertion and withdrawal. However, when used through vascular prosthetic grafts, sheaths frequently kink and may be difficult to remove. For this reason, a guidewire should always be maintained within the sheath when changing catheters to avoid weakening and kinking of the sheath.

Catheter size. The smallest catheter that provides the necessary data should be used in either venous or prosthetic grafts. This is usually a 5 or 6 Fr angiographic catheter.

ARTERIAL CUTDOWN

Although percutaneous arterial cannulation is the preferred route of catheterization for most physicians, others prefer to catheterize the arterial system via an arteriotomy of the surgically exposed vessel, followed by meticulous repair of the artery to minimize thrombosis and reestablish adequate blood flow.

Brachial artery cutdown

Catheterization of the brachial artery via a cutdown is a common approach to coronary arteriography and was first described and popularized by Dr. F. Mason Sones at the Cleveland Clinic. This method is also useful for coronary angioplasty or studies of the left heart in patients with peripheral vascular disease of the lower extremities when femoral artery cannulation has failed. Brachial artery cutdown is not recommended for placement of long-dwelling intra-arterial catheters for hemodynamic monitoring or blood sampling.

Anatomy

For description of the basic anatomy of the brachial artery, see p. 74.

Equipment

The equipment needed for cutdown of the brachial artery includes a basic cutdown tray plus a selected catheter.

Patient preparation

1. Begin patient preparation by following the steps described on pp. 32 to 33.

2. Secure an IV route or heparin lock.

3. Abduct the selected arm and secure it on a flat, padded surface.

4. Shave the antecubital area.

Procedure

1. Palpate and locate the direction of the brachial artery just above the antecubital crease.

2. After local infiltration, make a small (2.5 cm) transverse skin incision over the brachial artery pulsation just proximal to the antecubital crease, using a #15 scalpel.

3. Follow steps 3 through 8 of the basic cutdown technique on p. 43.

Catheter removal. On completion of the procedure, the catheter is removed in the manner described below.

1. Remove the catheter while maintaining tension on the proximal and distal tapes around the artery.

2. Momentarily release the tension on the distal tape to check blood flow, which should be brisk. If flow is minimal, insert the closed tips of a blunt curved forceps or a small hemostat into the distal artery to dislodge any small thrombi that may be present (Fig. 3-8). Be certain to insert the forcep tips beyond the site of occlusion by the distal tape. If retrograde blood flow does not appear, perform a Fogarty embolectomy (p. 81).

3. Momentarily release the tension on the proximal tape and verify abundant forward blood flow. If the flow is sluggish, follow the directions in step 2 above to establish brisk antegrade blood flow.

4. With tension on both ties, hold the artery near the skin level and flush the surface with heparinized saline so all edges of the artery are visible.

5. Place a small pillow under the patient's hand to remove tension from the vessel.

6. Suture the arteriotomy with 6-0 monofilament sutures on a cutting needle. Place and tie the first suture while incorporating the lateral edge of the arteriotomy. Carefully position the remaining stitches across the incision, lifting on the suture after each placement. (Take special care to avoid including the posterior wall of the artery in the stitch.) After the last stitch is placed (usually about four), pull the sutures taut and double-tie them.

7. Release the ties and check for bleeding.

8. Flush the wound with heparinized sterile saline.

9. Check the quality of the radial pulse.

10. If the radial pulse is adequate, close the skin with three or four interrupted mattress sutures using 4-0 silk (or use a subcuticular stitch of absorbable 4-0 suture material.)

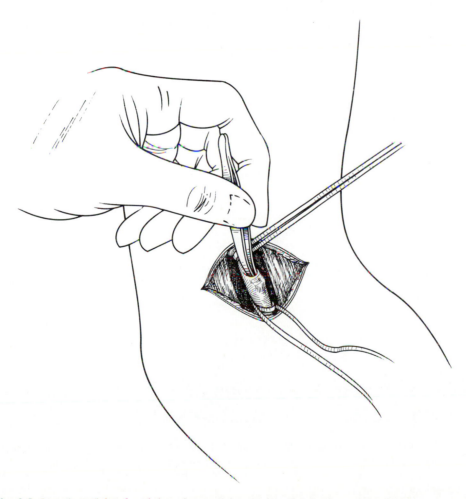

Fig. 3-8. Insertion of the closed tips of a small forceps into the distal artery to dislodge any small thrombi that may be present.

11. Cleanse the skin with sterile water and apply iodophor ointment and a small sterile dressing to the site.

Catheter introducer sheath with pneumatic seal

Some laboratories routinely utilize a catheter introducer sheath with a pneumatic seal and a side arm through a brachial arteriotomy to facilitate catheter exchange, minimize trauma to the arteriotomy, improve arteriotomy repair, and reduce the incidence of post-catheterization thrombosis.[24]

1. Introduce the guidewire/dilator/sheath as a unit through a small arteriotomy. Administer 3000 to 5000 units of heparin.

2. Advance the unit until the sheath hub reaches the wall of the vessel, and then remove the guidewire and dilator, leaving only the sheath in place.

3. Aspirate, discard the aspirate, flush the side arm, and connect it to a heparinized and pressurized flush solution.

4. Suture the side arm of the sheath to the edge of the cutdown. This is necessary because the sheath is not secured by any surrounding tissue and could easily be dislodged during catheter manipulation.

5. Insert the catheter(s) through the sheath and proceed in the usual manner.

6. At the end of the procedure, remove the sheath and administer additional heparin distally into the artery.

7. Flush the incision with heparinized sterile saline.

8. Close the artery with interrupted 6-0 monofilament sutures.

9. If the radial pulse is adequate, close the skin with three or four 4-0 interrupted mattress sutures.

10. Cleanse the skin with sterile water and apply iodophor ointment and a small sterile dressing to the site.

Special precautions

Avoiding arterial spasm. All catheters inserted through an arteriotomy should be premoistened with heparinized saline to reduce friction and the possibility of arterial spasm. If spasm should occur, follow the same directions given for venospasm on p. 46.

Incision size. Creating too small an incision in the artery results in a sharper angle of catheter insertion, increasing the risk of injury to the posterior intima of the vessel and subsequent thrombus formation (Fig. 3-9, *A*). Performing an adequate-size arteriotomy and using a vascular clamp to grasp a full thickness of the lateral portion of the arteriotomy during catheter insertion permit passage of the catheter at a much shallower angle (10° to 15°), avoiding damage to the posterior intima.

Arterial closure. Several vascular complications can be avoided by performing an accurate and careful arterial closure. Precise placement of each stitch through the full thickness of the intima, approximating the intimal margins, is imperative to avoid the development of an intimal flap. Such a flap could lead to thrombus for-

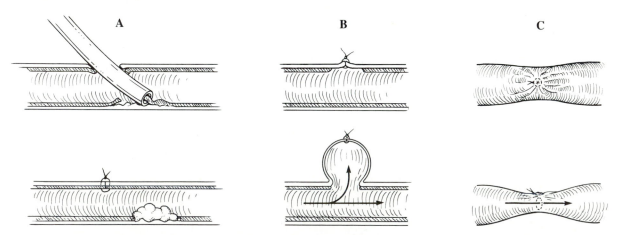

Fig. 3-9. Common technical complications associated with arterial cutdown. **A,** An arterial incision of inadequate size causes the catheter to enter at a sharper angle, resulting in damage to the posterior intima of the vessel with thrombus formation. **B,** Failure to approximate intimal margins by full-thickness suture placement can result in development of an intimal flap, causing a pseudoaneurysm. **C,** Use of a purse string suture to close the arterial incision may cause anteroposterior narrowing of the lumen.

mation or a pseudoaneurysm (Fig. 3-9, *B*). Use of a purse string suture for arterial repair is not recommended because the tension created on the vessel when the suture is tightened may cause the vessel to narrow. This is not always appreciated in the anteroposterior view (particularly if the skin incision is small) but becomes apparent when viewed laterally (Fig. 3-9, *C*). In addition, because the purse string suture does not approximate the intimal margins, an intimal flap is created that may cause thrombus or pseudoaneurysm formation or both. If a longitudinal rather than a transverse arteriotomy is performed, it is still necessary to repair the artery in a transverse fashion to avoid narrowing of the vessel.

Fogarty embolectomy. If poor blood flow is noted from the proximal or distal artery after catheter removal, or if pulsation from the radial artery is weak or absent, the artery should be explored with a Fogarty embolectomy catheter. Some physicians routinely perform a Fogarty artery embolectomy after cutdown, but most do so only if needed. Fogarty embolectomy is performed both proximally and distally in the following manner.

1. Check the patency of the balloon of the Fogarty catheter by filling it with the specified amount of sterile saline (never fill the balloon with air!).

2. Remove the fluid from the balloon.

3. Temporarily release the tension on one of the arterial ties and insert the tip of the Fogarty catheter (usually 3 or 4 Fr) into the artery, gently advancing it past the area of obstruction. *Never force the catheter if resistance is met.*

4. Expand the balloon by filling it with the specified amount of sterile normal saline.

5. Slowly withdraw the balloon, using a forceps to extract any withdrawn clot. If any resistance is met during withdrawal, *do not use force* to withdraw the catheter. Instead, reduce the volume of fluid in the balloon and again attempt to gently pull back the catheter. (Resistance may be encountered in areas of vessel narrowing.)

6. Repeat step 5 until no clots are obtained and vigorous blood flow is apparent.

7. Repair the vessel and close the skin as described in steps 4 to 11 on pp. 79 to 80.

Radial artery cutdown

A surgical cutdown of the radial artery may be required in critical care or emergency settings when percutaneous cannulation fails. Generally, a small catheter-over-needle unit is inserted directly into the exposed radial artery (see p. 69).

Anatomy

The anatomy of the radial artery is described on p. 67.

Equipment

The equipment used in cutdown of the radial artery includes a basic cutdown tray and a 20-gauge Teflon catheter-over-needle unit.

Patient preparation

Begin patient preparation by following the procedure described on pp. 32 to 33; in addition, secure the wrist and hand (palm side up) on an arm board.

Procedure

1. Locate the position and direction of the radial artery.

2. With a #15 scalpel, make a small incision (1.5 to 2 cm) over the radial artery.

3. Follow steps 2 through 5 of the basic cutdown technique on p. 43.

4. Puncture the exposed artery with the 20-gauge catheter-over-needle unit and advance it fully into the lumen of the artery.

5. Remove the needle and make sure the catheter remains fully advanced.

6. Connect the catheter to a pressurized and heparinized IV solution.

7. Remove the proximal and distal ties around the artery and apply slight compression for several minutes.

8. Close the skin around the catheter with two or three 4-0 silk sutures; also place sutures around the catheter hub.

9. Suture the hub of the catheter to the skin.

10. Cleanse the site with sterile water and apply iodophor ointment and a sterile dressing secured with tape.

REFERENCES

1. Hales, S.: Statistical essays: Hemostaticks, vol. 2, ed. 3, London, 1738, W. Innys & R. Manby.
2. Russell, J.A., et al.: Prospective evaluation of radial and femoral artery catheterization sites in critically ill adults, Crit. Care Med. **11:**936-939, 1983.
3. Bedford, R.F., and Wollman, H.: Complications of percutaneous radial artery cannulation in objective prospective study in man, Anesthesiology **38:**228-236, 1973.
4. Kelly, J., Braverman, B., Land, P.C., and Ivankovich, A.D.: Comparison of Allen test, Doppler and finger-pulse transducer to assess patency of ulnar artery, Anesthesiology **59**(supp.):A178, 1983.
5. Jones, R.M., Hill, A.B., Nahrwold, M.L., and Bolles, R.E.: The effect of the method of radial artery cannulation on post cannulation blood flow and thrombus formation, Anesthesiology **55:**76-78, 1981.

6. Davis, F.M.: Methods of radial artery cannulation and subsequent arterial occlusion, Anesthesiology **56:**331, 1982.

7. Shenoy, P.N., Leaman, D.M., and Field, J.M.: Safety of short-term percutaneous arterial cannulation, Anesth. Analg. **58:**256-258, 1979.

8. Soderstrom, C.A., et al.: Superiority of the femoral artery for monitoring: a prospective study, Am. J. Surg. **144:**309-312, 1982.

9. Thomas, F., et al.: The risk of infection related to radial vs. femoral sites for arterial catheterization, Crit. Care Med. **11:**807-811, 1983.

10. Rapoport, S., et al.: Pseudoaneurysm: a complication of faulty technique in femoral arterial puncture, Radiology **154:**529-530, 1985.

11. Pepine, C.J., Von Gunten, C., and Hill, J.A.: Percutaneous brachial catheterization using a modified sheath and new catheter system, Cathet. Cardiovasc. Diagn. **10:**637-642, 1984.

12. Maouad, J., Herbert, J.L., Fernandez, F., and Gay, J.: Percutaneous brachial approach using the femoral artery sheath for left heart catheterization and selective coronary angiography, Cathet. Cardiovasc. Diagn. **11:**539-546, 1985.

13. Campeau, L. Percutaneous brachial catheterization (letter), Cathet. Cardiovasc. Diagn. **11:**443-444, 1985.

14. Fergusson, D.J.G., and Kamada, R.O.: Percutaneous entry of the brachial artery for left heart catheterization using a sheath, Cathet. Cardiovasc. Diagn. **7:**111-114, 1981.

15. Gurman, G.M., and Krierman, S.: Cannulation of big arteries in critically ill patients, Crit. Care Med. **13:**217-220, 1985.

16. Valeix, B., et al.: Selective coronary arteriography by percutaneous transaxillary approach, Cathet. Cardiovasc. Diagn. **10:**403-409, 1984.

17. Abrams, H.L.: Angiography, Boston, 1983, Little, Brown & Co.

18. Eisenberg, R.L., Mani, R.L., and McDonald, E.J. Jr.: The complication rate of catheter angiography by direct puncture through aortofemoral grafts, AJR **126:**814-816, 1976.

19. Smith, D.C.: Catheterization of prosthetic vascular grafts: acceptable technique (editorial), AJR **143:**1117-1118, 1984.

20. Zajko, A.B., et al.: Percutaneous puncture of venous bypass grafts for transluminal angioplasty, AJR **137:**799-801, 1981.

21. Schatzki, S.C.: Catheter angiography through prosthetic vascular grafts using a Teflon sheath, Radiology **148:**565, 1983.

22. Mani, R.L., and Costin, B.S.: Catheter angiography through aortofemoral grafts: prevention of catheter separation during withdrawal, AJR **128:**328-329, 1977.

23. Weinshelbaum, A., and Carson, S.N.: Separation of angiographic catheter during arteriography through vascular graft, AJR **134:**583-584, 1980.

24. Folland, E.D., et al.: Brachial artery catheterization employing a side arm sheath, Cathet. Cardiovasc. Diagn. **10:**55-61, 1984.

25. Shenoy, P.N., Leaman, D.M., and Field, J.M.: Safety of short-term percutaneous arterial cannulation, Anesth. Analg. **58:**256-258, 1979.

26. Bryan-Brown, C.W., et al.: The axillary artery catheter, Heart Lung **12:**492-497, 1983.

27. Brown, M., Gordon, L.H., Brown, O.W., and Brown, E.M.: Intravascular monitoring via the axillary artery, Anesth. Intensive Care **13:**38-40, 1984.

Chapter Four

Hemodynamic monitoring

ELAINE K. DAILY
ARA G. TILKIAN

Invasive hemodynamic monitoring dates from 1758, when Rev. Stephen Hales cannulated the carotid artery of his horse and, with the use of a 12-foot brass rod, measured the height to which the column of blood rose.[1]

The introduction of the auscultatory method for blood pressure measurement by Korotkoff in 1905 offered a technique for simple, rapid determination of systolic and diastolic blood pressure. This noninvasive auscultatory method continues to be the primary method of blood pressure determination.

As early as 1953, Lategola and Rahn[2] from the University of Rochester described catheterization of the pulmonary artery (PA) in animals using a flow-directed, balloon-tip catheter. However, the clinical significance of this finding was not appreciated at the time because the experiment was designed to occlude the PA.

In 1962 Wilson et al.[3] described the value of central venous pressure (CVP) measurements for monitoring optimal blood volume levels, thus popularizing this tool for monitoring the critically ill patient.

For many years the basic "tools" of hemodynamic monitoring consisted of the monitoring of blood pressure via Korotkoff sounds, CVP monitoring, and ECG monitoring. This approach is still favored today for patients who are hemodynamically stable.

The armamentarium of monitoring techniques and capabilities was revolutionized with the development of the Swan-Ganz balloon-tip flotation catheter in the late 1960s. In 1970 Swan et al.[4] published the results of their catheter use in 100 critically ill patients, indicating the usefulness of hemodynamic monitoring in defining pathophysiologic conditions. Since that time technical improvements have resulted in the ability to measure cardiac output, perform atrial or ventricular pacing, and continuously measure the oxygen saturation of mixed venous blood (SvO_2) in the critically ill patient.

However, along with increased usage of these catheters are reports of increased complications, some of them life threatening. Although it is clear that invasive hemodynamic monitoring is helpful in the management of certain clinical disorders, the overall benefits must be carefully weighed against the risks.

Bedside hemodynamic monitoring employs the basic procedures used in the cardiac catheterization laboratory. This chapter includes a discussion of the indications, contraindications, complications, and techniques involved in hemodynamic monitoring. Chapter 1 includes a discussion of available catheters and accessory equipment. Chapters 2 and 3 include detailed descriptions of catheter insertion and removal techniques. Because placement of a catheter in the PA is an extension of central venous pressure catheterization techniques, discussion is limited to PA catheterization. Because of the recent availability and relative paucity of information on continuous SvO_2 monitoring, the principles and techniques of this procedure are discussed in some detail.

INDICATIONS

Hemodynamic monitoring is an invasive method of monitoring that imposes certain risks on the patient. Therefore it should only be used in high-risk, hemodynamically unstable patients who are not responding well to therapy or whose care would be improved by more exact data. Its greatest clinical usefulness lies in its ability to identify the course and the appropriate management of patients with low cardiac output and/or pulmonary congestion.

In general, indications for use of hemodynamic monitoring include complicated myocardial infarction, shock, respiratory failure, intraoperative and postoperative monitoring and management of the high-risk patient, and fluid management of the trauma patient. In many of these instances hemodynamic monitoring not only provides diagnostic or trend data but also allows rapid assessment of the patient's response to therapy, permitting better titration of specific therapies.

CONTRAINDICATIONS

Although there are no absolute contraindications to hemodynamic monitoring, relative contraindications include bleeding disorders (especially severe thrombocytopenia), immunosuppression (or severely compromised host), and terminal disease states. Lack of appropriate equipment and knowledgeable personnel (physicians, nurses, biomedical engineers) should also preclude invasive hemodynamic monitoring.

RISKS

The risks involved in either arterial or PA pressure (PAP) monitoring are those that are associated with the insertion of the catheter and those that occur once the catheters are in position for monitoring. The initial complications that can occur during catheter insertion are frequently related to the specific site of insertion and are discussed in Chapters 2 and 3. A comprehensive review of pulmonary artery catheterization in more than 6000 patients in a 5-year period revealed a low incidence (0.2%) of serious complications associated with PA catheterization.[5]

Complications that occur later during pressure monitoring in the PA are[5,6]:
- Cardiac arrhythmias
- Thrombosis of cannulated vein
- Pulmonary infarction
- Sepsis

Other complications include PA rupture, cardiac tamponate, catheter coiling or knotting, balloon rupture, hemorrhage, endocarditis (rare), and damage of the tricuspid or pulmonic valve.

EQUIPMENT

Hemodynamic monitoring of peripheral arteries, RA, PA, and PA wedge pressures requires the following equipment:
- Catheter of choice (e.g., four or five-lumen thermodilution PA catheter for PA catheterization; 20-gauge Teflon catheter for arterial catheterization)
- Catheter/sheath introducer (venous cannulation)
- Cutdown or percutaneous insertion tray with necessary instruments (see pp. 34 and 43)
- Pressure transducer (disposable or reusable)
- Sterile transducer dome (if reusable transducer is used)
- Electronic monitor and oscilloscope
- Heparinized infusion fluid in a plastic bag
- Pressure tubing
- IV tubing with pediatric drip chamber
- Three-way stopcocks
- Continuous flush device
- Pressurized IV cuff or pump
- Catheter sleeve
- Fluoroscope (optimal)
- Paper recorder (optimal)
- Cardiopulmonary resuscitation equipment

PERSONNEL

The personnel required for this procedure include a physician experienced in PA or arterial catheterization and a nurse to set up hemodynamic monitoring equipment, monitor the patient and the hemodynamic waveforms, and assist.

LOCATION

Hemodynamic monitoring can be initiated in the cardiac catheterization laboratory or in any of the critical care units, operating room, or emergency department.

PATIENT PREPARATION

1. Explain the procedure to the patient and the patient's family, if available.
2. Obtain informed consent.
3. Attach ECG electrodes for continuous monitoring.
4. For specific sites of cannulation see the discussion in Chapters 2 and 3.

EQUIPMENT PREPARATION

Before catheter insertion and hemodynamic monitoring, the catheter and monitoring equipment should be prepared as described below.

Assembly of intravenous tubing, transducer, and monitor

1. Plug the transducer cable into the pressure monitor.
2. Plug the monitor into a grounded electric outlet.
3. Turn the monitor power switch to "on."
4. Add heparin to the medication cutdown port of an IV solution in a collapsible bag (usually 1 to 2 units of heparin/ml of 0.9% saline solution). Label the infusion bag with date, time, and contents.
5. Remove all air from the infusion bag via a 22-gauge needle inserted into the medication port. Withdraw the needle after all air is removed.
6. Insert the spiked end of the IV tubing drip chamber into the outlet port of the infusion bag. (A second IV tubing and drip chamber can be inserted into the medication port of the infusion bag, permitting two monitoring lines from one fluid source.)

7. Open the IV roller clamp and lightly squeeze the drip chamber to fill it approximately 0.5 inch.

8. Close the roller clamp and insert the IV infusion bag into a pressure cuff and hang it on an IV pole.

9. Replace all vented caps on the stopcocks with nonvented ones.

10. Attach the IV tubing to a continuous flush device (if not preassembled).

11. Momentarily open the IV roller clamp and run a few drops of IV solution onto the diaphragm of a sterile transducer (only if a reusable transducer is used).

12. Attach a sterile disposable transducer dome to the head of the reusable transducer, taking care to prevent the entrapment of any air bubbles between the transducer and the membrane of the dome.

13. Attach a stopcock to each arm of the transducer dome (if not preassembled).

14. Attach the female end of the continuous flush device to one of the stopcocks on the transducer dome (Fig. 4-1).

15. Remove one of the dead-ender caps from the remaining stopcock on the transducer dome and open it to air.

16. Open the IV roller clamp and activate the fast-flush device to completely purge the tubing, stopcocks, flush device, and transducer dome of any air (to avoid formation of small air bubbles; this should not be done while the fluid is under pressure). It may be necessary to tap the dome or rotate the transducer to remove all air bubbles from the dome.

17. Close the roller clamp and the air vent stopcock on the dome. Replace the dead-ender cap on the side arm of the stopcock.

18. Attach pressure tubing to the continuous flush device (if not preassembled).

19. Attach a three-way stopcock to the Luer end of the pressure tubing.

20. Open the stopcock at the end of the pressure tubing and activate the fast-flush device to fill the tubing and added stopcock.

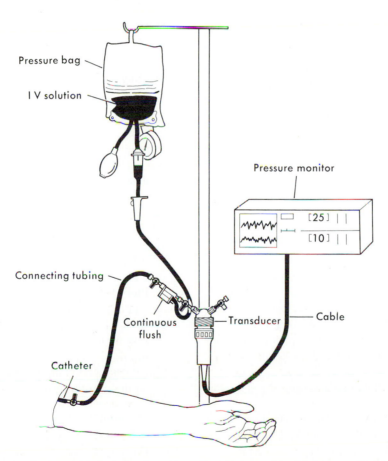

Fig. 4-1. Schematic illustration showing connections between the catheter, continuous flush device, transducer, IV solution, and pressure monitor. (From Daily, E.K., and Schroeder, J.S.: Techniques in bedside hemodynamic monitoring, ed. 3, St. Louis, 1985, The C.V. Mosby Co.)

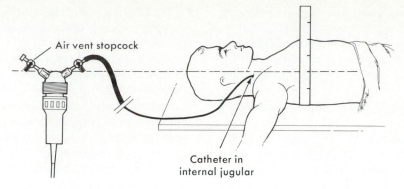

Air vent stopcock

Catheter in
internal jugular

Fig. 4-2. The air-reference port of the stopcock is positioned at the patient's midchest level. (From Daily, E.K., and Schroeder, J.S.: Techniques in bedside hemodynamic monitoring, ed. 3, St. Louis, 1985, The C.V. Mosby Co.)

21. Pressurize the cuff to 300 mm Hg. (Make sure the drip chamber does not fill completely!)

Most transducer manufacturers package a sterile preassembled disposable kit that greatly facilitates transducer set-up and reduces errors in equipment set-up.

Transducer/monitor zero and calibration

Set-up of the transducer and monitor should be performed 15 to 20 minutes in advance to allow a sufficient warm-up period for stabilization.

All transducers are affected by temperature changes, resulting in some drift of the zero baseline. Zero drift may also occur within the monitor itself. For these reasons, rezeroing should be performed before infrequent or critical measurement readings, if there is a discrepancy between readings, whenever there is a change in transducer level or a large environmental temperature shift, or at least every 4 hours. This is true for both disposable and reusable transducers.[7]

1. Position the *air-reference stopcock* at the patient's midchest level (Fig. 4-2) or at the phlebostatic axis. The transducer may be placed on an IV pole, on an arm board next to the patient, or directly on the patient's arm or chest. The transducer itself does not need to be placed precisely at the midchest or zero reference level. During the zeroing process, any fluid pressure on the transducer caused by the difference in height is cancelled out.

2. Remove the dead-ender cap and open the side arm of the air-reference stopcock.

3. Select the appropriate scale on the monitor to correspond to the anticipated pressure range.

4. Turn or press the zero control knob on the monitor to obtain a zero reading.

5. Adjust the tracing on the oscilloscope (or paper write-out) to the correct zero position.

6. Press and hold the calibration knob on the monitor to read the precalibrated value (e.g., 40, 100, or 200 mm Hg). Adjust the calibration knob, if necessary, to obtain the correct reading.

7. While depressing the calibration knob, adjust the tracing on the oscilloscope (or paper write-out) to the appropriate scale position.

8. Close the air reference stopcock on the transducer dome and replace the dead-ender cap.

Transducer calibration

To be assured of obtaining accurate pressure measurements, it is necessary to check the calibration of the transducer in addition to the monitor by applying a known pressure (either mercury or water) to the transducer and correlating it with the pressure read-out. Transducer calibration should be performed before patient use and anytime suspicion exists regarding the accuracy of the transducer. To do this, use a mercury manometer as follows (Fig. 4-3):

1. Attach a disposable dome to the transducer. (Do not use the dome that is or will be attached to the patient.)

2. Press the zero control knob on the monitor to obtain a zero reading.

3. Attach a mercury manometer to one of the Luer-Lok fittings of the transducer dome, using a short plastic tubing.

4. Attach a hand bulb to the second Luer-Lok fitting on the transducer dome.

5. Squeeze the hand bulb to 200 mm Hg and hold it. The digital readout should display 200 mm Hg.

6. Release the hand bulb and check for a return of the digital readout to zero.

7. Repeat step 5 at lower pressure levels (20, 50, and 100 mm Hg).

8. Remove the calibrating equipment and dome and

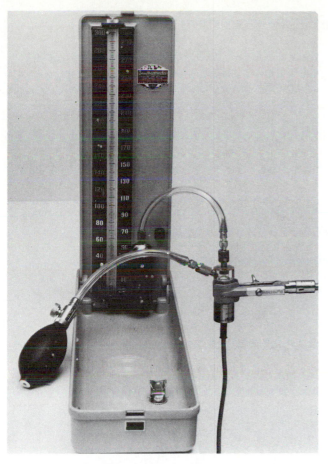

Fig. 4-3. The calibration of the transducer is checked against a known pressure using a mercury manometer. (From Daily, E.K., and Schroeder, J.S.: Techniques in bedside hemodynamic monitoring, ed. 3, St. Louis, 1985, The C.V. Mosby Co.)

attach the patient's dome or a new sterile dome to the transducer.

Pulmonary artery catheter preparation

All preparation for PA catheterization should be performed under sterile conditions.

1. Test the integrity of the balloon by inflating it with the designated volume of air using a 3 cc plastic syringe. The catheter tip should be immersed in water to detect any leakage. Faulty catheters, the result of either a ruptured balloon or an incompetent inflation lumen, have been found in up to 3% of catheters before insertion.[8]

2. If a thermodilution catheter is being used, test the integrity of the thermistor wires by connecting the cardiac output cable to the thermistor hub of the catheter and depressing the "SELF-TEST" button on the cardiac output computer. The cardiac output computer will flash "FAULTY CATHETER" if there is some fault with the catheter. A new catheter should then be used.

3. Connect the catheter hub(s) to the IV tubing while an assistant activates the fast-flush device; completely fill the catheter with IV fluid.

4. Connect the distal lumen of the catheter to a continuous flush and a transducer system.

5. Insert the catheter through a sterile catheter sleeve.

PROCEDURE
Pulmonary artery catheter insertion

The procedure for PA catheter insertion is described below; arterial catheter insertion is described in Chapter 3.

1. Perform a percutaneous venous catheterization or a vein cutdown under sterile conditions as described in Chapter 2.

2. Insert the catheter into the vein and gently advance the catheter.

3. If an internal jugular, subclavian, or antecubital approach is used, partially inflate the balloon of the PA catheter on reaching the superior vena cava. The pressure tracing in this position will begin to show respiratory variations. To confirm catheter location within the thoracic cavity, have the patient cough. If the catheter is in the thoracic cavity, a large pressure change will be recorded during the cough. This assures intrathoracic location when the catheter is advanced without fluoroscopy.

4. On reaching the right atrium, the balloon can be inflated with 0.8 to 1.0 cc of air. The hemodynamic waveform on the monitor will be characteristic of an atrial pressure with an *a* wave (if the patient is not in atrial fibrillation), a *v* wave, and perhaps a *c* wave (Fig. 4-4). Right atrial pressure (RAP) should be recorded on a paper write-out at this time.

5. Gently advance the catheter into the right ventricle while closely monitoring the ECG for signs of ventricular irritability. The right ventricular pressure waveform should be seen on the monitor (Fig. 4-5). Avoid entering the right ventricle with the balloon deflated, as this will cause frequent PVCs.

6. Continue advancing the catheter until a PAP waveform appears on the monitor (Fig. 4-6). Record this pressure. If a PAP waveform does not appear after advancing the catheter approximately 15 cm, it is probably coiling in the right ventricle. Slowly withdraw the catheter to the right atrium, as indicated by the RAP, and readvance it no more than 15 cm. This procedure prevents catheter knotting. Difficulty advancing the catheter out to the PA may occur in patients with atrial fibrillation, dilated right ventricle, or low cardiac output.

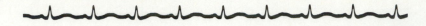

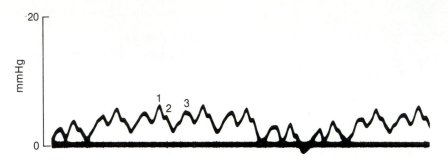

Fig. 4-4. Normal right atrial pressure waveform with an *a* wave *(1)*, *c* wave *(2)*, and *v* wave *(3)*.

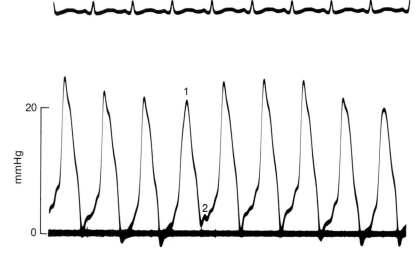

Fig. 4-5. Normal right ventricular pressure waveform showing *(1)* systole and *(2)* diastole.

7. With the balloon still inflated, advance the catheter further until the PA waveform changes to a PA wedge waveform (Fig. 4-7). At this point the balloon has obstructed a medium-size pulmonary artery and the catheter cannot be advanced further.

8. Remove the inflating syringe and allow the balloon to *passively* deflate. The waveform should change to a PA waveform at this time.

9. To obtain a PAWP, reinflate the balloon while continuously observing the PAP waveform. Discontinue inflation of the balloon as soon as a PA wedge waveform appears. This procedure prevents PA rupture from overinflation of the balloon. If necessary, withdraw the catheter so that the PA wedge waveform is obtained only when the balloon is inflated with 0.8 to 1.5 cc of air. A PA wedge waveform with inflation of less than 0.8 cc of air indicates that the catheter tip is located too far distally, as does spontaneous recording of PAWP with the balloon deflated.

10. Verify the relationship between the PA end-diastolic pressure (PAEDP) and the PAWP (see p. 93).

11. With fluoroscopy or a chest radiograph, determine the exact location of the catheter tip and the presence of excessive catheter loops within the heart. Ex-

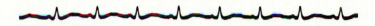

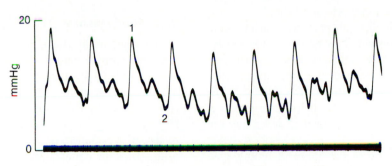

Fig. 4-6. Normal PAP waveform showing systole *(1)* and diastole *(2)*.

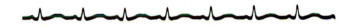

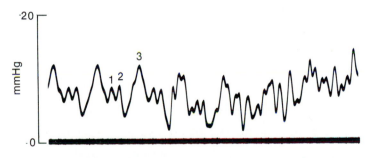

Fig. 4-7. Normal PAWP waveform showing *a* wave *(1)*, *c* wave *(2)*, and *v* wave *(3)*.

cessive catheter lengths should be withdrawn to reduce the hazard of forward migration or ventricular irritability.

12. Aspirate and flush the proximal lumen of the catheter; connect it to a continuous flush system and a transducer if desired.

13. Secure the sterile catheter sleeve to the hub of the sheath.

14. Suture the sheath, catheter, and sleeve to the skin near the insertion site.

15. Apply iodophor ointment and a sterile dressing secured with tape.

Pressure monitoring

Monitoring of hemodynamic pressures provides valuable information only when obtained in a technically accurate manner. This includes correct positioning of the air-reference point at the midchest or phlebostatic axis (fourth intercostal space at the midaxillary plane) and measurement of all hemodynamic pressures at end-expiration when pleural pressure is close to the reference atmospheric pressure.[9] This requires the use of a paper write-out, or calibrated oscilloscope, ideally one with a "freeze-sweep" mechanism for correct identification of end-expiration.[10,11] Because the digital readout provides an average of any number of previous pressures, it is not accurate for obtaining a pressure recording at the end-expiratory phase of the patient's respiratory cycle. Recently, monitoring equipment has become available that utilizes an algorithm to identify end-expiratory pressure using constant weight averaging of systemic arterial pressure beats and variable weight filtering of pulmonary arterial pressure beats.[12]

To optimize the fidelity of pressure transmission through a fluid-filled system, it is necessary to employ rigid, short-length pressure tubing, minimize the length of tubing and number of stopcocks used, and meticulously remove all air bubbles from the system.[14,15] If the natural frequency of the system is low, the pressure signal can be attenuated or accentuated, depending on the frequency level.

The frequency response of the entire plumbing system can be easily evaluated at the bedside with the use of a continuous flush device. While recording on graph paper, activate the fast-flush device and hold it open for approximately 1 second, then sharply release it. The waveform produced should look similar to that in Fig. 4-8 and will show the system's response to a rapid

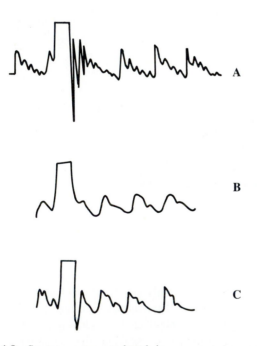

Fig. 4-8. Square waves produced in response to a rapid change in pressure produced by activating the fast flush device. **A,** Numerous oscillations before return to baseline indicating an underdamped system. **B,** A damped response indicating an overdamped system. **C,** A normal response with an adequately damped system. Following release of pressure the system quickly returns to baseline.

change in pressure. If the square wave has a damped appearance (Fig. 4-8, *B*), or if numerous oscillations are noted before it returns to baseline (Fig. 4-8, *A*), corrective steps should be taken.

Table 4-1 lists problems commonly encountered in hemodynamic monitoring and preventive and remedial measures.

Right atrial pressure

The right atrial (RA) pressure waveform normally has three positive waves, an *a* wave, a *c* wave, and a *v* wave, followed by the *x, x', and y* descents, respectively. Because the *a* and *v* waves in this low-pressure chamber are usually about the same (within 1 to 2 mm Hg), a mean pressure is usually recorded. The *a* wave is absent in patients with atrial fibrillation and may be exaggerated in patients with atrioventricular dissociation.

Normal RAP

Mean pressure: 2 to 6 mm Hg

Right ventricular pressure

As the catheter crosses the tricuspid valve into the right ventricle (RV) during its passage to the PA, the pressure will rise abruptly. The RV waveform consists of systolic and diastolic phases. In the absence of outflow obstruction, the peak systolic pressure is normally the same as the PA systolic pressure, whereas the diastolic pressure falls to zero ($\pm$ 5 mm Hg).

Normal RV pressures

Systolic pressure:	20 to 30 mm Hg
Diastolic pressure:	0 to 5 mm Hg
End-diastolic pressure:	2 to 6 mm Hg

Because of the risks of ventricular irritability, the RV pressure is usually not monitored for any length of time. The appearance of an RV waveform after catheter placement in the PA requires prompt manipulation of the catheter back out to the PA (if sterility has been maintained) or withdrawal back into the right atrium if sterility has not been maintained. The best procedure is to inflate the balloon of the catheter, which reduces the risk of catheter-induced PVCs and permits it to float out to the PA.

Pulmonary artery pressure

The PA waveform is the right-sided circulation's arterial pressure waveform and is comparable to the arterial waveform, consisting of systole, the dicrotic notch, and diastole. Pressure readings obtained are usually the peak systolic, end-diastolic, and mean pressures.

Normal PAP

Systolic: 20 to 30 mm Hg
End-diastolic: 8 to 12 mm Hg
Mean: 10 to 20 mm Hg

Pulmonary arterial wedge pressure

The PAWP is obtained during balloon inflation, which occludes a PA branch and interrupts forward blood flow. Thus the tip of the catheter only measures that pressure distal to it, generated retrograde by the left atrium (LA). Therefore the PAWP reflects LA pressure and is morphologically identical to the RA pressure waveform, consisting of an *a* wave, a *v* wave, and occasionally a *c* wave. The *a* wave is absent in patients with atrial fibrillation. The *a* and the *v* waves are normally within 1 to 3 mm Hg of each other, and when

Table 4-1. Trouble-shooting intravascular catheters

Problem	Possible cause	Prevention	Remedy
Overdamped waveform	Clot at catheter tip	Use continuous flush device Use heparinized IV solution Use heparinized catheters Hand-flush occasionally	Aspirate, then flush catheter with heparin solution (*not* in PA wedge position) Remove catheter if unable to clear
	Air bubble(s)	Care and attention to remove all air bubbles during equipment setup, particularly in the pressure transducer Use macrodrip vs. pedidrip	Flush system carefully (*not* to patient)
	Leak at some connecting point	Use Luer-Lok connectors and stopcocks Tighten securely	Check all connections and tighten if necessary
	Kink in catheter	Loosely coil excess catheter Immobilize arm, if arm insertion Exercise caution during patient movement	Try to straighten kink Replace catheter if necessary
	Use of soft compliant tubing	Use stiff connecting tubing	Replace soft tubing with stiff connecting tubing
"Noisy" waveform (with fling)	Use of lengthy tubing	Use no more than 2 or 3 ft of connecting tubing (preferably 18 inches or less) Use stiff connecting tubing	Decrease tubing length. Use stiff connecting tubing
	Catheter tip near valve with turbulent blood flow	Position catheter distal to valve	Check catheter position by radiograph and reposition if necessary Use commercial damping device
	Very rapid heart rate		Slow heart rate, if possible
Abnormally low or high pressures	Improper air-reference level	Place air-reference at midchest level	Remeasure phlebostatic axis or midchest and reset air reference level accordingly
	Incorrect zero or calibration	Zero and calibrate monitor correctly	Recheck zero and calibration of monitor
	Faulty transducer	Calibrate transducer with known pressure; replace if necessary	Recheck transducer calibration with mercury or water manometer

Continued.

Table 4-1. Trouble-shooting intravascular catheters—cont'd

Problem	Possible cause	Prevention	Remedy
"Over-wedged" or damped, elevated PAWP	Overinflation of the balloon	Slowly inflate balloon while closely observing waveform; inflate *only* enough to obtain PAWP; use a 3 ml plastic syringe with holes punctured at 1.5 ml to avoid injecting >1.5 cc air	Deflate balloon; reinflate slowly with only enough air to obtain a PA wedge waveform
	Eccentric inflation of the balloon	Check balloon inflation before insertion Do not inflate 7 Fr catheter with more than 1.0 to 1.5 cc air	Deflate balloon· reposition catheter and slowly reinflate
	Location of catheter tip in zone I or II of the lung	Position catheter in zone III below the left atrium Maintain adequate LA pressure through volume administration Reduce airway pressure	Obtain lateral chest film to confirm catheter tip location; if in zone I or II, reposition in zone III, administer volume, or reduce airway pressure
PAWP with balloon deflated	Forward migration of catheter tip 2° to excessive looping in RV or RA; inadequate suturing of catheter at insertion site; or excessive arm movement of catheter in antecubital vein	Advance catheter carefully avoiding excessive catheter insertion Check catheter position on radiograph Suture catheter securely at insertion site Insert catheter in vein proximal to shoulder	Slowly withdraw catheter until PA waveform appears Obtain chest radiograph to determine excessive looping of catheter in RV or RA
PA balloon rupture	Overinflation of the balloon	Inflate slowly with only enough air to obtain PAWP	Remove syringe and apply tape over stopcock to prevent further air injection
	Frequent balloon inflation	Monitor PAEDP as reflection of PAWP and LVEDP	Monitor PAEDP
	Active balloon deflation by withdrawing air into syringe	Allow balloon to deflate passively through stopcock Remove syringe after inflation	
Drastic change in pressure	Actual change in hemodynamic state		Carefully assess patient
	Air-reference or transducer level changed	Maintain air-reference at midchest level; rezero before each reading	Reposition air-reference at midchest level; rezero
	Air or blood in transducer dome	Carefully remove all air bubbles during initial set-up; maintain adequate pressure (300 mm Hg) in infusion bag	Carefully flush system to remove all air or blood (not into patient)
	Change in temperature of environment or IV solution	Use room temperature flush solution	Rezero and calibrate

Table 4-1. Trouble-shooting intravascular catheters—cont'd

Problem	Possible cause	Prevention	Remedy
	Broken transducer cable	Carefully handle transducer and cable	Check transducer with known pressure of mercury or water; replace if faulty
No pressure	Power off	Check power	Turn power on
	Stopcock open to air	Always turn stopcock off to air after zeroing	Turn stopcock off to air, open to catheter/transducer
	Transducer dome loose	Carefully tighten dome during set-up and check periodically	Tighten transducer dome
	Tubing connections loose	Carefully tighten all connections during set-up and check periodically	Tighten all connections
	Loose cable connections between transducer/monitor/oscilloscope	Carefully and firmly insert all connecting jacks during initial set-up	Check all connecting jacks
	Transducer attached to wrong module or monitor	Careful and accurate transducer and monitor set-up	Attach transducer to appropriate module
	Gain setting too low	Correctly adjust gain setting of oscilloscope during initial monitor calibration	Reset gain on the oscilloscope
	Incorrect scale selection	Select appropriate scale to correspond to the monitored pressure	Select appropriate scale
	Faulty transducer	Check transducer with known pressure of mercury or water before patient use	Check transducer with known pressure of mercury or water; if faulty, replace

this is the case, a mean of the PAWP is recorded.

Normal PAWP

Mean pressure: 4 to 12 mm Hg

In patients with normal heart rate and pulmonary vascular resistance, the PAEDP is usually within 1 to 3 mm Hg of the PAWP. If such a close relationship exists, it is prudent to monitor the PAEDP rather than routinely measuring the PAWP. This reduces the risk involved in recording the PAWP. However, in certain clinical conditions (primary pulmonary hypertension, pulmonary embolism, pulmonary disease, or severe hypoxia) the difference between the PAEDP and PAWP is large and mandates measuring the PAWP as a reflection of LVEDP. Rapid heart rates (>125 bpm) can also produce a PAEDP/PAW gradient, necessitating measurement of the PAWP.

Arterial pressure

Intra-arterial pressure is most commonly monitored from the radial artery, although the femoral artery is being used with increasing frequency. As the pressure pulse travels peripherally, the wave is reflected and summated. The peak pressure thus becomes delayed and increased in amplitude.[16] Therefore the more distal the catheter is from the aorta, the higher the recorded systolic pressure (by as much as 15 to 20 mm Hg), and the lower the diastolic pressure; however, the mean pressure remains the same. Despite artifactual alterations in the arterial pressure waveform (caused by damping, overshoot, or rapid heart rates), the mean arterial pressure remains reliable.[17] Like the PAP, the arterial waveform consists of systole, dicrotic notch, and diastole (Fig. 4-9).

Normal arterial pressure

Peak systolic pressure: 100 to 140 mm Hg
End-diastolic pressure: 60 to 80 mm Hg
Mean arterial pressure: 70 to 90 mm Hg

Blood sampling

Blood samples may be obtained from the PA for

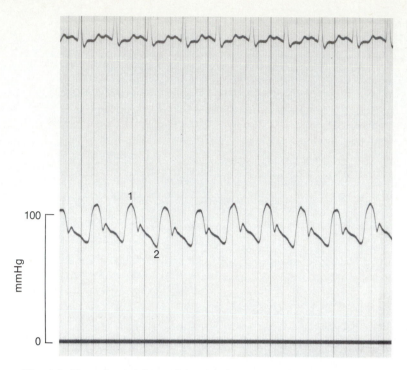

Fig. 4-9. Normal arterial waveform showing systole *(1)* and diastole *(2)*.

measurement of central venous oxygen saturation as well as other routine laboratory analyses. However, to increase the longevity of the catheter and reduce the risks of clotting or infection, blood should be withdrawn from the catheter for blood gas analysis only. If there is any suspicion of the existence of a left-to-right shunt, simultaneous blood samples should be withdrawn from the PA and RA to check for an oxygen step-up.

Before obtaining blood samples, it is necessary to completely rid the line of the IV fluid in the manner described below.

1. Withdraw and discard 5 ml of blood from the PA catheter, or 1 to 2 ml of blood from the peripheral artery catheter. (This is assuming that the sample is withdrawn directly from the stopcock at the hub of the catheter and not through extension tubing.)

2. To avoid hemolysis, slowly withdraw the blood sample into a second syringe. Immediately disconnect the syringe, expel any air, and cap it. (If the sample is for blood gas analysis, heparinize the syringe before sampling and after capping immediately place it in a bed of ice to reduce oxygen metabolism.)

3. Activate the fast-flush device to remove all traces of blood from the withdrawal port of the stopcock.

4. Replace a sterile dead-ender cap over the side-port of the stopcock.

5. Turn the stopcock to resume IV flow to the catheter and activate the fast-flush to flush the catheter.

Cardiac output determination

The thermodilution method for cardiac output measurement was first described by Fegler in 1954.[18] This adaptation of the indicator-dilution principle utilizes a known temperature as the indicator. The change in PA blood temperature induced by the indicator is recorded by a thermistor near the tip of the PA catheter. The change in temperature over time is inversely proportional to blood flow. A cardiac output computer determines the area beneath the temperature/time curve and applies appropriate constants to determine flow according to the Stewart-Hamilton indicator-dilution equation. The thermodilution determination correlates closely with both the Fick and dye dilution methods of determining cardiac output, except in the presence of intracardiac shunts or tricuspid regurgitation. Studies have demonstrated that both room temperature and ice temperature cardiac output measurements correlate closely with each other and with the Fick method of cardiac output measurement.[19-21]

Room temperature technique

Equipment
- Thermodilution catheter
- Sterile IV solution (saline or 5% dextrose in water) in a collapsible bag
- IV tubing
- 10 ml syringe
- Temperature probe
- Cardiac output computer

Preparation. Specific instructions given in this section relate to the American Edwards cardiac output computer model 540A. Follow specific manufacturer's directions for use of another cardiac output computer.

1. Insert the spiked end of the IV tubing into the solution bag and hang it from an IV pole.

2. Run some of the IV solution into a 10 ml test tube and tape the tube securely to the outside of the solution bag. (*Not* necessary if an in-line thermistor [the preferred method] is used.)

3. If an in-line thermistor is not used, place the temperature probe inside the filled test tube and tape securely. (Various other methods may be used to provide a way for the temperature probe to continuously monitor the temperature of the injectate. The important point is that it be *in* identical fluid of the same temperature.)

4. Connect the cable end of the temperature probe to the cardiac output computer connector cable labeled "injectate/needle probe." (This is usually done in the initial set-up of the computer and kept connected thereafter.)

5. Attach the IV tubing to a three-way stopcock at the hub of the proximal lumen of the catheter.

6. Attach a 10 ml syringe to the side port of the stopcock at the hub of the proximal lumen.

7. Attach the female end of the cardiac output computer connecting cable to the thermistor connector hub of the catheter.

8. Plug the cardiac output computer into a grounded outlet and depress the "ON/OFF" switch to turn on the computer. A "RDY" (ready) signal should be displayed after approximately 2 seconds.

9. Once each day perform the self-test: Depress the "SELF-TEST" button on the cardiac output computer. When the display shows "RDY," press the "START" button on the computer. The display will show a "0.00" reading, and then an "OK" within 15 seconds. If not, the cardiac output computer is not within calibration and requires manufacture maintenance. This self-test need only be performed once each day, and is not necessary before each set of cardiac output measurements.

10. Push the "INJECT TEMP" button on the cardiac output computer to obtain the temperature of the injectate solution. This display should be between 19° and 25° C.

11. Push the "BLOOD TEMP" button on the cardiac output computer to obtain the patient's core blood temperature. This display should be between 27° and 43° C.*

12. Enter the correct computation constant by turning the thumb wheel switches on the side panel of the cardiac output computer. The correct computation constant is included in the package insert of each catheter. Most

---

*For accurate cardiac output measurements, it is essential that the difference between the injectate temperature and the blood temperature be at least 12° C. In some instances (e.g., hypothermia), this may necessitate the use of iced injectate.

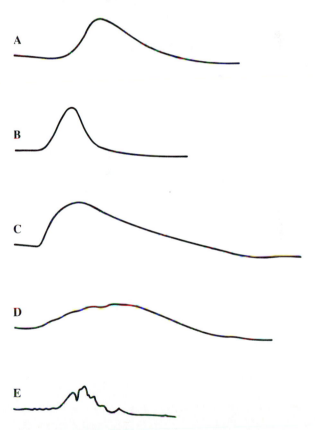

Fig. 4-10. Schematic representation of various thermodilution cardiac output curves. **A,** Normal cardiac output curve showing smooth upstroke. **B,** Small area beneath the curve as seen in patients with high cardiac outputs. **C,** Large area beneath the curve as seen in patients with low cardiac outputs. **D,** Uneven injection indicated by uneven upstroke on curve. **E,** Artifact in both upstroke and decline of curve resulting in erroneous cardiac output measurement.

Table 4-2. Cardiac output trouble-shooting

Problem	Cause(s)	Prevention	Remedy
Cardiac output (CO) reading higher than expected	Inaccurate injectate volume caused by air bubbles or loss of injectate	Carefully check for bubbles and expel, if any	Check for *exact* volume of injectate before injection
	Wrong computation constant (CC)	Check appropriate CC on catheter insert and set correctly on computer	For cardiac outputs already done: Correct CO = Wrong CO × Correct CC ÷ Wrong CC Enter correct CC
	Warming of iced injectate in syringe before injection	If syringe method is used, handle syringe briefly and hold only plunger and syringe flanges during injection	Perform outputs rapidly with minimal handling of syringe Use CO-SET with in-line temperature probe
	Migration of catheter tip toward PA wedge	Ascertain catheter tip position with radiograph Closely monitor PA pressure	Withdraw catheter few centimeters
	Thermistor against wall of artery		Withdraw catheter few centimeters
	Uneven injection	Use 2 hands to deliver fast, even bolus Use automatic injector.	Use automatic injector Analyze curve on strip-chart recorder
	Right-to-left shunt	None	Use another method of cardiac output determination (such as Fick)
	Low stroke volume with long lag time before onset of curve	None	Press "START" button *after* complete injection of indicator
Cardiac output reading lower than expected	Inaccurate injectate volume (more than indicated)	Use syringe of size that corresponds to injectate volume Exercise care in filling syringe	Check for *exact* volume of injectate before injection
	Wrong computation constant (CC)	Check appropriate CC on catheter insert and set correctly on computer	For cardiac outputs already done: Correct CO = Wrong CO × Correct CC ÷ Wrong CC Enter correct CC
	Iced injections spaced <1 min apart	Wait approximately 1 min between injections	Wait approximately 1 min between injections
	Catheter kinked or partially obstructed by clot	Careful protection of catheter during patient movement Occasional aspiration and manual flushing	Try to straighten catheter Aspirate and gently flush catheter Remove catheter if necessary

Table 4-2. Cardiac output trouble-shooting—cont'd

Problem	Cause(s)	Prevention	Remedy
Scattered CO readings (poor reproducibility)	Cardiac arrhythmias (ventricular ectopic beats, atrial fibrillation, etc.)	None	Try to inject during quiet period (i.e., without ventricular ectopic beats) Increase number of determinations (e.g., 5 or 6) and average readings
	Tricuspid regurgitation	None	Use another method of CO determination (e.g., Fick)
	Wide swings in intrapleural pressure (spontaneous respiration or mechanical ventilation)	Inject at same point in respiratory cycle Increase number of determinations (e.g., 5 or 6) and average readings Use iced injectate	Inject at same point in respiratory cycle Increase number of determinations (e.g., 5 or 6) and average readings Use iced injectate
	Electromagnetic interference	Isolate computer from other electromagnetic sources	Isolate computer from other electromagnetic sources Change power source (AC to battery or vice-versa) Wipe CO computer with damp cloth
	Migration of catheter tip toward PAW or thermistor against artery wall	Ascertain catheter tip location with radiograph Closely monitor PAP	Withdraw catheter several centimeters to position in main PA
	Catheter looped in RV	Advance catheter carefully, avoiding excessive catheter insertion Confirm catheter position with radiograph	Withdraw and reposition catheter

institutions tape one of these inserts to the top of the cardiac output computer. If the wrong computation constant is used, the data may still be saved (Table 4-2).

Procedure

1. Close the stopcock to the proximal lumen and carefully fill the syringe with *exactly* 10 ml from the IV solution bag. (Slow-filling of the syringe minimizes the occurrence of any air bubbles, which must be purged before injection.)

2. Push the "CARDIAC OUTPUT" button "2" on the front of the cardiac output computer. Wait for the "RDY" signal to appear on the left side of the display.

3. Start the strip-chart recorder.

4. Check the pressure from the distal lumen of the catheter to verify a good PA waveform.

5. Turn the stopcock closed to the IV solution and open from the syringe to the proximal lumen of the catheter.

6. Press the "START" button on the front of the cardiac output computer (or depress the auxilliary foot pedal) and immediately inject the contents of the syringe within 4 seconds. The injection must be rapid and even. The cardiac output should be displayed in approximately 10 to 30 seconds. Check the paper write-out from the strip-chart recorder to verify a fast, even injection by the presence of a smooth and rapid upstroke of the thermodilution curve (Fig. 4-10).

7. Repeat steps 1 through 6 for repeated cardiac output measurements.

At least three cardiac output determinations should be performed to obtain an average reading. If these readings vary significantly, up to five or six determinations may be necessary to obtain a more accurate mean value. Improved reproducibility may be obtained by always injecting at the same point in the patient's respiratory cycle.[19]

Iced injectate technique

Iced injectate can be injected from prefilled syringes placed in an ice bath or preferably, from a closed system utilizing a prechilled bag of IV solution whose tubing is coiled inside an ice bath (Fig. 4-11). With this technique the temperature probe is attached to a special flow-through housing component that is placed between the syringe and the stopcock at the proximal lumen. This system offers the advantage of being a closed system utilizing only one syringe, thereby reducing the risks of contamination with multiple entries.

The same steps for room temperature technique are followed except that the injectate temperature display will be between 0° and 4° C and the computation constant will be different as indicated on the catheter insert.

Preparation of iced injectate requires a longer period of time for complete cooling and stabilizing of the injectate temperature (from 5 to 45 minutes if the injectate solution has not been prechilled).

Table 4-2 lists some of the problems encountered in cardiac output measurement as well as possible causes and remedies.

From the above-measured parameters, other important hemodynamic parameters can be derived. Appendix G lists formulas used to calculate various hemodynamic parameters useful in the management of critically ill patients.

OXYGEN TRANSPORT, TISSUE DEMANDS, AND ADEQUACY OF CARDIAC FUNCTION

Although continuous monitoring of hemodynamic parameters provides useful information regarding preload, afterload, cardiac output, and heart rate, the adequacy of cardiac function is better evaluated by assessment of oxygen transport in relation to the oxygen demands of the body (i.e., the adequacy of tissue oxygenation). The following concepts are fundamental to an understanding of this relationship.

Oxygen transport

The amount of oxygen that is delivered to the tissues is determined by the flow rate (cardiac output), the oxygen saturation of arterial blood (SaO_2), and the hemoglobin concentration of blood.

Oxygen transport = Cardiac output
  × Arterial oxygen saturation
    × Hemoglobin (gm/dl) × 1.34

Oxygen saturation of blood

Oxygen, taken up in the lungs, combines chemically and reversibly with the hemoglobin in the blood (oxy-

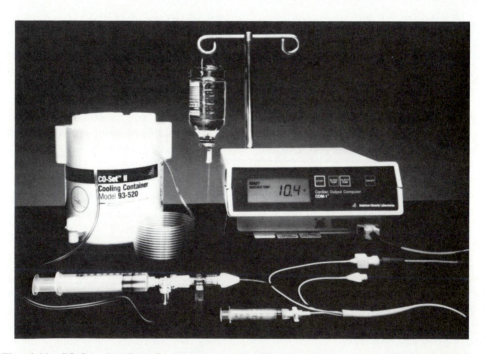

Fig. 4-11. CO-Set closed cardiac output system with connections to the catheter and cardiac output computer. (Copyright 1985, American Edwards Laboratories, American Hospital Supply Corporation. Reprinted with permission.)

hemoglobin). Approximately 1.34 cc of oxygen can combine with every gram of saturated hemoglobin. Although a small amount of oxygen (2% or less) also dissolves in the plasma of blood, its contribution is minimal and for trend monitoring is usually ignored. (Major exceptions to this include severe anemia and carbon monoxide poisoning.) The percentage of total available oxyhemoglobin is referred to as the oxygen saturation of blood. Normally, arterial blood is fully saturated, with an oxygen saturation of 95% to 99%. Venous blood is normally 65% to 75% saturated with oxygen.

Oxygen content of blood (CaO₂ or CvO₂)

The actual amount of oxygen that combines with hemoglobin to form oxyhemoglobin is a product of the total oxygen-carrying capacity (grams hemoglobin × 1.34 ml oxygen/gm hemoglobin) and the percent of hemoglobin that is saturated with oxygen (S_{O_2}). This is referred to as the oxygen content of 100 ml of blood (vol%) and can be calculated as follows:

$$\text{Oxygen content (vol\%)} = \text{Hemoglobin (gm/dl)} \times 1.34 \text{ ml/gm} \times S_{O_2} (\%)$$

The oxygen content of fully saturated arterial blood (Ca_{O_2}) in a patient with a 15 gm hemoglobin is:

$$15 \text{ gm/dl} \times 1.34 \text{ ml/gm} \times 0.97 = 19.5 \text{ ml/100 ml (vol\%)}$$

The oxygen content of mixed venous blood (PA sample) (Cv_{O_2}) would be:

$$15 \text{ gm/dl} \times 1.34 \text{ ml/gm} \times 0.75 = 15.07 \text{ ml/100 ml (vol\%)}$$

The normal value of Ca_{O_2} is 19 to 20 vol%; the normal value of Cv_{O_2} is 12 to 15 vol%.

Thus oxygen transport can be more simply calculated as the product of cardiac output and arterial oxygen content (vol%):

$$\text{Oxygen transport (ml/minute)} = \text{Cardiac output (L/minute)} \times \text{Arterial oxygen content (vol\%)} \times 10$$

For example, the oxygen delivery or transport in a patient with a cardiac output of 5 L/minute and an arterial oxygen content of 20 vol% would be:

$$5 \text{ L/minute} \times 20 \text{ ml/100 ml} \times 10 = 1000 \text{ ml/minute}$$

This represents a normal quantity of oxygen delivered to the tissues and is a commonly used index of the performance of the cardiopulmonary transport system. However, it does *not* indicate the adequacy of oxygen delivery in relation to tissue oxygen demands. Although low oxygen transport values are usually associated with tissue hypoxia, normal or high values do not assure that there is adequate oxygen delivery.[22]

Oxyhemoglobin dissociation curve

The oxygen saturation (%) and partial pressure of oxygen (p_{O_2}) are related via the oxyhemoglobin dissociation curve (Fig. 4-12). The p_{O_2} plays a major role in determining the affinity of hemoglobin for oxygen (association) and the ability of oxygen to be released from hemoglobin to the tissues (dissociation). Changes in oxygen affinity occur with right or left shifts of the oxy-

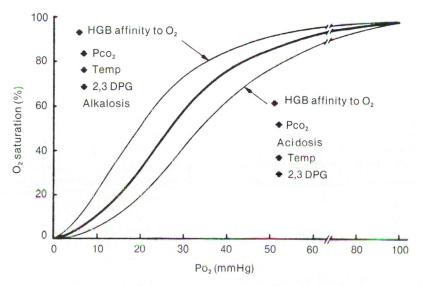

Fig. 4-12. Normal oxyhemoglobin dissociation curve showing the relationship between saturation and P_{O_2}.

Table 4-3. Various causes of alterations in SvO_2

	SvO_2 Reading	Physiologic alteration	Clinical causes
(High)	80%-95%	↓ O_2 Consumption	Hypothermia Anesthesia Induced muscular paralysis Sepsis
		↑ O_2 Delivery Mechanical interference	Hyperoxia Catheter wedged Left-to-right shunt
(Normal)	60%-80%	O_2 Supply = O_2 Demand	Adequate perfusion
(Low)	<60%	↑ O_2 Consumption	Shivering Pain Seizures Activity/exercise Hyperthermia Anxiety
		↓ O_2 Delivery	Hypoperfusion (↓ cardiac output) Anemia Hypoxemia

hemoglobin dissociation curve secondary to changes in temperature, pH, carbon dioxide, 2,3-DPG, and carbon monoxide. As can be seen in Fig. 4-12, on the flat ("arterial") part of the curve, at normal pO_2 levels (> 90 mm Hg), changes in pO_2 result in very small changes in percent saturation. The lower portion of the curve represents release of oxygen to the tissues. On this steep ("venous") side of the curve, small changes in pO_2 result in large changes in oxygen saturation. For example, at a pO_2 of 40 mm Hg, the hemoglobin is about 75% saturated, whereas a pO_2 of 10 mm Hg represents an SvO_2 of 9.6%. For this reason the saturation rather than the pO_2 of *venous* blood provides a closer look at the amount of oxygen released to the tissues.

Oxygen demand of tissues

The amount of oxygen released to the tissues is determined by the pO_2 of the tissues. This is determined by the basal metabolic rate, which is in turn affected by changes in temperature, metabolic condition, physical activity, and stress. Increased tissue demands of oxygen require increased oxygen transport to maintain adequate tissue oxygenation and sustain necessary metabolic functions.

Oxygen consumption ($\dot{V}O_2$)

The amount (ml) of oxygen actually diffused into the body's tissues per minute is referred to as the oxygen consumption (ml oxygen/minute). Under most conditions, oxygen consumption reflects the tissues' demand for oxygen. For the average person at rest, oxygen con-

sumption is approximately 230 to 250 ml/minute (or 125 ml/minute/M^2). With a normal oxygen delivery of 1000 ml/minute, an oxygen consumption of 250 ml/minute would result in an oxygen return in the venous blood of 750 ml/minute (15 vol%). This represents the venous oxygen reserve, which is only used under exceptional circumstances.

Oxygen consumption varies directly with alterations in metabolic rate, temperature, and physical work. When cardiac output and hemoglobin remain unchanged, oxygen consumption changes inversely with SvO_2. Significant changes in oxygen consumption should be clinically discernible. Table 4-3 lists some causes of increased or decreased oxygen consumption (demand) as well as alterations in the determinants of oxygen supply.

Oxygen consumption can be measured by having the patient breathe into a Douglas bag and analyzing the amount of oxygen in the patient's expired air. Computerized on-line computation of oxygen consumption can also be performed in intubated patients through the use of a pneumotachometer and a mass spectrometer, which measure flow and fractional oxygen concentration of inspired and expired gas.[23] Oxygen consumption can also be calculated as the product of cardiac output and arterial-venous oxygen (a-vO_2) difference according to the Fick formula (Appendix G). This requires measurement of thermodilution cardiac output and a-vO_2 difference.

Because resting oxygen consumption tends to remain fairly constant, estimates of the patient's oxygen consumption are commonly performed, using the value of

Table 4-4. Mean oxygen consumption data grouped by age and heart rate in adults

Age (yrs)	Heart rate (bpm)					
	<50	51-60	61-70	71-80	81-90	91-100
Females						
<35			128 ± 2.0	136 ± 5.4	136 ± 18.6	136.5 ± 16.4
36-45		119.7 ± 4.8	124.5 ± 9.5	142.1 ± 9.5	128.4 ± 9.4	
46-55		124.5 ± 8.4	113.1 ± 5.2	117.6 ± 9.2	124.7 ± 6.9	130 ± 12.4
56-65		104.2 ± 4.5	106 ± 7.9	111.4 ± 5.0	124.5 ± 2.9	134.3 ± 15.1
66-75		102.1 ± 6.0	105 ± 9.8	124.3 ± 8.8	117.6 ± 10.3	107.7 ± 8.4
Males						
<35				158.8 ± 7.3	160 ± 9.4	146 ± 16
36-45		122.9 ± 4.5	135.3 ± 6.3	138.9 ± 11.4	150.9 ± 8.7	134.4 ± 6.4
46-55	119.8 ± 6.8	120.3 ± 2.6	122 ± 3.6	130.6 ± 5.1	134.3 ± 8.6	134.7 ± 5.6
56-65	117.9 ± 8.6	121.6 ± 3.5	121.8 ± 3.8	125 ± 4.4	125.8 ± 7.4	125.4 ± 10.4
66-75	104.8 ± 2.0	113.8 ± 5.7	116.4 ± 6.1	124.1 ± 6.2	124.1 ± 9.2	

From Crocker, R.H., et al.: Determinants of total body oxygen consumption in adults undergoing cardiac catheterization, Cathet. Cardiovasc. Diagn. **8**:363, 1982.

125 ml oxygen/M^2 or according to a nomogram such as the one listed in Table 4-4.[24]

Fick equation

Rearrangement of the Fick formula describes the relationship between the oxygen consumption of the body as a product of the a-vO_2 difference and cardiac output and can be viewed in terms of demand and supply:

$$\underset{\text{Oxygen consumption } (\dot{v}O_2)}{\textbf{Demand}} = \underset{\text{Cardiac output} \times (\text{Arterial } O_2 \text{ content} - \text{Venous } O_2 \text{ content})}{\textbf{Supply}}$$

Arterial-venous oxygen difference

Subtraction of the oxygen content of venous blood from the oxygen content of arterial blood provides the a-vO_2 difference. Normally, the tissues extract approximately 25% to 30% of available oxygen from hemoglobin. Therefore the oxygen saturation of mixed venous blood (SvO_2) is normally between 65% and 75% when arterial blood is almost fully saturated. This results in a venous oxygen content of approximately 14% to 15vol% which, when subtracted from a normal arterial oxygen content of 19 vol%, gives an a-vO_2 difference of 4 to 5 vol%. The normal difference between arterial and venous oxygen content is 3.0 to 5.5 vol%. An a-vO_2 difference greater than 5.5 vol% is associated with reduced oxygen delivery (usually from reduced cardiac output) and/or an increased oxygen extraction by the tissues, producing a low SvO_2.

The a-vO_2 difference reflects the adequacy of cardiac output to match tissue oxygen demands and has long been used clinically to reflect directional changes in cardiac output. Under conditions in which arterial oxygen content (saturation and hemoglobin) and oxygen consumption remain relatively stable, changes in a-vO_2 difference are inversely related to changes in cardiac output. The a-vO_2 difference is a useful check of questionable thermodilution cardiac output readings. If the a-vO_2 difference is normal despite very high or very low thermodilution cardiac output readings, troubleshooting should be performed to correct the erroneous readings.

Oxygen supply and demand imbalance

The function of the cardiopulmonary system is to ensure a balance between oxygen supply and demand. However, this balance can be disrupted by factors affecting both the supply and demand of oxygen. The tissues' demand for oxygen, as reflected by the oxygen consumption, can be increased or decreased. Increases in oxygen consumption can occur with hyperthermia, shivering, pain, increased activity, etc. (Table 4-3). Reduced oxygen consumption is seen with hypothermia, anesthesia, sepsis, and induced muscular paralysis.

Compensatory mechanisms

A review of the components of the oxygen transport formula indicates the factors that can reduce oxygen *supply* or delivery, namely: reductions in cardiac output, hemoglobin (anemia), and arterial oxygen saturation (hypoxemia).

The body compensates for inadequate oxygen delivery in two important ways: first, by increasing cardiac output and second, by increasing oxygen extraction from the blood by the tissues. The cardiac output can triple, as can the amount of oxygen extracted by the tissues.[25] In patients with advanced heart disease who have limited ability to increase cardiac output, the only compensatory mechanism available to provide adequate tissue oxygenation is to increase oxygen extraction. A fall in venous oxygen saturation (SvO_2) to levels below 60% is therefore usually indicative of cardiac decompensation.[26] As the SvO_2 continues to fall to 50% or less, lactic acidosis occurs as a result of anaerobic metabolism. Increases in blood lactate are associated with permanent cellular damage and an ominous prognosis. Thus therapeutic interventions are directed toward restoration of adequate oxygen delivery. Table 4-3 lists various clinical conditions responsible for alterations in SvO_2.

MIXED VENOUS OXYGEN SATURATION AS INDEX OF TISSUE OXYGENATION
Principle

Causative factors changing the oxygen consumption or demand (either an increase or a decrease) are usually apparent clinically, particularly in the inactive, critically ill patient. Changes in oxygen consumption reflect changes in the *demand* for oxygen. On the other side of the equation, changes in cardiac output, hemoglobin, or SaO_2 reflect changes in the *supply* of oxygen. A decrease in hemoglobin and SaO_2 reduce oxygen supply unless cardiac output increases sufficiently to maintain the balance between supply and demand. A decrease in cardiac output, however, poses a more serious threat to the oxygen supply and demand balance because it eliminates one of the major compensatory mechanisms the body has to affect an adequate balance.

Another compensatory mechanism the body uses is to extract more oxygen from the blood at the tissue level and thus to decrease SvO_2. Marked decreases in the SvO_2 are the result of tissue hypoxia. Generally, an SvO_2 of less than 30% (20 torr), indicates insufficient oxygen availability to the tissues.[27] Clinically, this degree of tissue hypoxia is usually accompanied by coma. The precise level of SvO_2 at which anaerobic metabolism and lactic acidosis begin varies, but an SvO_2 of less than 40% likely represents the limits of compensation and impending lactic acidosis.[28]

Continuous monitoring of SvO_2 with a fiberoptic catheter provides immediate information on changes in cardiopulmonary function and the balance between oxygen demand and supply. A decrease of any of the determinants of oxygen supply (cardiac output, hemoglobin, or arterial saturation) is usually associated with a

decrease in SvO_2. On the other hand, any change in oxygen consumption is associated with an inverse change in SvO_2.

If the SvO_2 begins to decline (no matter what the value) immediate assessment must be performed to determine the cause. As discussed earlier, increase in oxygen consumption can usually be readily determined as the cause if the patient has just become active, had a seizure, spiked a temperature, developed pain, etc. If no apparent increase in oxygen consumption is noted, assessment must be made of the determinants of oxygen supply.

A reduction in hemoglobin, unless associated with massive bleeding, is usually a slowly changing determinant and is less frequently responsible for sudden decreases in SvO_2.

Hypoxemia, with a low SaO_2, can be evaluated by arterial blood gas determination. However, SaO_2 and CaO_2 rarely change more than 10% in most clinical situations.[17]

Hypoperfusion is the most common cause of decreasing SvO_2. To confirm this cardiac output determination should be performed. In this way, cardiac output measurements are made when hemodynamically indicated, rather than at some routine or preset time. Use of continuous SvO_2 monitoring has also reduced the need for routine arterial blood gas sampling.[29]

Sustained reductions in SvO_2 of 10% or greater over a 3 to 5 minute period should prompt the above assessment, as this finding frequently warns of impending deterioration.[30-33] Therapy should then be directed toward controlling the oxygen demands or correcting the decrease in oxygen supply. A rapid improvement in SvO_2 confirms the appropriateness of the chosen therapy.

Brief, minor changes in SvO_2 (5% or less) are clinically insignificant and are likely caused by some type of interference rather than changes in cardiac output.[34]

Technique of continuous SvO_2 monitoring

Continuous measurement of the saturation of venous blood (SvO_2) is available via a modified 7.5 or 8 Fr thermodilution PA catheter (Fig. 4-13). In addition to the standard features, this catheter has a lumen containing optical fibers that transmit light to and from the bloodstream. The light source consists of three diodes that emit alternating pulses of three different wavelengths of red light through one of the optical fibers. This light is absorbed, refracted by the hemoglobin constituents of the blood, and reflected back through the second optical fiber to a light detector. It is then converted to an electric signal and transmitted to a remote data processor. The computed oxyhemoglobin satura-

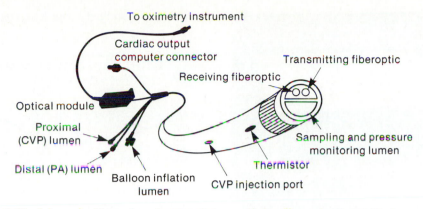

Fig. 4-13. Schematic illustration showing features of the fiberoptic thermodilution catheter. (Courtesy Oximetrix, Inc.)

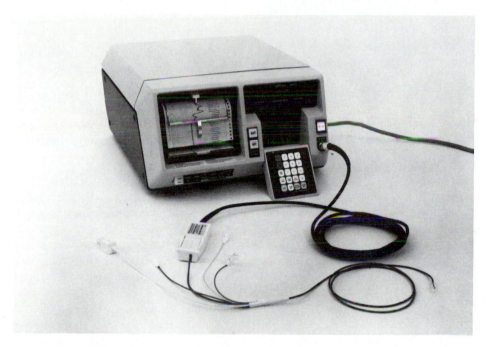

Fig. 4-14. Svo₂ thermodilution catheter connected to a microprocessor with a slow paper write-out. (Courtesy Oximetrix, Inc.)

tion is averaged over a 5-second interval, updated every 1 to 2 seconds, and displayed digitally on an oscilloscope, a slow-speed paper recorder (Fig. 4-14), or an LCD screen. The recorded output also indicates the light intensity at the tip of the catheter. Changes in the light intensity signify a change in catheter position (i.e., against the wall of the vessel or spontaneous wedging), inadequate blood flow (thrombus at the tip of the catheter), or damage to the fiberoptic fibers. The most recent oxymetric monitor is combined with a cardiac output computer to provide combined processing of Svo₂ and cardiac output (Fig. 4-15). This system also stores data over a 24-hour period.

Equipment

A fiberoptic thermodilution PA catheter and a microprocessor with a strip-chart recorder or data display and storage system are needed for this procedure.

Preparation of the fiberoptic pulmonary artery catheter

Follow each manufacturer's recommendations for preparation of the fiberoptic catheter before patient insertion. Handle the catheter gently, avoiding any sharp bending of the catheter to prevent damage to the optical fibers. The balloon and thermistor wires of the catheter should also be checked as discussed on p. 87. For

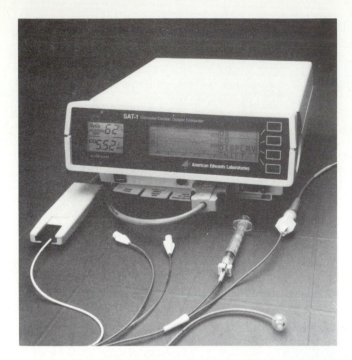

Fig. 4-15. Combined oximeter and cardiac output computer with attached fiberoptic thermodilution catheter. (Copyright 1985, American Edwards Laboratories, American Hospital Supply Corporation. Reprinted with permission.)

instruction on catheter insertion, follow the steps on pp. 87 to 89 for insertion of a standard flow-directed PA catheter. Although the fiberoptic PA catheter is somewhat stiffer than the standard PA catheter, it compares favorably in ease of insertion and complication rates.[35]

Svo₂ measurements

Normal saturation of mixed venous blood ranges from 65% to 77%. Table 4-3 lists the probable causes and clinical states associated with high and low Svo₂ readings. A fall in Svo₂ below 60% lasting for 5 minutes or longer indicates a compromise in at least one of the determinants of oxygen transport—cardiac output, hemoglobin, or arterial oxygenation. Figs. 4-16 and 4-17 show examples of the use of continuous Svo₂ monitoring in directing patient care and management.

Calibration

Calibration of the oximeter with a blood sample of known oxygen saturation should be performed daily or whenever there are doubts regarding the displayed Svo₂ reading. Calibration with a known saturation should be carried out when the patient's saturation values are relatively stable according to the specific manufacturer's instructions.

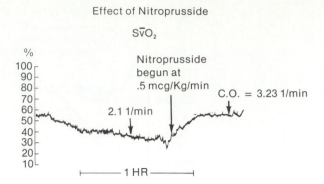

Fig. 4-16. Example of continuous $S\bar{v}o_2$ recording showing corresponding cardiac output readings and response to nitroprusside infusion. (Courtesy Oximetrix, Inc.)

Variations

A 4 Fr double-lumen fiberoptic catheter is also available for continuous monitoring of Sao₂. This catheter has been successfully used in neonates to monitor the rapid changes in oxygen saturation characteristic of hypoxic episodes.[36,37]

COMPLICATIONS OF HEMODYNAMIC MONITORING

Reported overall complication rates for PA catheters are as high as 75%.[5,6] However, this high rate relates to the frequent occurrence of transient and clinically benign arrhythmias. The majority of complications that occur with PA catheterization are minor, although fatalities may be associated with major complications. Potentially life-threatening complications have been reported to occur in approximately 4% of patients who have undergone PA catheterizations.[38]

The overall reported incidences of complications from arterial catheterization range from 0% to 8.8%; complications are directly associated with the duration of catheterization.

Cardiac arrhythmias

Either atrial or ventricular arrhythmias frequently occur during right heart catheter insertion and are usually transient and benign, subsiding with completion of catheter passage out to the PA. Transient PVCs and nonsustained ventricular tachycardia are the most common arrhythmias, but occasionally sustained ventricular tachycardia develops, requiring drug therapy or prompt cardioversion or both. Rarely, ventricular fibrillation may occur and is treated by immediate defibrillation. The occurrence of ventricular arrhythmias is highly correlated with the presence of shock, acute myocardial ischemia or infarction, hypokalemia, hypocalcemia, hypox-

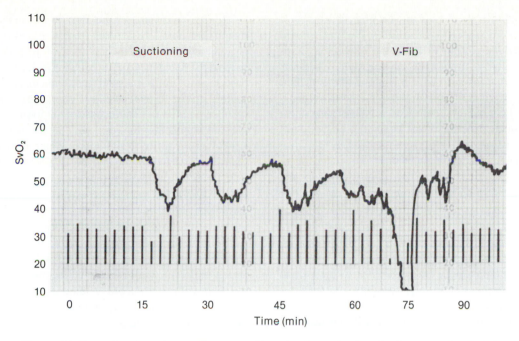

Fig. 4-17. Example of continuous Svo_2 recording showing reductions in Svo_2 associated with repeated suctioning. Note that the Svo_2 did not return to baseline between suctioning procedures. Ventricular fibrillation occurs as the Svo_2 falls to 40% and lower.

emia, acidosis, and prolonged catheter insertion times.[39]

The prophylactic use of lidocaine to control cardiac arrhythmias has been reported. This is not routinely used, but may be of some value in selected high-risk cases.[40,41]

Bundle branch block

Right bundle branch block may occur during manipulation of the catheter in the right ventricle. This is generally not a problem unless the patient has preexisting left bundle branch block (LBBB), resulting in complete AV block. In patients with preexisting LBBB, it may be prudent to insert a PA catheter with pacing electrodes to prevent ventricular asystole. If a pacing catheter is not inserted, transvenous or transcutaneous pacing equipment should be readily available.

The best prevention of the development of any cardiac arrhythmia or conduction abnormality is rapid placement of the catheter tip in the PA with minimal manipulation in the right ventricle or right atrium. In addition, the balloon should be fully inflated before entering the right ventricle to prevent catheter tip–induced arrhythmias.

Thrombus formation

Although thrombus formation may occur with any intravascular catheter, the polyvinylchloride material of the PA catheter has been shown to be highly thrombogenic, with formation of a fibrin sleeve around the catheter within 60 to 130 minutes of catheter insertion.[42] Small thrombi with erosion of the endothelium of the vein, endocardium, or valves along the course of the catheter have been found on autopsy.[43] This same study revealed a significant increase of blood vessel thrombosis (from 41% to 79%) after 2 days of catheterization despite anticoagulation.

Thrombus can also develop at the insertion site. In venographic autopsy examination, Chastre et al.[44] found thrombosis of the internal jugular veins (the catheter insertion site) in 66% of patients despite lack of clinical evidence of thrombosis. The presence of a PA catheter has been shown to correlate with a continuing reduction in platelet count, likely caused by increased platelet consumption associated with aggregation along the catheter. The platelet count usually returns to normal within 2 to 4 days after catheter removal.[45,46]

The incidence of thrombus formation is increased in patients with low cardiac output, disseminated intravascular coagulation, or congestive heart failure.[47]

Reduction of the risk of thrombosis may occur with a continuous flush of heparinized saline or use of a catheter bonded with heparin.[48] Use of a Teflon sheath with a side arm for continuous infusion may also reduce thrombus formation.[49] Manual flushing of either the PA or arterial catheter should always be preceded by aspiration to remove any clots, if present. Flushing should then be performed gently with a small volume of fluid. This is particularly important with the arterial catheter because vigorous flushing with as little as 7 ml of fluid into a radial artery catheter can reach the aorta and possibly result in cerebral embolization.[50] Because most continuous flush devices allow rapid delivery of fluid (0.75 to 1.5 ml/second) it is recommended to fast-flush arterial catheters for no longer than 2 seconds or to manually flush the catheter by gently tapping the plunger of the syringe with no more than 2 to 4 ml of fluid.

Pulmonary infarction

Pulmonary infarction may occur as a result of embolization of thrombus from the catheter or as a result of catheter migration and prolonged wedging. Forward migration of the catheter occurs primarily during the first 24 hours as the catheter loop tightens with repeated RV contractions.

Prevention of this complication includes a review of a chest radiograph in the first 12 hours, continuous display of the pressure from the distal lumen of the catheter, wedging of the catheter only for a very brief time, monitoring of the PAEDP rather than PAW pressure (if a close correlation is established), and, perhaps, use of heparin-bonded catheters to reduce thrombolic occlusions. Chest radiographs should be repeated if catheter migration is suspected.

Infection

Infection secondary to PA catheterization can range from contamination to colonization to sepsis. Contamination, with a positive culture of the catheter tip, or colonization, with growth of the same organisms from both the catheter tip and another site (e.g., sputum, urine), has been shown to occur in 5% to 35% of cases.[51]

Colonization with bacteria (most commonly coagulase-negative staphylococci) has been shown to occur more frequently with polyvinylchloride PA catheters than with Teflon intravascular CVP catheters.[52] Sepsis, in which the same pathogen is grown from the blood and the catheter tip, has been reported to occur in 1% to 8% of PA catheter placements.[53,54] Septic endocarditis involving the right side of the heart is a rare complication of prolonged PA catheterization.

Prevention of infection includes meticulous aseptic technique during catheter insertion, daily care of the insertion site (including cleansing with a bactericidal agent and application of iodophor ointment and a new

sterile dressing), and a short duration of catheter placement. Catheters left in place longer than 4 days are associated with a higher incidence of infection.[51,55] To reduce the incidence of infection the Centers for Disease Control (CDC) recommends changing the IV solution, tubing, stopcocks, and transducer dome every 48 hours, utilizing nonglucose IV solutions, and removing and replacing the catheter, if necessary, after 4 days.[56] A recent bacteriologic evaluation of disposable pressure transducers showed no increase in contamination rates of disposable transducers changed every 4 days or every 2 days (3%).[56a] Advancement of PA catheters after initial placement should only be done if the proximal portion of the catheter has been maintained sterile inside a sleeve. In one study, short-term sterility was provided by catheter sleeves for 1 to 2 days if inserted under meticulous aseptic technique.[57] All intravascular catheters should immediately be removed if colonization or sepsis develops, and appropriate antibiotic therapy instituted.

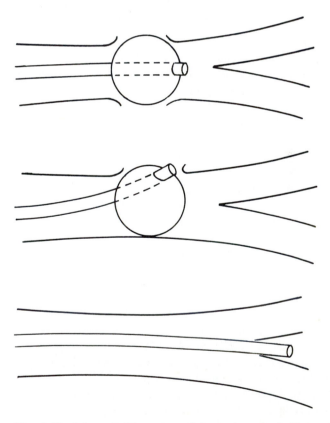

Fig. 4-18. Schematic illustration of the various mechanisms responsible for catheter-induced rupture of the PA: overinflation of the balloon, eccentric balloon inflation, and distal migration of the catheter tip.

Pulmonary artery rupture

Rupture of the PA is a dramatic and usually fatal complication that occurs infrequently with the use of PA catheters. Because this complication is often associated with pulmonary hypertension, advanced age (>60 years), anticoagulation, and cardiopulmonary bypass surgery,[58,59] PAWP measurements should be performed with caution in this subgroup of patients. In all patients, PAWP should be obtained with *continuous* visualization of the PAP during balloon inflation. Inflation should be discontinued immediately on visualizing a PA wedge waveform. Should the PA wedge waveform become nonphasic, the balloon should immediately be deflated because this may represent overinflation or eccentric inflation, with the balloon extending around the catheter tip.

Although pulmonary hypertension, per se, may not render the arteries more fragile, the higher PAP tends to drive the catheter further distally into smaller vessels, thereby increasing the risk of perforation.[59] Changes in the vessel wall that occur in patients over the age of 60 years also result in lower rupturing pressures. The use of hypothermia, which stiffens the catheter, and manipulation of the heart during cardiac surgery also increase the risk of PA rupture. The four causes of PA rupture are distal migration of the catheter tip, overinflation of the balloon, eccentric inflation of the balloon, and manual flushing of a wedged catheter. Fig. 4-18 illustrates some of the mechanisms responsible for rupture of the PA.

To prevent this frequently fatal complication, the following procedures should be performed:

1. Monitor the distal lumen pressure continuously.
2. Radiographically confirm catheter tip location in the central PA.
3. Inflate the balloon slowly, using only that amount of air necessary to achieve a PAWP tracing, while constantly monitoring the pressure.
4. Perform infrequent balloon inflations (monitor PAEDP, if possible).
5. Always deflate the balloon before performing a manual flush. If necessary, withdraw the tip of the catheter slightly to prevent forceful flushing in the wedge position.
6. Never inflate the balloon with an excessive volume of air (greater than the recommended volume of air). If a PAWP is obtained with less than the usual volume of air, check the catheter position for migration.
7. Never inflate the balloon with fluid. Carefully identify infusion ports before injections to avoid injecting fluid into the balloon lumen.

If PA rupture is small, as indicated by a small amount of hemoptysis, the patient should be placed in a lateral recumbent position with the affected side down and closely monitored and observed. Anticoagulation should be stopped and reversed. Hemoptysis of 15 to 30 ml should prompt consideration of a "wedge" angiographic study to determine the amount and location of extravasation of dye.[60] Massive hemoptysis can be controlled with insertion of a double-lumen endotracheal tube to prevent bleeding into the unaffected lung and aid ventilation.[61] Prompt surgical repair may be necessary, along with pneumonectomy or lobectomy.

Cardiac tamponade

Cardiac perforation resulting in cardiac tamponade can occur during manipulation of any catheter placed in the heart. This rare complication is associated with central venous (RA) catheters more commonly than PA catheters and may occur anywhere from minutes to days after catheterization. Clinical manifestations of cardiac tamponade in conjunction with low cardiac output and elevated RA and CVP pressures in patients with a right heart catheter should prompt suspicion of this complication.

Immediate decompression by pericardiocentesis (Chapter 10) is necessary to prevent a fatal outcome. Aspiration from the tip of the catheter may be performed in the possible event that the tamponade is a result of cardiac penetration and infusion of IV fluid into the pericardial sac.[62] This maneuver can be performed until pericardiocentesis is carried out, but should not delay the pericardiocentesis.

Table 4-5. Guidelines for pulmonary catheter length estimations

Desired catheter tip location	Insertion site	Approx. length of insertion
Superior vena cava—right atrium	Right antecubital fossa	40 cm
	Left antecubital fossa	50 cm
	Internal jugular vein	15-20 cm
	Subclavian vein	10-15 cm
	Femoral vein	30-40 cm
Right ventricle	Right antecubital fossa	55-60 cm
	Left antecubital fossa	65-70 cm
	Internal jugular vein	30-40 cm
	Subclavian vein	25-30 cm
	Femoral vein	45-55 cm
Pulmonary artery	Right antecubital fossa	65-75 cm
	Left antecubital fossa	75-85 cm
	Internal jugular vein	40-55 cm
	Subclavian vein	35-45 cm
	Femoral vein	55-70 cm

Table 4-6. Complications of PA catheters, possible causes, prevention, and interventions

Complication	Possible cause	Prevention	Interventions
Arrhythmias	Irritation of endocardium by unprotected catheter tip	Keep balloon inflated during advancement; advance gently	Administer lidocaine if necessary Defibrillate if ventricular fibrillation occurs Insert pacemaker for complete heart block
	Excess catheter loop in RV or RA	Obtain chest radiograph	Withdraw catheter to remove loop
	Prolonged catheterization procedure with much manipulation	Insert catheter quickly, gently, and with minimal manipulation; use fluoroscopy, if possible	
	Catheter tip withdrawn or fallen back into RV	Situate catheter well into main PA	Inflate balloon to encourage catheter passage out to PA
Thrombus/embolism	Clot from fibrin sheath around catheter	Use heparin-bonded catheters Use sheath with side arm infusion of heparin solution	
	Clot from within catheter	Maintain continuous flush with heparinized solution; manually flush every 4 to 6 hours	Anticoagulation and possible thrombolysis
	Occlusion of branch of PA by catheter	Systemic heparinization in high-risk patients Maintain catheter tip in main PA	
Pulmonary infarction/PA rupture	Distal catheter tip migration (especially during first 24 hr)	Check radiograph immediately after catheter insertion and 12 hours later; remove catheter loop in RV or RA Continuously monitor PA waveform	Withdraw catheter tip to PA
	Prolonged wedging of catheter	Wedge very briefly (<30 sec); leave balloon deflated with stopcock open and syringe removed; monitor PAEDP instead of PA (if close relationship)	Supportive care Surgical repair if necessary
	Embolization of thrombus from catheters	Use heparin-bonded catheters; maintain adequate flush with heparinized solution	

Table 4-6. Complications of PA catheters, possible causes, prevention, and interventions—cont'd

Complication	Possible cause	Prevention	Interventions
Infection	Break in aseptic technique during catheter insertion, equipment set-up, blood sampling, or tubing change	Use careful aseptic technique	Remove all catheters if sepsis develops; administer antibiotics as indicated by culture and sensitivity
		Place sterile deadender caps on all stopcocks	
		Use sterile sleeve over catheter	
	Contamination via flow in transducer dome	Carefully check domes before use; never reuse disposable domes	
		Sterilize transducer between patients	
		Change disposable domes after defibrillation	
		Do not use 5% dextrose in water on transducer head or as IV flush solution	
	Prolonged catheterization	Change all equipment every 48 hrs	Apply iodophor ointment and sterile dressing to insertion site daily
		Inspect and cleanse wound with bactericidal daily	
		Minimize time catheter is in place	Remove catheter as soon as possible (replace after 4 days if necessary)
Cardiac tamponade	Perforation by catheter tip (usually during insertion)	Gently manipulate and advance catheter with balloon inflated	Pericardiocentesis
		Never advance catheter against resistance	Reverse anticoagulation
Catheter coiling or knotting	Dilated RA or RV	Advance catheter gently but swiftly before softening occurs; flush catheter with iced saline or insert 0.025-inch guidewire to stiffen	Replace with new catheter (see Chapter 17)
	Softening of catheter secondary to prolonged insertion time with much manipulation		
	Use of small (5 Fr) catheter		
Balloon rupture	Excessive number of balloon inflations	Monitor PAEDP instead of PAWP (if close relationship); wedge catheter infrequently	Turn off stopcock of air lumen; place tape over stopcock to prevent further use
	Overinflation of balloon	Inflate balloon only with amounts of air indicated on catheter (1.5 ml for 7 Fr)	Monitor PAEDP
	Inflation of balloon with fluid	Inflate balloon only with air or carbon dioxide	
	Active deflation of balloon by withdrawing air back into syringe	Deflate balloon by removing syringe and allowing air to escape passively	

Prevention of this serious complication includes never using force during catheter passage, inflation of the balloon before RV entry, and radiologic confirmation of the location of the catheter tip immediately after insertion and as needed thereafter.

Catheter coiling or knotting

Coiling or knotting of the PA catheter during catheter insertion is often associated with prolonged insertion time. This occurrence is considered a complication because it prevents correct catheter tip positioning and it can cause arrhythmias or endocardial trauma. Coiling can occur in either an enlarged RA or in the RV. If advancement of 15 cm of catheter does not result in a pressure change either from RA to RV or from RV to PA, the catheter should be slowly withdrawn and then readvanced to prevent knotting. Table 4-5 lists the approximate catheter length required to correctly place the catheter from various insertion sites. Stiffening of the catheter by immersing it in or flushing it with iced saline or inserting a 0.025-inch (0.64 mm) guidewire may decrease the tendency for catheter coiling and enhance forward passage.

Knotting of the catheter can be handled in a variety of ways, as discussed in Chapter 17. Surgical removal may at times be necessary if intracardiac structures are involved in the knot.

Balloon rupture

Balloon rupture after catheter insertion is usually a minor and infrequent complication that occurs as a result of improper technique. This may include overinflation of the balloon (more than 1.5 cc air for a 7 Fr catheter), inflation of the balloon with fluid instead of air, and active rather than passive deflation of the balloon. The balloon should only be passively deflated by removing the syringe and allowing the balloon to deflate. If the balloon air is actively withdrawn into the syringe, the latex of the balloon may be pulled into the side holes of the catheter, thus damaging the balloon.

Rupture of the balloon is indicated by a lack of feeling of resistance during inflation, failure of the bevel of the inflation syringe to spring back during passive inflation, and the inability to obtain a PA wedge waveform after inflation. The appearance of blood in the balloon lumen also indicates balloon rupture. Should this occur, the stopcock of the air lumen should be turned off, tape placed over the stopcock, and the message "do not inflate" inscribed on the tape. Table 4-6 summarizes the complications of PA monitoring along with causes, preventive measures, and appropriate interventions.

SPECIAL PRECAUTIONS
Choosing the insertion site

Choice of insertion site varies according to physician preference and experience. Internal jugular and subclavian routes are frequently used via the percutaneous technique. Insertion of PA catheters via the antecubital veins is very safe but some difficulty may occur in catheter positioning without fluoroscopy. This method is also associated with an increased incidence of infection and inadvertent advancement of the catheter caused by movement of the patient's arm. Insertion of PA catheters via the femoral vein requires the use of fluoroscopy and is associated with an increased risk of embolic complications.

Choosing the catheter

The choice of catheter type for insertion into the PA depends on the clinical needs of the patient.

The four-lumen thermodilution catheter, which offers the capability of cardiac outout measurement in addition to RAP, PAP, and PAWP monitoring, is most commonly used.

The five-lumen thermodilution catheter is also commonly used and offers an additional port in the RA for fluid or drug administration (Fig. 4-19). This added feature permits cardiac output measurements without interruption of fluid or drug administration. (Viscous solutions should not be administered through the PA catheter because of the reduced lumen size.)

The four-lumen PA catheter is also available with pacing wires. Use of this catheter should be considered in patients with a high risk of developing complete heart block, including patients with preexisting left bundle branch block (LBBB), inferior wall infarction, or trifascicular block. This may save the time of having to insert a temporary pacemaker, although the PA pacing catheter is somewhat more difficult to precisely position for consistent capture.

The fiberoptic thermodilution PA catheter is useful for continuous monitoring of Svo_2 in addition to RA, PA, PAW pressures and cardiac output determinations in select high-risk patients.

Insertion of pulmonary artery catheter without fluoroscopy

Pulmonary artery flotation catheters can be passed quickly at the bedside without fluoroscopy, using the hemodynamic pressure waveforms as a guide (Fig. 4-20). If fluoroscopy is available, it may facilitate a more rapid catheter insertion and improve the safety of the procedure. If fluoroscopy is not available, the femoral vein should not be used as the insertion site because its

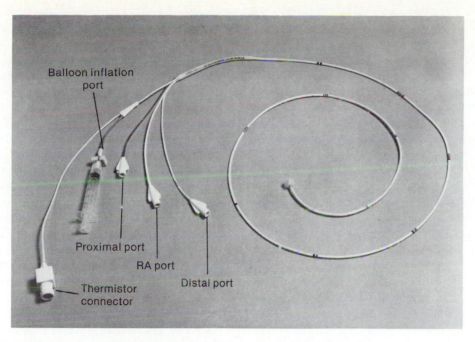

Fig. 4-19. The VIP Swan-Ganz thermodilution catheter. (Copyright 1985, American Edwards Laboratories, American Hospital Supply Corporation. Reprinted with permission.)

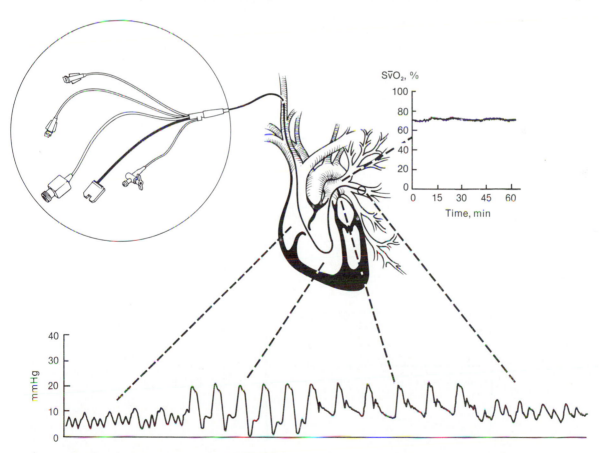

Fig. 4-20. Composite illustration showing normal hemodynamic waveforms obtained as a fiber-optic balloon flotation PA catheter is advanced from the RA to the PAW position. An example of a continuous $S\bar{v}O_2$ reading in the PA is shown on the right.

route up from the inferior vena cava requires some visualization and its passage from the inferior vena cava into the right atrium, the right ventricle, and then the PA requires careful manipulation. Regardless of insertion site or use of fluoroscopy, a chest radiograph should be obtained after final positioning of the catheter tip.

Balloon inflation in the presence of a shunt

If there is suspicion of an intracardiac shunt, carbon dioxide, rather than air, should be used for balloon inflation. This reduces the risk of a right-to-left embolism should balloon rupture occur.

PAWP interpretation with PEEP

Intrapleural pressure affects PAWP readings in two ways: (1) by direct transmission of intrapleural pressure to the cardiac and intrathoracic vascular pressures and (2) by the effects of pleural pressure on the collapsible pulmonary capillaries. These effects require particular caution in interpreting PAW pressures in patients with elevated airway or intrathoracic pressures. West et al.[63] described the regional pressure-flow relationships in three major zones of the lung. Zone I is that physiologic area in which the alveolar pressure is equal to or greater than both the PA and pulmonary venous (LA) pressures. There is basically no flow in this area, which anatomically approximates the upper one third of the lung (Fig. 4-21).

In zone II, the middle zone, the PAP is greater than both the alveolar pressure and the pulmonary venous pressure. The amount of blood flow into this zone is determined, of course, by the difference between the PA and alveolar pressures. However, when the balloon of the PA catheter is inflated, interrupting blood flow in that vessel, the pulmonary capillary is likely to collapse because of the higher alveolar pressure (Fig. 4-21). The PAWP obtained from this position will reflect alveolar and *not* pulmonary venous or LA pressure.

In zone III, the dependent zone, the PAP exceeds pulmonary venous (LA) pressure, which in turn exceeds alveolar pressure (Fig. 4-21). Balloon occlusion in this area does not result in vessel collapse because the higher pulmonary venous pressure maintains the vasculature open. Therefore PAW pressure accurately reflects pulmonary venous pressure only in zone III position. Vertical location of the catheter tip in the pulmonary vasculature can only be determined by lateral chest radiography, which should be performed if there is any suspicion regarding the PAW pressure reading. The

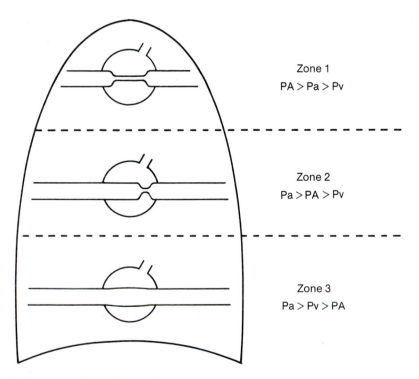

Fig. 4-21. Schematic illustration of the pressure/flow relationships in zones 1, 2, and 3 of the pulmonary circulation. (*Pa*, Pulmonary arterial pressure; *PA*, alveolar pressure; *Pv*, venous pressure.)

higher the catheter tip is above the left atrium, the greater the likelihood of being in zone I or II.[64,65]

It is important to remember that the zones of the lung represent physiologic and *not* anatomic areas, although related anatomic areas can be approximated. Therefore alterations in any of the three pressures (alveolar, PA, or LA) can change the size of a zone or convert one zone to another.[66] For example, zone I, which for practical purposes does not exist in the upright normal lung, can develop if PAP falls or alveolar pressure rises, or both, such as in the use of high levels of PEEP. Likewise, the size of zone II can increase (and zone III decrease) as a result of diuresis, hemorrhage, or the use of positive end-expiratory pressure (PEEP).[67] The size of zone III can be increased by volume administration or decreasing airway pressure.

Fortunately, most PA balloon catheters tend to float to areas with greatest blood flow (zone III).[65,68] In addition, PAWPs are not usually measured with the patient in an upright position. Therefore the hydrostatic pressure gradient and the amount of lung located above the LA are reduced, thus favoring a larger zone III area.[67] Both of these factors favor accurate reflection of pulmonary venous pressure or LAP. However, suspicion regarding the vertical location of the catheter tip should exist when the PAWP exceeds the PAEDP, when the PAWP increases proportionately with stepwise increments in PEEP level, or when the characteristic PAW waveform morphology is absent and marked respiratory variation is present. When the lateral chest film reveals that the PA catheter tip is outside of zone III, it can be repositioned, *or* zone III can be established through volume administration or decreasing airway pressure.

Because all vascular pressures are measured relative to atmospheric pressure, all readings should be obtained at end-expiration, when pleural pressure is closest to atmospheric pressure.[69] However, with the use of PEEP, pleural pressure remains positive at end-expiration and falsely elevates the measured PAWP. The amount of PEEP that is transmitted to the pleural space, and therefore added to the pressure reading, depends on lung compliance and is difficult to determine precisely. At end-expiration, pleural pressure is probably less than half of the PEEP in patients with poor lung compliance.[70] Interpretation of the PAWP in patients on PEEP should take into consideration the level of PEEP and its influence on the vascular pressure. Subtraction of airway pressure from the measured PAWP provides a more accurate reflection of actual transmural pressure. It is usually not recommended to disconnect PEEP to obtain PAWP readings.

Removal of pulmonary artery catheter

Removal of the PA catheter is performed by a physician or a critical care nurse in the following way:
1. Explain the procedure to the patient, including possible sensations that may be experienced.
2. Place the patient in a supine position. (The Trendelenburg position should be used for catheter removal from subclavian or internal jugular veins.)
3. Assure ECG stability.
4. With a syringe, aspirate air from the balloon lumen to ensure balloon deflation. (Active rather than passive deflation should be performed at this time.)
5. Remove the dressing and cut the sutures from the sheath and catheter.
6. Rapidly pull the catheter back to the approximate level of the introducer sheath (30 to 40 cm from the internal jugular vein and 25 to 35 cm from the subclavian vein).
7. Remove the catheter and the sheath as a unit (ask the patient to stop breathing or gently hum during this time).
8. Immediately apply light pressure to the site using a sterile 4 × 4-inch gauze pad to seal the opening.
9. Cleanse the skin with sterile water and dry it with gauze.
10. Apply iodophor ointment and an adhesive bandage to the site. If the catheter has been in place for a prolonged period, apply an occlusive dressing of gauze with petroleum jelly to adequately seal the tract and prevent air embolism.

Ventricular arrhythmias commonly occur during removal of the catheter, particularly if the catheter is removed slowly, and in patients with low cardiac index.[71] For this reason the ECG should be monitored during catheter removal, with lidocaine and a defibrillator close at hand. PVCs are usually transient and spontaneously resolve with removal of the catheter (Fig. 4-22). However, ventricular tachycardia may develop, requiring prompt treatment.

FUTURE DEVELOPMENTS

Technologic advances will continue to expand the abilities of bedside hemodynamic monitoring. On the forefront are a modified PA catheter with a rapid-response thermistor for calculation of ventricular ejection fraction by thermal techniques, a transducer-tip PA catheter that measures pressures directly without the use of a fluid-filled system, and the use of double indicator techniques (indocyanine green and thermodilution) for estimation of lung water to aid in the diagnosis and

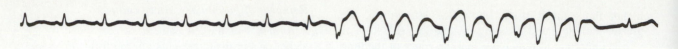

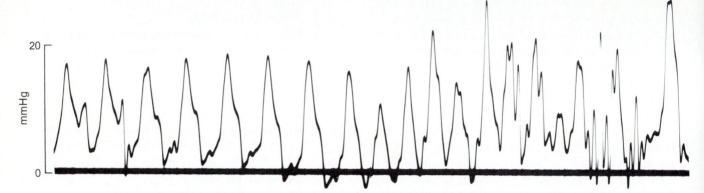

Fig. 4-22. Withdrawal of the PA catheter from the PA to the right ventricle. Note the occurrence of multiple (11) PVCs as the catheter tip comes in contact with the right ventricle. There is spontaneous resolution upon removal of the catheter.

treatment of pulmonary edema and adult respiratory distress syndrome.[72,73]

The use of on-line computers in the biomedical field will aid in calculating derived parameters and plotting hemodynamic trends as well as beat-to-beat analysis.

Of greatest need in terms of future applications of hemodynamic monitoring are carefully controlled prospective studies to clearly define those groups of patients in whom invasive hemodynamic monitoring is most helpful.[74,75]

REFERENCES

1. Hales, S.: Statistical essays: Hemostaticks, vol. 2, ed. 3, London, 1738, W. Innys & R. Manby.
2. Lategola, M., and Rahn, M.: A self-guiding catheter for cardiac and pulmonary arterial catheterization and occlusion, Proc. Soc. Exp. Biol. Med. **84**:667-668, 1953.
3. Wilson, J.N., et al.: Central venous pressure in optimum blood volume maintenance, Arch. Surg. **85**:563, 1962.
4. Swan, H.J.C., Ganz, W., and Forrester, J.S.: Catheterization of the heart in man with the use of a flow-directed balloon-tipped catheter, N. Engl. J. Med. **283**:447-451, 1970.
5. Shah, K.B., Rao, T.L.K., Laughlin, S., and El-Etr, A.A.: A review of pulmonary artery catheterization in 6,245 patients, Anesthesiology **61**:271-275, 1984.
6. Duncan, J.W., and Powner, D.J.: Complications associated with the use of pulmonary artery catheters, Arizona Med. **39**:433-435, 1982.
7. Disposable pressure transducers, Health Devices **13**:268-289, 1984.
8. Sise, M.J., Hollingsworth, P., and Brimm, J.E.: Complications of the flow-directed pulmonary artery catheter: a prospective analysis in 219 patients, Crit. Care Med. **9**:315-317, 1981.
9. Kaye, W.: Invasive monitoring techniques: arterial cannulation, bedside pulmonary artery catheterization, and arterial puncture, Heart Lung **12**:395-427, 1983.
10. Cenzig, M., Crapo, R.O., and Gardner, R.: The effect of ventilation on the accuracy of pulmonary artery and wedge pressure measurements, Crit. Care Med. **11**:502-507, 1983.
11. Berryhill, R.E., Benumof, J.L., and Rauscher, L.A.: Pulmonary vascular pressure reading at the end of exhalation, Anesthesiology **49**:365-368, 1978.
12. Ellis, D.M.: Interpretation of beat-to-beat blood pressure values in the presence of ventilatory changes, J. Clin. Monitoring **1**:65-70, 1985.
13. Whalley, D.G.: Hemodynamic monitoring: pulmonary artery catheterization, Can. Anesth. Soc. J. **32**:299-305, 1985.
14. Gardner, R.M.: Direct blood pressure measurement: dynamic response requirements, Anesthesiology **54**:227-236, 1981.
15. Boutros, A., and Albert, S.: Effect of the dynamic response of transducer-tubing system on accuracy of direct blood pressure measurement in patients, Crit. Care Med. **11**:124-127, 1983.
16. Scott, W.A.C.: Hemodynamic monitoring: measurement of systemic blood pressure, Can. Anesth. Soc. J. **32**:294-298, 1985.
17. Gore, J.M., et al.: Handbook of hemodynamic monitoring, Boston, 1985, Little, Brown & Co.
18. Fegler, G.: Measurements of cardiac output in anesthetized animal by a thermodilution method, Q. J. Exp. Physiol. **39**:153-164, 1954.

19. Shellock, F.G., and Riedinger, M.S.: Reproducibility and accuracy of using room temperature vs. ice temperature for thermodilution cardiac output determination, Heart Lung **12**:175-176, 1983.

20. Daily, E.K., and Mersch, J.: Comparison of Fick method of cardiac output with thermodilution method using two indicators, Heart Lung (in press).

21. Stetz, C.W., Miller, R.G., Kelly, G.E., and Raffin, T.A.: Reliability of the thermodilution method in determination of cardiac output in clinical practice, Am. Rev. Respir. Dis. **126**:1001-1004, 1982.

22. Miller, M.J.: Tissue oxygenation in clinical medicine: an historical review, Anesth. Analg. **61**:527-534, 1982.

23. Carpenter, J.P., Sreedhar, N., and Staw, I.: Cardiac output determination: thermodilution versus a new computerized Fick method, Crit. Care Med. **13**:576-579, 1985.

24. Crocker, R.H., et al.: Determinants of total body oxygen consumption in adults undergoing cardiac catheterization, Cathet. Cardiovasc. Diag. **8**:363, 1982.

25. Aberman, A.: Fundamentals of oxygen transport physiology in a hemodynamic monitoring context. In Fahey, P.J. (editor): Continuous measurement of blood oxygen saturation in the high risk patient, vol. 2, San Diego, 1985, Beach International, Inc.

26. McMichan, J.C.: Continuous monitoring of mixed venous oxygen saturation. In Schweiss, J.F. (editor): Continuous measurement of blood oxygen saturation in the high risk patient, vol. 1, San Diego, 1983, Beach International, Inc.

27. Bryan-Brown, C., Baek, S., Makabali, G., and Shoemaker, W.: Consumable oxygen: availability of oxygen in relation to oxyhemoglobin dissociation, Crit. Care Med. **1**:17-21, 1973.

28. Kandel, G., and Aberman, A.: Mixed venous oxygen saturation: its role in assessment of the critically ill patient, Arch. Intern. Med. **143**:1400-1402, 1983.

29. Divertie, M.B., and McMichan, J.C.: Continuous monitoring of mixed venous oxygen saturation, Chest **85**:423-428, 1984.

30. Jaquith, S.M.: Continuous measurement of SvO2: clinical applications and advantages for critical care nursing, Crit. Care Nurse **5**:40-44, 1985.

31. Jamieson, W.R.E., et al.: Continuous monitoring of mixed venous oxygen saturation in cardiac surgery, Can. J. Surg. **25**:538-549, 1982.

32. Schmidt, C.R., Frank, L.P., Forsythe, S.B., and Estafanous, F.G.: Continuous SvO2 measurement and oxygen transport patterns in cardiac surgery patients, Crit. Care Med. **12**:523-527, 1984.

33. White, K.M.: Completing the hemodynamic picture: SvO2, Heart Lung **14**:272-280, 1985.

34. Hoyte, J.W., et al.: Continuous SvO2 as a predictor of changes in cardiac output: clinical observations. In Schweiss, J.F. (editor): Continuous measurement of blood oxygen saturation in the high risk patient, vol. 1, San Diego, 1983, Beach International, Inc.

35. McMichan, J.C., Baele, P.L., and Wignes, M.W.: Insertion of pulmonary artery catheters—a comparison of fiberoptic and nonfiberoptic catheters, Crit. Care Med. **12**:517-519, 1984.

36. Krousop, R.W., Cabatu, E.E., and Chelliah, B.P.: Accuracy and clinical utility of an oxygen saturation catheter, Crit. Care Med. **11**:744-749, 1983.

37. Rao, K.H., Dunwiddie, W.C., and Lower, R.R.: A method for continuous postoperative measurement of mixed venous oxygen saturations in infants and children after open heart procedures, Anesth. Analg. **63**:873-881, 1984.

38. Horst, H.M., Obeid, F.N., Vij, D., and Bivins, B.: The risks of pulmonary arterial catheterization, Surg. Gynecol. Obstet. **159**:229-232, 1984.

39. Iberti, T.J., Benjamin, E., Gruppi, L., and Raskin, J.M.: Ventricular arrhythmias during pulmonary artery catheterization in the intensive care unit, Am. J. Med. **78**:451-454, 1985.

40. Salmenpera, M., Peltola, K., and Rosenberg, P.: Does prophylactic lidocaine control cardiac arrhythmias associated with pulmonary artery catheterization? Anesthesiology **56**:210-212, 1982.

41. Sprung, C.K., et al.: Prophylactic use of lidocaine to prevent advanced ventricular arrhythmias during pulmonary artery catheterization, Am. J. Med. **75**:906-910, 1983.

42. Hoar, P.F., et al.: Thrombogenesis associated with Swan Ganz catheters, Anesthesiology **48**:445-447, 1978.

43. Lange, H.W., Galliani, C.A., and Edwards, J.E.: Local complications associated with indwelling Swan-Ganz catheters: autopsy study of 30 cases, Am. J. Cardiol. **52**:1108, 1983.

44. Chastre, J., et al.: Thrombosis as a complication of pulmonary artery catheterization via the internal jugular vein, N. Engl. J. Med. **306**:278-281, 1980.

45. Richman, K.A., Kim, Y.L., and Marshall, B.E.: Thrombocytopenia induced by Swan-Ganz catheters (abstract), Anesthesiology **51**:5161, 1979.

46. Vincente Rull, J.R., et al.: Thrombocytopenia induced by pulmonary artery floatation catheters. A prospective study, Intensive Care Med. **10**:29-31, 1984.

47. Goodman, D., Rider, A.K., Billingham, M.E., and Schroeder, J.S.: Thromboembolic complications with the indwelling balloon-tipped pulmonary arterial catheter, N. Engl. J. Med. **291**:777-778, 1974.

48. Hoar, P.F., et al.: Heparin bonding reduces thrombogenicity of pulmonary artery catheters, N. Engl. J. Med. **305**:993-995, 1981.

49. Perkins, N.A.K., et al.: Internal jugular vein function after Swan-Ganz catheterization, Anesthesiology **61**:456-459, 1984.

50. Lowenstein, L., Little, J.W., and Lo, A.H.: Prevention of cerebral embolization from flushing radial-artery cannulas, N. Engl. J. Med. **285**:1414-1415, 1971.

51. Michel, L., March, H.M., and McMichan, J.C.: Infection of pulmonary artery catheters in critically ill patients, J.A.M.A. **245**:1032-1036, 1981.

52. Sheth, N.K., et al.: Colonization of bacteria on polyvinylchloride and Teflon intravascular catheters in hospitalized patients, J. Clin. Microbiol. **18**:1061-1063, 1983.

53. Boyd, K.D., Thomas, J., Gola, J., and Boyd, A.D.: A prospective study of complications of pulmonary artery catheterizations in 500 consecutive patients, Chest **84**:245-249, 1983.

54. Singh, J., et al.: Catheter colonization and bacteria with pulmonary and arterial catheters, Crit. Care Med. **10**:736-739, 1982.

55. Applefield, J.J.: Sterility and repositioning of the Swan-Ganz catheter, Chest **75**:743, 1978.

56. Centers for Disease Control: Guidelines for prevention of infections related to intra-vascular pressure–monitoring systems, Infect. Control **3**:68, 1982.

56a. Luskin, R.L., et al.: Extended use of disposable pressure transducers, J.A.M.A. **255**:916-920, 1986.

57. Johnston, W.E., et al.: Short-term sterility of the pulmonary artery catheter inserted through an external plastic shield, Anesthesiology **61**:461-464, 1984.

58. Stone, J.G., Khambatta, H.J., and McDaniel, D.D.: Catheter induced pulmonary artery trauma: can it always be averted? J. Thorac. Cardiovasc. Surg. **86**:146-155, 1983.

59. Hardy, J.F., Morissette, M., Taillefer, J., and Vauclair, R.: Pathophysiology of rupture of the pulmonary artery by pulmonary artery balloon-tipped catheters, Anesth. Analg. **62:**925-930, 1985.

60. Berg, R.A., Chiu, L.C., and Boutros, A.R.: Bedside pulmonary angiography in the diagnosis of complications of Swan-Ganz catheters, Crit. Care Med. **4:**99-100, 1976.

61. Barash, P.G., et al.: Catheter-induced pulmonary artery perforation: mechanisms, management and modifications, J. Thorac. Cardiovasc. Surg. **82:**5-12, 1981.

62. Edwards, H., and King, T.C.: Cardiac tamponade from central venous catheters, Arch. Surg. **117:**965-967, 1982.

63. West, J.B.: Regional differences in lung, New York, 1977, Academic Press, Inc.

64. Tooker, J., Huseby, J., and Butler, J.: The effect of Swan-Ganz catheter height on the wedge pressure–left atrial pressure relationship in edema during positive-pressure ventilation, Am. Rev. Respir. Dis. **117:**721-726, 1978.

65. Shasby, D.M., et al.: Swan-Ganz catheter location and left atrial pressure determine the accuracy of the wedge pressure when positive end-expiratory pressure is used, Chest **80:**666-670, 1981.

66. Wiedmann, H.P., Matthay, M.A., and Matthay, R.A.: Cardiovascular-pulmonary monitoring in the intensive care units, Chest **85:**537-549 and 656-668, 1984.

67. Marini, J.J.: Pulmonary artery occlusion pressure: clinical physiology, measurement and interpretation, Am. Rev. Respir. Dis. **128:**319-326, 1983.

68. Kronberg, G.M., et al.: Anatomic locations of the tips of pulmonary artery catheters in supine patients, Anesthesiology **51:**467-469, 1979.

69. Eaton, R.J., Taxman, R.M., and Avioli, L.V.: Cardiovascular evaluation of patients treated with PEEP, Arch. Intern. Med. **143:**1958-1961, 1983.

70. Marini, J.J., O'Quin, R., Culver, B.H., and Butler, J.: Estimation of transmural cardiac pressures during ventilation with PEEP, J. Appl. Physiol. **53:**384-391, 1982.

71. Damen, J.: Ventricular arrhythmias during insertion and removal of pulmonary artery atheters, Chest **88:**190, 1985.

72. Sibbald, W.J., et al.: Thermal dye measurements of extravascular lung water in the adult respiratory distress syndrome, Chest **87:**585-592, 1985.

73. Baudenstel, L.J., Kaminski, D.L., and Dahms, T.E.: Evaluation of extravascular lung water by single thermal indicator, Crit. Care Med. **14:**52-56, 1986.

74. Robin, E.D.: A critical look at critical care, Crit. Care Med. **11:**144-147, 1983.

75. Brandstetter, R.D., and Gitter, B.: Thoughts on the Swan-Ganz catheter, Chest **89:**5-6, 1986.

Chapter Five

Cardiac catheterization and coronary arteriography

ARA G. TILKIAN
ELAINE K. DAILY

The history of the development of cardiac catheterization and angiography may be summarized chronologically by the following landmarks[1]:
- Discovery of the x-ray by William Roentgen, 1895
- First documented human right heart catheterization (of his own heart) by Werner Frossman, 1929
- Attempt of cardiac angiography by Werner Frossman, 1930 and 1931
- Introduction and early development of cardiac angiography and intracardiac hemodynamic studies, 1940s and 1950s
- Attempts at *indirect* coronary arteriography by many investigators, 1945 to 1960
- Development of percutaneous catheter techniques by S.I. Seldinger, 1953
- Selective coronary arteriography via the transbrachial method developed by Mason Sones, 1960
- Selective coronary arteriography via the percutaneous femoral technique developed by Ricketts and Abrams, 1962; Melvin Judkins, 1967; and Kurt Amplatz, 1967

The techniques of cardiac catheterization and angiography, developed in the 1940s and 1950s, and coronary arteriography developed in the 1960s, have not changed substantially and are in widespread use today. Appreciable improvements in equipment have occurred during the past 20 years. Catheters and guidewires have been refined, procedural details have been streamlined, and procedure safety has improved. Contrast agents are better, and newer and safer agents are in development. Radiographic equipment provides better resolution and reduced radiation exposure. Computerized radiographic image processing has been introduced.

In addition, cardiac catheterization techniques have been further developed for *treatment* of cardiovascular disease. Andreas Gruentzig introduced the technique of percutaneous transluminal coronary angioplasty (Chapter 15). Catheter techniques are being investigated to permit visualization of the inside of vessels (angioscopy) and with the use of laser beams to remove obstruction in these vessels.

In this chapter we will review the indications and contraindications of cardiac catheterization studies as well as the complications and how to minimize them. We will discuss patient preparation and aftercare and present an outline of basic catheterization techniques. Details relating to special techniques of cardiac catheterization, coronary arteriography, ventriculography, aortography, hemodynamic studies, and interpretation of findings will not be discussed here. Excellent books covering these topics have already been written.[2-7]

No amount of written material can actually teach one the proper and safe performance of cardiac catheterization and angiography or the interpretation of findings. This chapter and the accompanying references can only supplement teaching by an experienced angiographer in a "hands-on" teaching program.

INDICATIONS

Indications[8,9] for cardiac catheterization and coronary arteriography are continuously changing, given the increasing safety of the procedure and the increasing utility of the angiographic information.

Generally accepted indications

Generally accepted indications for left heart catheterization and selective coronary arteriography are as follows:
- Suspected or known coronary artery disease with unstable, new-onset, or progressive angina

- Suspected or known coronary artery disease with angina pectoris not responding well to medical treatment
- Myocardial infarction complicated by ventricular septal rupture, acute mitral regurgitation, refractory arrhythmias, or unrelieved recurrent chest pain
- Variant angina
- Valvular heart disease or congenital heart disease being evaluated for surgical correction
- Sustained ventricular tachycardia or resuscitation from cardiac arrest (usually ventricular fibrillation) without definite myocardial infarction
- Following myocardial infarction, especially in younger patients, particularly if graded exercise testing or other studies reveal evidence of myocardial ischemia
- Recurrent, poorly controlled angina following coronary artery bypass grafting or balloon angioplasty
- Stress test results that are very suggestive of myocardial ischemia in patients who are free of symptoms, especially if radionuclide studies are also positive
- Recurrent chest pain of undetermined cause (atypical chest pain) when definitive diagnosis has not been made and coronary artery disease has not been excluded, especially in patients with a risk factor for coronary artery disease
- Miscellaneous conditions such as aortic dissection or suspected pericardial constriction.
- Suspected coronary artery disease in patients who are free of symptoms but for whom accurate diagnosis is important for employment (e.g., airline pilots) or for insurability
- After heart transplant, where clinically silent severe coronary atherosclerosis may develop rapidly

Controversial indications

Cardiac catheterization and coronary arteriography are sometimes performed in the following circumstances. These indications are not universally accepted.
- Acute myocardial infarction: Until 10 years ago acute myocardial infarction was considered a contraindication to the performance of selective coronary arteriography. Currently, coronary arteriography is sometimes performed within the first hours of acute myocardial infarction with the intention of initiating transcatheter intracoronary thrombolytic therapy (Chapter 16) or performing balloon angioplasty (Chapter 15). This type of treatment for acute myocardial infarction remains controversial (as of 1986), and the overall risks and benefits have not yet been adequately tested.
- Coronary artery disease with *stable* angina (good or excellent control with medication) and without major ischemic response on exercise testing: The issue as to

the need for coronary arteriography in all patients with known or suspected coronary artery disease remains controversial. There is a lack of hard scientific data and an abundance of philosophic and personal bias, as well as diverse and sometimes opposing economic incentives affecting the decision-making process in the individual case.
- Chronic congestive cardiomyopathy: Coronary arteriography is sometimes performed to diagnose or exclude ischemic cardiomyopathy and evaluate the prognosis.

Uncomplicated, suspected, or known coronary artery disease may be adequately studied by left heart catheterization with left ventricular and coronary arteriography. In cases of myocardial infarction, congestive heart failure, associated valvular or pericardial heart disease, cardiomyopathy or left ventricular aneurysm, right heart catheterization with complete hemodynamic evaluation should also be performed at the time of the coronary arteriographic study.

Further studies proving or disproving the benefits of surgical or catheter revascularization in various coronary artery disease subgroups will undoubtedly modify this list of indications.

Indications for right heart catheterization

The indications for right heart catheterization are as follows:
- Congenital heart disease, including atrial septal defect, ventricular septal defect, patent ductus arteriosus
- Pulmonary thromboembolic disease
- Suspected pericardial tamponade or constriction
- As part of endomyocardial biopsy or electrophysiologic studies (see Chapters 8 and 9)
- As part of left heart catheterization and coronary arteriography in complicated cases with left ventricular failure, previous myocardial infarction, or cardiomyopathy
- Valvular heart disease

CONTRAINDICATIONS

There are no absolute contraindications to the performance of cardiac catheterization and angiography. Relative contraindications for *elective* study include the following:
- Uncontrolled congestive heart failure, arrhythmias, renal dysfunction, electrolyte imbalance, drug toxicity, infection, or other uncontrolled systemic disease
- Pregnancy: If possible, studies requiring radiation exposure should be deferred until the completion of pregnancy

- Anticoagulants: The effect of warfarin sodium (Coumadin) may be reversed or administration stopped; when continued anticoagulation is needed, heparin can be used
- A poor record of morbidity and mortality or high incidence of nondiagnostic studies at a particular angiographic facility or associated with a particular angiographic team

In general, if information gained at cardiac catheterization and angiography will not be used to determine the method of treatment or change in treatment, then the study should not be done. This includes patients with known coronary artery disease who will not consider revascularization surgery or balloon angioplasty.

RISKS

Table 5-1 demonstrates that the serious risks[10-15] of cardiac catheterization and coronary arteriography have decreased appreciably during the past 20 years. In more than 250,000 reported cases, morbidity was 1.2% and the mortality 0.1% to 0.2%, with most of the deaths occurring in patients with severe coronary artery disease or advanced LV dysfunction. For these patients the mortality approached 1%.

Other complications that are infrequent or generally not reported include nondiagnostic study, cardiac puncture or tamponade, embolic events (systemic or pulmonic—thrombus, air, cholesterol, or catheter fragments), retroperitoneal or pelvic hemorrhage, contrast material toxicity, contrast material reaction, acute congestive heart failure, supraventricular tachycardia, aortic dissection, pyrogen reaction, infection at the site of cutdown or systemic infection, endocarditis, and heart block or bradycardia/asystolic cardiac arrest.

In experienced hands, and via either the femoral or transbrachial approach, the mortality of cardiac catheterization can be kept at less than 0.1% and serious morbidity at less than 1%. In the interest of economy as well as patient convenience, the procedure can be performed on an outpatient basis in selected patients (see p. 149).

Minimizing complications

The complications of cardiac catheterization relate to the cardiac catheterization team, patient preparation, high-risk subgroups, and maintenance of an adequate caseload.

Table 5-2 summarizes methods of avoiding specific complications as well as methods of treating them should they occur.

The cardiac catheterization team

An experienced operator working with an efficient team using quality imaging equipment in good repair is the best guarantee that a diagnostic study will be done gently (with the least amount of vascular, cardiac, or psychologic trauma to the patient) and in the shortest amount of time. Physicians performing cardiac catheterization should be experienced in the procedure and should demonstrate good judgment. Hospital requirements for credentials need to be uncompromising in this. The team assisting the physician should include an experienced nurse (preferably two), a radiology technologist, and a cardiovascular technologist who work well as a team during routine studies as well as emergencies. To compromise at this level—that is, to use poorly trained personnel, inadequate staffing, or obsolete equipment for reasons of economy—is to court medical disaster and legal liability.

Correction of preexisting abnormalities

The safety of the procedure is enhanced when congestive heart failure and myocardial ischemia are adequately treated and arrhythmias, renal dysfunction,

Table 5-1. Risks of cardiac catheterization and coronary arteriography

Complication or fatality	Baltaxe[4] (1965-1970)	Adams[10] (1973) (n = 46,904)	Davis[15] (1979) (n = 7553)	Kennedy[11,12] (1982) (n = 53,581)	Kennedy[14] (1983) (n = 200,000)
Death	0.1%-1%	0.45%	0.2%	0.14%	0.15%
Myocardial infarction	0.3%-2.6%	0.61%	0.28%	0.07%	0.09%
Stroke		0.23%	0.03%	0.07%	0.07%
VT/VF	0.72	1.3%	0.6%	0.6%	
Serious vascular complication (thrombosis, hematoma, pseudoaneurysm)	0.41%-1.4%	1.6%	0.7%	0.6%	0.5%* 2-3%†

VT/VF, Ventricular tachycardia/ventricular fibrillation; *n,* number of patients.
*Percutaneous femoral (Judkins) approach.
†Brachial artery cutdown (Sones) approach.

Table 5-2. Methods for avoiding and treating complications of cardiac catheterization

Methods for avoiding complication	*Treatment*
Myocardial infarction (0.2%)	
Systemic heparinization	Visualize coronary artery involved
Heparinized flush solution	Intracoronary nitroglycerin
Meticulous cleaning of guidewires before each introduction	If a major vessel thrombus is suspected, consider intracoronary thrombolysis or possible coronary angioplasty
Limit time of guidewire insertion (<2 min)	In selected cases consider emergency aortocoronary bypass
If arterial sheath is not used, aspirate and flush arterial catheter in descending aorta and before crossing the arch	Supportive care
With catheters with sharply angled tips (Amplatz, graft catheters), use guidewire to cross aortic arch, especially in atherosclerotic aortas	
Aspirate and flush catheters frequently, especially if polyurethane catheters are used	
Carefully observe for and remove air bubbles in any of the tubing, solution, or injection syringe	
Make certain all connections are tight	
Always use Luer-Lok connections for injection syringe	
Cerebrovascular accident (0.1%)	
Methods as for myocardial infarction	Supportive care
Dissection (0.1%)*	
Never advance guidewire or catheter against resistance; inject contrast if in doubt regarding catheter tip location	No further coronary injections
Manipulate catheter in coronary ostium very gently	Consider emergency aortocoronary bypass
Continuous pressure monitoring of catheter tip; do not inject unless good pressure is seen and catheter tip is free	It is not clear if heparin should be continued or stopped
Use of flexible-tip coronary catheters may be helpful, but experience is limited	Anecdotal positive experience has been reported for treatment of coronary artery dissection with balloon angioplasty
	Supportive care
Acute congestive heart failure (CHF), pulmonary edema	
Treat preexisting CHF optimally before elective angiography	Elevate patient's trunk 30°-45°
Limit volume of contrast medium in high-risk patients avoid LV angiography in patients with severe aortic stenosis, marked CHF, or pulmonary hypertension; consider alternate methods of two-dimensional echocardiography and radionuclide wall motion study	Administer oxygen, morphine, nitrates (sublingually or IV), diuretics
Consider use of nonionic or low osmolar contrast agents	Control hypertension with nitroprusside
Space the frequency of coronary injections so that myocardial depression is reversed before injections	Phlebotomy
Carefully monitor and control volume of fluid administered during study	Intra-aortic balloon pumping (rarely required)
Fever	
Meticulous aseptic technique	Morphine (2-4 mg IV)
Use of disposable catheters, stopcocks, etc.	Blood cultures
Strict protocol and careful quality control for cleansing of reusables	Remove catheters and send tips to laboratory for culture and sensitivity testing
	If fever occurred after injection of contrast medium, culture this and send remaining medium in bottle to manufacturer for complete analysis

*May occur with all catheters but highest risk with preformed Judkins or Amplatz coronary artery catheters.

Table 5-2. Methods for avoiding and treating complications of cardiac catheterization—cont'd

Methods for avoiding complication	*Treatment*
Nondiagnostic study	Consider alternate methods of obtaining missing data
Adequate precatheterization clinical evaluation and testing	Consider repeat study
Test fluoroscopy and cine camera equipment before starting procedure	
Use only high-quality equipment in good repair	
Review video playback to ensure adequacy of study before termination	
Cardiogenic shock, death (0.1%-0.2%)	If patient is not responding and there is documented severe coronary artery disease, proceed to emergency balloon angioplasty or surgical revascularization, whichever can be performed promptly; revascularization should include attempt to bypass all major coronary artery branches
Careful patient selection: patients with left main coronary artery stenosis or aortic stenosis are at risk	
Use of prophylactic IABP for high-risk patients	
Inject at or near coronary ostium in suspected cases of left main coronary artery stenosis	
Identify left main coronary artery or ostial stenosis early in study; minimize number of injections; avoid and promptly treat hypotension	
Do not continue procedure if patient remains hypotensive	
If atropine and adequate volume expansion do not correct hypotension promptly, use intra-aortic injection of 0.125-0.250 mg Aramine and proceed to intra-aortic balloon pumping; adequate arterial (coronary) perfusion is essential for reversal of shock	
Rule out pericardial tamponade by immediate measurements of RA and RV pressures; if in doubt, obtain echocardiogram immediately	
Air embolism	
For prevention and treatment see p. 47	
Ventricular tachycardia, ventricular fibrillation (0.6%)	Initiate cough CPR immediately
Use nonionic contrast agents in high-risk patients; use conventional radiocontrast agent with disodium calcium–EDTA (Angiovist), which reduces incidence from 0.6% to 0.1%	Remove catheter from RV, LV, or coronary ostium
	Prompt defibrillation (200 joules)
Do not wedge catheter following coronary artery injection; permit prompt washout of contrast material; permit ECG and blood pressure to return to baseline before next injection	Chest compression is obviated by proper use of cough CPR followed by prompt defibrillation
	Lidocaine, if ventricular ectopy persists or recurs
Avoid hypotension; use atropine and volume expansion for vasovagal reaction or metaraminol (Aramine) as needed	Ventricular fibrillation that cannot be reversed usually reflects profound myocardial ischemia secondary to left main coronary artery disease or severe three-vessel coronary artery disease: emergency aortocoronary bypass should be considered
Avoid marked increases in heart rate or blood pressure; use adequate sedation, nitroglycerin, oxygen, or IV propranolol (Inderal)	
Limit volume of contrast medium injected into coronary arteries to necessary amount for adequate visualization; avoid overzealous and prolonged injections	
Do not inject when catheter tip pressure is damped	
Avoid using temporary RV pacemakers during coronary injection; If pacer is used, ensure that it is in demand mode or on standby	

For prevention and treatment see p. 47

Table 5-2. Methods for avoiding and treating complications of cardiac catheterization—cont'd

Methods for avoiding complication	Treatment
Asystole	
In high-risk patients (LBBB with right heart catheter, or preexisting A-V block) use prophylactic pacing (see Chapter 13)	Cough CPR
	Atropine and transvenous pacemaker; if bradycardia/asystolic cardiac arrest is irreversible, consider emergency revascularization
Do not wedge catheter; permit prompt contrast material washout	
Avoid hypotension	
Initial right coronary artery injection of 3-4 ml of contrast material only	
Use atropine promptly for bradyarrhythmias	
Permit time between contrast medium injections for heart rate stabilization	
Supraventricular tachycardia	
Control supraventricular arrhythmias prior to elective angiography	Atrial flutter: rapid atrial pacing with/without verapamil, propranolol, and digoxin
Electrolyte balance (potassium and magnesium)	Atrial fibrillation: digoxin, verapamil, propranolol
Avoid excessive catheter manipulation in RA	Paroxysmal supraventricular tachycardia: initiate vent ectopic beat by catheter manipulation to interrupt the reentry circuit; verapamil
Use flow-directed right heart catheters	
Thrombosis of brachial artery (2%)	
Meticulous attention to technique and avoidance of intimal injury	Surgical exploration is required in almost all cases (usually not emergency); wait for 4-12 hr to eliminate artery spasm or promote spontaneous lysis of thrombus; if not successful, proceed to thrombectomy
Avoid using transbrachial approach in women with small arteries	If there is vascular stenosis, resection and end-to-end anastomosis are required
Adequate systemic heparinization	No need for preoperative arteriography
Use Fogarty catheter if back-bleeding is not prompt	Maintain heparin treatment during waiting period
Limit number of catheter exchanges and procedure time; use arterial sheath with hemostatic valve to reduce trauma to vessel; use safety wire during all catheter exchanges	
Thrombosis of femoral artery (0.2%)	
Meticulous attention to femoral puncture and compression technique (see text); avoid catheterization of the superficial femoral artery	Prompt vascular surgery consultation; rule out spasm, inject 25 mg tolazoline (Priscoline) intra-arterially
Use systemic heparin administration during study	Early exploration and Fogarty catheter thrombectomy are usually successful
Check pedal pulses frequently during femoral compression; avoid obstructing vessel totally for any length of time	In patients with distal vascular disease or suspected distal emboli, an arteriogram is usually needed
Reduce time of procedure and number of catheter exchanges	
Use smaller catheters in patients with small arteries; avoid totally occluding vessel with large sheath or catheter	

electrolyte and fluid imbalance, and coagulopathies are corrected before the study.

High-risk subgroups

Most deaths that occur during cardiac catheterization and coronary arteriography occur in patients with left main coronary artery disease, high-grade three-vessel coronary artery disease, severe aortic stenosis, or severe LV dysfunction. It is important to identify these patients before or early during angiography. It is crucial to tailor the study so that the necessary information is obtained with minimal risk. For example, in a patient with unstable angina, the coronary study should be performed before ventriculography. In dealing with a case of suspected critical aortic stenosis, coronary arteriography should precede introduction of the catheter into

Table 5-2. Methods for avoiding and treating complications of cardiac catheterization—cont'd

Methods for avoiding complication	*Treatment*
Hematoma in femoral artery (0.1% major, 1%-2% minor)	
Femoral artery puncture should be below inguinal ligament	Generally conservative; surgical exploration and evacuation are rarely required; when necessary usually a tear in the artery is found
Attention to technique of compression; prolonged compression if protamine is withheld or if patient has recurrent coughing, aortic insufficiency, or hypertension	
Use of smaller sheaths and catheters in patients with aortic insufficiency	
False aneurysm	
Methods as for hematoma	Surgical correction
Attention to technique	
Avoid puncture of superficial femoral artery; special precaution in patients with aortic insufficiency or chronic anticoagulation	
Retroperitoneal bleeding	
Avoid femoral artery puncture high at iliac crest; recognized by hypotension, acute anemia, and low abdominal or flank pain within 2-12 hr of procedure	Discontinue or reverse anticoagulants Supportive care Follow hematocrit Usually self-limited
Cardiac puncture—tamponade	
Avoid straight-tip, severely tapered, or stiff catheters in RA or RV; be especially careful with pacing catheters	If tamponade: prompt pericardiocentesis with catheter drainage (Chapter 10)
Be very gentle in all catheter manipulations in the RA and RV	Cardiovascular surgery consultation
Radiographic confirmation of correct catheter tip location	Prompt surgical intervention for continuous bleeding
Contrast agent nephrotoxicity	
See p. 441	Supportive care for 2-4 days; generally self-limited; dialysis rarely needed
Hydration, mannitol, furosemide (Lasix), and nonionic contrast agents	
Contrast agent reaction	
Careful review of history and use of premedication (p. 444)	See p. 445
Vasovagal reaction	
Careful patient preparation, including sedation	Volume expansion (IV fluids), elevate legs
Adequate local anesthesia	Atropine (0.5-1.0 mg IV)
Gentle technique	Discontinue catheter manipulation until blood pressure and heart rate return to baseline
Correct hypovolemia: use normal saline infusion if RA pressure <3-4 mm Hg	

the LV. After determination of the aortic valve gradient and left ventricular end-diastolic pressure (LVEDP), a decision can be made as to the safety and advisability of proceeding with ventriculography. It is important to limit the duration of the study in such patients. The number of contrast medium injections should be minimized, and the patient should be closely observed for 6 to 10 hours after the procedure.

Caseload and surveillance

An adequate caseload for each laboratory and physician seems important in maintaining the skills of the cardiac catheterization team. What constitutes an adequate caseload continues to be debated.[3,16,17] Generally, cardiac catheterization laboratories with large caseloads tend to have lower rates of complications, but many facilities that handle 100 to 200 studies/year maintain excellent records of morbidity and mortality.[13,14] Irrespective of the caseload size, each facility should keep a detailed record of the quality of the studies and the associated mortality and morbidity; it should carefully analyze its own record and use this information in obtaining informed consent. Corrective action is necessary when morbidity and mortality are unexpectedly high.

EQUIPMENT

Equipment[3,18] required for cardiac catheterization and angiography includes the following:
- Fully equipped radiography room capable of cineangiography with a rotational device, serial radiography, and fluoroscopy with video monitoring
- Multichannel (8- to 12-channel) physiologic recorder capable of three simultaneous pressure recordings, two- to three-channel electrocardiogram (ECG) recordings, and cardiac output curve display (thermodilution or dye dilution); a remote oscilloscope to permit the cardiovascular technologist to remain out of the radiation field
- Emergency cart with drugs, IV solutions, airway equipment, and defibrillator
- Power injector
- Complete set of diagnostic catheters, special function catheters, guidewires, needles, introducers, transducers, trays of equipment for percutaneous catheterization as well as arterial and venous cutdown, and related items
- Equipment for oxymetry, blood gas level determination, determination of oxygen consumption, and hydrogen shunt study
- Pacemaker (transvenous and transcutaneous) and associated equipment
- Cine film processor and viewer
- Computers for on- or off-line analysis of the data and preparation of the report are helpful in a high-volume laboratory but are not essential
- Digital subtraction angiography capability (desirable but not essential)
- Pericardiocentesis tray and thoracotomy tray for the rare complication requiring emergency pericardial drainage or thoracotomy

PERSONNEL

The *minimal necessary personnel* for an adequate study includes one physician, one assisting nurse, and two technologists who are cross-trained for cardiopulmonary and radiology procedures. The optimal cardiac catheterization team would include six people.
- Physician performing the procedure, trained in cardiovascular medicine and radiographic techniques
- Assisting physician, usually in the cardiac catheterization room for complex procedures or for unstable patients, otherwise immediately available
- Nurse(s): scrub nurse to assist the physician with sterile field; circulating nurse for patient care and monitoring, administration of drugs, and handling of emergencies
- Radiologic technologist to operate radiographic equipment and power ejector and to assist in radiation safety and patient monitoring
- Monitoring and recording technician to perform ECG and pressure recording and monitoring, determination of thermodilution or dye dilution cardiac output, hydrogen study, and other technical tasks
- Cardiopulmonary technician for blood gas analysis, oxymetry, and estimation of cardiac output (Fick method)

The functions of the circulating nurses, radiology technologist, and cardiopulmonary monitoring technicians can be carried out by two to three people with cross-training.

PATIENT PREPARATION

Performing a diagnostic-quality cardiac catheterization study with minimal risk starts with careful patient preparation. Adequate psychologic and emotional preparation of the patient will contribute to the success and safety of the study. The patient should be fully informed of the intended procedure as well as the risk of complications. Discussion of the risks of cardiac catheterization should relate to the experience of the specific hospital and the catheterization team and should take into account the patient's medical condition. A description of the procedure (including sensations the patient may expect to experience and the anticipated duration of the procedure) can help relieve the patient's anxieties. Written material should be made available to the patient but should not be considered "required reading." A precatheterization visit by one or more members of the catheterization team not only provides an opportunity for the patient to ask questions not previously asked of the physician, but also allows the patient the comfort of seeing a familiar face in the laboratory the next day. If possible, a brief tour of the catheterization laboratory some time before the study is beneficial to the patient because it allays fear of the unknown.

PLANNING THE STUDY

Incomplete familiarity with the patient's medical condition and failure to tailor the study to the individual case court a nondiagnostic or incomplete study as well as higher complication rates. The following questions are suggested as a means of preparing for the procedure:

1. Has the patient been examined and have all pertinent laboratory data been reviewed? Have congestive heart failure, uncontrolled arrhythmias, electrolyte and fluid disorders, and renal dysfunction been corrected?

2. Have the history and the physical examination findings been reviewed to determine if the study is clearly indicated and if the patient is taking Coumadin, aspirin, or heparin? Has there been excessive bleeding following operation or trauma in the past? Careful review of the history is far more valuable than the ritualistic ordering of laboratory coagulation studies.

3. Does the patient have peripheral vascular disease? If so, is it symptomatic? In the interests of safety, should the study be performed from a femoral, brachial, or axillary approach? Should the study include peripheral arteriography?

4. Does the patient have diabetes or renal disease? If so, the volume of contrast material should be monitored carefully to avoid nephropathy. Hydration and the use of mannitol or furosemide (Lasix) may be needed during and after the procedure (p. 441). Has the patient been taking NPH insulin? If so, protamin reversal of heparin anticoagulation is best withheld (see p. 147).

5. Is there a history of multiple allergies or reaction to contrast material? Special preparation may be required (see p. 444).

6. Is there evidence of cerebrovascular disease? Perhaps the study should include an arch angiogram.

7. Does the history suggest coronary artery spasm? If no major obstructive coronary artery disease is found, should ergonovine provocation be used (see Chapter 6)? Discuss this with the patient and include it in the informed consent.

8. Does the patient have valvular heart disease? Will exercise during the cardiac catheterization be needed?

9. Is dyspnea an unexplained symptom? Should the study include evaluation of both right and left heart hemodynamic pressures and possibly pulmonary angiography and blood gas analysis?

10. Is pericardial constriction a real possibility? Study may require *simultaneous* right and left heart pressure measurements before and after fluid challenge and volume expansion.

11. Is there a high probability that emergency coronary angioplasty or cardiac operation will be required? Has the patient been informed and adequate preparation been made?

12. Is the use of intra-aortic balloon pumping (Chapter 11) desirable or likely to be required?

PRECATHETERIZATION ORDERS

A standard set of orders is helpful to ensure that important details are remembered and that the correct information is passed on to the nursing staff, the patient, and the cardiac catheterization team. Information on this form should (1) confirm the date and time of the cardiac catheterization study and the type of study to be performed; (2) ensure that informed consent is obtained; and (3) detail instructions for the nursing staff concerning the patient's IV fluids, catheter insertion site and preparation, meals, hydration, and medications in relation to the catheterization time. The patient should be fasting but well hydrated. The form should also include a section on precatheterization medications and laboratory studies. Other details can be included to meet the needs of different facilities.

PRECATHETERIZATION MEDICATIONS

Sedation is recommended to reduce the patient's anxiety and increase comfort, and it may also reduce the incidence of venous spasm. The medications used should not alter cardiovascular or pulmonary function. Adequate use of local anesthesia during the procedure is perferable to premedication with high doses of narcotics or barbiturates. A comfortable, well-informed adult with little or no apprehension may not require premedication. Oral administration of 10 mg of diazepam seems adequate for most patients. Heavy sedation and use of narcotics may be required for apprehensive patients who will not tolerate much discomfort, especially if the procedure is to be long. In adults, the study rarely must be performed with the use of general anesthesia.

Antibiotics are not routinely required, as the procedure is sterile and the risk of endocarditis is remote. Antibiotics may be used prophylactically in patients who are at high risk for infective endocarditis (history of subacute bacterial endocarditis, prosthetic valves) or if a break occurs in sterile technique during the procedure (see Appendix C).

PRECATHETERIZATION LABORATORY STUDIES

The laboratory tests required before cardiac catheterization study should be individualized. For a routine cardiac catheterization study in an otherwise well person, minimal laboratory tests should include ECG; serum creatinine, electrolytes (at least potassium), and hemoglobin; and possibly chest x-ray examination.

PREPARATION OF THE CARDIAC CATHETERIZATION LABORATORY

Before the patient is brought to the catheterization laboratory, all equipment should be checked and the items that will be used during the study prepared:

1. Test the radiographic equipment and the cine cam-

era. Expose the patient's name and the date of the study on cine film.

2. Check the defibrillator and place it in a position for use.

3. Check the multichannel recorder for calibration and settings.

4. Prepare the pressure injector and fill the syringe with contrast medium so that it is ready for use.

5. Prepare the sterile table. Place all sterile equipment to be used on this table (there are many types of equipment, both disposable and nondisposable, and the specific choice will vary in different institutions) (see box below).

6. Place the catheters and guidewires on the table. The choice of these is based on physician preference and the type of study to be performed.

7. Pour 1000 ml of normal saline with 5000 units of heparin into a large, sterile basin and immerse the catheters and guidewires in the solution. Flush all catheters. Use a smaller basin for flushing solution and a second small basin for discarded solutions.

8. Under sterile conditions, assemble the manifold with pressure line, saline flushing line, and contrast material line. Clear air from all the lines and syringes (Fig. 5-1).

9. Fill the 12 ml flush syringes with saline from the smaller basin and clear them of air.

STERILE EQUIPMENT FOR CARDIAC CATHETERIZATION

Eight 12 ml syringes for flushing
Four heparinized syringes for blood samples
Three-port manifold with distal rotator and proximal Luer-Lok
Syringe for contrast agent injection with Luer-Lok connection
Lidocaine 1% plain (20 ml)
Pressure tubing
Contrast material tubing
Saline flush tubing
Vascular needle
Heparin (5000 units)
Arterial cutdown tray for brachial artery approach
Large basin for soaking catheter and guidewire
Two small basins
#11 scalpel
Curved Kelly clamp
Drapes, towels, and towel clips
Needles: 25 gauge × 1 inch, 21 gauge × 1½ inches
Suture material and needle holder
Catheter of choice, dilator, and guidewire

---

10. Draw the lidocaine and heparin into marked syringes and attach the appropriate needle to the lidocaine syringe.

11. Cover the table with a sterile drape until the patient arrives.

PATIENT PREPARATION IN THE LABORATORY

When the patient is brought into the room, all personnel should be introduced by both name and function. At all times during the preparation it is important to answer the patient's questions and to strive to reduce his or her anxiety. Each step of preparation should then be explained to the patient as it is being done:

1. Review the patient's chart and complete the preexamination checklist. Before starting the examination, bring to the physician's attention all abnormal laboratory values or changes in the patient's condition.

2. Place the patient on the radiography table and provide a blanket as the gown is removed. If a rotating cradle is used, explain this to the patient. Cover the patient's chest with a small towel and secure the table straps.

3. Apply the ECG electrodes and secure them with tape to prevent dislodgment during the procedure. Avoid electrodes or wires in the radiographic field.

4. Take the anteroposterior measurement of the chest and level the transducer air reference port at midchest.

5. Note and mark pulses in the extremities, record the blood pressure, and generally observe the patient's condition.

6. Wash the groin insertion area with povidone-iodine solution and cover the patient with sterile drapes, leaving only the insertion site exposed. Cover the image intensifier and the table control panel with a clear plastic, sterile drape.

7. Pass the free ends of the manifold lines from the sterile field to the circulating nurse for connection of the pressure line to the transducer, the flush line to a heparin-saline pressure bag, and the contrast agent tubing to the contrast solution. Again clear air from the system.

8. Fill the control syringe with contrast medium and clear all air from the syringe.

9. Place the instruments in order according to use (Fig. 5-2).

10. Instruct the patient regarding coughing and deep breathing on command and repeat the basic elements of the procedure.

RIGHT HEART CATHETERIZATION

Right heart catheterization studies consist of right heart hemodynamic pressure readings (during rest and exercise), angiography (RA, RV, and PA), oxymetry, hydrogen shunt study, and determination of cardiac output. Only selected topics are discussed here. These studies are necessary in patients with valvular heart disease, myocardial dysfunction, pulmonary vascular disease, suspected intracardiac shunt, or pericardial constriction. The approach may be via a basilic vein (percutaneous or cutdown technique) or femoral vein (percutaneous technique), as discussed in Chapter 2.

Angiographic examination of the RA is infrequently performed in adults with cardiac disease, although it may be useful in defining the separation between the RA and the pericardium in patients with pericardial thickening or effusion.

Right ventriculography is performed in adults with cardiac disease to define the RV outflow tract and pulmonic valve in cases of pulmonic stenosis and to evaluate the degree of tricuspid regurgitation. Positioning of the ventriculography catheter depends on the area to be defined (i.e., catheter tip in the outflow tract to define it; catheter tip in the middle of the RV to define the RV).

Pulmonary angiography is the most frequently performed right heart angiographic procedure in adults with cardiac disease and is discussed in depth in Chapter 7.

Catheter selection

Catheter selection for right heart catheterization depends on the purpose of the study and certain anatomic

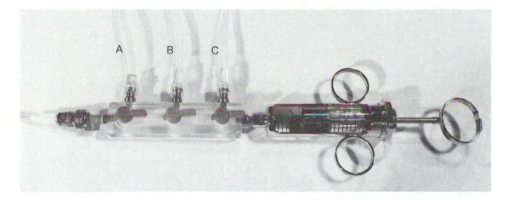

Fig. 5-1. Injection syringe and manifold with lines for (*A*) pressure measurements, (*B*) saline flush, and (*C*) introduction of contrast material. The injection syringe is connected to the proximal end of a three–side port manifold with Luer-Lok fittings. The distal end has a rotator, which attaches to the catheter with Luer-Lok fittings. All other connections are also Luer-Lok.

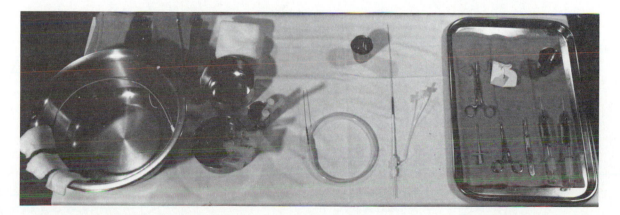

Fig. 5-2. Table set-up for cardiac catheterization (*right to left*): Tray containing lidocaine in syringes (with needle), #11 scalpel, Kelly clamp, disposable vascular needle, suture material, needle holder. On the table: vascular introducer, guidewire, cup with contrast agent, small basin with six to eight syringes filled with saline, another basin for discard solution, four 3 ml heparinized syringes in a cup, large basin with saline and catheters, extra towels, 4 × 4-inch sponges.

considerations. If measurement of right heart pressures is the primary purpose, a catheter with only an end hole is most satisfactory. However, if multiple blood samples or injections of contrast material are anticipated, a catheter possessing side holes would be more suitable. If thermodilution cardiac output determinations are to be performed, a thermodilution PA catheter must be used. If pacing may be required, a thermodilution pacing catheter or a Zucker catheter may be used for right heart catheterization. In patients with preexisting left bundle branch block a pacing catheter should be inserted. Angiography of the right side of the heart is performed through catheters with multiple side holes for rapid injection of large volumes of contrast medium. The most commonly used catheters for this purpose include the Grollman, Berman, NIH, and Eppendorf catheters (see Chapters 1 and 7 for more complete descriptions of catheters).

Basic procedure

The specific manner in which right heart catheterization is performed depends on the purpose of the study and, to a certain extent, the dictates of the catheter. The basic procedure is as follows:

1. After the catheter has been percutaneously or surgically inserted into the selected vein (see Chapter 2), advance it as quickly and gently as possible; the longer the catheter remains in the bloodstream, the softer and less manageable it becomes. Also, venous spasm may occur if an arm vein is used.

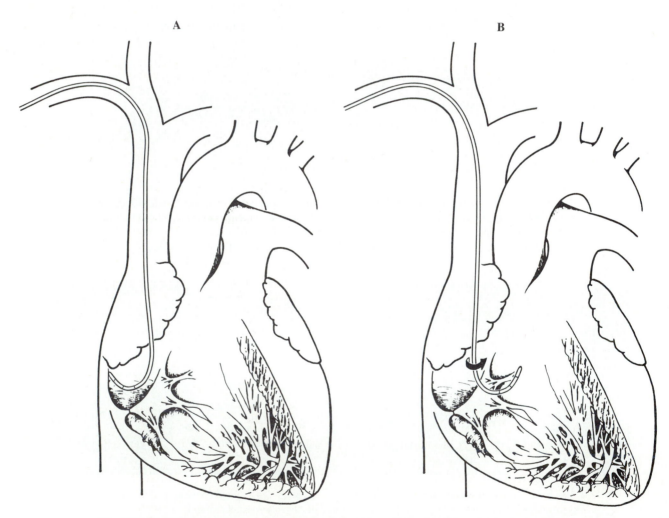

Fig. 5-3. A, Catheter forming J curve in the right atrium. Note that the catheter tip catches on the lateral wall of the atrium. **B,** Counterclockwise rotation of the catheter brings its tip anterior. The catheter then flips across the tricuspid valve and into the right ventricle.

2. Upon reaching the superior vena cava, slowly withdraw a blood sample into a syringe containing heparin for analysis of oxygen saturation.

3. Flush the catheter and connect it to a heparin flush system and transducer. Slight advancement will place the catheter in the RA, where pressure measurements should be obtained over several respiratory cycles (see Fig. 4-4).

4. After the completion of RA pressure measurements, advance the catheter and rotate it, if necessary, to form a J curve in the RA with the catheter tip catching on the lateral wall of the atrium (see Fig. 5-3, *A*). Keeping the catheter in this position for 15 to 20 seconds will facilitate retention of this curve. Counterclockwise rotation of the catheter will then bring its tip anterior, and it will flip across the tricuspid valve (see Fig. 5-3, *B*). An RV pressure waveform, as well as some premature ventricular contractions (PVCs), will be evident on the oscilloscope at this time. Some catheter tip manipulation away from the apex of the ventricle may be necessary to find a "quiet place" in the RV, where multiple PVCs are not provoked. If ventricular tachycardia occurs, either advance the catheter to the PA or withdraw to the RA.

5. Record the RV pressure (systolic and diastolic) over several respiratory cycles (see Fig. 4-5). With the catheter tip still retaining its J curve and directed toward the RV outflow tract, gently advance the catheter out to the PA; deep inspiration may help this maneuver. Do not force or push the catheter, as it may double up on itself and could become knotted.

6. When the catheter tip lies in the PA, slowly withdraw a PA blood sample into a glass syringe containing heparin for oxygen analysis.

7. Record a PA pressure (systolic, diastolic, and mean) over several respiratory cycles (see Fig. 4-6). Rule out the presence of an unsuspected intracardiac shunt by comparing the superior vena cava and PA oxygen saturation. If the PA oxygen saturation is substantially higher than that of the superior vena cava (Appendix D), perform complete oxymetric analysis, with oxygen analysis of blood samples successively obtained from the right, left, and main PAs; RV; RA; and superior and inferior (below the diaphragm) vena cavae.

8. If no abnormal step-up in oxygen saturation exists (Appendix D), between the PA and superior vena caval blood samples, advance the catheter until the tip will go no farther and becomes wedged in a small branch of the PA. Having the patient hold his or her breath or cough during advancement often aids in obtaining a wedge position. This procedure is not necessary if a balloon flotation PA catheter is used, as inflation of the balloon with only slight advancement produces the same effect of stopping blood flow in that vessel. Fluoroscopy should be used to make certain that the catheter tip is not moving and to withdraw any excess catheter loops that may be present in the RV. A PAWP should be evident on the oscilloscope (see Fig. 4-7). The pressure should be equal to or lower than the PA end-diastolic pressure (PAEDP) and should have the morphologic characteristics of an atrial pressure.

9. Record the mean PAWP over several respiratory cycles.

10. After satisfactory pressures are obtained, withdraw the catheter (or deflate the balloon) to allow the catheter tip to rest in the right or left PA while left heart catheterization is performed. The catheter should not be left in the wedge position for any length of time.

Alternate procedure

An alternate method of right heart catheterization favored by many physicians includes rapid passage of the catheter out to the PA wedge position. Pressures and blood samples are then obtained during catheter pullback from the PA wedge position to the PA, RV, and RA. This technique reduces the time of catheter manipulation and therefore softening, and it provides right heart pressures that are more closely related in time.

Measurement of cardiac output

Determination of cardiac output and right heart pressures is performed during a stable period of rest and, if necessary, during exercise by the thermodilution or Fick method. The thermodilution technique is discussed in detail on p. 94. Cardiac output determination by the Fick method requires collection of the patient's expired gas over a stable 5- or 6-minute period for calculation of oxygen consumption. Simultaneous blood samples are slowly withdrawn from the PA and a systemic artery midway during the gas collection for oxygen analysis and calculation of arteriovenous oxygen difference. Cardiac output is calculated by means of the Fick principle (see Appendix G).

Detection of intracardiac shunts

If an intracardiac shunt is suspected, multiple blood samples should be drawn from various locations within the heart and great vessels for determination of oxygen saturation and content. An abnormal increase in the oxygen saturation of blood from one intracardiac site to another indicates a left-to-right shunt. Appendix D lists (1) normal oxygen saturations in different cardiac chambers, (2) the saturation change between cardiac chambers suggesting a left-to-right shunt, and (3) variations in oxygen content that typically occur with specific left-to-right shunts. However, very small intracardiac shunts can be overlooked by the oxymetric technique, particularly if the catheter tip is not located at or near the exact area of shunting. Hypoxia, valvular incompetence, and alterations in the patient's metabolic, respiratory, or circulatory state also complicate interpretation of apparent differences. In such instances the use of the indicator dilution technique is a more sensitive method of detection and localization of an intracardiac shunt. Injection of indocyanine green dye into the right side of the heart with photoelectric detection of the appearance of the dye in the systemic blood has traditionally been the method of shunt detection.

Hydrogen curve technique

A faster and simpler method of indicator dilution is the hydrogen curve technique, in which a platinum-tip catheter is inserted into the right side of the heart and the patient inhales a breath of hydrogen. A small ($\leq$500

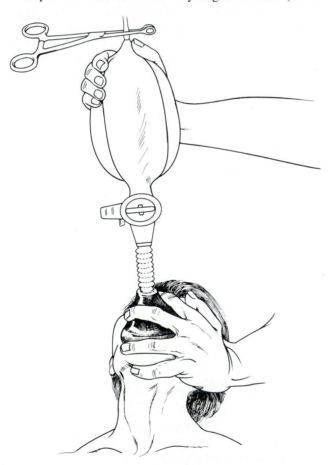

Fig. 5-4. Mask, valve, and gas bag used for inhalation of the hydrogen during the hydrogen curve technique for shunt detection.

ml) rubber bag connected to an oronasal mask or mouthpiece via a one-way valve is used for inhalation of the hydrogen gas (Fig. 5-4). Since hydrogen produces a significant potential when it comes into contact with platinum, its appearance time can be measured and evaluated in various locations within the heart. Early detection of hydrogen is seen in patients with left-to-right shunt.

Before the performance of hydrogen curve analysis, the procedure should be explained to the patient and the patient should practice it. The gas bag should be filled with room air for this trial run. The mouthpiece is placed in the patient's mouth (or the mask over the nose and mouth), and the patient is instructed to breathe quietly. After several seconds, the patient is asked to inhale deeply as the one-way valve is opened. If a mouthpiece rather than a mask is used, the nostrils should be pinched during inhalation to ensure complete inhalation from the bag. The actual test is as follows:

1. Insert a plantinum-tip catheter (6, 7, or 8 Fr) into the PA wedge position (verify by fluoroscopy and pressure).

2. With an alligator connecting cable, connect the metal hub of the catheter to the V lead of an ECG cable.

3. Connect the ECG cable to an ECG amplifier.

4. Select the V lead on the ECG amplifier and adjust the sensitivity to obtain a suitable response.

5. Flush the air out of the bag by filling and emptying it at least three times with hydrogen. (*Note:* Because hydrogen is flammable, the gas tank should be stored outside the catheterization laboratory and the hydrogen expelled from the bag into an outside area.)

6. Fill the gas bag with hydrogen and close the clamp.

7. Place the mouthpiece in the patient's mouth or place the mask over the nose and mouth.

8. Record a baseline intracardiac signal.

9. While recording, open the one-way stopcock (pinch the patient's nose, if necessary) and instruct the patient to take a single, deep breath of hydrogen. The recorder should mark the moment of inhalation, as timing is obtained from the calibrated recording. In the PA wedge position, the intracardiac signal should deflect very quickly ($<$5 seconds) after inhalation of hydrogen. If this does not occur, a new alligator connector or a new platinum-tip catheter should be used and retested in the wedge position.

10. If this is successful, withdraw the catheter to the PA and repeat steps 8 and 9 using fresh hydrogen in the gas bag.

11. Withdraw the catheter to the RV, RA, and supe-

rior vena cava, performing hydrogen curve test in each location. Early detection of hydrogen in any site indicates left-to-right shunt. To limit the number of inhalations and recordings, the first determination may be done with the plantinum-tip catheter just distal to the site of suspected left-to-right shunt. A positive response (early hydrogen appearance time) establishes the diagnosis, and further determinations may not be necessary. This shortcut is not feasible when more than one left-to-right shunt is suspected. Fig. 5-5 shows representative hydrogen potential curves from various parts of the circulation.

LEFT HEART CATHETERIZATION

Left heart catheterization studies consist of aortic and left heart hemodynamic pressure recording and angiography (coronary arteries, grafts, aortic root, and LV).

Catheterization is performed either via the transbrachial method of Sones[19,20] with brachial artery cutdown or via the percutaneous Seldinger technique with the femoral artery approach.[21,22] Other approaches include percutaneous entry via the axillary or brachial artery. Transseptal entry or direct LV puncture can also be per-

formed in unusual cases. Table 5-3 summarizes the characteristics of the catheters commonly used for left heart catheterization and coronary arteriography. Only selected topics are discussed here.

Transbrachial approach of Sones

The technique of arteriotomy has already been discussed (p. 78), and the Sones catheter has been described (Chapter 1). The Sones catheter has a stiff shaft (7 or 8 Fr), but its tapered tip (5 Fr) with two side holes is quite flexible, permitting gentle entry into a coronary artery ostium. It is also suitable for selective catheterization of aortocoronary vein bypass grafts. For internal mammary artery grafts, the polyurethane Cordis brachial artery catheter is used with preforming.

1. After arteriotomy, introduce the catheter into the brachial artery.

2. Use systemic administration of heparin in addition to injection of 3000 to 4000 units of heparin into the distal portion of the brachial artery.

3. Connect the catheter to the manifold system, fill the catheter with contrast material, and advance it through the subclavian and innominate arteries and into

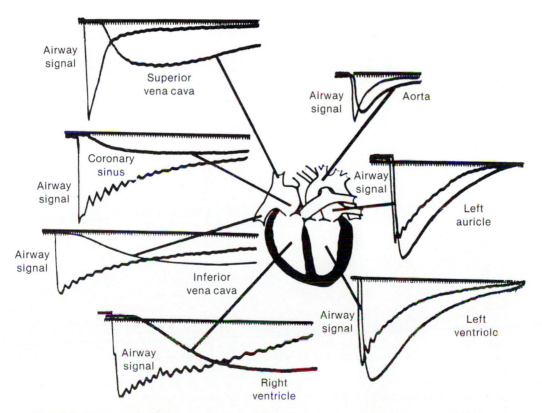

Fig. 5-5. Hydrogen potential curves from various parts of the circulation. (From Zimmerman, H.A.: Intravascular catheterization, 1966. Courtesy of Charles C Thomas, Publisher, Springfield, Ill.)

Table 5-3. Left heart catheters in common use for selective coronary arteriography and ventriculography*

Catheter (year introduced)	Vascular entry	Catheter design	Catheter sizes

Sones (1960)	Brachial artery cutdown	Woven Dacron; end hole; two small side holes close to tip (original)	7 & 8 Fr
			Type I: 80 & 100 cm
			  Tapered tip: 3.8 cm, 5 Fr
			  Style: A or B curve†
			Type II: 80 & 100 cm
			  Tapered tip: 2.5 cm, 5 Fr
			  Style: B curve

		Cordis brachial coronary catheter; polyurethane; end hole & 4 side holes	7 & 8 Fr, 80 and 100 cm

Judkins (1967)	Percutaneous (femoral or axillary)	Polyurethane or polyethylene; metal braided: end hole only
		Primary curve 90° (right & left catheter); secondary curve 180° (left coronary catheter); 30° (right coronary catheter)
		Gentle tertiary reverse curve on right coronary catheter
			5, 6, 7, & 8 Fr
			Tip: 5 Fr, 18 mm
			Length: 100 cm
			Secondary curve‡
			  Left catheter: 3.5, 4, 5, & 6 cm
			  Right catheter: 3.5, 4, & 5 cm

Amplatz (1967)	Percutaneous (femoral or axillary); may also be used via brachial artery cutdown (Castillo modification, see below)	Polyurethane or polyethylene; preformed with end hole only; various curve sizes	5, 6, 7, & 8 Fr
			Tip: 5 Fr
			Length: 100 cm
			Curve size§
			  Left: 1, 2, 3, 4
			  Right: 1 & 2

Castillo‖ (1973)	Brachial artery cutdown	Polyurethane preformed; end hole only; varying curves	7 & 8 Fr, 80 cm; sizes I, II, III
Schoonmaker (1974)	Percutaneous (femoral or axillary)	Polyurethane with wire mesh; end hole & 2 side holes.	7 & 8 Fr Length: 100 cm 45° Curve, slightly tapered flexible tip
El Gamal (1980)	Same as above	Similar to Schoonmaker but with variable tip lengths	7 & 8 Fr Length: 100 cm 80° curve, tapered tip; tip length varies 40-45-50 mm¶

*For discussion see text.
†Style A: Preformed curve of 7.5 cm from the tip; available in 80, 100, and 125 cm lengths. Style B: Preformed curve of 3.8 cm from the tip; with narrow aortic root.
‡For Judkins catheters the numbers refer to the length (cm) of the secondary arm. For the left coronary catheter it refers to the length of the primary and secondary curves. For the right coronary catheter, the size reflects the distance (cm) from the primary curve to the midpoint of the is 4 cm.
§For Amplatz catheters the numerical designation refers to the overall size of the curved portion of the catheter.
‖Amplatz catheter has been modified (Castillo, 1973) to facilitate its use via the brachial artery approach. It has a smaller main curve and a with a side hole, these catheters now have only end holes.
¶For El Gamal catheters the tip length is the distance from the shaft of the catheter to end opening, measured perpendicularly.

Choice of catheter	Comments	
Same catheter for right & left coronary, graft, & LV angiography	Proven record of 25 years; requires surgical exposure of artery & ability to form & direct catheter in aortic root See references 19,20	**Curve Style A** 1 ½ inch Tip
Same	Flexible; can be preshaped	**Curve Style B** 1 ½ inch Tip
See text	Catheter is preformed Shape can be changed by reforming with steam See references 21, 22, 24	
AR & AL1 & 2 (most cases); AL3 or AL4 for patients with dilated roots; separate catheter for each coronary artery	Catheter is preformed Shape can be changed by reforming with steam See references 4, 23	Right I Right II Left I Left II
Brachial coronary II: normal aortic root Brachial coronary I: narrow aortic root Brachial coronary III: dilated aortic root Same catheter for both right & left coronary arteries	Permits use of preformed catheter for brachial artery approach See references 25, 26	Type I Type II Type III
Right & left coronary artery, LV, & vein bypass graft, all with one catheter	Multipurpose catheter requiring forming and maneuvering in aortic root See reference 27, 28	
Right & left coronary artery, vein bypass graft	Multipurpose catheter similar to above See reference 29	

available only in 80 and 100 cm. Most procedures can be performed with type I catheter using style B curve. Type II catheters are used in patient

segment between the primary curve and the secondary curve. Thus JL4 refers to a Judkins left coronary catheter with a 4 cm arm between the secondary curve. Thus JR4 is a Judkins right coronary catheter where the distance from the primary curve to the midpoint of the secondary curve

reduced hooklike shape distally, facilitating right and left coronary catheterization via the brachial approach with one catheter. Originally designed

Table 5-3. Left heart catheters in common use for selective coronary arteriography and ventriculography—cont'd

Catheter (year introduced)	Vascular entry	Catheter design	Catheter sizes
Coronary vein bypass graft catheter I (left or right)	Percutaneous	Polyurethane or polyethelene Right vein bypass: 110°-120° primary curve, 30° secondary curve Left vein bypass: 90° primary curve, 30° secondary curve	7 & 8 Fr Length: 100 cm
II (B₁)	Same as above	2 Circular bends in opposite directions 90° Curved tip	7 & 8 Fr Length: 100 cm
Internal mammary catheter	Same as above May be used via brachial cutdown	Polyurethane with wire mesh; similar to right coronary Judkins catheter with primary curve 80°-85° & tip length 1.5-2.0 cm	7 & 8 Fr Length: 100 cm
Pigtail ventriculography catheter (1967-1968)	Same as above	Polyurethane, 5 cm tapered terminal segment curled to loop; 4 or more side holes & end hole	5-8 Fr Length: 110 cm Van Tassel modification: 145° & 155° curve

the aortic arch, using fluoroscopy and pressure monitoring. The pressure waveform will be slightly damped because of the dye-filled catheter.

4. Advance the catheter to the central aorta. If the subclavian artery is tortuous, ask the patient to take a deep breath, raise the shoulder, or turn the head to the left while you gently manipulate the catheter. If this is not promptly successful, insert a flexible J-tip safety guidewire (0.035 inch, 0.9 mm) to negotiate the vessel without causing vascular injury. *Never apply force* in advancing the catheter, as this will risk vascular dissection.

5. Administer 0.3 mg of nitroglycerin sublingually.

6. Advance the catheter tip to the left sinus of Valsalva in the left anterior oblique projection and press it against the aortic valve, forming a J loop approximately 1½ inches long in the right aortic cusp (Fig. 5-6).

7. Attempt to engage the left coronary ostium by moving the catheter up and down in an alternating advancement and withdrawal motion, while maintaining its J-tip configuration. Having the patient take a deep breath helps this maneuver.

8. Inject small amounts of contrast medium to confirm the position of the catheter tip and its relation to the left coronary ostium. When the catheter tip engages the left coronary ostium, tip motion is reduced. Stabilize the catheter tip in the coronary ostium by gently advancing the catheter. If a long loop is present, slight retraction of the catheter may be needed.

9. Inject small amounts of contrast medium to confirm proper and stable positioning.

10. Check aortic pressure at the catheter tip to ensure the absence of damping.

11. Proceed with selective arteriography of the left coronary artery in various rotations and angulations with a rapid (2- to 3-second) manual injection of radiocontrast material (5 to 7 ml/injection). Injections are made during full inspiration to avoid imaging of the diaphragm. Have the patient cough and take a deep breath after each injection. Allow the ECG and blood pressure to stabilize and check the catheter tip pressure before each injection.

12. If left main coronary artery or ostial stenosis is suspected, repeat the injection as the catheter is pulled

Choice of catheter	Comments	
Selective catheterization of aortocoronary vein graft, right & left coronary artery	Judkins or Amplatz right coronary catheters, also suitable for graft angiography See references 22, 29, 30	
Right coronary bypass grafts with superior origin	Used infrequently	
Selective catheterization of internal mammary grafts	Judkins right coronary catheter, JR4 can also be used for internal mammary grafts See references 22, 30, 31	
Left ventriculography & aortography	Nontraumatic design Reduced chance of arrhythmias during ventriculography Excellent contrast delivery See references 22, 24	

back into the left coronary sinus. After stabilization, follow this with a nonselective injection in the left sinus of Valsalva.

13. After satisfactory completion of the left coronary arteriogram, remove the catheter from the left ostium back into the left coronary sinus, maintaining a smaller loop at the catheter tip.

14. Rotate the catheter shaft clockwise (Fig. 5-6) while slowly withdrawing it to displace the catheter tip anteriorly and into the right sinus of Valsalva (a counterclockwise rotation will displace the catheter tip posteriorly and to the left into the noncoronary sinus). A rapid in-and-out motion of the catheter over a few millimeters helps in transmitting this torque. As the catheter tip enters the right coronary sinus, it usually falls in the right coronary ostium; further rotation is not applied and the initial torque is partially reversed to prevent "overshoot." Having the patient take a deep breath will help this maneuver.

15. Observe the aortic pressure at the catheter tip. If the pressure appears damped, withdraw the catheter, because the catheter tip may be selectively in the conus artery or may have advanced deep into the right coronary artery, occluding the vessel with its 7 or 8 Fr shaft.

16. Complete the right coronary arteriogram in multiple views, manually injecting 5 to 6 ml of radiocontrast agent.

17. After satisfactory completion of the right coronary arteriogram, draw the catheter backward above the sinus of Valsalva.

18. Advance the catheter across the aortic valve to the LV, avoiding the right and left coronary arteries. To do this, form a long loop with the catheter by pushing its tip against the aortic valve and then gently and rapidly moving the catheter up and down against the aortic valve while rotating it clockwise. This can be done in the left or right anterior oblique projection.

19. For crossing tight aortic stenosis, advance the catheter tip straight, without a loop, through the aortic valve; a guidewire may be required.

20. After the catheter enters the LV, direct its tip toward the LV apex and confirm its position in both left and right anterior oblique projections.

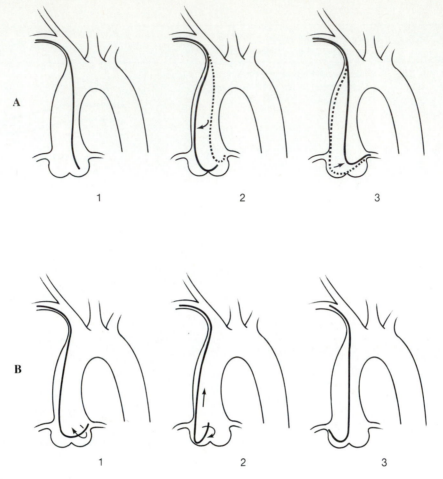

Fig. 5-6. Catheterization of the left **(A)** and right **(B)** coronary arteries in the left anterior oblique projection using the Sones technique.

The Sones catheter is adequate (but not ideal) for ventriculography, as the tapered (5 Fr) tip limits the volume of contrast material delivered and the end hole causes the catheter to recoil. Ectopic beats are routinely seen during LV angiography. Ventriculography can be performed with a power injection of 30 to 40 ml of contrast agent at a rate of 10 to 15 ml/second.

This brief description of the Sones method of coronary arteriography may make the technique appear deceptively simple. Experience and subtle catheter manipulation are required for the safe and satisfactory use of the technique, especially in difficult cases. Hands-on experience with close supervision is required to master the technique. The reader is referred to the superb illustrations and the detailed description of this technique as found in the report by Huepler.[20]

Femoral artery approach of Judkins

Three catheters are usually needed for a complete diagnostic study—a left coronary artery catheter, a right coronary artery catheter, and a pigtail angiographic catheter.[21,22] The sequence in which the study is performed is up to the angiographer. A good general policy is to obtain the most important information first and then proceed, leaving the least critical study for last. With this approach, we usually perform the left coronary arteriogram first, followed by right coronary arteriogram, and finally the left ventriculogram.

1. Choose the correct-size left coronary artery catheter based on review of the patient's chest radiograph, age, and body size and the presence or absence of aortic valve disease or hypertension (see Table 5-3). Success of selective coronary arteriography with use of the Jud-

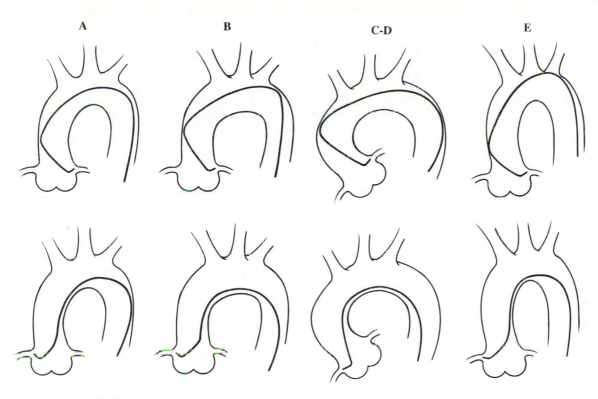

Fig. 5-7. Choice of proper catheter size for selective coronary arteriography via the Judkins technique. Catheter sizes (cm) refer to the secondary bend (see Table 5-3). **A,** Normal-size aorta without dilatation or distortion (4L, 4R). **B,** Rounded and unfolded aorta: hypertension, advanced age, aortic stenosis with mild poststenotic dilatation (5L, 4R). **C,** Significant aortic stenosis with definite poststenotic dilatation (5-6L, 5R). **D,** Severe aortic dilatation, ascending aortic aneurysm, Marfan's syndrome (7-9L [special order], 5R). **E,** Small aortic arch in small women and children (3.5L, rarely 3.0 [special order], 3.5R).

kins-type catheter is predicated on selection of correct catheter size (Fig. 5-7).

2. Catheterize the femoral artery as described on p. 71.

3. If an arterial sheath is used, institute systemic administration of heparin after the sheath is securely in place. Insert the coronary artery catheter through the sheath with a safety guidewire (with the guidewire leading) and advance it with the aid of fluoroscopy via the femoral and iliac arteries up the thoracic aorta until the tip of the guidewire reaches the distal aortic arch. Hold the guidewire and advance the catheter over it to a neutral position in the aortic arch.

If resistance is met and gentle guidewire manipulation does not overcome it, remove the guidewire and inject a small amount of contrast medium through the catheter both to confirm the intravascular location of the catheter tip and to outline the vascular anatomy around the catheter tip as an aid in guidewire and catheter manipulation.

4. Remove the guidewire, aspirate the catheter, discard the aspirated fluid, manually flush the catheter with heparin-saline solution, and connect it to the contrast-filled manifold and syringe.

5. Record the catheter tip aortic pressure.

6. Fill the catheter with contrast medium.

7. Slowly advance the catheter down the medial wall of the ascending aorta. If the correct catheter size has been chosen, the catheter will rotate slightly and seek and engage the left coronary ostium without requiring any manipulation (Fig. 5-8).

8. Advance the catheter a few millimeters farther to

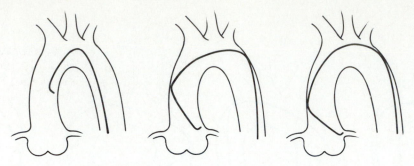

Fig. 5-8. Catheterization of the left coronary artery (Judkins method, left anterior oblique projection). The correct-size Judkins catheter, when advanced down the medial wall of the ascending aorta, rotates slightly, seeks, and engages the left coronary ostium.

relieve any tension on it. The catheter position is usually very stable with the tip in the left coronary artery orifice and the secondary bend resting on the medial aortic wall.

9. Inject a small amount of contrast medium to check catheter position and correct tip alignment. The catheter tip should be free, pointing in the direction of blood flow and not directly at the artery wall. There should be no pressure damping.

10. Perform left coronary arteriograms in various projections with a hand injection of 6 to 8 ml of contrast medium over 2 to 3 seconds. Check the catheter tip pressure before each injection. Permit enough time between injections for heart rate, ECG, and blood pressure changes to stabilize. We ask the patient to cough twice, follow this with a deep breath, and then continue breathing normally. This maneuver seems to shorten the period of hypotension and bradycardia following coronary artery injections. The catheter is not withdrawn during this time as long as tip pressure is not damped.

11. After completion of the left coronary arteriogram, withdraw the catheter to the abdominal aorta at a level below the renal arteries.

12. If an arterial sheath has been used, pull out this catheter (a guidewire for removal of the catheter is not necessary) and introduce the right coronary artery catheter in a manner similar to that for the left coronary artery catheter. *Note:* If an arterial sheath has been used but tortuous iliac vessels were encountered with insertion of the first catheter, requiring guidewire and catheter manipulation, then introduce a guidewire through the left coronary artery catheter and position it in the abdominal aorta, remove the catheter, wipe the guidewire clean, and introduce the right coronary catheter over the guidewire into the abdominal aorta and up to the aortic arch. You may need to pinch the introducer during this exchange to prevent back-bleeding. An alternate approach would be to use a 25 cm long introducer that will bypass the iliac tortuosity and will improve catheter torque control (Fig. 5-9).

If an arterial introducer is not used, it may be safer to first position the coronary catheter in the abdominal aorta below the renal arteries, flush the catheter clear, and then advance it across the aortic arch, preferably with the help of a guidewire. A J-curve guidewire should be used in all cases where atherosclerotic involvement of the aorta is present or suspected.

13. Fill the right coronary artery catheter with contrast medium and advance it under fluoroscopic and pressure monitoring to the central aorta. This catheter (unlike the left coronary artery catheter) will not head directly for the appropriate coronary ostium and must be directed.

14. Advance the catheter to 1 to 2 cm above the level of the left coronary artery orifice and 2 to 4 cm above the level of the aortic valve (Fig. 5-10).

15. *Very slowly* apply clockwise rotation (torque) to the catheter hub. Do not use excessive torque. As the clockwise rotation approaches 60°, the catheter tip will rotate anteriorly and to the right and will fall 2 to 3 cm into the right sinus of Valsalva. Continue slow clockwise rotation and observe the catheter tip as it drops into the right coronary artery orifice. If the catheter rotates properly but does not drop in the right coronary orifice (seen in patients with high aortic arches), advance the catheter during subsequent rotation to facilitate its correct entry. If rotation was started too low, the catheter tip will fall into the right sinus of Valsalva or across the aortic valve. If rotation was started too high, the catheter tip will flip in the ascending aorta.

16. Check the pressure at the catheter tip. If it is damped, gently withdraw the catheter until the pressure is satisfactory.

17. Inject a small amount of contrast medium to confirm proper catheter tip position.

18. Proceed with right coronary arteriography in mul-

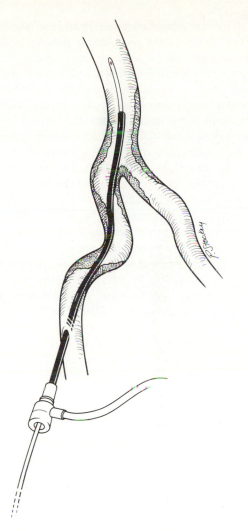

Fig. 5-9. Use of a 25 cm long introducer improves catheter torque control and facilitates passage through an atherosclerotic and tortuous artery.

tiple projections, rapidly and manually injecting 4 to 6 ml of contrast material.

19. If easy selective catheterization is not accomplished early in the study, do not waste time trying to manipulate this preformed catheter. Recognize and correct the mistake by changing to a proper catheter size. Catheter maneuvers used for the Sones or multipurpose Schoonmaker-King catheter are entirely inappropriate for these preformed catheters.

20. Withdraw the right coronary artery catheter to the abdominal aorta below the level of the renal arteries. Follow step 12 in removing this catheter and introducing the pigtail ventriculographic catheter over a guidewire.

21. Remove the guidewire and advance the pigtail catheter to the aortic root and across the aortic valve, and position it in the LV. Check pressures. If the catheter does not directly cross the aortic valve, a simple maneuver will help its passage: In the anteroposterior or 15° right anterior oblique projection advance the pigtail to the aortic valve area. Apply firm, sustained, but gentle pressure, causing the distal catheter to form a wide loop of 2 to 3 cm just above the aortic valve, and then gently withdraw the catheter until its pigtail tip drops into the sinus of Valsalva. Withdraw the catheter 1 to 3 cm and then advance it across the open valve during systole.

22. If this is not helpful, insert a guidewire to help guide the catheter across the aortic valve. Judkins advocates positioning the coiled loop of the pigtail catheter in the LV inflow tract to permit optimal mixing of contrast agent with blood and reduce ventricular ectopic beats. This is achieved by withdrawing the catheter from its neutral position 2 to 3 cm, rotating it 70° to 90° counterclockwise, and advancing it until a stable

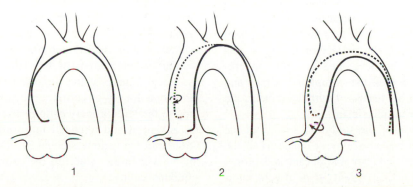

Fig. 5-10. Catheterization of the right coronary artery (Judkins method, left anterior oblique projection). The catheter is advanced to 1 to 2 cm above the left coronary orifice *(1)*. The catheter hub is slowly rotated clockwise *(2)*, and the catheter tip falls into the right coronary artery orifice *(3)*.

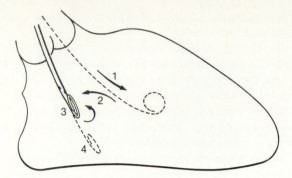

Fig. 5-11. Judkins method of left ventricular catheterization. Having crossed the aortic valve, the pigtail catheter will be in position *(1)*. The catheter is withdrawn 2 to 3 cm and rotated 70° to 90° counterclockwise *(2)*. The coiled loop will be in the inflow tract of the mitral valve *(3)*. If the catheter moves excessively in this position, it should be advanced until it is stable *(4)*. (From Judkins, M.P., and Judkins, E.: Coronary arteriography and left ventriculography: Judkins technique. In King, S.B. III, and Douglas, J.S., Jr.: Coronary arteriography and angioplasty, New York, 1985, McGraw-Hill Book Co., p. 201. Reproduced with permission.)

position is obtained above the base of the LV (Fig. 5-11).

23. Perform a test injection with 5 to 8 ml of contrast agent to confirm satisfactory catheter position.

24. Proceed to left ventriculography in the 30° right anterior oblique projection (and 60° left anterior oblique if necessary) with a power injection of 30 to 45 ml of contrast agent at 12 to 15 ml/second.

25. Obtain left ventricular pressures before and after the ventricular injections.

26. Pull the catheter back to the aorta while recording a pullback pressure, then pull the catheter to the abdominal aorta below the renal arteries.

27. Review the entire study on videotape playback to ensure that all necessary information is obtained. It is a good policy not to immediately discuss the preliminary (videotape) findings with the patient or family at this stage. Cine films may be developed promptly and reviewed with care, and then the complete findings and recommendations can be discussed with the patient, the family, and the referring physician.

28. After completion of the study and review of the preliminary data, the decision may be made as to the removal of the arterial catheter and sheath and proper location for monitoring the patient. If no urgent intervention is planned and if the patient's condition is stable, the catheter and sheath can be removed in the cardiac catheterization laboratory or adjacent holding area. High-risk patients (e.g., those with severe coronary dis-

ease or critical aortic stenosis) should be moved to a monitored special care unit. Stable patients with noncritical disease can be observed in a general recovery area or regular hospital bed. If the patient's condition is unstable, early intervention is anticipated (angioplasty, operation), or the cine films need to be scrutinized before a decision is made, secure the arterial catheter/ sheath unit with sutures, continue systemic administration of heparin, and transfer the patient to a closely monitored area. This permits hemodynamic monitoring and continuation of heparin treatment and leaves the options open for prompt angioplasty or use of a thrombolytic agent. Such catheters may be kept in place for 24 to 48 hours or longer, if necessary. Heparin is discontinued 2 to 3 hours before their removal.

29. After catheter and sheath removal, establish adequate hemostasis with 10 minutes of *manual* pressure. This will be time well invested, as it will help prevent puncture site complications. Compression that is too forceful will occlude the flow and risk femoral artery thrombosis, whereas inadequate compression will risk bleeding. Check distal pulses to confirm flow. Once hemostasis is established by manual compression, you can delegate this function to an assistant. Mechanical devices (sandbags, clamps) should not be used for compression of the femoral artery at this stage. For use of protamine see p. 147.

Variations of the femoral artery approach

Table 5-3 outlines other catheters that use modifications of this basic theme. Complete description of each technique and variation is beyond the scope of this discussion. The reader should consult the cited references for details.

Amplatz technique

Amplatz catheters, first used in 1967, offer an alternative to coronary arteriography via the femoral approach.[4,23] This catheter is also suitable for selective catheterization of aortocoronary vein grafts.

For catheterization of the left coronary artery, the secondary curve of the catheter (AL1 to AL4) rests on the noncoronary posterior aortic cusp, with its tip pointing to the left coronary ostium (Fig. 5-12). The catheter is advanced and retracted in an alternating gentle motion until the ostium is engaged. Slight retraction at this point will further stabilize the catheter tip. As with the Judkins catheter, it is necessary to use a proper-size catheter to match the size of the aortic root.

The right coronary artery catheter (AR1 or AR2) initially may point to the left coronary sinus (Fig. 5-12). It should be withdrawn slightly and rotated clockwise

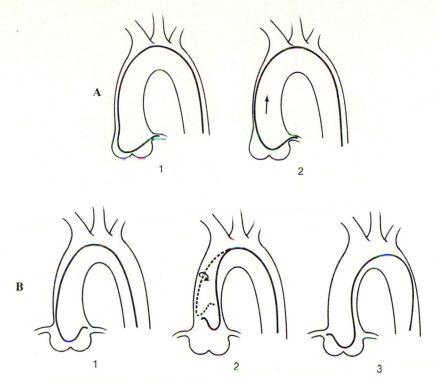

Fig. 5-12. Catheterization of the coronary arteries (Amplatz technique, left anterior oblique projection). **A,** Catheterization of the left coronary artery. (*1*) The left coronary catheter is advanced until the secondary curve rests in the noncoronary posterior aortic cusp and its tip points to the left coronary ostium. (*2*) The catheter is gently advanced and retracted until the left coronary ostium is engaged. **B,** Catheterization of the right coronary artery. (*1*) The right coronary catheter may initially point to the left coronary sinus. (*2*) It is withdrawn slightly and rotated clockwise until the tip points toward the right coronary artery and the secondary curve rests against the left aortic cusp. (*3*) The right coronary artery is engaged as the catheter is advanced and withdrawn.

(similar to the Judkins right coronary artery catheter) until the tip points toward the right coronary artery and the secondary curve rests against the left aortic cusp. Slight advancement and withdrawal will engage the right coronary ostium.

Castillo modification of the Amplatz technique

Wells et al.[25] and Zir et al.[26] modified the Amplatz catheter by using a smaller curve and reduced hooklike shape toward the tip, making it suitable for use via the brachial artery approach (Fig. 5-13). Usually the same catheter is used for the right and left coronary arteries.

Catheter manipulation, seating, and tip positioning are similar to those used for the Amplatz catheter. Again the catheter curve size (I to III) must be matched with the size of the aortic root and sinus of Valsalva. Once this is achieved, stable catheter position requires minimal manipulation. If a rotating cradle is used and the catheter is introduced via the right brachial artery,

the catheter is advanced slightly when the patient is rotated into the right anterior oblique position so that it will not fall out of the coronary ostium, and it is then withdrawn slightly while the patient is rotated to the left anterior oblique position to prevent advancement of the catheter deep into the coronary artery. If the catheter is introduced via the left brachial artery, these maneuvers are reversed.

Schoonmaker-King technique

The Schoonmaker-King multipurpose catheter technique was described in 1974.[27,28] A single catheter is used for left and right selective coronary arteriography, vein graft angiography, and ventriculography via the femoral artery approach. This is not a preformed catheter, and manipulation and forming of its flexible tip are required for selective catheterization of the coronary arteries. This technique offers the advantage of one-catheter use and the ability to form the catheter curve and

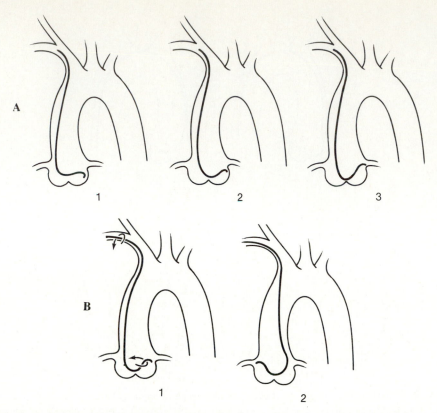

Fig. 5-13. Castillo modification of the Amplatz technique. **A,** Catheterization of the left coronary artery. (*1*) The Castillo catheter is advanced until the secondary curve rests in the noncoronary posterior aortic cusp and its tip points to the left coronary ostium. (*2 and 3*) The catheter is gently advanced and retracted until the left coronary ostium is engaged. **B,** Catheterization of the right coronary artery. (*1*) Initially the catheter points to the left coronary sinus. (*2*) It is withdrawn slightly and rotated until the tip points toward the right coronary artery. The right coronary ostium is engaged as the catheter is advanced and withdrawn.

thus be able to handle anatomic variations. Consistent, selective, and stable catheterization of the left coronary artery is not always possible (as with the Sones catheter), and subselective injections in the left coronary cusp are sometimes used. This catheter is frequently used as a second-choice catheter when the preformed catheters have not been satisfactory.

Coronary vein grafts

The Judkins and Amplatz right coronary artery catheters as well as the Schoonmaker-King multipurpose and Sones catheters are frequently successful for selective catheterization of vein grafts.[22,30] Special graft catheters are available, facilitating graft angiography. The Judkins right vein bypass catheter is similar to the right coronary artery catheter, but its tip (primary curve) is modified from 90° to 100° to form a smooth, downward-pointing 3 cm curve. This catheter can also be used to catheterize the right coronary artery. This graft catheter is rotated in a manner similar to that for the right coronary artery catheter (clockwise catheter hub rotation, left anterior oblique projection), but rotation is started 2 to 3 cm higher and continued until its tip is superior to the anticipated site of the graft orifice (Fig. 5-14). The catheter is then advanced down the aortic wall to the orifice of the graft. If the rotation is started lower, the catheter may be slowly withdrawn during the rotation, permitting entry into the graft.

The Judkins left vein bypass graft catheter has a 90° primary curve similar to that of the right coronary artery catheter, but it has a 70° secondary curve. Thus it has an upward-pointing tip and is more suitable for grafts to the left anterior descending and left circumflex arteries, where the initial segment of the graft frequently points upward. These left vein grafts may be sought in the left or right anterior oblique projection where the left vein bypass catheter is rotated clockwise and advanced into the graft.

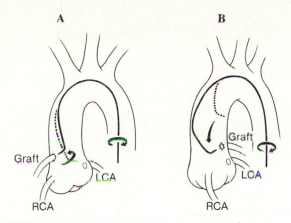

Fig. 5-14. Use of the Judkins right and left vein bypass catheters. **A,** For right coronary artery *(RCA)* grafts, the catheter is rotated clockwise in the left anterior oblique projection until its tip is superior to the graft orifice. It is then advanced down the aortic wall to the orifice of the graft. **B,** For left coronary artery *(LCA)* grafts, clockwise rotation is applied in the left or right anterior oblique projection.

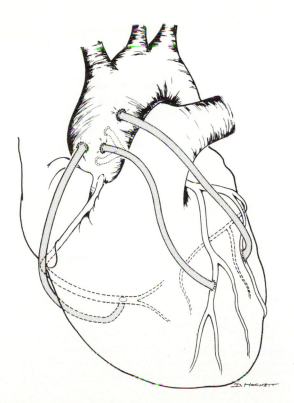

Fig. 5-15. Usual insertion sites of vein grafts to coronary arteries. The proximal (aortic) anastomosis site of the graft to the right coronary artery is most anterior and usually the lowest. Grafts to the branches of the left coronary artery are usually inserted in a progressively higher and more posterolateral position. Variations frequently occur.

The aortic insertion (origin) of these grafts is to the anterolateral surface of the ascending aorta, 2 to 3 cm above the origin of the native coronary arteries. Usually the graft to the right coronary artery is lowest. Above and to its left is the origin of the graft to the left anterior descending artery, and most superior and leftward in origin is usually the graft to the diagonal and marginal arteries (Fig. 5-15).

Metal clips or rings are frequently used during surgery to mark these grafts and facilitate angiography. These markers can be misplaced or may migrate and cannot be consistently relied on. A helpful initial approach may be to perform an aortic root angiogram, with the pigtail catheter positioned 3 to 4 cm above the aortic valve. This may help locate the origin and the course of the graft and can be used as a "map" for subsequent selective graft angiography. Digital subtraction techniques can further improve graft visualization.

Internal mammary artery grafts

Internal mammary artery grafts have become popular because of demonstrated superiority of their long-term patency rates.[31-33] Selective catheterization of these arteries is best achieved in the anteroposterior projection by means of a specially designed, preformed catheter, which resembles a Judkins right coronary artery catheter except at its tip, which has a primary curve of 80° to 85° and a length of 1.5 to 2.0 cm. This sharply angled tip facilitates selective entry into the origin of the internal mammary artery, which branches off from the subclavian artery at an acute angle. This catheter should be handled gently, as it has a stiff tip and can cause trauma or dissection. The standard Judkins right coronary catheter is sometimes suitable but frequently not optimal for this purpose, whereas the Amplatz and multipurpose catheters are unsuitable. For catheterization of the left internal mammary artery, the catheter is first placed in the aortic arch in a neutral position with its tip pointing downward (Fig. 5-16). It is then rotated counterclockwise until it falls into the left subclavian artery. It is advanced with a slight anterior rotation of its tip until it engages the origin of the left internal mammary artery, just distal to the origin of the left vertebral artery.

Entry into the right internal mammary artery is accomplished by counterclockwise rotation of the catheter just at the orifice of the right innominate artery, past the origin of the right internal carotid artery, followed by advancement until it engages the orifice of the internal mammary artery (Fig. 5-16). At this stage it helps to point the catheter tip in a lateral direction. A guidewire may be used to facilitate entry to the left subclavian or

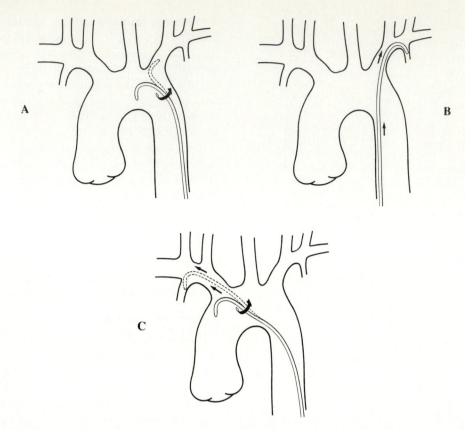

Fig. 5-16. Catheterization of the internal mammary arteries. **A,** To catheterize the left internal mammary artery, the catheter is located in the aortic arch in a neutral position, with its tip pointing downward. The catheter is then rotated counterclockwise until it falls into the left subclavian artery. **B,** The catheter is then advanced with a slight anterior rotation until it engages the origin of the left internal mammary artery. **C,** The right internal mammary artery is entered by counterclockwise rotation of the catheter at the origin of the right innominate artery and advanced until the origin of the internal mammary artery is engaged.

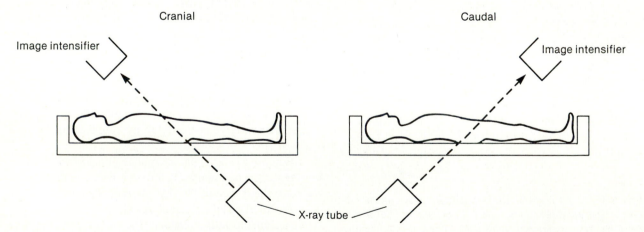

Fig. 5-17. Position of the x-ray tube relative to the image intensifier for cranial and caudal angulations.

right innominate artery. Before full injection and cine filming are done, test injections should be performed to confirm satisfactory catheter position. The contrast agent may be diluted to reduce the patient's discomfort and avoid delivery of concentrated contrast material to the vertebral circulation.

ANGLED PROJECTIONS IN CORONARY ARTERIOGRAPHY

During the 1960s and early 1970s coronary arteriography was performed with use of a fixed x-ray tube perpendicular to the long axis of the patient. Oblique projections in the transverse plane were made by rotating the patient. A complete study generally included projections in the anteroposterior, steep (60° to 70°) left anterior oblique, and shallow (20° to 30°) and steep (60° to 70°) right anterior oblique positions.

During the past 10 years the clinical value of adding angulation of the x-ray beam to the transverse oblique projections has been amply illustrated.[34-36] Modern radiographic equipment used for coronary arteriography uses x-ray tubes and image intensifiers mounted on modified U- or C-shape arms with triaxial motion capability. This permits the equipment to be rotated around the patient, with the heart in the isocentric part of the radiographic system. This system permits both cranial and caudal angulation projections in various degrees of obliquity.

With a *cranial angulation* the image intensifier and the cine camera are tilted toward the patient's head; the x-ray beam enters at the patient's back and exits through the front, while being inclined toward the patient's head. The picture obtained would be as if the viewer were in the position of the image intensifier looking down into the chest from an angle (Fig. 5-17).

With *caudal angulation* the image intensifier and cine camera are tilted toward the patient's feet; the x-ray beam enters at the patient's back and exits through the front while being inclined toward the feet. The image obtained would be as though the viewer were looking up into the chest from an angle (Fig. 5-17).

The capability of increased projections and angulations has done away with the concept of the "standard" examination. The correct and complete examination is the one that permits clear visualization of the coronary anatomy and overcomes problems of overlap, eccentric lesions, and foreshortening of arteries.

Guidelines

The majority of the studies will be complete if the left coronary artery is recorded in shallow (10° to 15°),

moderate (30°), and steep (45° to 50°) right anterior oblique projections with a 15° to 20° cranial and caudal angulation, as well as steep (50° to 60°) left anterior oblique projection with 0° up to 30° cranial angulation. The right coronary artery is best visualized in moderate right and steep left anterior oblique projections. To tailor the study to the needs of the patient, additional views may be taken based on the observations made on the routine study and using the following guidelines:

1. Left anterior oblique projection with cranial angulation is best for the visualization of the distal left main coronary artery (also seen well in 10° right or 30° to 45° left anterior oblique), proximal left anterior descending coronary artery, origin and proximal segment of the circumflex coronary artery, origin of the diagonal branches (also seen well in steep left or 30° to 40° right anterior oblique), and distal right coronary artery, separating posterior descending and posterior left ventricular branches (Fig. 5-18, *B* and *I*).

2. Right anterior oblique projection with cranial angulation is best for visualization of the origin of diagonal branches, separation of proximal circumflex branches, and assessment of the mid–left anterior descending artery (distal portion is foreshortened) and distal right coronary artery branches (Fig. 5-18, *E* and *K*).

3. Left anterior oblique projection with caudal angulation is best for visualization of left main coronary artery with cephalad orientation, and, especially in the horizontal heart, the origin and proximal portion of the circumflex coronary artery, as well as the proximal portion of the left anterior descending artery (Fig. 5-18, *C*).

4. Right anterior oblique projection with caudal angulation is best for visualization of the left main coronary artery especially when it is short, separate left anterior descending artery, diagonal and circumflex arteries, proximal and distal circumflex arteries, origin of the diagonal artery, and proximal and middle sections of the left anterior descending artery (Fig. 5-18, *F*).

5. Left lateral projection without cranial or caudal angulation shows the proximal left anterior descending artery and avoids overlap with the diagonal vessels (Fig. 5-18, *G*).

Considerable variations in coronary anatomy and position of the heart will require individual tailoring of the study and prohibit following any rigidly preconceived plan. For laboratories using a fixed x-ray tube and a cradle to rotate the patient, limited cranial angulation can be obtained by propping up the patient's chest 20° to 30° with a radiolucent pillow.

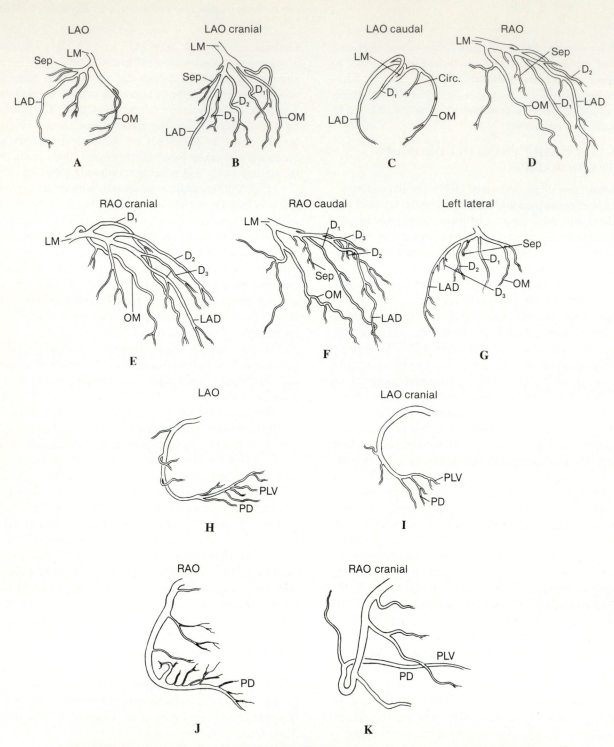

Fig. 5-18. Diagram of the left (**A** to **G**) and right (**H** to **K**) coronary arteries in different projections and various angulations. **A,** Steep left anterior oblique *(LAO)*. **B,** LAO with cranial angulation. **C,** LAO with caudal angulation. **D,** Right anterior oblique *(RAO)*. **E,** RAO with cranial angulation. **F,** RAO with caudal angulation. **G,** Left lateral (90°) projection. **H,** Right coronary artery in LAO projection. **I,** Right coronary artery in LAO projection with cranial angulation. **J,** Right coronary artery in steep RAO projection. **K,** Right coronary artery in RAO projection with cranial angulation. (*LAD,* Left anterior descending; *LM,* left main coronary artery; *D,* diagonal(s); *OM,* obtuse marginal; *Sep,* septals; *PD,* posterior descending; *PLV,* posterior left ventricular branches.) (Adapted from Douglas, J.S. Jr., and King, S.B. III: New radiographic views for imaging the coronary anatomy. In King, S.B. III, and Douglas, J.S., Jr.: Coronary arteriography and angioplasty, New York, 1985, McGraw-Hill Book Co. Reproduced with permission.)

DRUGS USED DURING CORONARY ARTERIOGRAPHY

Heparin

Widespread use of systemic heparinization during coronary arteriography was begun in the early 1970s. Until then, heparin had been used only for coronary arteriography using the transbrachial (Sones) approach. There are no randomized studies proving the benefit of systemic heparinization, but careful analysis of morbidity and mortality data since the general use of heparin in all forms of coronary arteriography has convinced most investigators that the risk of thromboembolic complications (cerebrovascular accident, myocardial infarction, femoral artery thrombosis) is appreciably reduced with heparin without any increased risk of bleeding complications. Use of heparin during cardiac catheterization in children has markedly reduced the incidence of neurologic complications in this group.[37]

Heparin is administered via the first arterial catheter, usually in doses of 4000 to 5000 units. This may be repeated during a prolonged study, approximately one-half the initial dose every hour.

Protamine sulfate

The effects of heparin are usually reversed with protamine sulfate at the end of the study just before removal of the percutaneous arterial catheter or sheath. This is prompted by concern about the risk of femoral puncture site bleeding. There are no controlled studies concerning the need, benefit, and risks of using protamine reversal.

Recent reports estimate the risk of anaphylactic reaction to protamine to be 0.5% in the general population and 25% in patients with diabetes who have been taking insulin preparations containing protamine (NPH).[38,39] Death has occurred from these reactions.[40] Also, experience has shown that adequate femoral hemostasis can frequently be achieved without the use of protamine sulfate. Actual practice varies in different laboratories and there are no firm standards concerning the use or nonuse of protamine. We have routinely used protamine reversal until recently and have witnessed two major acute anaphylactic reactions in more than 3000 coronary arteriographic studies.

A reasonable policy may be to use protamine sulfate more selectively. Specifically, it may be prudent to avoid the use of protamine in patients who are at high risk of having allergic reaction (diabetes mellitus on insulin preparations containing protamine), patients with repeated past exposures to protamine, or patients with a definite history of fish allergy. Protamine may be used in others, especially those who are at high risk of femoral puncture site bleeding (i.e., those with hypertension, marked obesity, or aortic insufficiency or those using aspirin) or when 10 to 15 minutes of adequate manual pressure does not achieve hemostasis. More data are needed before firm recommendations can be given.

The recommended dose is 10 mg of protamine sulfate for every 1000 units of heparin used. This is given intravenously, slowly over 2 to 3 minutes. This dose may be reduced by 50% if more than 1 hour has elapsed since the previous dose of heparin was given. It should not be injected via the arterial catheter or mixed with contrast material. Some contrast materials and protamine sulfate will cause a precipitate.

Other alternatives to the use of protamine that have been proposed[38] include the following:

1. Hexadimethrine is also used for reversal of heparin effect. Hexadimethrine is not commercially available in the United States and must be prepared from the powder form by the pharmacist.

2. If patients are known to be allergic to protamine or are at high risk for this and protamine is to be used, premedication with prednisone and diphenhydramine similar to that used in preparation of patients who are allergic to radiocontrast material (Chapter 19) is to be used.

We have no experience in the use of these two alternatives.

Atropine

Atropine is routinely used in many laboratories immediately before coronary arteriography with the aim of preventing vasovagal reaction or marked bradycardia secondary to coronary artery injections. These reflexes are most pronounced with injections into a dominant right coronary artery or a dominant circumflex artery supplying the inferior LV wall. There are no controlled studies evaluating the benefits or risks of using atropine routinely in all coronary artery studies. Undesirable effects are increased heart rate, possibility of precipitating angina, and some difficulty in adequate opacification of the coronary artery in patients during sinus tachycardia and large runoff. We do not use atropine routinely in all patients but follow these guidelines:

1. Use atropine early in suspected vasovagal reactions with bradycardia or hypotension (or both) followed promptly with volume expansion. Hypotension with minimal or no bradycardia can be caused by vasovagal reaction and responds promptly to atropine.

2. Use atropine prophylactically in patients with

demonstrated tendency to a vasovagal reaction or those who are at high risk of bradyarrhythmias, as well as those undergoing pericardiocentesis.

3. Have a transcutaneous pacer and capability of transvenous pacing immediately at hand.

The recommended dose is a bolus IV injection of 0.5 to 1 mg. It may be repeated once if needed.

Nitroglycerin

The routine use of nitroglycerin during coronary arteriography has been controversial. Controlled studies are lacking. Proponents claim increased safety, avoidance of catheter spasm, and better visualization of coronary arteries. Opponents worry about missing the diagnosis of coronary artery spasm.

In our practice, in the absence of hypotension, hypovolemia, or suspected vasospastic angina, we routinely administer nitroglycerin 0.3 or 0.4 mg sublingually before selective coronary arteriography. In cases where the history suggests a major element of vasospastic angina—and ergonovine provocation is a consideration—nitroglycerin is withheld until after the first set of coronary injections. The study is continued without nitroglycerin if no obstructive coronary artery disease is found. (See the discussion of ergonovine provocation, Chapter 6). Nitroglycerin is used as treatment of coronary artery spasm. It is also effective treatment for acute pulmonary edema. Intracoronary administration of nitroglycerin can also be used to reverse coronary artery spasm. Recent reports implicate potassium-containing nitroglycerin preparations as causing coronary artery spasm and ventricular fibrillation.[41] For intracoronary injection, a preparation that has no potassium should be used. In the United States most parenteral nitroglycerin preparations are free of potassium.

The recommended doses are as follows:
- Sublingual: 0.3 to 0.4 mg
- Intravenous: 100 to 400 μg; may be repeated in 10 to 20 minutes
- Intracoronary injection: 100 to 200 μg; used for coronary artery spasm not promptly responding to sublingual or IV nitroglycerin
- Continuous IV drip infusion: 20 to 200 μg/minute; for recurrent coronary artery spasm or acute pulmonary edema

PACING

Bradycardia during coronary arteriography is not rare. Causes are vasovagal reaction or contrast material injection into the coronary artery supplying the inferior LV wall (usually dominant right coronary artery), previous use of drugs (beta blockers, some calcium block-

ers), preexisting sinus node disease, or conduction system disease. Most episodes of bradycardia are brief and self-limited and can be prevented by or respond well to atropine. Prolonged and symptomatic asystole or atrioventricular block requiring a pacemaker during cardiac catheterization and angiography is rare. Thus, the routine use of prophylactic temporary transvenous pacing in all cases is not advised. It adds to the complexity of the procedure and increases the risk (ventricular tachycardia, ventricular fibrillation, RV perforation) and the cost of the procedure.

We use the following guidelines:
1. All patients are instructed in the performance of cough CPR (see p. 430) at the beginning of the procedure.
2. Atropine (0.6 to 1.0 mg administered intravenously) is used early in vasovagal reactions or prophylactically in patients with marked sinus bradycardia or high risk of developing bradycardia.
3. An external transcutaneous pacer is available at all times.
4. A temporary transvenous pacer is available but used prophylactically only for patients considered to be at high risk for major bradycardia. These include patients with the following:
   a. Left bundle branch block undergoing right heart catheterization
   b. High doses of beta blockers and calcium blockers with bradycardia
   c. Right bundle branch block with aortic stenosis
   d. Sick sinus syndrome
   e. Trifascicular block or transient complete heart block
   f. Right coronary artery angioplasty
   g. Angiography during acute inferior wall myocardial infarction
   h. Ergonovine stimulation tests in patients suspected of right coronary artery spasm, especially if there is a history of syncope

Remember that the reflex bradycardia triggered by injection of contrast agent in the dominant right coronary artery is accompanied by vasodilatation and hypotension. Pacing will prevent the bradycardia but not the hypotension, which will require atropine and sometimes volume expansion.

ETIQUETTE IN THE CARDIAC CATHETERIZATION LABORATORY

The cardiac catheterization laboratory is an operating suite where complex diagnostic and therapeutic procedures are performed on awake patients who are generally concerned and apprehensive. It is important to maintain a high level of professional decorum during the entire procedure. Treating the patient with respect and compassion will greatly minimize his or her emotional distress.

The following guidelines are offered:

1. All personnel—physicians and technicians—should introduce themselves to the patient and explain briefly what they will be doing.

2. Observers and curious onlookers do not belong in the cardiac catheterization room. A remote television can be used for observation and teaching purposes.

3. All conversations must keep the patient in mind. Instructions should be given clearly. Small talk may help to put the patient at ease, but garrulous chitchat is inappropriate. Especially inappropriate are comments about the findings and their significance during the study. Music can be soothing and helpful. It should be low-volume, background, noncontroversial music.

4. The patient's family should be advised to wait in a special area where they will be contacted after the study.

5. In the cardiac catheterization laboratory dress code must comply with both infection control as well as proper function. Generally, all personnel in contact with the sterile field and the catheters wear a sterile gown and gloves, cap and mask. The circulating personnel should be either in surgical scrub suits or their functional clothing. It appears that in procedures involving venous or arterial cutdown, the incidence of infection is reduced when all personnel wear a surgical scrub suit. In percutaneous techniques this does not seem to be important.[42]

6. Remember, the patient is naked, horizontal, strapped on a cradle or a table, and apprehensive and is feeling very vulnerable.

PATIENT AFTERCARE

Proper patient aftercare is important for reducing the chance of late complications and increasing patient comfort. The patient is probably tired, cold, thirsty, and hungry, although happy and relieved that the study is over.

1. Give clear instructions to the patient as to activity, diet, fluid intake, and voiding.

2. Postcatheterization orders should clearly specify duration of bedrest, type of monitoring, and frequency of vital signs. They should include provisions for treatment of chest pain or late-appearing nausea and vomiting as well as clear instructions regarding what to do for any bleeding problems or inability to void. Continuation or changes of IV fluid should be addressed.

3. If an unexpected problem arises the nursing staff should be able to reach the operating cardiologist or a designated alternative immediately.

4. Precatheterization orders may be resumed or altered.

OUTPATIENT CATHETERIZATION

In the pioneer days of cardiac catheterization and coronary arteriography, studies were performed with use of general anesthesia with cardiovascular surgeons at hand to deal with complications. In the ensuing 20 years, tremendous advances and improvements in safety allow many of these studies to be performed safely in an outpatient setting. Economic motivation, improvement in catheter design such as high-flow 5 Fr catheters, and patient preference have encouraged this. The feasibility and general safety of outpatient cardiac catheterization in carefully selected patients have been well demonstrated for both the transbrachial (cutdown or percutaneous) and the femoral approach.[43-52]

It is estimated that 20% to 40% (and possibly as high as 80%) of all studies can be performed without an overnight hospital stay with savings of 25% to 50% on hospital-related expenses. Outpatient cardiac angiography studies should be limited to *low-risk* patients who are clinically stable and who have the support of family or a friend who will help with the transportation and stay with them overnight following the study. Patients with suspected critical aortic stenosis or left main or severe triple-vessel coronary disease, congestive heart failure, recent myocardial infarction, severe pulmonary hypertension, uncontrolled angina, or arrhythmias are not suitable for outpatient cardiac catheterization. Also, any patient who is at high risk for a late puncture site bleeding should be observed overnight. The physician who will perform the cardiac catheterization study and will be responsible for the patient immediately after catheterization must determine the advisability of outpatient catheterization study in the individual patient.

Patients can be admitted to a day care area 1 hour before the study, prepared, and then observed (for 1 to 2 hours after the procedure for the brachial approach and 4 to 5 hours for the femoral approach) and discharged to continue resting at home, barring any complications. If a critical abnormality is discovered, such as high-grade narrowing of left main coronary artery, severe three-vessel coronary artery disease, or severe aortic stenosis, then overnight hospital observation is advisable. *To be able to cope with all possible emergencies, the resources of a complete hospital must be immediately available to the patient who undergoes such studies on an outpatient basis.*

It is necessary to give clear instruction to the patient before the study, obtain appropriate laboratory studies and informed consent, give clear oral and written instructions to the patient before release from the observation area, and arrange for follow-up of the patient and for review of the findings.

FUTURE DEVELOPMENTS

Cardiac catheterization and angiography have advanced from a high-risk and complex diagnostic study to a commonly performed and generally safe test. The technique has been expanded to include the intervention of coronary angioplasty. Anticipated future developments include the following:

• Newer contrast agents and smaller catheters will probably permit more of these studies to be done safely on an outpatient basis.

• Digital subtraction angiography application to coronary arteriography would permit use of less contrast agent, immediate playback, image enhancement, and greater ease of quantification of coronary obstructive lesions, coronary flow, and coronary reserve. Also, ventricular function could be quantitated.[53-55]

• The development of fiberoptics has permitted flexible angioscopes of 1.5 to 2.5 mm in diameter with a steering mechanism. Currently, angioscopy is applied experimentally to the pulmonary arteries, renal arteries, and, in a preliminary manner, the coronary arteries. It is possible that angioscopy will permit a three-dimensional view of coronary obstructive lesions, help determine the presence and age of a thrombus, aid in a more accurate diagnosis of arterial obstructive disease, and help in evaluation of results of angioplasty or other interventions. Coupled with laser techniques, angioscopy may facilitate laser angioplasty.[56,57]

• The feasibility of measuring gradients across coronary artery stenosis has been amply demonstrated and is routinely performed during coronary angioplasty. If the value of these pressure gradient measurements in the evaluation of coronary artery disease is confirmed,[58] then such measurements may be routinely performed in the future. Coronary blood flow velocity can be measured by means of a steerable Doppler coronary catheter.[59] Such techniques may be used to assess the physiologic significance of obstructive coronary artery disease.[60]

• Noninvasive coronary arteriography using intravenously injected contrast material and intense radiation produced by linear-accelerator and computer-imaging techniques is in early phases of investigation.

REFERENCES

1. Fye, W.B.: Coronary arteriography—it took a long time! Circulation **760:**781-786, 1984.
2. Grossman, W.: Cardiac catheterization and angiography, ed. 3, Philadelphia, 1986, Lea & Febiger.
3. Abrams, H.L.: Coronary arteriography: a practical approach, Boston, 1983, Little, Brown & Co.
4. Baltaxe, H.A., Amplatz, K., and Levin, D.C.: Coronary angiography, Springfield, Ill., 1973, Charles C Thomas, Publisher.
5. Silverman, J.: Coronary angiography, John Wiley & Sons, 1985.
6. King, S.B. III, and Douglas, J.S., Jr.: Coronary arteriography and angioplasty, New York, 1985, McGraw-Hill Book Co.
7. Miller, S.W.: Cardiac angiography, Boston, 1984, Little, Brown & Co.
8. Ambrose, J.A.: Unsettled indications for coronary angiography, J. Am. Coll. Cardiol. **3:**1575-1580, 1984.
9. Levin, D.C.: Invasive evaluation (coronary arteriography) of the coronary artery disease patient: clinical, economic and social issues, Circulation **66**(Supp III):71-79, 1982.
10. Adams, D.F., Fraser, P.B., and Abrams, H.L.: The complications of coronary arteriography, Circulation **48:**609, 1973.
11. Kennedy, J.W., et al.: Mortality related to cardiac catheterization and angiography, Cathet. Cardiovasc. Diagn. **8:**323-340, 1982.
12. Kennedy, J.W.: Complications associated with cardiac catheterization and angiography: from the Registry Committee of the Society for Cardiac Angiography, Cathet. Cardiovasc. Diagn. **8:**5-11, 1982.
13. Hansing, C.E.: The risk and cost of coronary angiography. II. The risk of coronary arteriography in Washington state, JAMA **242:**735-738, 1979.
14. Kennedy, J.W.: Report of the Registry Committee, Society for Cardiac Angiography, Annual meeting, Scottsdale, Ariz., May 12, 1983.
15. Davis, K., et al.: Complications of coronary arteriography from collaborative study of coronary artery surgery (CASS), Circulation **59:**1105-1112, 1979.
16. Hansing, C.E.: The risk and cost of coronary angiography. I. Cost of coronary arteriography in Washington state. JAMA **242:**731-734, 1979.
17. Fisher, M.L.: Coronary angiography: safety in numbers? Am. J. Cardiol. **52:**898-901, 1983.
18. Fresinger, G.C., et al.: Optimal resources for examination of the heart and lungs: cardiac catheterization and radiographic facilities. Examination of the chest and cardiovascular system study group, Circulation **68:**893A-930A, 1983.
19. Sones Jr., F.M., and Shirey, E.K.: Cine coronary arteriography. Mod. Concepts Cardiovasc. Dis. **31:**735-738, 1962.
20. Heupler, F. Jr.: Coronary arteriography and left ventriculography Sones technique. In King, S.B. III, and Douglas, J.S. Jr.: Coronary arteriography and angioplasty, New York, 1985, McGraw-Hill Book Co., pp. 137-181.
21. Judkins, M.P.: Selective coronary arteriography. I. A percutaneous transfemoral technic, Radiology **89:**815-824, 1967.
22. Judkins, M.P., and Judkins, E.: Coronary arteriography and left ventriculography: Judkins technique. In King, S.B. III, and Douglas, J.S. Jr.: Coronary arteriography and angioplasty, New York, 1985, McGraw-Hill Book Co., pp. 182-217.
23. Amplatz, K., Formanek, G., Stanger, P., and Wilson, W.: Mechanics of selective coronary artery catheterization via femoral approach, Radiology **89:**1040-1047, 1967.
24. Judkins, M.P.: Percutaneous transfemoral selective coronary arteriography, Radiol. Clin. North Am. **5:**467-490, 1968.

25. Wells, D.E., et al.: A simplified method for left heart catheterization including coronary arteriography, Chest **63**:959-962, 1973.

26. Zir, L.M., Dinsmore, R.E., Goss, C., and Harthorn, J.W.: Experience with preformed catheters for coronary angiography by the brachial approach, Cathet. Cardiovasc. Diagn. **1**:303-310, 1975.

27. Schoonmaker, R.W., and King, S.B. III: Coronary arteriography by the single catheter percutaneous femoral technique, Circulation **50**:735-740, 1974.

28. King, S.B. III, and Douglas, J.S.: Coronary arteriography and left ventriculography: multipurpose technique. In King, S.B. III, and Douglas, J.S. Jr.: Coronary arteriography and angioplasty, New York, 1985, McGraw-Hill Book Co.

29. El Gamal M.I.H., et al.: Selective coronary arteriography with a preformed single catheter: percutaneous femoral technique, A.J.R. **135**:630-632, 1980.

30. Guthaner, D.F., and Wexler, L.: Coronary arteriography following bypass surgery. In Abrams, H.L. (editor): Coronary arteriography: a practical approach, Boston, 1985, Little, Brown & Co.

31. Lytle, B.W., et al.: Long-term (5 to 12 years) serial studies of internal mammary artery and saphenous vein coronary bypass grafts, J. Thorac. Cardiovasc. Surg. **89**:248-258, 1985.

32. Loop, F.D., et al.: Influence of the internal-mammary-artery graft on 10-year survival and other cardiac events, N. Engl. J. Med. **314**:1-7, 1986.

33. Bashour, T.T., Hanna, E.S., and Mason, D.T.: Myocardial revascularization with internal mammary artery bypass: an emerging treatment of choice, Prog. Cardiol. **111**:143-151, 1986.

34. Douglas, J.S., and King, S.B.: New radiographic views for imaging the coronary anatomy. In King, S.B. III, and Douglas, J.S. Jr.: Coronary arteriography and angioplasty, New York, 1985, McGraw-Hill Book Co., pp. 275-287.

35. Sos, T.A., and Baltaxe, H.A.: Cranial and caudal angulation for coronary arteriography revisited, Circulation **56**:119-123, 1977.

36. Aldridge, H.E.: A decade or more of cranial and caudal angled projections in coronary arteriography—another look, Cathet. Cardiovasc. Diagn. **10**:539-542, 1984.

37. Weissman, B.M., Aram, D.M., Levinsohn, M.W., and Ben-Shachar, G.: Neurologic sequelae of cardiac catheterization, Cathet. Cardiovasc. Diagn. **11**:577-583, 1985.

38. Stewart, W.J., et al.: Increased risk of severe protamine reactions in NPH insulin–dependent diabetics undergoing cardiac catheterization, Circulation **70**:788-792, 1984.

39. Chung, F., and Miles, J.: Cardiac arrest following protamine administration, Can. Anaesth. Soc. J. **31**:314-318, 1984.

40. Sharath, M.D., et al.: Protamine-induced fatal anaphylaxis: prevalence of antiprotamine immunoglobin E antibody, Thorac. Cardiovasc. Surg. **90**:86-90, 1985.

41. Quigley, P.J., and Maurer, B.J.: Ventricular fibrillation during coronary angiography: association with potassium-containing glyceryl trinitrate, Am. J. Cardiol. **56**:191, 1985.

42. Leaman, D.M., and Zelis, R.F.: What is the appropriate "dress code" for the cardiac catheterization laboratory? Cathet. Cardiovasc. Diagn. **9**:33-38, 1983.

43. Mahrer, P.R., and Eshoo, N.: Outpatient cardiac catheterization and coronary angiography, Cathet. Cardiovasc. Diagn. **7**:355-360, 1981.

44. Rogers, W.F., and Moothart, R.W.: Outpatient arteriography and cardiac catheterization: effective alternatives to inpatient procedures, A.J.R. **144**:233-234, 1985.

45. Fierens, E.: Outpatient coronary arteriography, Cathet. Cardiovasc. Diagn. **10**:27-32, 1984.

46. Health and Public Policy Committee, American College of Physicians: The safety and efficacy of ambulatory cardiac catheterization in the hospital and freestanding setting, Ann. Intern. Med. **103**:294-298, 1985.

47. Diethrich, E.B., Kinard, S.A., Pierce, S.A., and Koopot, R.: Outpatient cardiac catheterization and arteriography: twenty-month experience at the Arizona Heart Institute, Cardiovasc. Dis. **8**:195-204, 1981.

48. Kahn, K.L.: The efficacy of ambulatory cardiac catheterization in the hospital and free-standing setting, Am. Heart J. **111**:152-167, 1986.

49. Lominack, E.K., Lutz, J.F., Douglas, J.S. Jr., and King, S.B.: Evaluation of 5 French catheters for outpatient coronary arteriography, Circulation **72**(Supp. III-457):1816, 1985.

50. Campeau, L.: Percutaneous brachial catheterization, Cathet. Cardiovasc. Diagn. **11**:443-444, 1985.

51. Cohen, M., Rentrop, P., and Cohen, B.: Percutaneous entry of the brachial artery versus cutdown/arteriotomy for left heart catheterization, Circulation **72**(Supp. III-455):1820, 1985.

52. Klinke, W.P., Kubac, G., Talibi, T., and Lee, S.J.K.: Safety of outpatient cardiac catheterizations, Am. J. Cardiol. **56**:639-641, 1985.

53. Hodgson, J.M., et al.: Validation in dogs of a rapid digital angiographic technique to measure relative coronary blood flow during routine cardiac catheterization, Am. J. Cardiol. **55**:188-193, 1985.

54. Bray, B.E., et al.: Digital subtraction coronary arteriography using high-pass temporal filtration: a comparison with cineangiography, Cathet. Cardiovasc. Diagn. **11**:17-24, 1985.

55. Vogel, R.: The radiographic assessment of coronary blood flow parameters, Circulation **72**:460-465, 1985.

56. Vincent, G.M., and Fox, J.: Cardiovascular endoscopy, Cardiovasc. Rev. Rep. **6**:1227-1234, 1985.

57. Spears, J.R., Spokojny, A.M., and Marais, H.J.: Coronary angioscopy during cardiac catheterization, J. Am. Coll. Cardiol. **6**:93-97, 1985.

58. Ganz, P., et al.: Usefulness of transstenotic coronary pressure gradient measurements during diagnostic catheterization, Am. J. Cardiol. **55**:910-914, 1985.

59. Sibley, D.H., Whitlow, P.L., Millar, H., and Hartley, C.J.: Use of a new steerable Doppler coronary catheter to subselectively measure coronary blood flow velocity, Circulation **72**(Supp. III-20):80, 1985.

60. Herrold, E.M., and Borer, J.S.: Efforts toward quantitation of coronary artery functional capacity (editorial), J. Am. Coll. Cardiol. **7**:114-115, 1986.

Chapter Six

Ergonovine provocative testing for coronary artery spasm

ARA G. TILKIAN

ELAINE K. DAILY

Coronary artery spasm is widely accepted as a cause of angina pectoris.[1-6] It may also be a contributing factor in acute myocardial infarction.[7] The syndrome ranges in varying degrees from patients with angiographically normal coronary arteries to those with severe, fixed anatomic coronary artery stenosis. In patients with coronary artery spasm but angiographically normal coronary arteries, the periodic, focal, spastic obstruction of the vessel causes chest pain and ST segment shifts. In patients with fixed coronary artery obstructive disease, spasm adds to the degree of obstruction and may cause ST segment elevation or depression. Chest pain may or may not accompany these events.

Coronary artery spasm can be the cause of chest pain during sleep, at rest, or during exercise. Causes and consequences of coronary artery spasm have been reviewed.[6] Accurate diagnosis is important because it determines the choice of treatment. If the dominant cause of angina and myocardial ischema is coronary artery spasm superimposed on mild to moderate coronary artery obstruction, vasodilators (nitrates and calcium entry blockers) are the treatment of choice. On the other hand, if the dominant cause of angina is fixed, high-grade coronary artery obstruction, and if vasospasm is a minor contributor, the choice of treatment, in addition to vasodilators, will include drugs that will reduce myocardial oxygen demand. Revascularization surgery or balloon angioplasty may also be used in patients with predominantly fixed coronary obstruction. Coronary artery spasm with variant angina has been reported in patients as young as 11 years,[8] although it is most frequent in women 30 to 50 years of age.

Provocation of coronary artery spasm with ergonovine maleate as an aid to the diagnosis of vasospastic angina has been used with some regularity for the past 10 years.[9,10] The test has been shown to be both sensitive and specific for the diagnosis of coronary artery spasm and vasospastic angina.[11,12] Although a recent report demonstrated ergonovine-induced spasm of a saphenous vein coronary bypass graft,[13] the test has rarely been performed after this operation, and the response of vein grafts to ergonovine provocation remains generally unknown. Although some questions have been raised about the clinical validity as well as the risk/benefit ratio, the ergonovine provocation test is generally accepted as a useful aid to the diagnosis of vasospastic angina.[12,14,15]

INDICATIONS

Ergonovine provocation testing is indicated for patients with suspected coronary artery spasm for whom the diagnosis remains in doubt. These include two basic groups of patients—carefully selected patients with mild to moderate one-vessel obstructive coronary artery disease in whom vasospastic angina is strongly suspected in noninvolved vessels, and patients who have angiographically normal coronary arteries or nonobstructive coronary atherosclerosis with the following findings:

• Clinically typical variant angina (rest or sleep angina) where there is no ECG documentation during the pain; if the ECG immediately preceeding or during the pain shows definite ST segment elevation or depression and response to nitroglycerin is prompt, then the clinical diagnosis would be secure and ergonovine provocation is generally not necessary and treatment can be instituted; in patients with a typical history of variant angina for whom it has not been possible to obtain ECG documentation during chest pain, the use of either Holter ECG recorders or ECG recorders with memory (Cardiobeeper [Survival Technology, Inc.], and others) or the use of continuous home ECG monitoring via telemetry (CELIA System, Cardiac Communications, Ltd.) may be helpful

- Rest or effort angina for which the ECG during pain shows nondiagnostic ST segment changes or no changes at all
- Rest pain with left bundle branch block or a ventricular paced rhythm
- Rest pain with syncope or major arrhythmias, either heart block or ventricular tachyarrhythmias (*Note:* Exercise caution during ergonovine provocative testing in these patients)

Ergonovine provocation testing has been recommended for evaluation of therapy for patients with proven coronary artery spasm. This is not a widely accepted indication.[16]

CONTRAINDICATIONS

Patients with the following conditions should not have ergonovine stimulation testing:

- High-grade obstruction in a major coronary artery, even if the obstruction is in only one vessel
- Multivessel obstructive coronary artery disease where the risk of complications is substantial, and where the test is of questionable value in the clinical management of these patients
- Uncontrolled hypertension, where provocative testing could precipitate a hypertensive crisis
- Recent myocardial infarction with some obstructive coronary artery disease: ergonovine may cause extension of the infarction; ergonovine testing has been safely done in patients with recent myocardial infarction and no coronary obstructive disease, with negative results[17]
- Poor-quality or nondiagnostic coronary angiogram or no current angiogram
- Uncontrolled congestive heart failure
- Pregnancy
- Increased risk of cerebral hemorrhage (aneurysms or anticoagulation)
- Allergy or hypersensitivity to ergonovine

RISKS

Ergonovine provocation tests are quite safe if proper indications, contraindications, and precautions are observed.[9,11,18-23]

In patients who have a negative response (i.e., those in whom coronary artery spasm is not provoked), adverse effects are limited to atypical chest pain (50% to 70%), nausea (40%), vomiting (13%), hypertension (diastolic blood pressure >100 mm Hg) (20%), and headaches (8%). Rarely, bronchospasm occurs in patients with a history of bronchial allergic response.

In patients with a positive response (i.e., those in whom coronary artery spasm is provoked and myocardial ischemia is precipitated), more serious complications may occur. These include severe hypotension (5% to 10%), major arrhythmias (ventricular tachycardia, ventricular fibrillation, complete heart block, sinus arrest), myocardial infarction (0.3%), and death (0.1% to 0.2%).

Given these risks, ergonovine provocation tests should be performed only on carefully selected patients when the diagnosis cannot be made by ECG monitoring, the indications are clear, there are no contraindications, and a positive or negative response will substantially contribute to the treatment plan. We perform this test only in the cardiac catheterization laboratory and following coronary arteriography. However, performance of the ergonovine stimulation test in a coronary care setting has been advocated and proven to be generally safe[15,24] (see p. 156).

EQUIPMENT

The equipment needed is the standard cardiac catheterization equipment, a multichannel ECG monitor and hemodynamic monitor, a stopwatch, and the following drugs: nitroglycerin* (800 μg diluted in 8 ml of 5% dextrose in water); nifedipine (10 mg capsules, given sublingually); IV verapamil; IV nitroprusside.

PROCEDURE

Ergonovine provocation testing is carried out as outlined below.[9,11,19-21,23]

1. Studies should be done after all vasoactive medications have been discontinued. Discontinue all nitrates for at least 4 hours, calcium entry blockers and other vasodilators for 24 hours, and beta blockers for 48 hours.
2. Obtain informed consent. This may be included in the consent for diagnostic coronary arteriography if ergonovine provocation testing is anticipated.
3. Complete right and left coronary arteriograms. Do not use nitroglycerin during coronary arteriography unless spontaneous coronary artery spasm is noted.
4. Review the arteriographic data by means of a high-quality video playback system or develop and re-

---

*Intracoronary injection of potassium-containing nitroglycerin has been implicated as a cause of coronary artery spasm and ventricular fibrillation.[25] Most preparations available in the United States do not contain potassium.

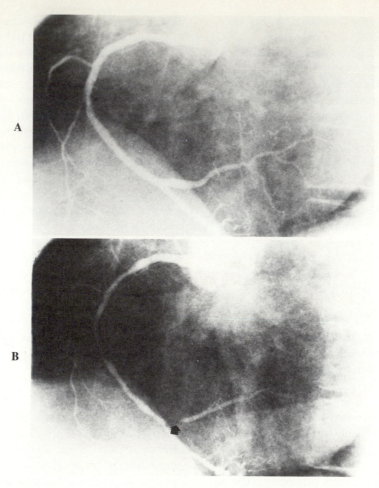

Fig. 6-1. Positive response to ergonovine provocation test (dominant right coronary artery, left anterior oblique projection) **(A)** before ergonivine infusion, **(B)** at the onset of ergonovine-induced spasm of posterior left ventricular branch.

view the cine films. *The possibility of severe coronary artery obstruction must be excluded before the ergonovine provocation study is done.*

5. Establish continuous multichannel ECG and pressure monitoring.
6. Have a RV pacer in position or immediately available. A standby transcutaneous pacer may also be satisfactory.
7. Establish the ability to obtain right and left selective coronary arteriograms in rapid sequence. This may involve use of one of the following methods:
   a. Sones or Schoonmaker-King multipurpose catheter
   b. Arterial introducer with ability for rapid exchange of preformed catheters
   c. The double catheter technique, with simultaneous use of right and left preformed coronary artery catheters[18,19]
8. Baseline hemodynamic pressure readings and 12-lead ECG recordings (use radiolucent electrodes [Hayes pediatric electrodes] and leave them on the patient)
9. Administer the initial dose of ergonovine maleate (Ergotrate Maleate) (0.05 mg intravenously, or 0.025 mg for the first dose in patients with frequent chest pain or suspected malignant arrhythmias). *Note:* The *onset* of the ergonovine effect, and therefore coronary artery spasm, usually occurs within 3 to 6 minutes after ergonovine infusion. The vasoconstrictive effect of ergonovine and the duration of spasm may last 10 to 15 minutes. Most positive responses occur with cumulative doses of

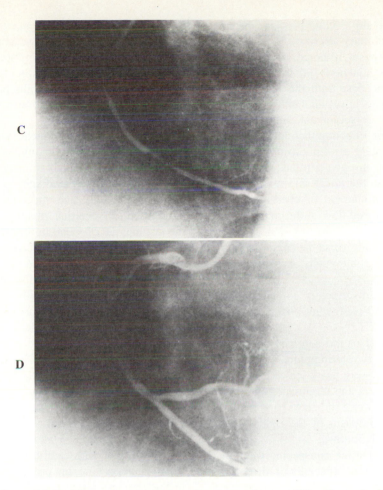

Fig. 6-1, cont'd. Positive response to ergonovine provocation test **(C)** at the peak of ergonovine-induced spasm with total occlusion of vessel and **(D)** following intracoronary nitroglycerin reversal of the coronary artery spasm.

less than 0.2 mg, although cumulative doses of 0.3 to 0.4 mg have been used.

10. Observe the patient for clinical response. Continue hemodynamic pressure and ECG monitoring. Visualize both coronary arteries within 3 to 5 minutes of ergonovine injection. If there is no ECG change to suggest which coronary artery may be in spasm, visualize the dominant right coronary artery first. In a nondominant coronary system, visualize the left coronary artery first.

11. Do not give additional ergonovine if a positive result is elicited or major adverse effects are noted. A positive result constitutes chest pain with ECG signs of ischemia, focal coronary artery spasm as shown by arteriography ($\geq 75\%$ lumen reduction) (Fig. 6-1), or major arrhythmias (ventricular tachy-cardia, ventricular fibrillation, complete heart block). Adverse effects include excessive hypertension, hypotension, severe nausea and vomiting, and severe headache.

12. If a positive result is not elicited and there are no major adverse effects:
   a. Give a second dose of ergonovine 5 minutes after the first injection (0.1 mg intravenously) and repeat steps 10 and 11)
   b. If there is no positive response after the second dose and no adverse effects, give a third and last dose of ergonovine (0.25 mg) 5 minutes after the second dose, repeat the sequence, and closely monitor the patient for 10 minutes

If there is a *positive response* (chest pain with ECG ST segment abnormality) proceed as follows:

1. Record the ECG, obtain a blood pressure recording, and visualize both coronary arteries.

2. If coronary artery spasm is noted, promptly reverse it by intracoronary injection 100 to 200 μg of nitroglycerin, repeating the dose until the spasm is reversed. Exercise care not to inject air bubbles! Follow this by administration of sublingual nitroglycerin, which has a longer duration of action than intracoronary nitroglycerin. Coronary artery air embolism during arteriography or infusion of nitroglycerin can cause temporary cessation of flow in the artery and mimic coronary artery spasm with production of chest pain, ST segment elevation, and delayed flow of the contrast material.[26]

3. If nitroglycerin does not reverse the spasm, administer 10 mg of nifedepine sublingually and repeat the dose if necessary.

4. In the unlikely event of refractory coronary artery spasm, IV nitroprusside (50 μg/minute titrated to clinical response) can be used.[20]

5. Document the reversal of the coronary spasm by repeat right and left coronary arteriography.

6. Monitor the patient closely for at least 15 minutes before removing the catheters and terminating the test.

If there is a *negative response* (no chest pain or ECG abnormalities and no focal spasm of the right or left coronary artery), proceed as follows:

1. It is advisable to reverse the nonspecific vasoconstrictive effect of ergonovine, especially if there has been a hypertensive response. Use 200 μg of nitroglycerin intravenously or 400 μg sublingually.

2. Monitor the patient for 5 more minutes and terminate the procedure.

Chest pain may occur without ECG abnormalities and without coronary artery spasm. This may suggest esophogeal motility disorder as the cause of chest pain.[27] Nitroglycerin is usually effective treatment.

Alternate method

An alternate schedule of ergonovine administration can be used. Ergonovine can be administered in individual doses of 0.05 mg 2 to 3 minutes apart to a maximal cumulative dose of 0.25 to 0.3 mg. The yield and safety of both methods are comparable.

TESTING IN THE CORONARY CARE UNIT

There have been reports indicating the feasibility and general safety of performing ergonovine provocation tests in the coronary care unit or in an outpatient setting in patients without documented obstructive coronary artery disease utilizing ECG and external blood pressure monitoring.[15,16,28] The advantages of this method are its simplicity, better patient acceptance, and reduced cost. Disadvantages can be detailed as follows:

• A current coronary arteriogram is required before proceeding to ergonovine stimulation. An arteriogram dated several weeks or months previously may not accurately reflect the coronary anatomy at the time of the provocation study.

• Coronary artery spasm can occur without chest pain and without ECG abnormality, whereas chest pain during ergonovine infusion can occur without coronary artery spasm. Thus, the diagnosis may remain unclear and the sensitivity and specificity of the test may be diminished. Myocardial imaging with thallium during the test may be of value in this setting.

• Coronary artery spasm can be refractory to sublingual or IV nitroglycerin, and the test can provoke prolonged spasm with obstruction of the artery and myocardial infarction with all of its complications, including death. Intracoronary administration of nitroglycerin would be more effective in dealing with such a complication.[29,30]

• Coronary artery spasm is diagnosed earliest with coronary arteriography. ECG changes and subsequent chest pain occur later. Thus, relying on these external signs and symptoms will delay the diagnosis of spasm and therefore the reversal or treatment of it.

Although these are valid considerations, experience has shown that with careful patient selection and close supervision, ergonovine provocation can be done safely in the coronary care unit setting with satisfactory sensitivity and specificity.[15,16,28]

Procedure

Ergonovine provocation testing in the coronary care unit consists of the following:

1. Review current coronary arteriograms and confirm that the patient has no obstructive coronary disease.

2. Secure an IV line including a three-way stopcock.

3. Institute 12-lead ECG monitoring.

4. Ensure that a cardiologist and coronary care unit nurse are at the bedside throughout the test.

5. Obtain baseline heart rate, blood pressure, and 12-lead ECG recordings.

6. Administer ergonovine IV according to the following protocol:

Time (min)	Dose* (mg)
0	0.0125
5	0.025

---

*A convenient preparation is 0.4 mg of ergonovine diluted to 16 ml, yielding a concentration of 0.025 mg/ml.

Time (min)	Dose* (mg)
10	0.05
20	0.10
30	0.20
40	0.30 (rarely needed)
50	0.40 (rarely needed)

7. Record heart rate, blood pressure, and 12-lead ECG at 2-minute intervals up to 10 minutes after the test.

8. Stop the test if a positive response is noted (≥ 1 mm of ST segment elevation with or without pain; ST segment depression, especially if accompanied by chest pain, is also considered a positive response) or if an adverse reaction occurs.

9. Give 200 to 400 µg of nitroglycerin intravenously as soon as a positive response is noted or at the completion of a negative test. The IV nitroglycerin may be repeated until a positive response is reversed. Sublingual nifedipine (10 mg) can be given if nitroglycerin is not effective.

10. Use myocardial imaging with thallium as a possible aid in evaluating a positive response and localizing the area of myocardial ischemia.

INTERPRETATION OF FINDINGS
Negative or nonspecific response

The following observations are consistent with a negative response: atypical chest pain, nausea, vomiting, headache, no ECG abnormalities, blood pressure elevation of 10 to 20 mm Hg, and mild to moderate (rarely marked) diffuse and concentric narrowing of coronary arteries.

Angiographically normal coronary arteries may have a 20% to 30% reduction of caliber. Arteriosclerotic coronary arteries may show a somewhat increased responsiveness to ergonovine, with diffuse concentric narrowing approximately 50% of luminal diameter (Fig. 6-2).

A false negative response may occur as a result of the variable clinical course in coronary artery spasm. The same patient can have a positive response at one time and a negative response at another time. Other causes of false negative response include the use of calcium blockers or nitroglycerin (the patient might be continuing medications) and the use of topical nitroglycerin, which may have been overlooked. If the clinical history is characteristic of coronary artery spasm and the ergonovine stimulation test result is negative or nonspecific, an empiric trial with the use of calcium blockers may be of value. In such circumstances, both the physician and the patient should understand that a definitive diagnosis has not been made.

Positive response

For a test to be interpreted as positive, there must be focal luminal narrowing of 75% or more (Fig. 6-1), usually with chest pain and ischemic changes as shown by ECG of either ST segment elevation or depression correlating with the area of myocardial ischemia. In unusual circumstances, chest pain may be absent (myocardial ischemia with no angina) or ECG changes may not be observed (ischemia in an electrocardiographically silent area).

Coronary artery spasm can involve, with decreasing frequency, the right coronary artery, the left anterior descending coronary artery, the circumflex artery, the left main coronary artery (rare), and saphenous vein grafts (very rare).

A positive test has been observed in the following conditions: cardiac myopathy or valvular heart disease, 0% to 2%; coronary artery disease with coronary atherosclerosis, less than 20%; coronary artery disease with predominant rest angina, approximately 40%; coronary artery disease with clinical syndrome of variant angina, 85% to 90%.[15,31]

COMPLICATIONS

Complications arising with a negative response include atypical chest pain (no treatment required), nausea and vomiting (usually self-limited), hypertension (administer sublingual or IV nitroglycerin or IV nitroprusside), and severe headaches (stop the test and administer IV nitroglycerin).

In patients with a positive response and documented coronary artery spasm, complications are limited by prompt relief of the coronary artery spasm. Chest pain, hypotension, and arrhythmias are caused by myocardial ischemia, and time should not be wasted controlling hypotension, using vasopressors, or using antiarrhythmic agents. The primary effort should be directed toward relief of spasm.

1. Inject 200 µg of nitroglycerin directly into the coronary artery and repeat as necessary.
2. Administer 10 mg of sublingual nifedipine and repeat as necessary.
3. Give IV nitroprusside (50 µg/minute titrated to clinical response).

PATIENT AFTERCARE

Ergonovine action may last 15 to 20 minutes. Coronary artery spasm may recur 10 to 15 minutes after nitroglycerin reversal. Thus, the patient should be monitored for 20 minutes after completion of the test, and nitroglycerin should be readministered in 10 to 15 minutes, especially if the initial reversal was accomplished

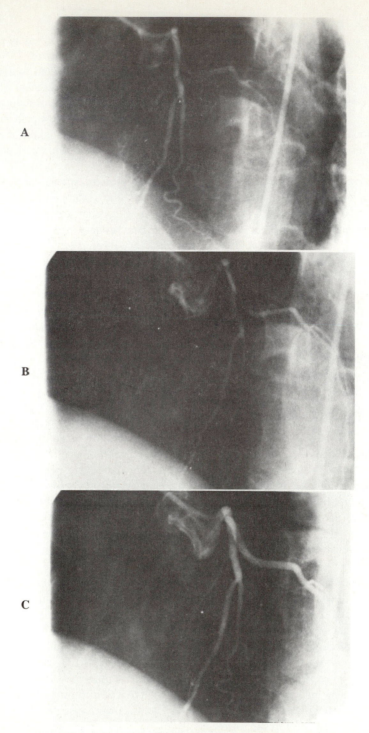

Fig. 6-2. Negative response to ergonovine provocation test (left coronary artery, left anterior oblique projection). **A,** No obstructive abnormalities before ergonovine infusion. **B,** Mild, diffuse narrowing of the left anterior descending coronary artery following ergonovine infusion (normal physiologic response). **C,** Reversal of this physiologic ergonovine effect with intracoronary nitroglycerin administration.

with intracoronary or IV nitroglycerin, which has shorter duration of action than sublingual nitroglycerin.

Patients who undergo the procedure in the coronary care setting may walk about in 1 to 2 hours and be discharged if their condition is stable.

PROCEDURE CHECKLIST

- ✔ Review indications and verify that the test is needed.
- ✔ Review contraindications.
- ✔ Obtain informed consent.
- ✔ Discontinue vasodilator drugs, calcium-blocking drugs, and beta blockers.
- ✔ Proceed with diagnostic coronary arteriography.
- ✔ Carefully review the videotape or the cinearteriogram before proceeding to ergonovine provocation testing.
- ✔ Check the availability of all necessary drugs.
- ✔ Proceed to ergonovine provocation.
- ✔ For a negative test, reverse the ergonovine effect.
- ✔ For a positive test and after the reversal of the ergonovine effect, observe the patient for 20 minutes.
- ✔ Return the patient to a monitored care unit.

REFERENCES

1. Prinzmetal, M., et al.: Angina pectoris: a variant form of angina pectoris. Preliminary report. Am. J. Med. **27:**375-388, 1959.
2. Maseri, A., et al.: Coronary artery spasm as a cause of acute myocardial ischemia in man, Chest **68:**625-633, 1975.
3. Chahine, R.A.: Coronary artery spasm: the pendulum continues swinging (editorial), J. Am. Coll. Cardiol. **7:**446-448, 1986.
4. Epstein, S.E., et al.: Dynamic coronary obstruction as a cause of angina pectoris: implications regarding therapy, Am. J. Cardiol. **55:**61B-68B, 1985.
5. Conti, C.R.: Large vessel coronary vasospasm: diagnosis, natural history and treatment, Am. J. Cardiol. **55:**41B-49B, 1985.
6. Shepherd, J.T., and Vanhoutte, P.M.: Spasm of the coronary arteries: causes and consequences (the scientist's viewpoint), Mayo Clin. Proc. **60:**33-46, 1985.
7. Conti, C.R.: Myocardial infarction: thoughts about pathogenesis and the role of coronary artery spasm, Am. Heart J. **110:**187-193, 1985.
8. Wilkes, D., Donner, R., Black, I., and Carabello, B.A.: Variant angina in an 11 year old boy, J. Am. Coll. Cardiol. **5:**761-764, 1985.
9. Schroeder, J.D., et al.: Provocation of coronary spasm with ergonovine maleate. New test with results in 57 patients undergoing coronary arteriography, Am. J. Cardiol. **40:**487-491, 1977.
10. Heupler, F.A., et al.: Ergonovine maleate provocative test for coronary arterial spasm, Am. J. Cardiol. **41:**631-640, 1978.
11. Heupler Jr., F.A.: Provocative testing for coronary arterial spasm: risk, method and rationale (editorial), Am. J. Cardiol. **46:**335-337, 1980.
12. Chahine, R.A.: The provocation of coronary artery spasm (editorial), Cathet. Cardiovasc. Diagn. **6:**1-5, 1980.
13. de la Alegria, E., et al.: Methylergonovine-induced spasm of saphenous vein coronary bypass graft, Chest **87:**545-547, 1985.
14. Fester, A.: Ergonovine maleate—a provocative test (editorial), Cathet. Cardiovasc. Diagn. **6:**217-223, 1980.
15. Crean, P.A., et al.: Ergonovine testing inside and outside the catheterization laboratory (abstract), J. Am. Coll. Cardiol. **5:**431, 1985.
16. Waters, D.D., et al.: Ergonovine testing to detect spontaneous remissions of variant angina during long-term treatment with calcium antagonist drugs, Am. J. Cardiol. **47:**179-184, 1981.
17. Salem, B.I., et al.: Acute myocardial infarction with "normal" coronary arteries: clinical and angiographic profiles, with ergonovine testing, Texas Heart Inst. J. **12:**1-7, 1985.
18. Abeytua, M., and Bescos, L.L.: Ergonovine provocative testing: a double catheter technique, Cathet. Cardiovasc. Diagn. **11:**335, 1985.
19. Nakhjavan, F.K., and Yazdanfar, S.: Ergonovine provocative testing: description of a "double catheter technique," Cathet. Cardiovasc. Diagn. **10:**195-198, 1984.
20. Hastey, C.E., Erwin, S.W., and Ramanathan, K.B.: Ergonovine-induced coronary spasm refractory to intracoronary nitroglycerin but responsive to nitroprusside, Am. Heart J. **107:**778-784, 1984.
21. Schroeder, J.S.: Provocative testing for coronary artery spasm. In Schroeder, J.S. (editor): Invasive cardiology, Philadelphia, 1985, F.A. Davis Co., pp. 83-96.
22. Talwar, K.K., Kothari, S.S., and Bhatia, M.L.: Bronchospasm following ergometrine testing for coronary spasm (letter), Am. Heart J. **109:**1415, 1985.
23. Kurnik, P.B., et al.: Prolonged coronary vasoconstrictor effect of ergonovine maleate, Cathet. Cardiovasc. Diagn. **10:**353-361, 1984.
24. Waters, D.D., et al.: Ergonovine testing in a coronary care unit, Am. J. Cardiol. **46:**922-930, 1980.
25. Quigley, P.J., and Maurer, B.J.: Ventricular fibrillation during coronary angiography: association with potassium-containing glyceryl trinitrate, Am. J. Cardiol. **56:**191, 1985.
26. Heupler Jr., F.A., Ferrario, C.M., Averill, D.B., and Bott-Silverman, C.: Initial coronary air embolus in the differential diagnosis of coronary artery spasm, Am. J. Cardiol. **55:**657-661, 1985.
27. Vaksmann, G., et al.: The ergometrine test: a provocative test for coronary artery spasm or esophageal motility disorders? (abstract), J. Am. Coll. Cardiol. **7:**215A, 1986.
28. Health and Public Policy Committee, American College of Physicians: Performance of ergonovine provocative testing for coronary artery spasm, Ann. Intern. Med. **100:**152-154, 1984.
29. Buxton, A., et al.: Refractory ergonovine-induced coronary vasospasm: importance of intracoronary nitroglycerin, Am. J. Cardiol. **46:**329-334, 1980.
30. Pepine, C.J., Feldman, R.L., and Conti, R.: Action of intracoronary nitroglycerin in refractory coronary artery spasm, Circulation **65:**411-414, 1982.
31. Bertrand, M.E., et al.: Frequency of provoked coronary arterial spasm in 1089 consecutive patients undergoing coronary arteriography, Circulation **65:**1299-1306, 1982.

Chapter Seven

Pulmonary angiography

ARA G. TILKIAN
ELAINE K. DAILY

Selective pulmonary angiography is a procedure whereby radiocontrast material is injected into the pulmonary artery (PA) or its branches to provide visualization of the vessels on radiographic film. Nonselective techniques were introduced in the early 1930s, when radiocontrast material was injected into a peripheral vein and the pulmonary vessels were visualized. Selective angiography was established by 1963[1] and during the ensuing 20 years has developed into a remarkably safe and useful diagnostic technique.[2-4] Pulmonary angiography is useful in the diagnosis of numerous types of congenital or acquired disease of the pulmonary vessels. By far the most common indication for this procedure is suspected pulmonary thromboembolic disease.

DIAGNOSIS OF PULMONARY EMBOLISM

Pulmonary embolism is frequently suspected in patients with cardiopulmonary disease and also in patients who have undergone surgery or trauma or have underlying neoplastic disease. The diagnosis of pulmonary embolism is easy to suspect but difficult to confirm. Clinical diagnosis based on the history and physical examination alone is unreliable. The mortality associated with this condition is estimated to be 50,000 to 200,000/year in the United States. This fact along with the risks associated with long-term anticoagulation mandate an accurate diagnosis for early and effective treatment.

Routine diagnostic tests

Routine blood count, enzymes, chemistry studies, ECGs, and even arterial blood gas studies are too insensitive or too nonspecific to be of value in confirming or excluding a diagnosis of pulmonary embolism. Of some value are the standard chest radiograph and the perfusion lung scan, preferably in conjunction with a ventilation scan.

The role of chest radiography

No specific abnormalities on the chest radiograph are diagnostic of pulmonary embolism or pulmonary infarction. A completely normal radiograph does not exclude the diagnosis of pulmonary embolism. However, the chest radiograph has two valuable contributions to the diagnosis of pulmonary embolism: it may reveal abnormalities that suggest an alternative diagnosis that may mimic pulmonary embolism, and it is necessary in the proper interpretation of a radioisotope lung scan.

Perfusion and ventilation radioisotope lung scans

The proper role of perfusion and ventilation radioisotope lung scans in the diagnosis of pulmonary embolism remains controversial.[5,6] The technique is quite sensitive, but its specificity has been seriously questioned, and efforts toward improvement by combining ventilation scans with perfusion scans have not been adequately validated.

An entirely normal multiple-view (usually six views) perfusion lung scan is generally considered satisfactory evidence against clinically significant pulmonary embolism. An exception may be a large central pulmonary embolism, which may cause symmetric reduction in perfusion of both lungs without total occlusion of any branch. An angiographically confirmed case of clinical pulmonary embolism with a normal lung scan is rare.

Attempts to classify lung scans into low-probability, high-probability, and indeterminate categories suffer from large degrees of overlap. It has been demonstrated that patients with lung scans indicating a high probability of pulmonary embolism had pulmonary emboli confirmed by angiography in 55% of cases, whereas patients with lung scans with low probability had confirmed emboli in 33% of cases.[7]

Numerous conditions that mimic pulmonary embolism clinically also reduce blood flow to a portion of lung and produce perfusion defects. Thus a diagnosis of pulmonary embolism based on clinical criteria and a positive perfusion lung scan is frequently wrong. Still, the pulmonary perfusion scan has a very definite role in the diagnosis of pulmonary embolism. If all the evidence (including the history and physical examination) points to a pulmonary embolism, then a perfusion defect (localized, segmental, or lobar) is good evidence for pulmonary embolic disease, especially if in conjunction with a normal chest radiograph and normal ventilation scan. In this situation the angiographic confirmation of the diagnosis may not always be necessary.

A lung scan is of greater value in planning a confirmatory angiogram. A "positive" lung scan can guide the angiographer to the proper area of interest and permit selective angiography in multiple projections, greatly enhancing the diagnostic yield and safety of angiography by confirming the presence of pulmonary emboli while limiting the amount of contrast agent injected. Thus an abnormal perfusion lung scan, although rarely adequate for a definitive diagnosis, is an invaluable aid in guiding the angiographer to a specific diagnosis with the least number of injections.[7-13]

Why pulmonary angiography is not performed more frequently

There are three major reasons why pulmonary angiography is not performed more frequently in suspected pulmonary embolism.

First, there is a misconception about the risk of angiography as compared to the risk of prolonged and possibly unnecessary anticoagulation. The risk of chronic anticoagulation in patients with cardiopulmonary disease, trauma, or neoplastic disease is high, especially in elderly people, whereas the risks associated with selective angiography using modern catheters and techniques and newer contrast agents are continually declining.

In the past, the complexity and invasive nature of selective angiography discouraged its wider use. However, improvements in catheter and imaging techniques have greatly simplified this procedure.

Another major factor discouraging performance of pulmonary angiography is its expense. Selective pulmonary angiography remains a costly procedure, utilizing expensively equipped and staffed facilities. Frequently the study can be performed on an outpatient basis, reducing its cost. Still, the cost in dollars of a wrong diagnosis is probably more than the cost of a diagnostic study.

Given all these considerations, it is likely that pulmonary angiography will be performed with increasing frequency for the diagnosis of pulmonary embolism.

INDICATIONS

Pulmonary angiography is indicated for the following conditions:
- Suspected pulmonary embolism that cannot be excluded or confirmed by other studies
- Surgical intervention for treatment of pulmonary embolism
- Suspected peripheral PA stenosis
- Suspected anomalous pulmonary venous drainage
- Suspected pulmonary arteriovenous fistulas

CONTRAINDICATIONS

There are no absolute contraindications for pulmonary angiography. Relative contraindications[2-4,14] include:
- Moderate to severe pulmonary hypertension, especially if accompanied by right ventricular failure (see p. 174)
- Severe hypoxemia
- Uncooperative or restless patient
- Left bundle branch block (LBBB) without a standby pacemaker (right heart catheterization and pulmonary angiography may precipitate complete heart block)
- Pregnancy: The risk of radiation exposure (approximately 70 times as much as with chest radiography) must be weighed against the risk of missing the diagnosis or using heparin or coumadin during pregnancy
- Right-sided endocarditis with risk of dislodging vegetations
- Amiodorone pulmonary toxicity, in which pulmonary angiography has been reported to precipitate acute respiratory distress syndrome[14]
- Relative contraindications for any angiography, including uncontrolled congestive heart failure, uncontrolled arrhythmias, renal dysfunction, multiple myeloma, sickle cell disease, or history of radiocontrast agent reaction

Systemic anticoagulation is not a contraindication for pulmonary angiography; an arm vein may be used for greater safety. Ultimately the informed clinician, with the aid of the angiographer, must weigh the risk of pulmonary angiography in the individual patient against the risk of possible incorrect diagnosis and inappropriate treatment.

RISKS

The risks of pulmonary angiography vary with patient selection and technique.[2,15,16] Almost all cases of death directly related to selective pulmonary angiography have occurred in patients with pulmonary hypertension and failure of the right side of the heart with a right ventricular end-diastolic pressure of greater than 20 mm

Hg. Overall morbidity of pulmonary angiography is 1% to 2%, and overall mortality is 0.2% to 0.4%. Risks are divided into three categories: those associated with (1) the radiocontrast material, (2) right heart catheterization, and (3) vascular injury at the entry site.

Risks associated with radiocontrast material include anaphylactic reaction, volume overload and congestive heart failure, acute right ventricular failure, and acute renal failure (see Chapter 19).

Risks associated with right heart catheterization include atrial and ventricular arrhythmias (atrial tachycardia, atrial fibrillation, ventricular tachycardia, and ventricular fibrillation), right bundle branch block (RBBB), complete heart block, bradycardia, cardiac perforation with or without cardiac tamponade, pyrogenic reactions, and catheter knotting.

Risks associated with vascular injury at entry site including bleeding, infection, and thromboembolic complications.

Methods of reducing the morbidity and mortality are discussed on p. 120.

EQUIPMENT

For the safe performance of diagnostic-quality pulmonary angiography, the following equipment is required:
- Standard cardiac catheterization facilities and equipment, including equipment for cardiopulmonary resuscitation and cardiac pacing
- Capability for intracardiac pressure monitoring and oxymetry
- Capability for measuring cardiac output (Fick or thermodilution method); such equipment is desirable but not necessary
- Capability for exposing large film with serial film changer—must be able to expose at least three films/second and preferably four films/second
- Other filming capability considered desirable but not necessary: Cineangiography with framing rates of 30 to 60 frames/second and digital radiography
- Power injector with ability to control volume and rate of injection of contrast material with specified pressure limits
- Specialized catheters: A choice of various types and sizes of catheters is required (see p. 166)

PERSONNEL

Selective pulmonary angiography involves right heart catheterization, hemodynamic measurements, some estimate of cardiac output, selective angiography of a complex vascular tree in multiple projections, and recording utilizing various filming techniques. The interpretation of the data requires a basic understanding of cardiovascular physiology and experience in the interpretation of cut-film angiography and cine angiography, with appreciation of oblique views.

Safety of the procedure in large part depends on appreciation of hemodynamic abnormalities of the right side of the heart during the study, recognition and prompt treatment of arrhythmias, and expert management of cardiopulmonary complications.

For the performance of pulmonary angiography under *optimal* conditions, the following personnel are needed:
- Cardiologist or cardiovascular radiologist or both working in close cooperation
- Assistant to angiographer (usually a nurse)
- Radiology technologist responsible for radiographic equipment
- Cardiovascular technologist for hemodynamic measurements and ECG monitoring
- Circulating nurse for patient care and administration of oxygen and drugs

Studies can be performed with less help but at the risk of some compromise in patient safety or technical quality of the studies. In high-risk patients or when emergency pulmonary embolectomy may be considered, the anesthesiologist and the cardiothoracic surgeon should be immediately available during and after the study.

PATIENT PREPARATION

Patient preparation for selective pulmonary angiography is similar to that of any cardiac catheterization with angiography.

1. Inform the patient regarding procedure, risks, and what to expect, and obtain informed consent.

2. The patient should have nothing by mouth for 4 to 6 hours except for sips of water.

3. Ensure that the patient has adequate hydration and IV fluids if necessary.

4. Review the patient's recent ECG and electrolytes, blood urea nitrogen (BUN), creatinine, and arterial blood gas levels. Correct any abnormalities if possible.

5. Shave and prepare the anticipated venous entry site.

TIMING OF PULMONARY ANGIOGRAPHY

Pulmonary angiography ordinarily is not an emergency procedure; however, once the decision is made to proceed, it should be done without much delay. Acute pulmonary emboli resolve with a variable rate, usually involving days to weeks. The sooner the study is performed, the better the chance for a definitive diagnostic study and earlier institution of definitive treatment. Delay of several hours (or overnight) is generally considered acceptable if that is the time required to obtain access to the angiographic facility. Starting antico-agulant treatment during this period is an individual clinical decision. Rarely, the study needs to be done as an emergency procedure in critically ill patients when emergency thrombolytic therapy or surgical intervention is contemplated.

PROCEDURE
Site of venous entry

Factors to consider when deciding which vein to use are operator experience, the condition of the patient and his or her veins, the choice and size of catheters, the state of anticoagulation, and the anticipated use of heparin or thrombolytic agents. Commonly used sites and their advantages and disadvantages are listed in Table 7-1. The advantages and disadvantages of the antecubital versus the femoral approach have not been compared in formal studies, and experienced angiographers differ in their view as to the preferred route.[2,17]

Guidelines

1. Do not compromise patient safety or diagnostic quality of the study for operating convenience or ease of access to the venous system.

2. Avoid the femoral venous route if there is clinical evidence of iliofemoral deep vein thrombophlebitis. The femoral route cannot be used in patients who have had inferior vena caval ligation, plication, or insertion of an umbrella.

3. If the femoral route is chosen:
   a. Inject 8 to 10 ml of contrast agent into the iliac vein and follow it on fluoroscopy to assure patency and absence of major clots.
   b. If there is suspicion of iliofemoral or inferior vena caval thrombus, or if the guidewire or the catheter does not advance easily, then interrupt the procedure to obtain a diagnostic venogram of the iliofemoral veins and the inferior vena cava.
   c. If clots are identified, and selective pulmonary angiography is still considered necessary, proceed from an antecubital or a jugular vein.

4. If there is severe thrombocytopenia or if thrombolytic therapy is to be used upon diagnosis of pulmonary embolism, avoid the femoral venous route. The internal jugular route should not be used either. Bleeding complications are easier to control in an arm vein using careful venous cutdown. Heparin therapy alone is not a contraindication for percutaneous study using the femoral, internal jugular, or an antecubital vein.

5. Use the antecubital approach if you are planning to leave the catheter in the right side of the heart (Swan-Ganz catheter) for hemodynamic monitoring or selective infusion of thrombolytic agents. The risk of thromboembolic complication is probably higher with long-term femoral venous catheters.

6. In difficult circumstances consider using the axillary or internal jugular venous approach. Both methods have the advantages of the femoral venous approach, and the only negative consideration is the bleeding complication. For details of anatomy and venous access see Chapter 2.

Hemodynamic measurements

Hemodynamic measurements are performed under continuous ECG and intermittent fluoroscopic monitoring. A balloon-tip Swan-Ganz pressure-monitoring catheter and systemic administration of heparin are rou-

Table 7-1. Advantages and disadvantages of commonly used venous sites

Entry site	Advantages	Disadvantages
Median basilic vein or cephalic vein	Less risk of dislodging clots	May require vein cutdown
	Less risk of bleeding if heparin or thrombolytic agent is used	May be difficult to find vein if patient has had several cutdowns
	Percutaneous entry frequently possible—right or left arm may be used	Veins may be small, requiring use of smaller catheters and compromising quality of study
		Difficult to manipulate catheter to superselective positions
Femoral vein	Easy and rapid access percutaneously	Bleeding risk if thrombolytic agents are used
	Repeated entry possible	May dislodge clots in pelvic veins
	Large catheters can be used, enhancing quality of study	May cause femoral venous thrombus and rarely pulmonary embolism
	Easier to manipulate catheter for superselective studies and therefore better chance of diagnostic study	Left side may make catheter manipulation difficult because of sharp angle of inferior vena cava with iliac vein

tinely used. Obtain the following measurements before any angiographic study.

1. Measure pressures in right atrium, right ventricle, PA, and PA wedge position. In the absence of left ventricular dysfunction and with a normal pulmonary artery diastolic pressure, obtaining PA wedge pressure (PAWP) is not mandatory because this is generally normal.

2. Assess cardiac output. This can be done most expediently by simply obtaining an oxygen saturation determination in the pulmonary artery. Mixed venous oxygen saturation is a reliable index of cardiac output, especially if systemic arterial oxygen saturation is also considered and the Fick principle is applied. Right atrial oxygen saturation is also obtained to exclude intracardiac shunts (see Appendix D). Formal measurements of cardiac output, using the thermodilution or dye dilution technique, or actual measurements of oxygen consumption are generally not necessary or useful; they prolong the procedure and add to its cost. If severe pulmonary hypertension is found, then a more complete hemodynamic study and calculation of pulmonary vascular resistance and a study of the effects of oxygen and drugs may be needed.

3. Measure systemic arterial pressure. This is usually monitored noninvasively with an external blood pressure cuff.

Use of hemodynamic data

1. If there is severe pulmonary hypertension (mean pulmonary artery pressure of 50 mm Hg) with elevated right ventricular end-diastolic pressure (>20 mm Hg), angiography is an extremely high-risk procedure. Use superselective angiography and a limited amount of nonionic or low osmolar contrast agents. Check PAWP to exclude left ventricular, mitral, or pulmonary venous disease.

2. If there is mild to moderate pulmonary hypertension, calculate pulmonary vascular resistance. This is an excellent index of the severity of the embolic obstruction and serves as a guide to the patient's response to treatment.

3. Check PAWP. Elevated PAWP usually indicates left ventricular dysfunction. Be sure that mitral stenosis has been excluded. Limit the total volume of contrast medium injected to prevent acute left ventricular congestive heart failure and pulmonary edema. IV diuretics may also be used and nonionic or low osmolar contrast agents may be preferred.

4. If there is evidence for hypovolemia and dehydration (reduced right atrial and pulmonary arterial pressure), infuse fluids to minimize the risk of acute renal failure, especially if there is preexisting renal disease (see p. 441).

5. Use the hemodynamic data and the cardiac output to gauge the "circulation time." This will help to determine the rate and duration of cut-film angiography. In a hyperdynamic circulation with an increased cardiac output, the entire study may be obtained in 4 to 5 seconds, whereas in low cardiac output states it may require 15 to 20 seconds to complete the full study (see p. 171). Observation of the rate of clearance of a test injection of contrast agent into the pulmonary artery can also be used to estimate the circulation time.

Catheter types

Several types of catheters (Fig. 7-1) are in general use. Each have their own advantages and disadvantages. Characteristics of the commonly used catheters are summarized in Table 7-2 and their advantages and disadvantages are summarized in Table 7-3. No single catheter is considered "best" by most angiographers; there are trade-offs in each catheter design. Thus it is important for the angiographer to be familiar with the design and characteristics of each catheter system and choose the catheter(s) to suit the study at hand.

Catheter manipulation and selective positioning
Grollman catheters

Grollman catheters[17,18] are popular for selective pulmonary angiography and are designed for the femoral route via direct percutaneous entry or via an introducer of proper size. The sequence for advancement into the pulmonary artery is illustrated in Fig. 7-2.

Procedure

1. Advance the catheter under fluoroscopy to the right atrium, with the pigtail facing the tricuspid valve (Fig. 7-2, *A*). Avoid excess manipulation of the catheter in the right atrium because the catheter may knot on itself.

2. Advance it across the tricuspid valve (Fig. 7-2, *B*). If this is not accomplished with simple manipulation, use a tip-deflecting wire to temporarily eliminate the reverse curve and direct the catheter toward and through the tricuspid valve.

3. As the catheter enters the right ventricle, release the tension on the deflecting wire but leave the wire in the catheter.

4. Once the catheter is in the right ventricle, it usually rotates by itself and moves toward the right ventricular outflow tract (Fig. 7-2, *C*). If this does not occur spontaneously, gently withdraw the catheter tip within the right ventricle and rotate it counterclockwise.

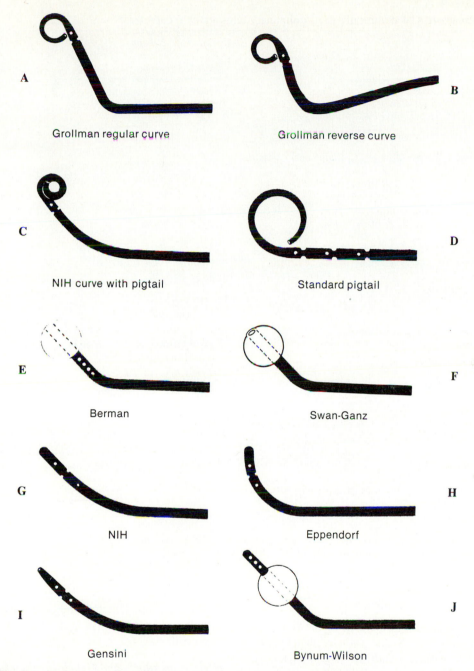

A Grollman regular curve

B Grollman reverse curve

C NIH curve with pigtail

D Standard pigtail

E Berman

F Swan-Ganz

G NIH

H Eppendorf

I Gensini

J Bynum-Wilson

Fig. 7-1. Catheters used in pulmonary angiography. See Tables 7-2 and 7-3 for characteristics of these catheters.

5. After directing the catheter into the right ventricle outflow tract, advance it into the main PA (Fig. 7-2, *D*). If the catheter loops in the right atrium, advance the relaxed deflecting wire up to the beginning of the pigtail to add stiffness. This permits easy advancement into the main pulmonary artery.

6. The catheter with the reverse curve (Fig. 7-1, *B*) seeks the left PA. A deflecting wire may be needed for selective entry into the right PA (Fig. 7-2, *E*). In such a case the reverse curve of the catheter causes it to seek the ascending branch of the right PA. Manipulation with a safety guidewire is frequently needed to direct this catheter into the descending branch. Substituting a catheter without the reverse curve facilitates its entry through the tricuspid valve and selective positioning in the branches of the right PA.

Table 7-2. Characteristics of commonly used pulmonary angiographic catheters*

Catheter	Manufacturer	External diameter	Length (cm)	Maximum pressure (psi)	Maximum volume (cc/sec)	Guidewire (inch)	Catheter tip configuration	Approx. price (1986)
Grollman (regular & reverse curve)	Cook	6.7 Fr 7.1 Fr 8.3 Fr	100 & 110	900 1000 1200	23 35 50	0.038†	Pigtail <1 cm diameter, 4 side holes, & end hole	$12.00
Pigtail pulmonary angiocatheter with NIH curve	Cook	Same characteristics as Grollman						
Pigtail angiocatheter (standard general purpose)	Cook, Cordis, USCI, & others	7 Fr 8 Fr	100 & 110	Approx. 1000	18-25 28-35	0.038	Pigtail 1.5-2.0 cm diameter	$15.00
Berman angiocatheter	Critikon & others	7 Fr 8 Fr	110 110	700 800	20 27	None	Eight side holes proximal to balloon at tip	$35.00
Swan-Ganz monitoring catheter	American Edwards and others	5-7 Fr	110	Hand injections only—balloon occlusion angiogram		0.018 (6 Fr) 0.028 (7 Fr)	End hole only with balloon proximal to it	$30.00
NIH	Cook, Cordis, USCI, & others	5-9 Fr	80-125	Approx. 1000	10-40	None	Closed end, six side holes	$45.00
Eppendorf	USCI	6-8 Fr	100-125	Approx. 1000	20-40	None	Closed end, six side holes	$45.00
Gensini	USCI	5-8 Fr	80-125	800-1100	5-40	0.025 0.035	End hole, six side holes	$40.00
Bynum Wilson‡	American Edwards	8 Fr	110	350	30	None	Six side holes distal to balloon	$60.00

*For specific catheter length, French size, and contrast medium delivery see specific product information.
†Tip-deflecting wire for 8.3 Fr catheter is 1.14 mm, and for the 6.7 Fr catheter 0.97 mm.
‡Special order item.

Other pigtail angiographic catheters

Similar maneuvers using a regular guidewire will give satisfactory results with the catheter that has an NIH type of curve with a pigtail tip (Fig. 7-1, *C*). A tip-deflecting wire is not needed. This catheter will not preferentially seek the left or the right pulmonary artery, but a guidewire can be used for selective positioning. A similar result can be achieved using a standard pigtail angiocatheter used for ventriculography or aortography (Fig. 7-1, *D*). The pigtail angiocatheter with the 155° curve (Van Tassel) will permit easier maneuvering across the tricuspid valve and to the right ventricular outflow tract. The large size of the pigtail makes this catheter unsuitable for superselective positioning.

The balloon-tip Berman angiographic catheter (Fig. 7-1, *E*) is flow directed and will advance to the PA (usually the right PA) in a manner similar to a Swan-Ganz catheter.

NIH, Eppendorf, and Gensini catheters

The NIH, Eppendorf, and Gensini catheters are designed for the brachial approach. A loop is formed in the right atrium against the right atrial wall and the catheter tip is rotated toward the tricuspid valve and advanced across the valve to the right ventricle, the right ventricular outflow tract, and the PA (see Fig. 5-3).

These catheters should not be used with the femoral approach. When using these catheters with the brachial approach, caution should be exercised. All intracardiac manipulation should be done gently because of the risk of cardiac perforation.

Table 7-3. Advantages and disadvantages of commonly used pulmonary angiographic catheters

Catheter	Advantages	Disadvantages
Grollman (with and without reverse curve)	Nontraumatic tight pigtail design; easy percutaneous entry; satisfactory contrast delivery, selective injections, & superselective placement with help of guidewire	Cannot record PAWP; passage through right side of heart may provoke arrhythmias, generally benign; reverse curve not satisfactory for brachial, axillary, or internal jugular approach; catheter manipulation in RA may form knot
Pigtail pulmonary angiographic catheter with NIH curve	Nontraumatic tight pigtail design; easy percutaneous entry via femoral, brachial, or internal jugular route; easy to maneuver to right & left PA; satisfactory contrast delivery & selective injections; superselective placement possible with guidewire	Cannot record PAWP; more difficult to enter PA from femoral approach; easier from brachial approach; passage through right heart may provoke arrhythmias, generally benign
Pigtail angiocatheters (standard general purpose)	Nontraumatic pigtail design; easy percutaneous entry via femoral or brachial route; easily available in all angiographic laboratories; satisfactory contrast delivery	Cannot record PAWP; absence of primary curve makes catheter manipulation difficult in PA; not satisfactory for superselective injections (pigtail diameter 1.5-2.0 cm); passage through right side of heart may provoke arrhythmias, generally benign
Berman angiocatheter	Flotation technique—atraumatic & nonarrhythmogenic; easy entry via femoral, brachial, or internal jugular route with use of venous introducer	Cannot record PAWP; limited rate of contrast delivery with increased risk of nondiagnostic study; not suitable for main PA injections; no guidewires: superselective placement not easy; increased catheter recoil during power injection
Swan-Ganz monitoring catheter	Nontraumatic & nonarrhythmogenic; permits wedge recording & balloon occlusion angiography	Only end hole; not suitable for power injection; cannot be used for angiography without balloon occlusion of vessel
NIH	High rate of contrast injection; suitable for main PA injection if 8 Fr used; minimal catheter recoil; designed for brachial approach	Stiff, straight tip with risk of RA or RV perforation; no PAWP recordings; no guidewires—not suitable for superselective injections; should not be used from femoral venous approach (increased risk of cardiac perforation)
Eppendorf	Similar to NIH	Similar to NIH
Gensini	Similar to NIH, but with end hole, therefore some catheter recoil	Similar to NIH but permits guidewire use; increased risk of intramyocardial or subintimal injection
Bynum-Wilson	Flotation technique—atraumatic & nonarrhythmogenic; one catheter for PAWP recording, power injection angiography, & balloon occlusion angiography	Limited rate of contrast delivery; increased catheter recoil during power injection; no guidewires; 9 Fr or 10 Fr sheath required for percutaneous entry; special order (American Edwards); expensive

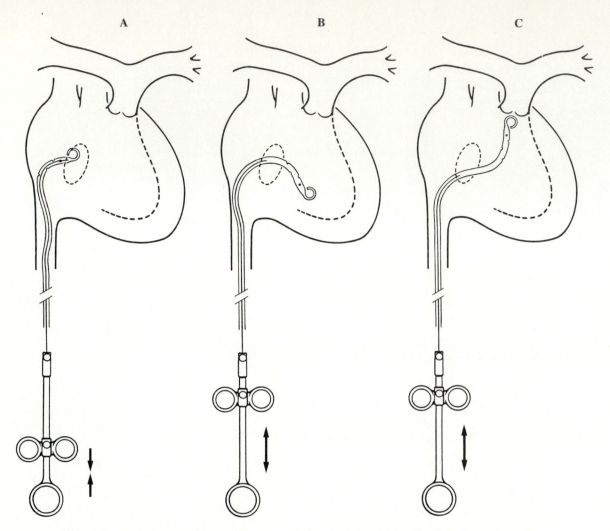

Fig. 7-2. A, Grollman catheter with a reverse curve introduced from the right femoral vein into the right atrium, pigtail facing the tricuspid valve. Tip-deflecting wire is used to eliminate the reverse curve and direct the catheter through the tricuspid valve. **B,** The catheter is advanced into the right ventricle. Tension on the tip-deflecting wire is released. **C,** Counterclockwise rotation and simultaneous advancement will direct the catheter to the right ventricular outflow tract and **D,** the main PA. **E,** Tip-deflecting wire helps direct the catheter into the right PA.

Catheter manipulation in patients with pacemakers

Special care is to be taken in patients with a permanent pacemaker, especially those with a dual-chamber pacemaker with both atrial and ventricular electrodes. Balloon-tip catheters (with minimal manipulation) seem to be the safest in these patients. If a pigtail catheter is used, special care should be taken so that catheter manipulation does not dislodge the atrial or ventricular electrodes. Catheter withdrawal from the PA should be done under fluoroscopic guidance and with the aid of a guidewire.

Projections
The first injection

Traditionally, the first injection is made into the main PA with film exposed in the anteroposterior (AP) projection, permitting visualization of both right and left PAs. However, this involves flooding both lung fields with large amounts of contrast agent (60 to 65 ml), which is rapidly diluted. Such an approach is associated with increased patient discomfort and increased risk of contrast material toxicity, especially in patients with cardiopulmonary disease.

D   E

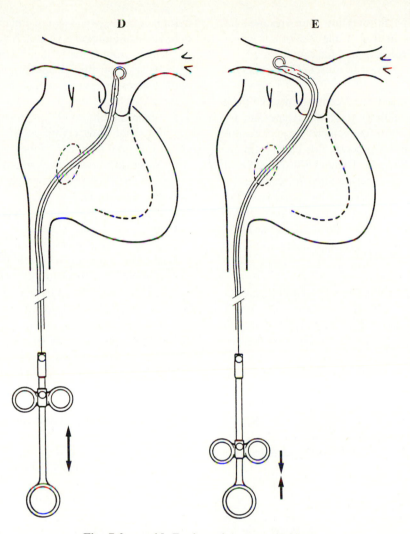

Fig. 7-2, cont'd. For legend see opposite page.

A more prudent approach is to use the chest radiograph and the perfusion lung scan as guides and to start the study with a selective injection. Thus, because it is not necessary to show every single thrombus on an angiogram, the right or left lung, whichever shows the largest perfusion defect on the perfusion lung scan, is studied first. This approach permits superselective and oblique views, enhances the likelihood of a diagnostic study, and still does not exceed the safe limits of the use of radiocontrast material. Catheters and films can be so positioned that the reflux will visualize the main PA and the proximal sections of the contralateral PA, thus avoiding the chance of missing a saddle pulmonary embolus on selective angiography. This approach presupposes the availability of a diagnostic-quality, multiple-view perfusion lung scan.

Additional injections

After the first study in the AP projection, additional selective injections may be made into the right or left PA with oblique projections; superselective injections can be made if there is an area of questionable abnormality on the initial study. Table 7-4 supplies information that may be used in choosing the proper oblique projections.[19]

Contrast injection

Contrast injection is normally performed in the manner described below.

1. Warm the radiocontrast material to body temperature and use a pressure injector under controlled conditions.

2. Deliver the desired volume in a specified period of

time without exceeding the pressure limit specified for the particular catheter in use. Table 7-5 offers guidelines for volume and injection rate for contrast material. The appropriate catheter must be selected, especially if a main PA injection is planned.

3. During pressure injection of contrast material there is a tendency for the catheter to recoil. Therefore, for main PA injection, position the catheter tip 1 cm to the right or left of the spinous process. For balloon-tip angiographic catheters (Berman, Bynum-Wilson), 2 cm is more appropriate. Similar consideration for catheter recoil should be given in superselective injections. For catheters inserted via the brachial approach, form a loop in the right ventricle so that the catheter does not recoil and fall into the right ventricle during injection.

Filming

Large film technique using a rapid serial film changer is the standard imaging method.

1. Take a scout film first to ensure that the area of interest is adequately included in the film and that the technique used is appropriate for the patient.

2. For selective right or left PA injections (the preferred method for starting a study), include the entire right or left side as well as the main PA and the proximal branches of the contralateral PA. For main PA injections include both right and left lung field.

3. Assure adequate penetration. Overpenetration risks

missing emboli, whereas underpenetration will not permit visualization of the vessel. A wedge filter will even the density from spine to lung periphery.

4. If the scout film is not fully satisfactory, repeat it with changes in patient position or technique (higher or lower kilovoltage) until a satisfactory film is obtained.

5. When moving to oblique or lateral projections, repeat the scout films before contrast material is injected and rapid serial filming is done.

6. When the proper angiographic catheter is in correct position, choose the appropriate projection and review the scout film.

7. Program the pressure injector and the rapid film changer.

8. Connect the catheter directly to the pressure injector and ensure that the system is free of air bubbles.

9. Remind the patient to follow instructions, to anticipate the warm and unpleasant sensation of the radiocontrast material, and to avoid coughing.

10. At this point all personnel should be behind adequate shields in the x-ray control room or behind lead or leaded glass partitions.

11. The radiographic technologist will turn on the x-ray rotor.

12. When the noise of the rotor is heard, prompt the patient to take a deep breath and hold it.

13. Proceed with the injection and the simultaneous filming.

14. Urge the patient to hold his or her breath as long as possible. After 6 to 8 seconds the patient may breathe while filming continues for the left atrial and left ventricular phase.

15. At completion of filming, the circulating nurse should pay attention to patient comfort and provide an emesis basin if needed.

16. Clear the catheter of any contrast material and discard; then connect the catheter to a pressure monitor to evaluate the effects of the contrast material on the patient's PA pressure.

17. Review the films and decide whether repeat or selective or oblique projections are needed and if the patient's hemodynamic status would permit this. Subtraction films are helpful in evaluating distal thrombi and should be immediately available.

Table 7-4. Optimal oblique projections[19]

Area of interest	Optimal projections
Proximal RPA	AP and LPO
RLL (well-expanded lung)	AP and RPO or LPO
RLL (atelectasis)	RPO
RML	AP and RPO or lateral
RUL	AP and RPO or lateral
Proximal LPA	AP and RPO or lateral
LLL and lingula	AP and LPO
LUL	AP and LPO or lateral

R and *LPA*, right and left pulmonary artery; *RLL,* right lower lobe; *RML,* right middle lobe; *RUL* right upper lobe; *LLL,* left lower lobe; *LUL,* left upper lobe; *AP,* anteroposterior; *R* and *LPO,* right and left posterior oblique.

Table 7-5. Guidelines for volume and injection rate for contrast material

Site of injection	Volume of contrast	Injection rate
Main PA	1 ml/kg, up to 70 ml max.	30-45 ml/sec over 1½ sec
Selective right or left PA	30-40 ml	20-25 ml/sec over ½ to 2 sec
Superselective (lobar or segmental)	15-30 ml	7-15 ml/sec over 2 sec
Balloon occlusion	5-10 ml	Hand injections

Filming rates

Adjust filming rates to the individual case and film during held respiration on end-inspiration. Record the pulmonary arterial phase at 2 to 4 films/second, the capillary and the venous phase at 1 film/second, and the left atrium and the aorta at 1 film/2 seconds. This is usually achieved by filming at:

2 films/second × 1 second
3 to 4 films/second × 3 seconds
1 film/second × 3 seconds
1 film/2 seconds × 4 seconds

For patients in congestive heart failure and long circulation time use:

2 films/second × 5 seconds
1 film/second × 4 seconds
1 film/2 seconds × 4 seconds

In superselective studies, filming may be carried only to the capillary phase (6 seconds).

This sequence of filming will achieve satisfactory results in most cases without excessive use of film or radiation exposure. In individual cases faster filming rates or longer duration of filming may be necessary.

Alternative imaging methods

Three alternate imaging methods—cineangiography, balloon occlusion angiography, and digital subtraction angiography—are discussed below.

Cineangiography

High-resolution cineangiography[20,21] is available in laboratories equipped for cardiac catheterization and angiography. Traditionally, it has not been used to record pulmonary angiographic studies. Although the size of the image intensifier limits the area that can be imaged, excellent detail can be observed with rapid rates of filming. Nine- to ten-inch image intensifiers are preferable and allow a good field of view.

Cineangiography, by its ability to delineate flow and motion, is of great help in clarifying questionable filling defects and overlap of adjacent structures. The sequential filling and the relative motion observed on cine film helps avoid the most common cause of difficulty in interpreting cut-film angiograms: addition or subtraction of radiodensity at critical points, which may simulate filling defects or vessel cut-off. An additional advantage is the ability to monitor fluoroscopically the catheter tip immediately before injections. Thus cineangiography is an excellent adjunct to cut-film pulmonary angiography and its use should substantially reduce the number of equivocal angiograms.

Cineangiography is best suited to selective injections into lobar or segmental vessels, with pressure injections

of 15 to 20 ml/second. The optimal framing rate is 60 frames/second, but 30 frames/second will yield satisfactory results. Adjust the camera shutters to exclude high-density structures, such as the heart, diaphragm, or spine. A wedge filter will help by evening the density from spine to lung periphery. One disadvantage of cineangiography is the time required to develop the film. Simultaneous recording on videotape recorders may obviate this. Cineangiography may be combined with balloon occlusion angiography.

Balloon occlusion angiography

Balloon occlusion angiography[12,22-24] has been rediscovered. The technique involves using a balloon-tip catheter to occlude a PA branch, injecting a small amount (approximately 10 ml) of contrast material by hand, and recording the results on cine film or cut film. Several variations of this procedure have been described.

The technique is best used as a *supplement* to the standard pulmonary angiogram, with the vessel to be visualized by balloon occlusion angiography selected on the basis of perfusion lung scan and the preliminary mainstream or selective right and left pulmonary angiogram.

Catheters used. Ordinary 7 Fr, two-lumen, flow-directed catheters (Swan-Ganz catheters) have been used with good results. These catheters ordinarily float to the right lower lobe vessels, which are the most common site of pulmonary emboli. Manipulation with the aid of a 0.018- or 0.028-inch guidewire permits the angiographer to direct the catheter tip into upper lobe vessels or left PA branches.

A special balloon catheter (Bynum-Wilson*) has been developed with six side holes distal to the balloon to permit PAWP recording, selective right or left pulmonary angiography with power injection (without balloon occlusion), and balloon occlusion angiography with hand injection (see Tables 7-2 and 7-3).

Vessels suitable for this technique should be 12 mm or less in diameter, given the size of the balloon on catheters in use today. However, if the demand is present, industry should be able to provide the angiographer with varying and larger balloon sizes.

Contrast injection. For balloon occlusion angiography, inject undiluted contrast material by hand (usually 10 ml) until adequate opacification of the occluded vessel is seen on fluoroscopy. If this provokes coughing or patient discomfort, the contrast medium may be diluted with saline (2:1 and 1:1).

---

*Available from American Edwards on special order.

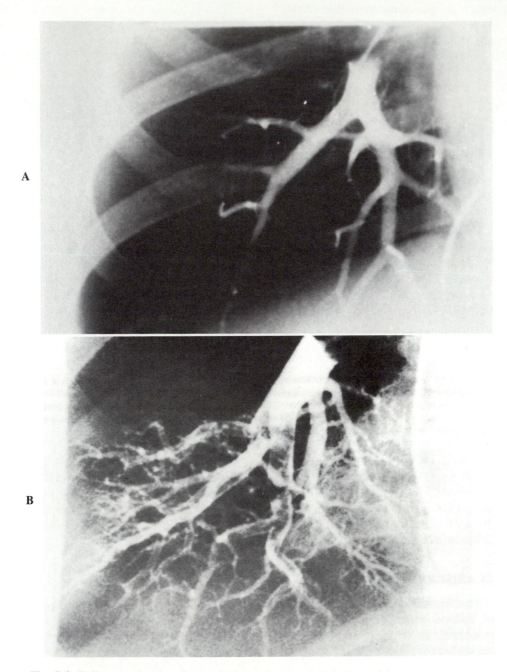

Fig. 7-3. Balloon occlusion pulmonary cineangiogram. A right lower lobe pulmonary angiogram is performed by manual injection of contrast medium. **A,** Normal study. **B,** Multiple intraluminal filling defects diagnostic of pulmonary embolism (from Benotti, J.R., Ockene, I.S., Alpert, J.S., and Dalen, J.E.: Balloon-occlusion pulmonary cineangiography for diagnosing pulmonary embolism, Cathet. Cardiovasc. Diagn. **10:**519-527, 1984).

Filming method. After balloon occlusion of a PA branch and adequate opacification of the vessel with contrast material injected under fluoroscopic monitoring, record the image on cine film at 30 to 60 frames/second with simultaneous videotape recording. Deflate the balloon before the end of filming to permit visualization of the washout phase of the study. The image can also be recorded on large film at 1 to 2 films/second, but fluoroscopic monitoring will be sacrificed. Fig. 7-3 compares a normal study *(A)* with an abnormal one *(B)*.

Advantages. There are several advantages to balloon occlusion angiography.

- It requires a limited amount of contrast material per injection. Thus it is useful for patients in whom volume of contrast material should be limited—patients with pulmonary hypertension, critically ill patients, and patients with renal disease, sickle cell disease, or congestive heart failure.
- It provides excellent opacification and definition of details in the selected vessel, overcoming problems of motion, vessel overlap, or poor contrast.
- It is of great value in clarifying questionable areas of pulmonary arteries observed on mainstream injections.

Disadvantage. Only a limited number of vessels are seen; therefore, unless a limited area of interest is being studied, the technique becomes very time consuming and exposes the patient to an excessive level of radiation.

Digital subtraction angiography

Digital subtraction angiography[25-27] was introduced clinically in late 1970; by early 1980 several investigators had applied this technique to pulmonary angiography, and there was hope that it would deliver diagnostic-quality angiograms with reduced amount of contrast material injected in the superior vena cava or right atrium, simplifying the procedure and enhancing its safety.

Preliminary studies using early generation equipment encountered serious difficulties, including poor resolution, limited field of vision, problems with motion of the heart and pulmonary vessels, and lack of complete patient cooperation for 10 seconds of held respiration. Thus early and overenthusiastic claims that digital subtraction angiography would replace selective pulmonary angiography as the definitive study for pulmonary embolism did not materialize.

Currently digital subtraction angiography can be a useful adjunct to selective pulmonary arteriography. In patients for whom the volume of contrast material injected is of concern, areas of interest can be recorded by this method using superselective injections and minimal amounts of contrast material.

The role of digital subtraction angiography in pulmonary angiography may expand as further technical improvements are made. Some of these forthcoming improvements include advances in image intensifier design (larger image intensifier with improved resolution),

Table 7-6. Comparison of three imaging methods

Imaging methods	Advantages	Disadvantages
Conventional cut-film changer	Excellent resolution Large field of view Rapidly developed film Magnification technique possible	Increased radiation exposure 2-4 films/sec only Large amount of contrast needed Catheter and injection cannot be monitored during filming
35 mm cineangiography	Reduced motion unsharpness (sharper image) Resolves overlap Sequential flow seen Very suitable for balloon occlusion angiography Permits simultaneous recording on videotape	Reduced spatial resolution More time needed to develop film Limited field of view—panning may be necessary Resolution reduced at periphery of field
Digital subtraction angiography	Less contrast needed Less invasive (right atrium) Possible post-processing to enhance images Higher density resolution	Needs cooperative patient (8-10 sec of breath holding) Increased motion unsharpness (blurred) Limited field—function of image intensifier size No panning possible

faster image acquisition to obtain framing rates of 30 or more/second, gating to the cardiac cycle (to end-diastole) to eliminate cardiac motion, biplane image capability, and improvements in video camera design and postprocessing techniques. Use of nonionic contrast agents, by enhancing patient comfort, will improve patient cooperation and permit more diagnostic studies.

It is possible that technical advances will permit digital subtraction angiography to be the diagnostic study of choice in many patients with suspected pulmonary embolism. Its value should be greatest in patients with pulmonary hypertension, renal disease, congestive heart failure, or sickle cell disease, where conventional pulmonary arteriography with currently available contrast agents carries appreciable risk of morbidity or even death.

Table 7-6 summarizes the advantages and disadvantages of cut-film, cine, and digital angiography.

SPECIAL PRECAUTIONS
Angiography and pulmonary hypertension

Most fatalities secondary to pulmonary angiography have occurred in patients with pulmonary hypertension and elevated right ventricular end-diastolic pressure. Pulmonary systemic pressures exceeding 70 mm Hg and right ventricular end-diastolic pressure over 20 mm Hg identify the subgroup of patients that are considered to be at high risk for major morbidity and death from this procedure. Systemic hypotension, cyanosis, acute right ventricular failure, ventricular arrhythmias, profound shock, and cardiac arrest can occur even with selective injections of 25 to 30 ml of contrast material. When angiography is clearly needed in this setting, the risk may be reduced by following these steps:

- Do not inject into the main PA.
- Avoid selective right and left mainstem injections.
- Use the perfusion lung scan as a "map" to start the study with a superselective injection with very limited volume of contrast material.
- Use balloon occlusion angiography to further reduce the volume of contrast material needed during each injection.
- Use nonionic or low osmolar agents (see Chapter 19).
- Be ready for intubation and assisted ventilation.

Pulmonary angiography in chronic pulmonary embolism

Acute pulmonary emboli frequently resolve with or without anticoagulant or thrombolytic therapy. However, in some patients this may not occur and in time may result in the clinical syndrome of chronic pulmonary embolism, presenting with pulmonary hyperten-

sion, respiratory insufficiency, and cor pulmonale. At this stage, addition of anticoagulant therapy has little to offer, and surgical embolectomy in selected patients is the treatment of choice.[28]

Before surgical treatment, hemodynamic and angiographic studies are necessary. Additionally, aortography or selective bronchial arteriography may be performed to evaluate the patency of the PA distal to the occlusion. This may help select patients who have the potential to benefit from surgery.[29] The value of preoperative bronchial arteriography is controversial and not universally accepted.[30]

COMPLICATIONS

The following complications arising from pulmonary angiography have been reported in several series comprising more than 4000 patients.[2,15,16]

Complications	Incidence
Fever	1%
Serious arrhythmias	0.7%
Cardiopulmonary arrest— successfully treated	0.2%
Cardiac perforation*	0.4%
Subintimal injection	0.2%
Bronchospasm	0.5%
Pulmonary edema	0.2%
Hypotension	0.2%
Anaphylaxis	0.1%
Death	0.2%

See p. 120 for methods of avoiding and treating complications relating to catheterization and angiography (Table 5-2).

PATIENT AFTERCARE

Care of the patient following uncomplicated pulmonary angiography is simple.

1. Keep the patient warm and comfortable.
2. Repair the venous entry site if there has been a cutdown.
3. Gently press until hemostasis is established for percutaneous method. Reversal of heparinization is not necessary.
4. Bed rest for 2 to 4 hours is advisable.

INTERPRETATION OF FINDINGS
Value of pulmonary angiography in diagnosing pulmonary embolism

Selective pulmonary angiography is the "gold standard" in the evaluation of pulmonary embolism. The

---

*Only with the use of NIH-type catheters. Should not occur with balloon-tip catheters or pigtail angiographic catheters.

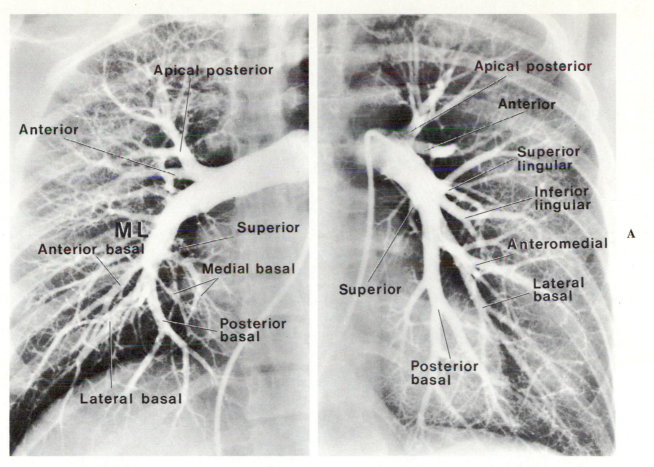

Fig. 7-4. A, Normal right and left selective pulmonary arteriograms in two different patients (anteroposterior projection). (From Dotter, C.T.: The normal pulmonary arteriogram. In Abrams, H.L. [editor]: Abram's angiography, ed. 3, Boston, 1983, Little, Brown & Co., pp. 715-722.)

Continued.

sensitivity and specificity of high-quality pulmonary angiography expertly interpreted are excellent. Emboli 2.5 mm or larger can be documented. Positive pulmonary angiographic findings correlate well with postmortem findings. Patients with suspicion of pulmonary emboli but with normal pulmonary angiograms who are not treated for pulmonary emboli generally have a benign clinical course and do not have the morbidity or mortality related to pulmonary embolic disease. Thus the idea that a pulmonary angiogram may not be sensitive enough and may miss clinical pulmonary embolism has not been validated.[8,10,31] This presupposes high-quality angiograms with appropriate oblique views, expertly interpreted.

The interpretation of the pulmonary angiogram can be difficult and requires experience. Although demonstration of one thrombus is generally enough to establish a diagnosis, and not all clots need to be documented angiographically, a definitive diagnosis may require multiple injections, oblique views, subselective injections, balloon injection angiography, and magnification angiography.

The normal pulmonary angiogram

Fig. 7-4, *A,* illustrates the normal pulmonary arteriogram, whereas Fig. 7-4, *B,* is a schematic diagram that outlines the main branches of the PA tree. For details of PA anatomy see the excellent description by Dotter.[32]

For a study to be considered definitely normal:

- Both right and left PAs, with their lobar branches and 1 to 3 subdivisions, should be well seen and noted to be free of any filling defects or vessel cutoff.
- Filling of the vessels should be prompt and symmetric.

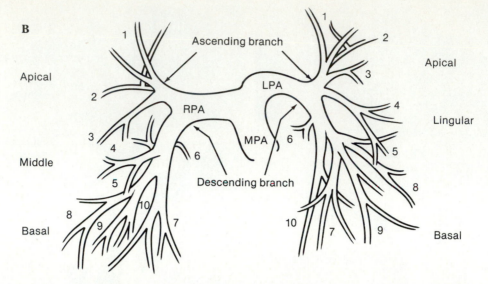

Fig. 7-4, cont'd. B, Diagram of a normal pulmonary arterial tree (anteroposterior projection). (*MPA,* Main pulmonary artery; *RPA,* right pulmonary artery; *LPA,* left pulmonary artery.)

Right pulmonary artery branch	Arises from	Supplies
1. Apical	Ascending branch	Upper lobe
2. Posterior	Ascending branch	Upper lobe
3. Anterior	Ascending branch	Upper lobe
4. Lateral	Ascending or descending branch	Middle lobe
5. Medial	Ascending or descending branch	Middle lobe
6. Superior	Descending branch	Lower lobe
7. Medial basal	Descending branch	Lower lobe
8. Anterior basal	Descending branch	Lower lobe
9. Lateral basal	Descending branch	Lower lobe
10. Posterior basal	Descending branch	Lower lobe
Left pulmonary artery branch		
1. Apical	Ascending branch	Upper lobe
2. Posterior	Ascending branch	Upper lobe
3. Anterior	Ascending branch	Upper lobe
4. Superior lingular	Ascending or descending branch	Lingula
5. Inferior lingular	Ascending or descending branch	Lingula
6. Superior	Descending branch	Lower lobe
7. Medial basal	Descending branch	Lower lobe
8. Anterior basal	Descending branch	Lower lobe
9. Lateral basal	Descending branch	Lower lobe
10. Posterior basal	Descending branch	Lower lobe

• There should be no areas of oligemia.

Abnormal pulmonary angiogram

Only two angiographic signs are considered diagnostic of pulmonary embolism: definite intraluminal filling defect and abrupt arterial cut-off. Unless one or the other of these is clearly observed, the diagnosis of pulmonary embolism cannot be definitely established. Superimposed structures and acute turns in vessels can mimic the signs, thus making the interpretation of these signs quite difficult. Also, a totally missing vessel (occlusion at the point of origin of the vessel) is difficult to detect, and a filling defect can be obscured by contrast medium flowing by it.

Equivocal pulmonary angiograms

Despite all efforts, some pulmonary angiographic studies will remain equivocal. Angiographic abnormal-

Table 7-7. Angiographic findings in suspected pulmonary embolism

	Intraluminal filling defect	Abrupt vessel cut-off	Oligemia	Asymmetry of flow
Definite pulmonary embolism	+	+	+/−	+/−
Equivocal for pulmonary embolism	−	−	*	*
Negative for pulmonary embolism	−	−	†	†

+, Present; −, absent.
*Not explained on the basis of existing cardiopulmonary disease.
†Explained on the basis of existing cardiopulmonary disease.

ities that may suggest pulmonary emboli but that are not diagnostic include:

- Oligemia of an area of lung: When seen in isolation, this has the same diagnostic significance as a perfusion defect on lung scan. A frequent nonembolic cause is bullous disease of the lung. In this setting, selective, oblique, balloon occlusion, magnification, and subtraction angiograms are of great help.
- Asymmetry of flow: Delay in filling or asymmetric filling of a vessel or a pruninglike effect of a vessel is frequently seen in association with an emboli, but in itself cannot be the basis of diagnosis. Atelectasis is another common cause. Special selective oblique or balloon occlusion angiographic views are required.

Other conditions that are frequently associated with oligemia or asymmetric flow and can mimic pulmonary emboli include pneumonia, bronchiectasis, pulmonary hypertension, congestive heart failure, emphysema, and carcinoma.

Thus, after best efforts, the final interpretation of a pulmonary angiogram may fall into the category of definite, equivocal, or negative. Table 7-7 summarizes the abnormalities characteristic of each category.

With nonselective mainstream angiograms, 15% to 30% of studies may fall in the equivocal category. With the use of selective and superselective injections, oblique views, balloon occlusion angiogram, and cineangiography, the incidence of equivocal angiogram may be reduced to 1%.

FUTURE DEVELOPMENTS
Pulmonary fiberoptic angioscopy

A flexible fiberoptic catheter (angioscope)[33,34] with a distal balloon has been used for direct visualization of the PA in dogs and in humans. Clots as small as 4 mm have been seen, as have other pathologic changes in PAs. Very preliminary studies have suggested that the angioscope may contribute to the diagnosis of chronic and acute pulmonary emboli and may have a role in the evaluation of intravascular tumors and masses. Further improvements in catheter design and further validation of the technique may be forthcoming.

Catheter pulmonary embolectomy

Aggressive medical treatment, including thrombolytic treatment, is sufficient for most patients with major pulmonary embolism. In a small minority, massive pulmonary embolism causes profound shock and rapidly leads to death. The approach in these patients has been surgical embolectomy, with variable and generally high (50%) surgical mortality. Percutaneous catheter embolectomy is a potential alternative. This technique was first described in dogs in 1969.[35] A 10 Fr catheter with suction cups is used to retrieve the clots. In humans, a retrieval rate of 90% with a mortality of 25% has been reported.[36] With renewed interest in interventional catheter techniques and improved catheter design, this approach may be further developed. If technology can develop a combined pulmonary fiberoptic angioscope and embolectomy catheter, then a real advance in the treatment of this difficult condition can be anticipated.

Magnetic resonance imaging

Computerized tomographic scanning has been disappointing for the diagnosis of pulmonary embolism. Magnetic resonance imaging is a newer technique. Case reports have documented the ability of this technique to detect pulmonary embolism.[37] The capability of this imaging method and its resolution for pulmonary emboli are under investigation. However, high cost and long scanning times may limit its application in this field.

PROCEDURE CHECKLIST

- Review the indications and contraindications of the procedure in relation to the specific patient.

✔ Obtain informed consent.

✔ Check equipment.

✔ Notify appropriate departments for a scheduled procedure (radiology, cardiology).

✔ Obtain and review laboratory results: recent ECG and electrolytes, BUN, creatinine, and arterial blood gases.

✔ Review the patient's status.

✔ Review chest radiograph and ventilation perfusion lung scan.

✔ Preplan the study. Determine the type of catheter and the site of venous entry to be used according to individual patient and purpose of the study.

✔ Prepare the patient: site of entry, premedication, appropriate instructions, and reassurance.

✔ Obtain necessary hemodynamic measurements and respond appropriately.

✔ Perform the angiogram.

✔ Review the films and determine adequacy of the study and need for additional injections or different techniques.

✔ Watch for possible complications.

✔ Document the procedure and the outcome in the medical record.

REFERENCES

1. Williams, J.R., Wilcox, W.C., Andrews, G.J., and Burns, R.R.: Angiography in pulmonary embolism, J.A.M.A. **184**:473-476, 1963.
2. Benotti, J.R., and Grossman, W.: Pulmonary angiography. In Grossman, W., editor: Cardiac catheterization and angiography, ed. 3, Philadelphia, 1986, Lea & Febiger, pp. 213-226.
3. Dotter, C.T., and Roche, J.: Pulmonary arteriography: technique. In Abrams, H.L., editor: Abram's angiography, ed. 3, Boston, 1983, Little, Brown & Co., pp. 707-713.
4. Goodman, P.C.: Pulmonary angiography, Clin. Chest Med. **5**:465-477, 1984.
5. Robin, E.B.: Overdiagnosis and overtreatment of pulmonary embolism: the emperor may have no clothes, Ann. Intern. Med. **87**:755-781, 1977.
6. Mercandetti, A.J., Kipper, M.S., and Moser, K.M.: Influence of perfusion and ventilation scans on therapeutic decision making and outcome in cases of possible embolism, West. J. Med. **142**:208-213, 1985.
7. Marsh, J.D., Glynn, M., and Torman, H.A.: Pulmonary angiography; application in a new spectrum of patients, Am. J. Med. **75**:763-770, 1983.
8. Greenspan, R.H.: Angiography in pulmonary embolism. In Abrams, H.L., editor; Abram's angiography, ed. 3, Boston, 1983, Little, Brown & Co., pp. 803-816.
9. Hull, R.D., et al.: Pulmonary angiography, ventilation lung scanning, and venography for clinically suspected pulmonary embolism with abnormal perfusion lung scanning, and venography for clinically suspected pulmonary embolism with abnormal perfusion lung scan, Ann. Intern. Med. **98**:891-899, 1983.
10. Heim, C.R., and Des Prez, R.M.: Pulmonary embolism: a review, Adv. Intern. Med. **31**:187-212, 1986.
11. Polak, J.F., and McNeil, B.J.: Pulmonary scintigraphy and the diagnosis of pulmonary embolism. A perspective, Clin. Chest Med. **5**:457-464, 1984.
12. Ferris, E.J., et al.: Radionuclide-guided balloon occlusion pulmonary cineangiography: an adjunct to pulmonary arteriography, Am. Heart J. **108**(3, Part 1):539-542, 1984.
13. Moses, D.C., Silver, T.M., and Bookstein, J.J.: The complimentary roles of chest roentgenography, lung scanning, and selective pulmonary arteriography in the diagnosis of pulmonary embolism, Circulation **49**:179-187, 1974.
14. Wood, D.L., Osborn, M.J., Rooke, J., and Holmes, D.R.Jr.: Amiodarone pulmonary toxicity: report of two cases associated with rapidly progressive fatal adult respiratory distress syndrome after pulmonary angiography, Mayo Clin. Proc. **60**:601-603, 1985.
15. Sasahara, A.A., et al.: The urokinase pulmonary embolism trial, Circulation **47**(suppl. II):1-103, 1973.
16. Mills, S.R., et al.: The incidence, etiologies, and avoidance of complications of pulmonary angiography in a large series, Diagn. Radiol. **136**:295-299, 1980.
17. Grollman, J.H., and Renner, J.W.: Transfemoral pulmonary angiography: update on technique, A.J.R. **136**:624-626, 1981.
18. Grollman, J.H.: Editorial: Pigtail catheters in pulmonary angiography, Cathet. Cardiovasc. Diagn. **10**:389-391, 1984.
19. Gomes, A.S., Grollman, J.H., Jr., and Mink, J.: Pulmonary angiography for pulmonary emboli: rational selection of oblique views, A.J.R. **129**:1019-1025, 1977.
20. Meister, S.G., et al.: Pulmonary cineangiography in acute pulmonary embolism, Am. Heart J. **84**:33-37, 1972.
21. Price, L., and Dunn, M.: Are modifications necessary in the performance of pulmonary angiograms? Chest **88**:1-2, 1985.
22. Benotti, J.R., Ockene, I.S., Alpert, J.S., and Dalen, J.E.: Balloon-occlusion pulmonary cineangiography for diagnosing pulmonary embolism, Cathet. Cardiovasc. Diagn. **10**:519-527, 1984.
23. Wilson, J.E. III, and Bynum, L.J.: An improved pulmonary angiographic technique using a balloon-tipped catheter, Am. J. Resp. Dis. **114**:1137-1143, 1976.
24. Bynum, L.J., Wilson, J.E. III, Christensen, E.E., and Sorensen, C.: Radiographic techniques for balloon-occlusion pulmonary angiography, Radiology **133**:518-520, 1979.
25. Goodman, P.C., and Brant-Zawadski, M.: Digital subtraction pulmonary angiography, A.J.R. **139**:305-309, 1982.
26. Reilley, R.F., et al.: Digital subtraction angiography: limitations for the detection of pulmonary embolism, Radiology **149**:379-382, 1983.
27. Pond, G.D.: Pulmonary digital subtraction angiography, Radiol. Clin. North Am. **23**:243-260, 1985.
28. Tilkian, A.G., Schroeder, J.S., and Robin, E.D.: Chronic thromboembolic occlusion of main pulmonary artery or primary branches, Am. J. Med. **60**:563-570, 1976.
29. Sabiston, D.C., et al.: Surgical management of chronic pulmonary embolism, Ann. Surg. **185**:699-701, 1977.
30. Utley, J.R., Spragg, R.G., Long, W.B. III, and Moser, K.M.: Pulmonary endarterectomy for chronic thromboembolic obstruction: recent surgical experience, Surgery **92**:1096-1098, 1982.
31. Novelline, R.A., et al.: The clinical course of patients with suspected pulmonary embolism and a negative pulmonary arteriogram, Diagn. Radiol. **126**:561-567, 1978.
32. Dotter, C.T.: The normal pulmonary arteriogram. In Abrams, H.L., editor: Abram's angiography, ed. 3, Boston, 1983, Little, Brown & Co., pp. 715-722.

33. Moser, K.M., Shure, D., Harrell, J.H., and Tulumello, J.: Angioscopic visualization of pulmonary emboli, Chest **77:**198-201, 1980.

34. Shure, D., Gregoratos, G., and Moser, K.M.: Fiberoptic angioscopy: role in the diagnosis of chronic pulmonary arterial obstruction, Ann. Intern. Med. **103:**844-850, 1985.

35. Greenfield, L.J., Kimmell, G.O., and McCurdy, W.C. III: Transvenous removal of pulmonary emboli by vacuum cup catheter technique, J. Surg. Res. **9:**347-352, 1969.

36. Dedrick, C.G., and Athanasoulis, C.A.: Transvenous pulmonary embolectomy. In Athanasoulis, C.A., Greene, R.E., Pfister, R.C., and Roberson, G.H.: Interventional radiology, Philadelphia, 1982, W.B. Saunders Co., pp. 370-373.

37. Fisher, M.R., and Higgins, C.B.: Central thrombi in pulmonary arterial hypertension detected by MR imaging, Radiology **158:**223-226, 1986.

Chapter Eight

Endomyocardial biopsy

ARA G. TILKIAN
ELAINE K. DAILY

Endomyocardial biopsy is the procedure by which tissue samples are obtained from the endomyocardium of the right or left ventricle. This involves the introduction of a biopsy forceps (bioptome) through a vein or an artery into the right or left ventricle of the heart.

Until the early 1970s, endomyocardial biopsy required either an open-chest or a transthoracic needle approach. Complications included the morbidity and mortality of a thoracotomy, or, in the case of needle biopsy, laceration of the heart or a coronary artery, ventricular fibrillation, and hemopericardium with tamponade.[1]

The modern era of endomyocardial biopsy dates back to 1962 with the introduction of the *Konno-Sakakibara* bioptome, permitting the *transvascular* approach to the heart.[2] By 1970 the safety and efficacy of this bioptome were conclusively demonstrated, making the more hazardous techniques obsolete.[3]

Researchers at Stanford University Medical Center have developed the *Stanford-Shultz* and the *Scholten* bioptomes,[4] the result of serial modifications on the original *Konno-Sakakibara* bioptome, modified for use via the internal jugular approach. These instruments are similar in design. The Scholten bioptome (Fig. 8-1) is in common use in the United States. Since the death of Werner Shultz in 1984, the Shultz bioptome has not been in production.

The *King* bioptome (Fig. 8-2), is another commonly used instrument. Developed in the early 1970s[5] as a modification of the Olympus bronchial biopsy forceps, it has proved to be both safe and useful for right and left heart endomyocardial biopsy.

These four bioptomes have moved the endomyocardial biopsy procedure from a position of rare usage and high risk to that of an established diagnostic procedure that may be performed with small risk in a cardiac catheterization laboratory, frequently on an outpatient basis.

INDICATIONS

Endomyocardial biopsy may be indicated for the diagnosis or clinical management of the following disorders or conditions.[6,7]

• Cardiac allograft rejection (the best established indication for endomyocardial biopsy).

• Doxorubicin (Adriamycin)–induced cardiomyopathy: For diagnosis, grading of severity, and monitoring of the clinical course. This is the only other well-established and noncontroversial indication for endomyocardial biopsy.

• Myocarditis: For the diagnosis, grading of severity, and monitoring of treatment. This category may include patients with a clinical diagnosis of peripartum and postpartum cardiomyopathy,[8] Kawasaki syndrome,[9] unexplained ventricular tachycardia or fibrillation,[10,11] or congestive heart failure of recent onset and undetermined origin. Accurate diagnosis and evaluation of response to treatment are possible only by endomyocardial biopsy. Treatment of myocarditis remains supportive, and therefore the value of biopsy-proved definitive diagnosis can be questioned in the routine (nonexperimental) care of patients (see p. 198).

• Restrictive or infiltrative cardiomyopathy, such as cardiac amyloidosis, sarcoidosis or hemochromotosis, endomyocardial fibrosis, scleroderma, radiation injury (myocardial fibrosis), carcinoid heart disease, glycogen storage disease, and tumor infiltration. These disorders can mimic pericardial constriction and cause diagnostic confusion. After a clinical and hemodynamic diagnosis of pericardial constriction is made and before surgical treatment is recommended, consideration should be given to endomyocardial biopsy if it is possible that any of the above-mentioned infiltrative or restrictive cardiomyopathies could be present. This is especially important in radiation heart disease in which both pericar-

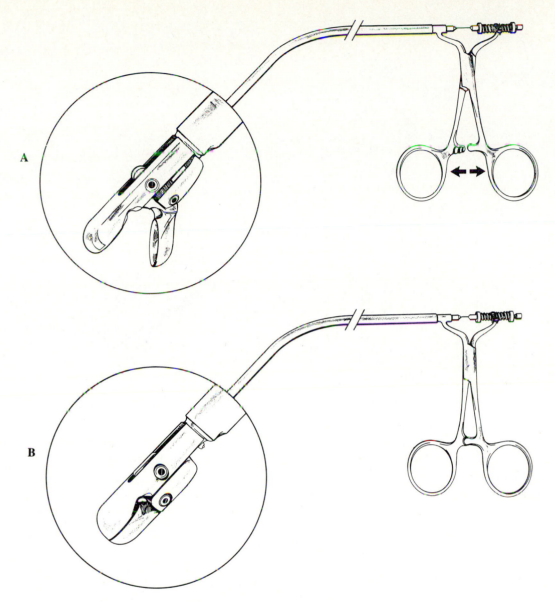

Fig. 8-1. Scholten bioptome, open (**A**) and closed (**B**).

dial constriction and restrictive cardiomyopathy may coexist.

• Miscellaneous: Vasculitis, toxoplasmosis, Chagas cardiomyopathy, rheumatic carditis. In these conditions endomyocardial biopsy can help in making a definitive diagnosis.

• Research: Biopsy in patients with suspected early cardiomyopathy is an area of active interest, as is a search for a better diagnostic criterion for "myocarditis." Endomyocardial biopsy techniques are also used in biochemical and enzymologic studies of cardiac tissue.

Rare indications

Endomyocardial biopsy is usually not indicated in the clinical care of patients with dilated chronic cardiomyopathy, since a specific biopsy diagnosis cannot be made in an overwhelming majority of such cases. Rarely, amyloidosis, sarcoidosis, or endocardial fibroelastosis may present as a dilated congestive cardiomyopathy. In these cases biopsy is useful for diagnosis.[6,7,12]

Other conditions in which endomyocardial biopsy is not usually indicated are hypertrophic cardiomyopathy, Wilson's disease, myotonic dystrophy, alcoholic car-

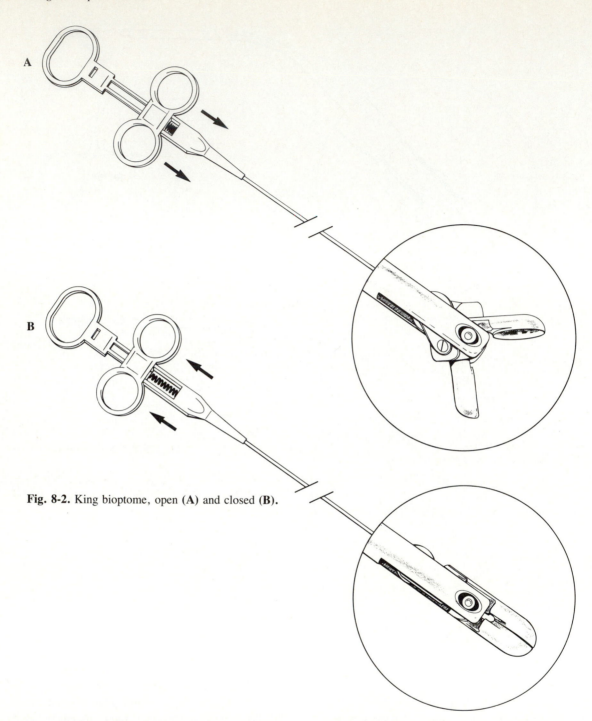

Fig. 8-2. King bioptome, open **(A)** and closed **(B)**.

diomyopathy, thyroid heart disease (hyperthyroid or hypothyroid), mitral valve prolapse, "small vessel disease," and diabetes with diabetic cardiomyopathy. If the procedure is performed for any of these conditions, nonspecific abnormalities will frequently be demonstrated. However, the information obtained does not help in making a specific diagnosis or prognosis, nor does it guide therapy.

CONTRAINDICATIONS

There are several contraindications for endomyocardial biopsy.

• Bleeding disorder, severe thrombocytopenia (platelets $<50,000/\mu L$), or systemic anticoagulation. In these conditions right ventricular endomyocardial biopsy, which carries a small risk of myocardial puncture or perforation, could precipitate a lethal hemopericardium.

For left ventricular biopsy, heparin is used during the procedure.

• Restless and uncooperative patients who cannot be sedated adequately.

• Left ventricular thrombus or prior myocardial infarction. In these conditions, *left ventricular* endomyocardial biopsy is contraindicated. In prior myocardial infarction the incidence of left ventricular thrombus is high, and left ventricular wall thinning in the infarct area may predispose to ventricular perforation.

• Shunt lesions are a relative contraindication. In this condition, *right ventricular* endomyocardial biopsy is best avoided because of the risk of paradoxic systemic embolization.

RISKS

In the past decade endomyocardial biopsy has evolved into a remarkably safe procedure, having an overall morbidity of 1% to 2% and a procedure-related mortality of less than 0.1%.[6,7,13] This remarkable safety record was accumulated in a few centers with extensive experience in the technique. This low risk frequently quoted in the literature assumes that the procedure will be performed by or under the close supervision of a physician experienced in the technique. Competence in this technique is generally acquired after performing approximately 50 procedures.

However, even in the most experienced hands endomyocardial biopsy may be associated with potentially life-threatening complications such as cardiac perforation, hemopericardium, and acute pericardial tamponade, as well as systemic or pulmonary embolization. Other complications may include atrial or ventricular tachyarrhythmias or heart block (especially if preexisting bundle branch block), vasovagal reaction (more common in left ventricular biopsies), disruption of mitral or tricuspid valve apparatus (inadvertent biopsy of papillary muscle or chordae tendineae), air embolism, and risks related to vascular injury or trauma at the site of bioptome introduction (see Chapters 2 and 3).

Clearly, this invasive procedure has the potential for major complications and should only be performed by experienced personnel for clearly defined indications.

EQUIPMENT

The procedure is usually performed in the cardiac catheterization laboratory with the capability of hemodynamic measurements, ECG monitoring, and fluoroscopy. Under special circumstances, the procedure can be performed at the bedside, using a radiolucent bed, portable fluoroscopy unit, and bedside hemodynamic monitoring. A fully equipped resuscitation cart, including a pericardiocentesis tray, should be available. Additional equipment includes:

• Percutaneous vascular access tray (see p. 34)
• Percutaneous vascular needle, 18 gauge, 7 cm
• 0.035-inch (0.9 mm) or 0.038-inch (1.0 mm) guidewire of appropriate length
• Catheter introducer set with side arm and hemostatic valve; use a 45 cm introducer for internal jugular approach, 90 to 100 cm sheath with a 110 cm ventricular catheter for the femoral approach, the sheath being one French size larger than the bioptome used
• Bioptome (see Table 8-1)
• Specimen containers and fixatives: 10% buffered formaldehyde and 2.5% buffered glutaraldehyde
• Sterile filter paper (for nontraumatic removal of biopsy specimen from bioptome)
• Portable echocardiograph (optional; see p. 200)

Fig. 8-3 illustrates the table set-up for endomyocardial biopsy.

Equipment for left ventricular endomyocardial biopsy

The following additional equipment is needed for left ventricular biopsy: Scholten left ventricular bioptome (7, Fr, 100 cm), with left ventricular pigtail catheter (6.7 Fr, 110 cm) and 90 cm radiopaque Teflon sheath with a special Luer-Lok adaptor, 7 or 8 Fr (SBS-1 Cook, Inc.).

The King bioptome (Cordis Corp.) used for right ventricular endomyocardial biopsy from the femoral approach is also suitable for left ventricular endomyocardial biopsy.

PERSONNEL

The endomyocardial biopsy team ideally includes the members described below.

• A physician experienced in cardiac catheterization and biopsy techniques, usually a cardiologist, sometimes a cardiothoracic surgeon.

• Catheterization laboratory personnel, including an assistant to the operating physician in the sterile field.

• Circulating nurse to monitor the patient, administer drugs, provide supplies, and receive the specimen.

• Cardiovascular technologist to obtain hemodynamic measurements. This function can be performed by the circulating nurse if appropriately trained.

• Radiology technician, responsible for the fluoroscopy equipment.

• Echocardiography technician, if echocardiogram is to be used in guiding the bioptome.

• Cardiac pathologist to process and interpret the tissue obtained.

• A cardiothoracic surgeon should be available (not

Table 8-1. Endomyocardial bioptomes

Features	Scholten bioptome*	King's endomyocardial bioptome†	Konno-Sakakibarra bioptome
Construction	Catheter over movable wire	Modification of Olympus bronchial biopsy forceps	Coiled wire and steel central wire
Handle	Modified mosquito hemostat with rachet, locking jaws; handle in same plane as distal curve of catheter	Three-ring plastic handle with spring keeping jaws closed; inner wire connects to jaws	Ringlike operating handle, sliding assembly controlling biopsy head, pushing the jaws open and pulling them closed
Catheter	Teflon covered, movable shaft; variable approx. 45° curve, 7 cm from the tip; controlled by handle; curve in same plane as handle	Teflon covering applied to the stainless steel 1.8 mm wire coil	2 mm diameter Teflon-coated coiled wire and stainless steel central core wire
Biopsy head (jaws)	Sharpened cutting jaws; two cups, one fixed, one mobile; 2.5 mm span; 2.1-2.8 mm diameter; controlled by opening and closing handle with adjustable spring mechanism	Scissor action; two sharpened heads, both mobile, stainless steel cutting jaws, 1.8 mm, opened by moving the double ring away from the thumb ring	Two cutting elliptic spoons; 2.5 mm diameter (small), 3.5 mm diameter (large)
Length	50 cm for RV biopsy 100 cm for LV biopsy‡	104 cm & 50 cm‡	100 cm
Diameter (outer)	8.5-9 Fr for RV biopsy (2.8 mm head); 7 Fr for LV biopsy (2.1 mm head)	6 Fr; requires 7 or 8 Fr sheath	8 Fr (small) 9 Fr (large)
Sampling mechanism	Cutting plus avulsion	Cutting plus avulsion	Cutting plus avulsion
Advantages	Large biopsy specimen at least 1.5 and usually 2-3 mm Multiple use possible Instrument very durable Cleaning and sterilizing not difficult Short and very maneuverable; no need for guiding catheter for RV biopsy	Very flexible and responsive Easy to use, safe Suitable for right or left endomyocardial biopsy May be introduced by arm, leg, or neck approach Disposable one-time use (Cordis); can be cleaned and reused (KeyMedical)	Introduced era of transvascular endomyocardial biopsy Adequate specimen usually 3-4 mm
Disadvantages	Stiff catheter; more experience needed in its use; RV endomyocardial biopsy only from internal jugular approach	Biopsy specimen smaller, usually 1-2 mm	Difficult to clean—blood trapped between Teflon coat and wire; rigid, difficult to manipulate; chance of trauma; susceptible to mechanical failure
Cost (approximate)	$1000 (reusable)	$150 (Cordis disposable bioptome)	

*Scholten Surgical Instruments, 707 Warrington Ave., Redwood City CA 94063, (415) 368-5426.
†Cordis Corp., PO Box 025700, Miami, FL 33102-5700, (800) 327-7714; KeyMedical House, Stock Rd., Southend-on-Sea, Essex, SF2 SQH, (0702) 616333.
‡SBS Cook supplies the ventricular catheter and sheath used for left ventricular biopsy using the Scholten bioptome. Cordis Corp. supplies the ventricular catheter and the sheath (Catalogue #502-617, 501-618) used with the disposable biopsy forceps.

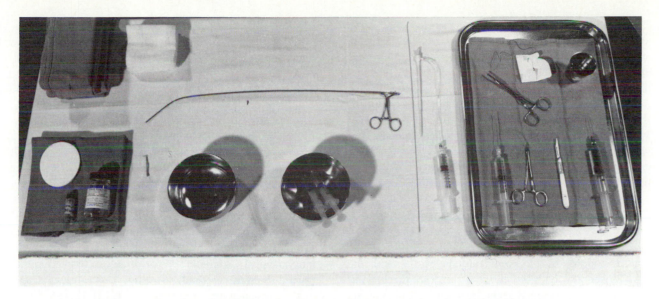

Fig. 8-3. Table set-up for endomyocardial biopsy. *Right to left:* Tray containing: lidocaine in a syringe, #11 scalpel, Kelly clamp, 18-gauge vascular needle with syringe and lidocaine (or saline), suture material, and needle holder. On the table: Vascular introducer with hemostatic valve and its guidewire, Scholten bioptome, two small basins (one with flush solution), plastic pick, 4 × 4-inch sponges, towels, specimen containers, and filter paper.

on standby!) for the rare instance of cardiac puncture and cardiac tamponade that does not resolve by percutaneous pericardial drainage.

Cross-training of personnel will help reduce the number of people needed to cover these functions.

PATIENT PREPARATION

The patient is prepared in a manner similar to that for cardiac catheterization.

1. Review the indication and possible contraindications for endomyocardial biopsy as it applies to the specific patient.

2. Explain the procedure to the patient. Emphasize the fact that this is basically a specialized form of cardiac catheterization. Avoid provoking additional anxiety.

3. Obtain consent for the procedure: this may include right and left heart catheterization and right and left endomyocardial biopsy.

4. Obtain results of studies, which may include ECG, chest radiograph, complete blood count, and coagulation studies (prothrombin time, partial thromboplastin time).

5. Keep the patient fasting for 6 hours. Small amounts of liquids may be taken by mouth. Maintain hydration intravenously, if needed.

6. Secure an IV line and keep it open with 5% dextrose in water.

7. Shave and cleanse the appropriate area.

8. Premedication is generally not required, although mild sedative may be used.

9. Transfer the patient to a special procedure room or cardiac catheterization room for the procedure.

PROCEDURES
Right ventricular approaches
Internal jugular approach

The following procedure describes the right ventricular endomyocardial biopsy using the Stanford-Shultz or Scholten bioptomes and the right internal jugular approach.[14]

1. Place the patient in the supine position on the catheterization table without the use of a cradle.

2. Attach ECG electrodes and monitor the patient's cardiac rhythm.

3. Place a cap over the patient's hair and a pillow under the shoulders and neck to hyperextend the neck.

4. Turn the patient's head to the left side and prepare the right side of the neck for internal jugular vein entry. The Trendelenburg position will help distend the vein, facilitate entry, and reduce the risk of air embolism.

5. Enter the internal jugular vein using a vascular needle (18 gauge, 7 cm), a 50 cm straight-tip flexible guidewire (0.038 inch [1.0 mm]), and a 9 Fr dilator and sheath with a hemostatic valve *with the side arm closed to the patient* (see p. 54).

6. Once inside the vessel, flush the side arm of the sheath and connect it to a heparinized saline infusion system. The valve on the introducer prevents any air embolization to the right side of the heart. Ensure that the seal is satisfactory.

7. Right heart catheterization may now be performed, if indicated, using a balloon-tip flotation catheter. Pressures and thermodilution cardiac output may be obtained at rest and during exercise. Save the right heart catheter, as hemodynamic measurements may be repeated at the completion of the biopsy procedure if complications occur.

8. Prepare the bioptome by bending it at a 45° angle, 6 to 7 cm from the tip in the same plane as the handles. Test the handle and the integrity of the cutting jaws.

9. Introduce the bioptome into the sheath with the jaws closed and with the tip (and therefore the handle) pointing to the patient's right. Monitor all movements of the bioptome with fluoroscopy.

10. Advance the bioptome to the superior vena cava and to the right atrium, keeping the tip pointing toward the lateral border of the heart (Fig. 8-4). Take care not to enter the right subclavian vein.

11. As the bioptome tip reaches the lower third of the right atrium, rotate the bioptome anteriorly using 180° counterclockwise rotation so that the tip points medially (Fig. 8-5). As the handle and tip of the bioptome point in the same direction, the direction of the handle in the operator's hand will indicate the direction of the bioptome tip; fluoroscopy will confirm this.

12. Approach the tricuspid valve and advance the bioptome across the valve into the right ventricle (Fig. 8-6). If difficulty is encountered in crossing the tricuspid valve, rotate the bioptome in the right atrium at a level slightly higher or lower than the initial attempt. It may be necessary to draw the bioptome out of the body and reshape the bend at its tip. Right ventricular entry is signaled by the appearance of premature ventricular contractions (PVCs).

13. Further rotate the bioptome handle (and the tip) to point posteriorly by additional counterclockwise rotation (Fig. 8-7). The bioptome tip will now be pointing toward the intraventricular septum.

14. Advance the bioptome to the right ventricular apex while pointing the tip of the bioptome toward the septum (Fig. 8-8). At this point, two-dimensional (2D) echocardiography may be used to direct the bioptome tip (p. 200).

15. The bioptome tip makes contact with the right ventricular septum at the apex; the operator will feel the cardiac impulses. PVCs will confirm presence in the right ventricular cavity, thus reassuring the operator that

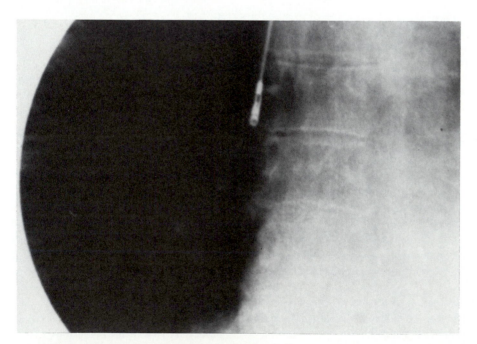

Fig. 8-4. Fluoroscopic view of the bioptome with its tip pointing toward the lateral border of the heart.

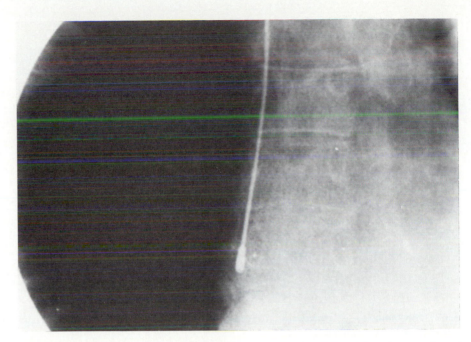

Fig. 8-5. Correct position of the bioptome tip in the lower third of the right atrium confirmed by fluoroscopy. The tip is being rotated anteriorly and medially, using a 180° counterclockwise rotation. The direction of the handle in the operator's hand indicates the direction of the bioptome tip.

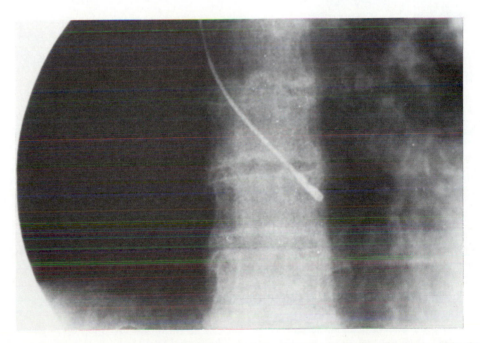

Fig. 8-6. Fluoroscopic view of the bioptome tip just across the tricuspid valve and within the right ventricle.

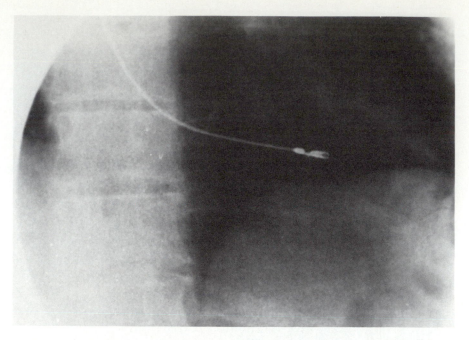

Fig. 8-7. The bioptome is rotated posteriorly by additional counterclockwise rotation and advanced into the right ventricle.

A

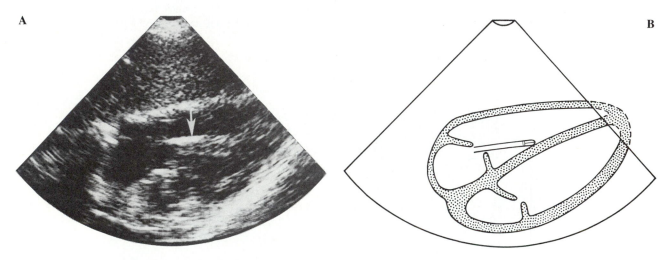

B

Fig. 8-8. Two-dimensional echocardiographic view of the bioptome being advanced into the right ventricular apex, while the tip of the bioptome (*arrow*) is pointed toward the septum.

the coronary sinus has not been entered. In this position, anteroposterior (AP) fluoroscopy will show the bioptome tip at or below the left diaphragmatic shadow, well past (4 to 7 cm) the left border of the spine (Fig. 8-9). The curve of the catheter will appear foreshortened. The bioptome tip is now in the right ventricular apex, pointing toward the interventricular septum (Fig. 8-10). If doubt exists, this final position can be confirmed again by fluoroscopy in the 45° left anterior

oblique (LAO) projection, showing the bioptome perpendicular to the septum. Echocardiography can also be used.

16. When the bioptome tip is properly positioned and the direction of the tip has been confirmed, obtain the biopsy specimen.

17. Withdraw the bioptome 1 to 2 cm and open the jaws (Fig. 8-11).

18. Readvance the bioptome without any rotation un-

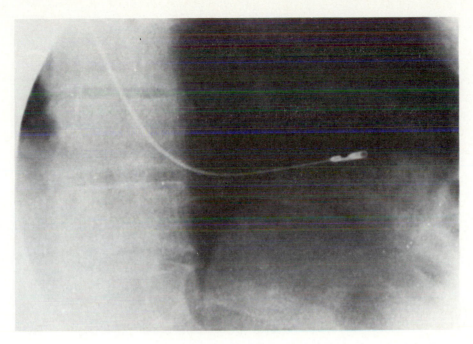

Fig. 8-9. Anteroposterior fluoroscopy shows the bioptome tip at or below the left diaphragm shadow well past (4 to 7 cm) the left border of the spine.

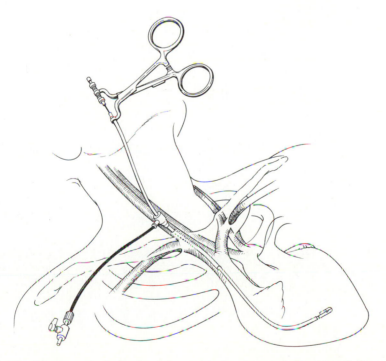

Fig. 8-10. The bioptome tip is in the right ventricular apex, pointing toward the ventricular septum.

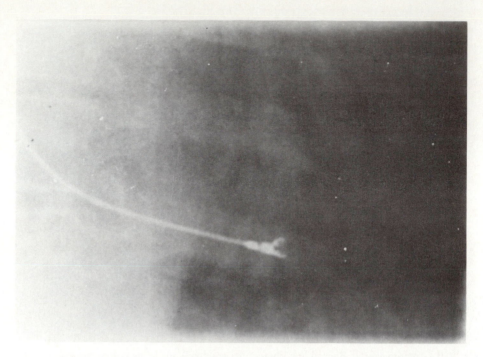

Fig. 8-11. The bioptome is withdrawn 1 to 2 cm and the jaws are opened.

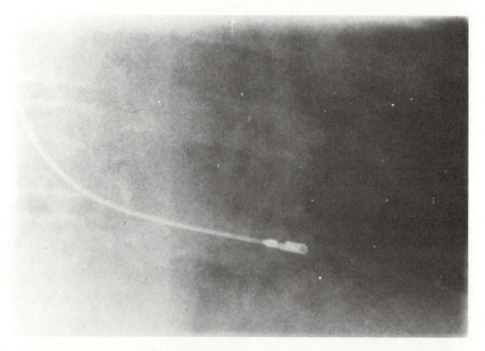

Fig. 8-12. The bioptome is gently advanced and pressed on the interventricular septum. The jaws are then closed and the bioptome is gently pulled free, with the specimen in its closed jaws.

til the interventricular septum is contacted. PVCs may be seen.

19. *Gently* press on the interventricular septum and close the handle of the bioptome (Fig. 8-12). This closes the cutting jaws, obtaining myocardial tissue.

20. Tug *gently* until the bioptome "gives." If two or three gentle tugs do not release the bioptome from the endocardial wall, open the bioptome handle, freeing the specimen, and proceed with a second attempt. The bite may have been too big, involving full thickness of the right ventricular wall, including the pericardium or chordae.

21. Once the bioptome is free, with the specimen in its closed jaws, rotate the bioptome clockwise while withdrawing it from the right ventricle to right atrium. Additional clockwise rotation will bring the bioptome tip to the right side of the patient (lateral border of the right atrium). *Do not reopen the jaws until the instrument has been fully withdrawn from the sheath, even if you think that no biopsy specimen has been obtained.*

22. Withdraw the bioptome from the sheath.

23. Open the jaws of the bioptome and remove the 1 to 3 mm sample *without crushing it*. The specimen may be removed by stroking it with a wet filter paper or teasing it with a needle. Very fine forceps may be used if necessary. Promptly place the tissue in the appropriate fixative (see p. 195). Gentle but prompt handling of the specimen is critical in minimizing artifact introduced by tissue trauma.

24. Wipe the bioptome with sterile heparinized saline before obtaining a second (or third or fourth) biopsy specimen. Clear the bioptome jaws of tissue or clots by swishing and opening and closing the jaws in a bowl of sterile heparinized saline. At least three specimens are generally obtained, however as many as five specimens may be taken, depending on the clinical indications and the size of the biopsy specimens.

Patient aftercare

1. With the internal jugular introducer still in place, observe the patient in the cardiac catheterization laboratory for 5 to 10 minutes. If the patient remains stable, pressure recordings of the right side of the heart are not routinely obtained at the end of the biopsy.

2. Check for pneumothorax or pleural effusion by fluoroscopy.

3. If the patient develops chest pain, hypotension, or dyspnea, immediately obtain pressure recordings of the right side of the heart. A diagnosis of cardiac tamponade can promptly be made or excluded on the basis of these recordings. Echocardiography is used to confirm suspected hemopericardium.

4. If there are no complications, sit the patient up at a 30° or 40° angle, remove the sheath, and apply gentle pressure for 5 minutes. Apply a sterile dressing.

5. Transfer the patient to a bed and observe for 2 to 4 hours. If there are no complications, the patient may be discharged the same day.

Precautions

• *Avoid air embolism:* Use of a venous introducer with a hemostatic one-way valve has significantly reduced the risk of air embolism. For added safety, the patient is asked to stop breathing (hum) during the introduction of the bioptome into the sheath, during its removal from the sheath, and during the removal of the sheath from the vein. For diagnosis and treatment of air embolism see Chapter 2.

• *Avoid the coronary sinus:* This structure is avoided by rotating the bioptome *anteriorly* and counterclockwise when moving from the right atrium to the right ventricle and reversing this motion when the catheter is moved back to the right atrium.

• *Heed warning signs of cardiac perforation:* Patients should experience no pain during the actual procedure. Any chest pain, especially if pleuritic or pericardial in nature, should be considered a warning of possible cardiac perforation. The procedure should be temporarily interrupted and the patient should be observed.

• *Do not hurry:* Speed is not of the essence, but proper catheter position is important before actual biopsy is undertaken. All the necessary time and effort should be expended to ensure proper bioptome position before the biopsy is attempted.

• *Be gentle:* All bioptome manipulations within the cardiovascular system should be performed with gentle motions under continuous fluoroscopic guidance.

When the King bioptome is used via the internal jugular vein, a 45 cm ventricular catheter sheath is used to guide the 50 cm bioptome to the right ventricular apical septum.

Femoral approach using a long sheath

The following procedure describes a right ventricular endomyocardial biopsy using the femoral approach and a long sheath.

1. Introduce the ventricular catheter into the sheath and prepare it for use.

2. Enter the right femoral vein using the Seldinger technique and insert a 0.038-inch (1.0 mm) safety J-curve guidewire into the inferior vena cava.

3. Pass the catheter/sheath assembly over the guidewire and position it in the right atrium.

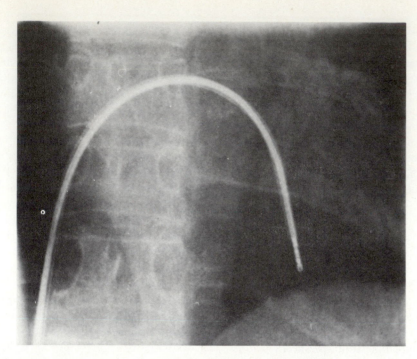

Fig. 8-13. The King (Cordis Corp.) bioptome introduced in the right ventricle from the right femoral vein with the help of a long sheath (anteroposterior projection).

4. Remove the guidewire, aspirate and flush the catheter, and connect it to a pressure transducer. Connect the side arm of the sheath to an IV infusion.

5. Advance the catheter under fluoroscopic and pressure monitoring to the right ventricle. Use a guidewire, if necessary, to position the pigtail catheter in the right ventricle. Now advance the sheath over the catheter and position it near the right ventricular apex.

6. Remove the catheter and aspirate and flush the sheath. Connect the sheath to a pressure transducer for monitoring. Free aspiration and undamped pressure recording indicate that the sheath is free in the right ventricle. Position may be confirmed by a small amount of contrast agent injected by hand.

7. Introduce the biopsy forceps (with jaws closed) through the sheath and pass it under fluoroscopic guidance to a point 1 cm proximal to the tip of the sheath.

8. Maintaining a clockwise rotation on the sheath and bioptome, hold the sheath in place, and gently advance the bioptome until it exits the sheath and makes contact with the right ventricular septum (Figs. 8-13 and 8-14). A slight bending of the sheath and bioptome will be noted in the right atrium. PVCs may be seen.

9. Withdraw the bioptome 0.5 to 1 cm, open the jaws, and readvance the bioptome in the same plane (without additional rotation) until contact with the septum is reestablished (Fig. 8-15). Gently press on the intraventricular septum and close the jaws.

10. Tug gently until the bioptome "gives"; withdraw it from the right ventricle into the sheath and remove it from the sheath.

11. Aspirate and flush the sheath and connect it to a pressure transducer to ensure its correct position in the right ventricle while an assistant removes the specimen from the bioptome.

12. Multiple specimens may be obtained from the right ventricular septum by gently moving the sheath—with the catheter in it—to different areas of the septum before reintroducing the bioptome.

Left ventricular approach
Long sheath technique

The following procedure describes a left ventricular endomyocardial biopsy using the long sheath technique with the Scholten or King bioptome.[14-16]

1. Prepare the patient in a manner similar to percutaneous left heart catheterization, using the Seldinger technique and the right or left femoral artery.

2. Insert a 7 Fr 110 cm left ventricular pigtail catheter into a radiopaque 90 to 100 cm sheath with an adaptor at its proximal tip.

3. Flush the catheters and prepare for use.

4. Enter the femoral artery using standard Seldinger technique and position a 0.038-inch (1.0 mm) safety J-curve guidewire in the aorta.

5. Administer 5000 units of IV heparin.

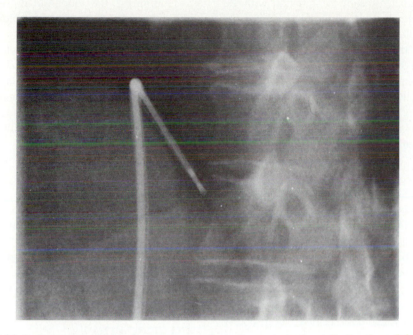

Fig. 8-14. Left anterior oblique fluoroscopy confirms the posterior (septal) direction of the bioptome.

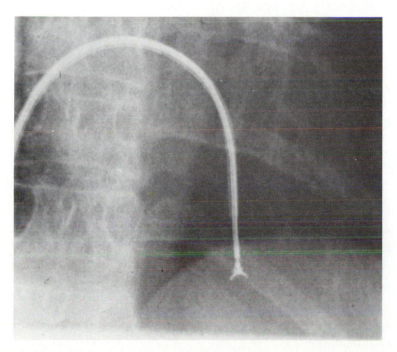

Fig. 8-15. The King (Cordis Corp.) bioptome, with the jaws open and advanced to the right ventricular septum (anteroposterior projection).

6. Advance the catheter/sheath combination with the pigtail end of the catheter out of the sheath over the guidewire and into the abdominal aorta. Remove the guidewire and flush the pigtail catheter. Advance the catheter and position it across the aortic valve into the left ventricle in the standard manner. If you encounter difficulty in crossing the aortic valve, you can use the guidewire.

7. After entering the left ventricle, advance the sheath over the catheter into the left ventricle and then withdraw the pigtail catheter. Aspirate and flush the sheath. Now only the sheath is in the left ventricle.

8. Connect the sheath to a continuous IV infusion, with an air trapper, under pressure.

9. Detach the sheath and permit brisk back-bleeding just before introducing the bioptome.

10. Introduce the bioptome and advance it through the sheath to the left ventricular apex or left ventricular lateral wall.

11. Confirm the location of the bioptome by fluoroscopy; echocardiography can also be used to properly position the bioptome.

12. Withdraw the bioptome 1 cm, open the jaws, and readvance the bioptome to the left ventricular apex. Promptly close the jaws.

13. Withdraw the bioptome with a firm tug until it is released.

14. Withdraw the bioptome through the sheath. *Do not reopen the jaws until the instrument has been fully withdrawn from the sheath, even if you think that no biopsy specimen has been obtained.*

15. Remove the specimen and transfer it into the appropriate fixative.

16. Keep the sheath well flushed and irrigated between biopsy procedures. Wash and clean the bioptome thoroughly with heparinized saline before reintroducing it into the left ventricle.

17. At completion of the procedure, remove the sheath and establish hemostasis. Heparin reversal is not routinely used but may be used if necessary (see Chapter 5 for details).

The Kono bioptome may be introduced into the right or left ventricle using a cutdown or percutaneous approach. We have no experience in its use. For details in technique the reader is referred to the original description.[3]

CARE OF THE BIOPTOME

Instructions for the care of the bioptome provided by the manufacturer should be followed. The bioptome made by Scholten Surgical Instruments, Inc., is a multiple-use catheter that is very durable but needs careful maintenance.

1. Immerse the bioptome in sterile saline immediately after each biopsy to clear blood from the catheter/bioptome interface.

2. Wash the bioptome thoroughly immediately on completion of the procedure.

3. After complete cleansing, introduce 0.5 ml of olive oil or instrument oil under pressure at the catheter/bioptome interface, using the special instrument provided by the manufacturer. Follow this with air under pressure to clear excess oil.

4. Use gas sterilization after mounting the bioptome on a firm protective surface. Autoclaving is also possible but not recommended.

5. Do not traumatize the jaws; they have sharp cutting edges. Periodic sharpening is necessary and is provided by the manufacturer.

The King endomyocardial bioptome (Cordis Corp.) is intended for one-time use. The Konno and Olympus bioptomes are multiple-use catheters. Follow the instructions provided by the manufacturer.

COMPLICATIONS
Cardiac perforation, hemopericardium, and tamponade

Cardiac perforation may occur with both right and left ventricular endomyocardial biopsy procedures and with any of the instruments described. In experienced hands the risk is 1% or less. The diagnosis is suspected if the patient develops chest pain, dyspnea, hypotension, bradycardia or tachycardia, or distended neck veins. The diagnosis of cardiac compression (tamponade) can be confirmed by measuring right atrial/right ventricle pressures with a flotation right heart catheter through the internal jugular or femoral sheath (kept in place for 5 to 10 minutes after the biopsy). An echocardiogram will show fluid (blood) in the pericardial space.

Treatment consists of close observation and monitoring, volume expansion (especially if the patient is hypovolemic), and prompt pericardiocentesis and drainage if the patient is hemodynamically unstable (Chapter 10). Very rarely, thoracotomy may be required for continuous bleeding.

Systemic embolization

Systemic embolization is limited to left ventricular endomyocardial biopsy or right ventricular endomyocardial biopsy when there is an intracardiac shunt. This risk is minimized by meticulous attention to technique of catheter flushing and to thorough cleansing of the bioptome with heparinized saline before each introduction. Systemic administration of heparin is used as part of the procedure of left ventricular endomyocardial biopsy but is not a substitute for meticulous technique.

Care of the patient with embolic complication is supportive. Frequently, the problem is self-limited. For diagnosis and treatment of air embolism see p. 48.

Arrhythmias

PVCs or nonsustained ventricular tachycardias are always seen as a result of catheter manipulation in the right ventricle and during the actual biopsy procedure. These require no treatment and serve the useful function of assuring the operator that the catheter is in the ventricle.

Sustained ventricular tachycardia rarely occurs. Treatment may require IV lidocaine or cardioversion (see Chapter 12).

Atrial fibrillation may be precipitated in right ventricular endomyocardial biopsy with catheter manipulation in the right atrium. Rate control is achieved with digoxin or verapamil, or both, and usually the arrhythmia is self-limited. If not, cardioversion can be done electively (see Chapter 12).

Finally, heart block may result from right ventricular endomyocardial biopsy in the presence of preexisting LBBB. Temporary pacing may be required in these instances (see Chapter 13).

TISSUE PRESERVATION

All biopsy specimens are fixed directly in the cardiac catheterization laboratory, with care being taken to transfer the specimen promptly and atraumatically to the fixative. At least three and sometimes five specimens are obtained.

The details of tissue handling (number of pieces obtained, fixative used, and method of biopsy processing) vary among laboratories. It is recommended that facilities where endomyocardial biopsy is performed establish specific procedure details with the pathology laboratory where the tissue will be examined. Appendix I lists laboratories experienced in the evaluation of endomyocardial biopsy. Facilities where endomyocardial biopsy is done but where experience in tissue analysis is limited may consult a center close to them. The following guidelines are suggested.

If the biopsy is performed for anthracycline (Adriamycin) cardiotoxicity, fix all specimens in 2.5% buffered (pH 7.35) glutaraldehyde at room temperature. This will permit subsequent processing for both light and electron microscopy. For all other biopsies (myocarditis, cardiac transplant rejection, cardiomyopathy, etc.), fix at least three pieces in 10% buffered formalin for light microscopy evaluation and fix another piece in glutaraldehyde for electron microscopy.

It is a good policy to quick-freeze one specimen. This can be done by placing the specimen in a plastic capsule filled with freezing mixture, closing the lid of the capsule, and immersing it in isopentane and dry ice or liquid nitrogen. It may then be stored indefinitely at $-70°$ C. This piece can be used for immunofluorescence or histochemistry studies, as a back-up for diagnostic histology, and for the instances when a frozen section is needed for rapid diagnosis, for example in acute cardiac rejection following transplantation. Except for research purposes the biopsy specimen is not put on culture medium for viral studies.

THE ENDOMYOCARDIAL BIOPSY SPECIMEN

What is an adequate specimen? Usually four biopsy specimens of at least 2 mm are considered necessary for a complete histologic evaluation. In conditions in which the pathologic process may be patchy and focal, as many as five (and sometimes up to 10) pieces may be required for adequate study. If histochemical or enzymatic studies (mostly experimental) are to be done, additional pieces may be required.

What are the generally observed abnormalities of the endomyocardial biopsy specimen? A detailed description of the histopathology of endomyocardial biopsy is outside the scope of this chapter. Tables 8-2 and 8-3 provide an overview of some of the commonly observed abnormalities seen with the light and electron microscope and the conditions they are frequently observed in, while Table 8-4 lists the special stains that may be used for the diagnosis of various conditions.

DIAGNOSING CARDIAC ALLOGRAFT REJECTION

The frequent use of endomyocardial biopsy in the cardiac transplant patient for early and definitive signs of rejection has contributed to the improved survival rate observed during the past decade. This is the most frequent indication for the procedure.[6,7]

At least three pieces of biopsy are taken. Electron microscopy is not performed routinely; therefore all specimens can be fixed in 10% buffered formalin (or 2.5% glutaraldehyde) and embedded in parrafin blocks. If an answer is urgently needed, rapid processing or frozen section analysis can be done. All sections are stained with hematoxylin and eosin as well as Masson's trichrome stain to detect inflammatory infiltrate and fibrosis and early myocyte necrosis. In addition, methyl green–pyronin stain is used to detect the pyroninophilic cytoplasm of immunoblasts, which marks acute rejection. To help the clinician in determining the intensity and duration of immunosuppressive therapy, the changes have been graded into four categories relative to the intensity of rejection (Table 8-5).

Table 8-2. Abnormalities observed with light microscopy

Abnormality	Cardiac transplant rejection	Doxorubicin cardiotoxicity	Inflammatory carditis	Cardiomyopathy dilated	Cardiomyopathy hypertrophic	Cardiomyopathy restrictive	Artifact
Endocardial fibrosis	Frequent	None	None	Frequent	Frequent	Frequent	None
Interstitial edema	Common	Common	Common	None	None	None	Frequent
Interstitial fibrosis	Late stages	Late stage	Variable (healing phase)	Common	Common	Common	Unlikely
Perivascular lymphocytic infiltrate	Common	None	Common	None	None	None	None
Polymorphonuclear leukocytes	In severe cases	Minimal or absent	Variable	None	None	None	Unlikely
Interstitial lymphocyte infiltration	Common (immunoblasts)	Uncommon	Common (hallmark)	Occasionally	Occasionally	Occasionally	Unlikely
Myocyte degeneration necrosis	Common in moderate-severe cases	In severe cases	Common	Unlikely	Unlikely	Unlikely	Possible
Myocardial cell atrophy/dropout	Rare	Frequent	Occasionally	Frequent	None	None	Occasionally
Myocardial cell hypertrophy	In later stages	None	Variable (chronic)	Common (varying cell sizes)	Common	Common	Unlikely

Table 8-3. Abnormalities observed with electron microscopy

Abnormality	Doxorubicin cardiotoxicity	Cardiomyopathy dilated	Cardiomyopathy hypertrophic	Cardiomyopathy restrictive	Artifact
Contraction bands	—	—	—	—	Frequent
Myofibrillar dropout	Characteristic	Occasionally seen	Usually increased myofibrils	Not seen	Not seen
Sarco-tubular swelling and cytoplasmic vacuolation	Characteristic	Occasionally seen	Occasionally seen	Unlikely	Occasionally seen
Cellular/capillary edema	None	Frequent	Frequent	Occasionally seen	Frequent
Mitochondrial changes	In severe cases	Frequent	Frequent	Unlikely	Occasionally seen
Nuclear changes	In severe cases	Very frequent	Very frequent	None	Occasionally seen
Myocyte degenerative changes	In severe cases	Frequent	Frequent	None	None
Membrane bound vacuoles	In severe cases	Frequent	Frequent	None	None
Fiber crossover (sarcomere crossover)	None	Infrequent	Frequent	None	None

Table 8-4. Stains used for light microscopic analysis of endomyocardial biopsy tissue

Tissue, condition or cells	Stain	Common associated disease(s)
Amyloid fibrillar protein	Congo red Thioflavin T.	Amyloidosis
Fibrous tissue	Masson's tri-chrome	Cardiomy-opathies, nonspecific but includes methysergid radiation damage, en-docardial fi-brosis, car-cinoid heart disease
Elastic tissue	Elastic Van Giesen	Fibroelastosis
Granulomatous tissue	Hematoxylin and eosin	Sarcoidosis
Iron deposits	Perl's iron	Hemachro-motosis
Lymphocytes	Hematoxylin and eosin Methyl green–pyronin	Myocarditis
Immunoblasts	Hematoxylin and eosin Methyl green–pyronin	Acute allograft rejection Acute allograft rejection
Myocytes	Hematoxylin and eosin Masson's tri-chrome	Doxorubicin-induced car-diomyopa-thy
Cellular necrosis	Masson's tri-chrome	Acute allograft rejection

Adapted from Billingham, M.E., et al.: Anthracycline cardiomyopa-thy monitored by morphologic changes, Cancer Treat. Rep. **62**:865-872, 1978.

Table 8-5. Endomyocardial biopsy grading of acute cardiac rejection

Intensity	Histopathologic observations	Clinical observations
Mild rejection	Interstitial and en-docardial edema; few perivascular lymphoblasts; endothelial cells show pyronino-philia	Early rejection; re-versible with therapy
Moderate rejection	Moderate intersti-tial infiltrate of lymphoblasts as well as focal myocyte dam-age	Degree of damage is reversible; longer therapy required
Severe rejection	Interstitial infil-trate with lym-phoblasts as well as neutro-phils; interstitial hemorrhage; myocyte and vascular necro-sis	Difficult to re-verse; agressive and long-dura-tion therapy re-quired
Resolving rejection	Fibrosis; residual lymphocytes; plasma cells and pigment	Seen after ade-quate treatment of rejection

Adapted from Billingham, M.E., et al.: Anthracycline cardiomyopa-thy monitored by morphologic changes, Cancer Treat. Rep. **62**:865-872, 1978.

DIAGNOSING ANTHRACYCLINE CARDIOTOXICITY
Safe use of anthracycline

Anthracycline (Adriamycin) is a potent antineoplastic agent with a broad spectrum of activity. A major limi-tation to its use is cardiotoxicity[17-19] with development of acute congestive heart failure, usually several months after use of the drug. A generally safe cumulative dos-age is 400 to 500 mg/m^2. Some patients develop cardio-toxicity with a lower dose, especially if they are in the older age group, have pre-existing heart disease, or have received mediastinal (cardiac) radiation. Other pa-tients will tolerate, and benefit from, higher doses.

Several diagnostic tests are available to aid the on-cologist in the safe use of anthracycline in patients at high risk of developing congestive heart failure (those receiving over 500 mg/m^2 or having had radiotherapy or preesixting heart disease). These include echocar-diography, systolic time intervals, nuclear wall motion studies, and endomyocardial biopsy. Of the noninvasive studies, the nuclear wall motion studies during exercise with determination of left ventricular ejection fraction is the most helpful in detecting early left ventricular dys-function.

Endomyocardial biopsy with electron microscopy has been most helpful in the diagnosis of anthracycline car-diotoxicity and avoidance of clinical cardiomyopathy. When doses in excess of 450 mg/m^2 are used, endo-myocardial biopsy is recommended before every addi-tional 150 to 200 mg/m^2 dosage.[18,19] In patients who are at higher risk of developing cardiotoxicity (cardiac irradiation, preexisting heart disease, older age group) biopsy monitoring may start earlier and be repeated af-

Table 8-6. Billingham scale of anthracycline cardiac damage

Grade	Characteristic	Usual clinical response
0	No change from normal	Additional anthracycline used
1	Minimal number of cells (less than 5% of total number of cells per block) with early changes of myofibrillar loss or distended cytoplasmic reticulum	Additional anthracycline used
1.5	Small group of cells involved (5%-15% of total number), some of which have definite myofibrillar loss and/or cytoplasmic vacuolization	Additional anthracycline given if clinically indicated
2	Groups of cells (16%-25% of total number), some of which have clear myofibrillar loss and/or cytoplasmic vacuolization	Further anthracycline is given only if strongly indicated, and patient is followed carefully
2.5	Groups of cells involved (26%-35%) some of which have definite myofibrillar loss and/or cytoplasmic vacuolization	No more than one further dose of anthracycline is generally given; if additional doses are absolutely required, patient is followed very carefully with follow-up biopsies
3	Diffuse cell damage, >35% of total number of cells with marked changes, total loss of contractile elements, loss of organelle, mitochondria, and nuclear degeneration	No additional anthracycline may be given; patient is observed for possible development of heart failure

Adapted from Billingham, M.E., et al.: Anthracycline cardiomyopathy monitored by morphologic changes, Cancer Treat. Rep. **62**:865-872, 1978.

ter every 100 to 120 mg/m^2 dosage. Except for advanced cases of cardiotoxicity, electron microscopy is needed for an accurate diagnosis; thus all the specimens are fixed in 2.5% glutaraldehyde. The abnormalities are listed and graded in Tables 8-3 and 8-6 in an attempt to guide the clinician. With this approach, total cumulative doses exceeding 1100 mg/m^2 have been used safely.[20]

DIAGNOSING INFLAMMATORY MYOCARDITIS

Endomyocardial biopsy remains the only reliable way of diagnosing inflammatory carditis, assessing its severity, and following its response to therapy.[21-23] The qualitative changes in inflammatory carditis, as seen with light microscopy, are listed in Table 8-2; the quantitative diagnosis is not as well defined.[24-28] It is not known how many mononuclear cells per high-powered field are required before a definitive diagnosis of inflammatory carditis can be made, nor is there agreement regarding the classification of inflammatory carditis into categories of acute, subacute, rapidly progressive, or chronic. The differentiation of infective myocarditis from allergic and toxic myocarditis is the subject of ongoing study.

Inflammatory involvement of the heart is not a well-defined entity and may be secondary to bacterial, fungal, viral, or rickettsial infection; however, most frequently no specific cause is found, and the diagnosis is one of idiopathic inflammatory carditis.

Therapy of myocarditis is commonly supportive and includes conventional treatment of congestive heart failure. Anecdotal reports have suggested that anti-inflammatory agents (azathioprine, prednisone) are helpful, but controlled studies are not yet available.[29] The possible benefit or harm of using anti-inflammatory or immunosuppressive agents in these patients is not known, and such therapy is considered experimental. Thus endomyocardial biopsy in the clinical care of these patients is limited to making a definitive diagnosis, but it does not aid in the choice of therapy.[30-32]

DIAGNOSING RESTRICTIVE HEART DISEASE

Unless the diagnosis of constrictive pericarditis is definitive (pericardial calcification; pericardial thickening on CT scanning or magnetic resonance imaging, with characteristic hemodynamic abnormalities), endomyocardial biopsy should be considered to exclude the possibility of restrictive cardiomyopathy.[33-36]

Restrictive cardiomyopathy (nondilated cardiomyopathy) may be primary or secondary to amyloidosis, sarcoidosis, endomyocardial fibrosis, or tumor infiltration. The clinical presentation is one of biventricular congestive heart failure; mitral or tricuspid valve regurgitation may also be present. Echocardiographic, cardiac catheterization, and angiographic studies may show abnormalities similar to those seen in constrictive pericarditis. Thus the differential diagnosis of constrictive pericarditis versus restrictive heart disease may not al-

Table 8-7. Diagnostic features of pericardial constriction and restrictive cardiomyopathy

	Constrictive pericarditis	*Effusive-constrictive pericarditis*	*Restrictive cardiomyopathy*
Hemodynamic features			
RVSP ≤40 mm Hg	Common	Common	Present in 50% of patients
RVEDP ≥⅓ RVSP	Common	Common	Present in 50% of patients
Diastolic pressure plateau	Almost always	Almost always	Present in 33% of patients
LVDV normal or reduced	Almost always	Almost always	Almost always
LVEF >0.40	Almost always	Almost always	Almost always
Signs that are not generally helpful in the differential diagnosis			
Diastolic dip-plateau in initial RV pressure	Common	Not common	May occur
Cardiac output normal	Common	Common	May occur
Equalization of ventricular diastolic pressure	Common	Common	May occur
Cardiomegaly	Uncommon, may occur	Common	Common
Atrial fibrillation	Present in 25% of patients	Occurs	Present in 25% or more
Low-voltage QRS	Common	Common	Common
Echocardiographic features			
Pericardial effusion	May occur	Present	Common
Pericardial thickening	50%-70% of patients		Uncommon
Abnormal septal motion	50% of patients		Common in amyloid
Flattened motion of diastolic LVPW	Perhaps 75% of patients		Uncommon (?)
Diastolic notch on septal motion	Common in few patients studied		Absent, but few studied
Biventricular ⁹⁹ᵐTc-pyrophosphate uptake	Not studied		Possibly common in amyloid
Thickened pericardium on CT	Probably common, not invariable		(?)Rare, but few studied
Right atrial angiogram: straightening of right border, poor pulsations	Not invariable		Uncommon (?)
PEP/LVET	Normal or nearly so		Sometimes increased, but few studied

SP, Systolic pressure; *EDP,* end-diastolic pressure; *DV,* diastolic volume; *EF,* ejection fraction; *PW,* posterior wall; *PEP,* preejection period; LVET, left ventricular ejection time. Adapted and reproduced with permission from Johnson, R.A., and Palacios, I.: Nondilated cardiomyopathies. In Stollerman, G.H., et al., editors: Advances in internal medicine, vol. 30. Copyright © 1984 by Year Book Medical Publishers, Inc., Chicago.

ways be possible, even with invasive studies[33] (Table 8-7).

The pathologic changes observed in some of the restrictive cardiomyopathies may not be specific, but the presence of extensive abnormalities will point away from a diagnosis of constrictive pericarditis. In this setting, if pericardial calcification is also absent, then the diagnosis of constrictive pericarditis can be seriously questioned. If this precaution is not taken, some patients sent for pericardiectomy will have the diagnosis of restrictive cardiomyopathy made at the operating table (approximately 10% in a recent series!).[35,36]

In radiation heart disease, both constrictive pericarditis and restrictive myocardial disease may coexist. Endomyocardial biopsy may help assess the presence and degree of myocardial involvement.

RIGHT VENTRICULAR VS. LEFT VENTRICULAR BIOPSY

Early in the development of techniques for endomyocardial biopsy, the right ventricle was biopsied more frequently than the left. With the current bioptomes, both ventricles are accessible for biopsy. Initial concern that left ventricular biopsy may carry high risk has not been confirmed by experience. Still, right ventricular biopsy remains the more frequently performed procedure. The following observations are made.

In experienced hands, right ventricular biopsy is safer than left ventricular biopsy. Risk of arterial complications and the potentially serious sequelae of embolization in left ventricular biopsy are always a concern, especially when repeated procedures are performed in the same patient.

Improper localization of the bioptome in the right ventricle and biopsy of the right ventricular free wall carries a greater risk of perforation and hemipericardium. Thus heparin is not used in right ventricular endomyocardial biopsy.

As long as the biopsy is obtained from the interventricular septum, the diagnostic information appears to be similar in both ventricular biopsies, except in the special conditions in which the pathologic process may predominantly or exclusively involve one or the other ventricle (e.g., cardiac tumors, localized radiotherapy, hypertrophic cardiomyopathy, and sclerodermal heart disease).

Right ventricular endomyocardial biopsy is usually done on an outpatient basis, with early postprocedure ambulation. Left ventricular endomyocardial biopsy requires a longer period of observation and rest because of the femoral artery puncture and the risk of hematoma. In selected cases, ambulation in 4 to 6 hours and same-day discharge are possible.

Because of these considerations, left ventricular biopsy should be reserved for patients in whom the disease process is thought to be localized in the left ventricle, or in situations in which right ventricular biopsy cannot be done for technical reasons.

THE ENDOMYOCARDIAL BIOPSY REPORT

The clinician should not always expect a definitive diagnostic label from the pathologist. More frequently a descriptive report is received that needs to be interpreted in the context of the specific case.

The clinician should provide the pathologist with key information, including the patient's age, sex, suspected diagnosis, medications used, and findings on radiographs, ECG, echocardiogram, and hemodynamic or angiographic studies. Tissue handling, staining, and the use of light and electron microscopy and special stains or special studies will be based on this information.

The pathologist will give a description of the biopsy covering gross tissue observation, microscopic observations, electron microscopic observations if applicable, and a summary of these observations into a pathologic diagnosis. A complete report will also attempt to

relate these observations to the patient's clinical and hemodynamic abnormalities.

A consultation between cardiologist and pathologist is frequently helpful in making a final evaluation and guiding treatment in cases of cardiac allograft rejection, doxorubicin (Adriamycin) toxicity, or inflammatory carditis.

Cardiac pathology is evolving as a subspeciality of general pathology. Experience in evaluation of endomyocardial biopsy is acquired over many years. For reference, we provide a list of centers in the United States, Europe, and Japan where experienced cardiac pathologists are available who have indicated willingness to assist cardiologists in their community in the evaluation of endomyocardial biopsies (see Appendix I).

ENDOMYOCARDIAL BIOPSY USING TWO-DIMENSIONAL ECHOCARDIOGRAPHY

Transvascular endomyocardial biopsy techniques were developed during 1962 to 1975 before the general availability of two-dimensional (2D) echocardiography. The technique of both right and left endomyocardial biopsy without the aid of 2D echocardiography has been widely applied, with over 90% to 95% success rate and with remarkable safety. Although it is clear that the procedure, as described, can be performed by an experienced cardiologist without the help of 2D echocardiography, it is likely that the use of echocardiography as an adjunct to fluoroscopy to guide the bioptome will further improve the diagnostic yield and the safety of the technique.[37-40]

The technique

2D echocardiography is performed in the manner described below.

1. Before the biopsy is underway, perform a preliminary 2D echocardiographic study to locate the proper transducer position and confirm the ability to obtain images of diagnostic quality.

2. Perform endomyocardial biopsy as described above, with no change in the basic technique.

3. Perform 2D echocardiography with the patient supine on the cardiac catheterization table, using the apical and subcostal windows.

4. Pass the bioptome through the tricuspid or aortic valve with fluoroscopic guidance. At this point the catheter bioptome is easily visualized in the ventricle, using the subcostal or apical four-chamber view (Fig. 8-8). The operator may use information obtained by fluoroscopy as well as echocardiography for optimal positioning of the *bioptome tip*. After optimal position is obtained, perform the biopsy in the standard manner

described above. Simultaneous use of fluoroscopy and echocardiography is technically feasible but is also cumbersome and thus not recommended.

5. It is best to use fluoroscopy to direct the bioptome through the tricuspid (or aortic) valve to the ventricular apex and to rotate it properly. After this, fluoroscopy is not required.

6. Confirm bioptome position by echocardiography and make corrections before proceeding with the biopsy.

7. After completion of the procedure, use fluoroscopy to check for the possible complication of pneumothorax (if the internal jugular approach is used) and use echocardiography to check for pericardial effusion.

Advantages

The use of 2D echocardiography to guide the bioptome appears to have the following advantages.

• 2D echocardiography provides independent confirmation of the *direction* of the biopsy tip and jaws immediately before the biopsy procedure. This additional aid is helpful to relatively inexperienced operators or when dealing with cardiac rotation or malposition in which the standard views and manipulations in locating the right ventricular apical septum may not be very accurate. Thus the risk of biopsy of the free wall of the right ventricle should be reduced.

• Radiation exposure is reduced with this procedure because catheter manipulation in the right ventricle is performed mostly with echocardiographic visualization.

• 2D echocardiography provides better definition of the precise location of the biopsy site. This is helpful in directing the biopsy tip so that multiple biopsy pieces are not obtained from the same spot and also may be valuable when it is necessary to obtain a specimen from a specific area in the ventricle, such as in asymmetrical hypertrophy, cardiac tumor, or endomyocardial fibrosis. Valvular structures are also easily avoided.

• Observation of the actual biopsy procedure on 2D echocardiography helps the operator evaluate the degree of septal pull and ventricular-pericardial separation, which are valuable indices of force applied, and aids the relatively inexperienced operator in avoiding the use of excessive force.

• In the rare case of ventricular perforation, echocardiographic monitoring helps in the immediate diagnosis of hemopericardium. In combination with hemodynamic monitoring, it is possible to make a precise diagnosis of pericardial tamponade and follow its progression. Echocardiography is also of value during pericardiocentesis (see p. 248).

Disadvantages

The disadvantages of using 2D echocardiography during fluoroscopically guided endomyocardial biopsy include those described below.

• The procedure involves added complexity and expense. Another instrument is introduced into the cardiac catheterization laboratory, there is an additional technician in the room, and another monitor scan must be watched.

• Misinterpretation of catheter location may occur as a result of reverberations and lateral beam spread but should pose no serious confusion if two different standard views are used for sampling and if fluoroscopy is also used to confirm initial catheter location.

Role

At this time the precise role of 2D echocardiography in endomyocardial biopsy is not clearly defined. Time and further experience will determine whether it should be applied routinely along with fluoroscopy and whether it will replace fluoroscopy as the primary mode of guiding the bioptome. Presently, it should be helpful to operators with limited experience in endomyocardial biopsy technique, especially if there is alteration in cardiac position or rotation or if a precise location in the ventricular chamber is to be biopsied, and in children and adults with abnormally shaped ventricles.

ENDOMYOCARDIAL BIOPSY IN INFANTS AND CHILDREN

The basic endomyocardial biopsy technique described here has been adapted for use in small children.[41,42] Small bioptomes (4 or 5 Fr) are guided to the right and left ventricular septum using guiding catheters. Endomyocardial biopsy has been performed safely in children as young as 4½ months and as small as 4.5 kg. Animal experiments have indicated that the procedure may also be feasible in infants. The value of endomyocardial biopsy in infants and children is being explored and at this time is mostly experimental.

FUTURE DEVELOPMENTS

The currently popular bioptomes may be considered second generation in the evolution of endomyocardial biopsy catheters. Newer catheters are in development and testing (e.g., the steerable bioptome of Kawai,[43] and further advances in bioptome technology are anticipated. Combining the steerable biopsy catheter with the angioscope may provide a whole new dimension to cardiac biopsy.

Myocarditis can usually be diagnosed with endomyocardial biopsy, but the value of specific anti-inflammatory therapy remains controversial. Controlled studies are in progress; if specific helpful treatment is found, the diagnostic role of endomyocardial biopsy will expand.[29]

Preliminary studies suggest a role for endomyocardial biopsy in assessing the prognosis of patients with congestive cardiomyopathy and hence determining whether a patient is a candidate for heart transplant. If these preliminary observations are confirmed, the role of endomyocardial biopsy in the evaluation of these patients would expand.[44]

Biochemical, pharmacologic, and enzymatic studies on endomyocardial biopsy tissue are currently research tools. Clinical applications may follow.

PROCEDURE CHECKLIST

✔ Review the indications and contraindications of the procedure in relation to the specific patient.

✔ Note special circumstances that may apply regarding right ventricular versus left ventricular endomyocardial biopsy.

✔ Determine need for 2D echocardiography.

✔ Obtain informed consent.

✔ Check equipment.

✔ Check to see that proper fixatives and materials for quick freeze are available.

✔ Notify appropriate departments for a scheduled procedure (radiology, cardiology, pathology).

✔ Obtain and review laboratory results (ECG, chest radiograph, complete blood count, and coagulation studies).

✔ Prepare the patient: IV route, routine cardiac catheterization preparations, appropriate instructions, and reassurance.

✔ Perform endomyocardial biopsy.

✔ Watch for possible complications.

✔ Deliver the specimen and pertinent clinical information to the pathology laboratory.

✔ Document the procedure and the outcome in the medical record.

REFERENCES

1. Shirey, E.K., et al.: Percutaneous myocardial biopsy of the left ventricle, Circulation **46:**112-120, 1972.
2. Sakakibara, S., and Konno, S.: Endomyocardial biopsy, Jpn. Heart J. **3:**537-542, 1962.
3. Kono, S., Sekiguchi, M., and Sakakibara, S.: Catheter biopsy of the heart, Radiol. Clin. North Am. **9:**491-510, 1971.
4. Caves, P.K., et al.: New instrument for transvenous cardiac biopsy, Am. J. Cardiol. **33:**264-267, 1974.
5. Richardson, P.J.: King's endomyocardial bioptome, Lancet, April 13, 1974, pp. 660-661.
6. Mason, J.W., and Billingham, M.E.: Myocardial biopsy. In Yu, P.N. and Goodwin, J.F., editors: Progress in cardiology, Philadelphia, 1980, Lea & Febiger, pp. 113-146.
7. Fowles, R.E., and Mason, J.W.: Role of cardiac biopsy in the diagnosis and management of cardiac disease, Prog. Cardiovasc. Dis. **27:**153-172, 1984.
8. Melvin, K.R., et al.: Peripartum cardiomyopathy due to myocarditis, N. Engl. J. Med. **307:**731, 1982.
9. Marcella, J.J., et al.: Kawasaki syndrome in an adult: endomyocardial histology and ventricular function during acute and recovery phases of illness, J. Am. Coll. Cardiol. **2:**374-378, 1983.
10. Vignola, P.A., et al.: Lymphocytic myocarditis presenting as unexplained ventricular arrhythmias: diagnosis with endomyocardial biopsy and response to immunosuppression, J. Am. Coll. Cardiol. **4:**812-819, 1984.
11. Sugrue, D.D., et al.: Cardiac histologic findings in patients with life-threatening ventricular arrhythmias of unknown origin, J. Am. Coll. Cardiol. **4:**952-957, 1984.
12. Ratner, S.J., and Ursell, P.C.: Utility of heart biopsy in diagnosis and management of cardiac sarcoid, Circulation **72**(supp III-158):629, 1985.
13. Sekiguchi, M., and Take, M.: World survey of catheter biopsy of the heart. In Sekiguchi, M., and Olsen, E.G.J., editors: Cardiomyopathy: clinical, pathological, and theoretical aspects, Baltimore, 1980, University Park Press.
14. Mason, J.W.: Techniques for right and left endomyocardial biopsy, Am. J. Cardiol **41:**887-892, 1978.
15. Brooksby, I.A.B., Coltart, D.J., Jenkins, B.S., and Webb-Peploe, M.M.: Left ventricular endoymocardial biopsy, Lancet, Nov. 23, 1974, pp. 1222-1225.
16. Brooksby, I.A.B., et al.: Left ventricular endomyocardial biopsy. I. Description and evaluation of the technique, Cathet. Cardiovasc. Diagn. **3:**115-121, 1977.
17. Bristow, M.R., Mason, J.W., Billingham, M.E., and Daniels, J.R.: Doxorubicin cardiomyopathy: evaluation by phonocardiography, endomyocardial biopsy, and cardiac catheterization, Ann. Intern. Med. **88:**168-175, 1978.
18. Kantrowitz, M.E., and Bristow, M.R.: Cardiotoxicity of antitumor agents, Prog. Cardiovasc. Dis. 27:195-200, 1984.
19. Billingham, M.E., et al.: Anthracycline cardiomyopathy monitored by morphologic changes, Cancer Treat. Rep. **62:**865-872, 1978.
20. Laser, J.A., Fowles, R.E., and Mason, J.W.: Endomyocardial biopsy. In Schroeder, J.S.: Invasive cardiology, Philadelphia, 1985, F.A. Davis Co.
21. Chi-Sung Zee, C., et al.: High incidence of myocarditis by endomyocardial biopsy in patients with idiopathic congestive cardiomyopathy, J. Am. Coll. Cardiol. 3:68-70, 1984.
22. Fenoglio, J.J. Jr., et al.: Diagnosis and classification of myocarditis by endomyocardial biopsy, N. Engl. J. Med. **308:**12-18, 1983.
23. Nippoldt, T.B.: Right ventricular endomyocardial biopsy, clinical pathological correlates in 100 consecutive patients, Mayo Clin. Proc. **57:**407-418, 1982.
24. French, W.J., et al.: Caution in the diagnosis and treatment of myocarditis, Am. J. Cardiol. **54:**445-446, 1984.
25. Shanes, J.G., et al.: Interobserver variability in the pathologic diagnosis of endomyocardial biopsies (abstract), J. Am. Coll. Cardiol. **7:**120A, 1986.
26. Dec, G.W. Jr., et al.: Active myocarditis in the spectrum of acute dilated cardiomyopathies: clinical features, histologic correlates, and clinical outcome, N. Engl. J. Med. **312:**885-890, 1985.
27. Cassling, R.S., et al.: Quantitative evaluation of inflammation in biopsy specimens from idiopathically failing or irritable hearts:

experience in 80 pediatric and adult patients, Am. Heart J. **110**:713-720, 1985.

28. Herskowitz, A., Beschorner, W.E., Soule, L.M., and Baughman, K.L.: The interpretation of the equivocal myocardial biopsy, Circulation **72**(suppl. III-346):1381, 1985.

29. Mason, J.W.: Endomyocardial biopsy: the balance of success and failure, Circulation **71**:185-186, 1985.

30. Hosenpud, J.D., McAnulty, J.H., and Niles, N.R.: Lack of objective improvement in ventricular systolic function in patients with myocarditis treated with azathioprine and prednisone, J. Am. Coll. Cardiol. **6**(4):797-801, 1985.

31. Sekiguchi, M., et al.: Natural history of 20 patients with biopsy proven acute myocarditis, Circulation **72**(suppl. III-109):433, 1985.

32. O'Connell, J.B., Reap, E.A., and Robinson, J.A.: The effects of cyclosporine or acute murine Coxsackie B3 myocarditis, Circulation **73**:353-359, 1986.

33. Johnson, R.A., and Palacios, I.: Nondilated cardiomyopathies. In Stollerman, G.H., editor: Advances in internal medicine **30**:243-274, Chicago, 1984, Year Book Medical Publishers.

34. Nishimura, R.A., Connolly, D.C., Parkin, T.W., and Stanson, A.W.: Constrictive pericarditis: assessment of current diagnostic procedures, Mayo Clin. Proc. **60**:397-401, 1985.

35. Seifert, F.C., et al.: Surgical treatment of constrictive pericarditis: analysis of outcome and diagnostic error, Circulation **72**(suppl. II):II264-II273, 1985.

36. Schoenfeld, M.H., et al.: Restrictive cardiomyopathy versus constrictive pericarditis: role of endomyocardial biopsy in avoiding unnecessary thoracotomy, Circulation **72**(suppl. III-355):1419, 1985.

37. French, W.J., Popp, R.L., and Pitlick, P.T.: Cardiac localization of transvascular bioptome using two-dimensional echocardiography, Am. J. Cardiol **51**:219-223, 1983.

38. Pierard, L.: Two-dimensional echocardiography: guiding of endomyocardial biopsy, Chest **85**:759-762, 1984.

39. Strachovsky, G., Zeldis, S.M., Katz, S., and McNulty-Mackey, M.: Two-dimensional echocardiographic monitoring during percutaneous endomyocardial biopsy, J. Am. Coll. Cardiol. **6**:609-611, 1985.

40. Mortensen, S.A., and Egeblad, H.: Endomyocardial biopsy guided by cross sectional echocardiography, Br. Heart J. **50**:246, 1983.

41. Lurie, P.R., Fujita, M., and Neustein, H.B.: Transvascular endomyocardial biopsy in infants and small children: description of a new technique, Am. J. Cardiol. **42**:453-457, 1978.

42. Lewis, A.B., Neustein, H.B., Takahashi, M., and Lurie, P.R.: Findings on endomyocardial biopsy in infants and children with dilated cardiomyopathy, Am. J. Cardiol. **55**:143-145, 1985.

43. Kawai, C., and Kitaura, Y.: New endomyocardial biopsy catheter for the left ventricle, Am. J. Cardiol. **40**:63-65, 1977.

44. Figulla, H.R., et al.: Spontaneous hemodynamic improvement or stabilization and associated biopsy findings in patients with congestive cardiomyopathy, Circulation **71**:1095-1104, 1985.

REVIEW ARTICLES AND TEXTS

Fenoglio, J.J. (editor): Endomyocardial biopsy: techniques and applications, Boca Raton, Fla. 1982, CRC Press, Inc.

Fowles, R.E., and Mason, J.W.: Role of cardiac biopsy in the diagnosis and management of cardiac disease, Prog. Cardiovasc. Dis. **27**:153-172, 1984.

Kawai, C., and Matsumori, A.: Myocardial biopsy, Ann. Rev. Med. **321**:139-157, 1980.

Mason, J.W., et al.: Myocardial biopsy. In Yu, P.N., and Goodwin, J.F., editors: Progress in cardiology, Philadelphia, 1980, Lea & Febiger, pp. 113-146.

Przybzojewski, J.Z.: Endomyocardial biopsy: a review of the literature, Cathet. Cardiovasc. Diagn. **11**:287-330, 1985.

Chapter Nine

Electrophysiologic studies

ISAAC WIENER

The modern era of intracardiac electrocardiography (ECG) began in the late 1960s with the demonstration by Scherlag et al.[1] that the His bundle potential could be reliably recorded in humans. The introduction of programmed stimulation by Wellens and Durrer[2] greatly expanded the potential of this technique. Early studies exhaustively analyzed the conduction system and its abnormalities. Attention then passed to the Wolff-Parkinson-White (WPW) syndrome and other supraventricular arrhythmias. Most recently, ventricular tachycardia (VT) and the problem of sudden cardiac death have become the major focus. During this evolution electrophysiologic study (EPS) has developed from a research tool to a practical clinical procedure.

This chapter reviews the indications and techniques for performing EPS. Theory of arrhythmias is not discussed. A complete discussion of the interpretation of intracardiac recordings is beyond the scope of this chapter, and the reader is referred to selected studies.[2-3]

INDICATIONS

EPS has been used in the evaluation of a wide variety of cardiac arrhythmias.[4-7] The relative frequencies of indications in this author's laboratory are cited in Table 9-1.

Sinus node disease

For most patients with sinus node disease, the decision regarding whether to implant a pacemaker can be made on the basis of the history and ambulatory ECG monitoring; electrophysiologic testing of the sinus node is not necessary. However, in some patients persistent symptoms may be associated with only mild ECG abnormalities. In these cases determination of sinus node recovery time may be helpful, as a markedly prolonged sinus node recovery time is an indication for implantation of a permanent pacemaker.[8] However, a normal sinus node recovery time does not exclude symptomatic sick sinus syndrome, and the significance of a mildly

Table 9-1. Indications for intracardiac EPS in the author's laboratory

Indication	Frequency
Cardiac arrest	30%
Unexplained recurrent syncope	25%
Recurrent sustained ventricular tachycardia	25%
WPW syndrome with symptomatic tachycardia	10%
Other supraventricular tachycardias	8%
Bradycardias	2%

abnormal sinus node recovery time is not established. The sinoatrial (SA) conduction time (p. 212) is a sensitive but nonspecific indication of sinus node dysfunction and has not been shown to be of clinical value.

Atrioventricular block

For most patients with atrioventricular (AV) block the decision regarding whether to implant a pacemaker can be made on the basis of history and the surface ECG without intracardiac recordings. Patients who have symptoms require a pacemaker. Patients who have no symptoms require pacemakers only for high-grade infranodal block. The Mobitz II pattern during second-degree block and the rate and morphologic characteristics of the escape rhythm during complete heart block are quite accurate in predicting the level of block.[9] However, for some patients the diagnosis is not clear from the surface ECG. Specifically, intracardiac recordings may be helpful in patients with AV Wenckebach block associated with bundle branch block, apparent Mobitz II pattern in the setting of a narrow QRS segment, and apparent Mobitz II pattern with frequent junctional extrasystoles, suggesting concealed junctional extrasystoles mimicking Mobitz II pattern.[10]

Intraventricular conduction delay

Patients who are free of symptoms who have bifascicular block have demonstrated slow progression to high-degree block and do not require specific therapy.[11,12]

Patients with symptomatic (syncope or presyncope) bifascicular block may have intermittent complete heart block that has escaped detection on monitoring. For these patients, demonstration during EPS of pacing-induced infranodal block or of a markedly prolonged HV interval is an indication for pacemaker implantation.[13,14] Some electrophysiologists would consider pacemaker implantation for more modest degrees of HV prolongation. A normal study does not exclude the possibility of intermittent heart block but makes it much less likely. For some of these patients with bifascicular block and symptoms, EPS will reveal causes for syncope other than heart block (e.g., inducible sustained VT).

Supraventricular tachycardia

Patients with supraventricular tachycardia (SVT) that is only mildly symptomatic may be treated with empiric drug therapy, if treated at all. EPS is needed for patients with rapid tachycardia (> 200 bpm) associated with severe symptoms and patients with recurrent symptomatic bouts of tachycardia refractory to empiric therapy. In such cases EPS allows selection of drug therapy, and in cases refractory to drug therapy, it allows the selection of nonmedical forms of therapy such as specific antitachycardia pacemakers and antitachycardia surgery.[15]

Wolff-Parkinson-White syndrome

Patients with WPW syndrome constitute a significant portion of patients with SVT requiring study. Because of the complex interactions of drugs on the normal and anomalous pathways, I prefer to study all patients with WPW in whom drug therapy is being started for tachycardias. Clearly, all patients with a very rapid ventricular response to atrial fibrillation require EPS. Complete EPS is a prerequisite to nonmedical therapy.

Patients with WPW who are free of symptoms may also have the potential for very rapid conduction during atrial fibrillation, but the risk of this appears to be quite small.[16] I do not routinely perform EPS in these patients.

Differential diagnosis of wide QRS tachycardia

EPS is the only definitive way to differentiate SVT with aberrancy from VT. In most patients, the tachycardia in question can be reproduced in the electrophys-iology laboratory. Careful documentation of the relationship of the His bundle and the atrial electrograms to the ventricular electrograms allows a definitive diagnosis of the nature of the tachycardia.

Ventricular tachycardia

EPS is indicated for all patients with recurrent, sustained VT (i.e., lasting more than 30 seconds). This arrhythmia can be reproduced in the electrophysiology laboratory in 90% of patients using the techniques of programmed stimulation. Moreover, drug testing during EPS predicts the clinical response to medications, with the possible exception of amiodarone.[17-19] EPS is mandatory if a pacemaker, the automatic implantable cardioverter/defibrillator (AICD), or surgical therapy is being considered. The role of EPS for patients with nonsustained VT is not established.

Out-of-hospital cardiac arrest

EPS is indicated for all patients who survive a cardiac arrest that is not related to acute factors such as myocardial infarction or electrolyte imbalance. EPS can induce VT or ventricular fibrillation (VF) in close to 70% of survivors of cardiac arrest. Patients without inducible arrhythmias may not require antiarrhythmic therapy and may do well with therapy directed at the underlying heart disease. In patients with inducible arrhythmias, drugs that prevent arrhythmia induction in the laboratory may be clinically effective. However, both of these findings are disputed.[20-22] EPS is necessary to evaluate patients for the AICD or EPS-guided surgery. Currently EPS is not useful for predicting the risk of sudden death in survivors of myocardial infarction.[22-23]

Syncope

For most patients with syncope, a careful history, physical examination, and ECG will establish a diagnosis. However, when syncope remains unexplained after noninvasive evaluation, and particularly when syncope is recurrent, EPS is indicated. EPS may detect bradycardias or tachycardias requiring therapy in up to 60% of such patients.[24] The yield of EPS is lower in patients without evidence of organic heart disease.[25]

CONTRAINDICATIONS

EPS is contraindicated (1) when acute factors make the findings unrepresentative of the patient's usual state (e.g., electrolyte abnormality, acute ischemia, and drug toxicity) and (2) when the patient's underlying cardiac disease makes it likely that induced arrhythmias will be extremely difficult to terminate and carry a high risk of death (e.g., acute myocardial infarction, unstable angina, hemodynamic instability such as persistent class IV heart failure, and critical aortic stenosis).

RISKS

Risks[26] of EPS include those related to cardiac catheterization (thromboembolism, cardiac perforation and tamponade) and infection (see Chapters 2 and 5). Risks specifically associated with electric stimulation include induction of atrial fibrillation, VT requiring cardioversion, and VF.

Induction of atrial fibrillation

Atrial stimulation may induce atrial fibrillation. In patients with WPW and a very rapidly conducting accessory pathway, ventricular response may be extremely rapid, hemodynamic deterioration may occur, and urgent cardioversion may be required. However, in most patients, atrial fibrillation is well tolerated but precludes further atrial stimulation. Atrial fibrillation induced in the electrophysiology laboratory usually converts spontaneously within several hours. It is our policy not to cardiovert these patients as a routine. Ventricular stimulation may still be performed during atrial fibrillation. After the study we allow sufficient time for spontaneous conversion before considering cardioversion.

Induction of hemodynamically unstable VT or VF

Induction of unstable ventricular arrhythmias is the major risk associated with EPS. This risk is small for patients studied for supraventricular arrhythmias but is 30% to 40% for patients with sustained VT or survivors of cardiac arrest. Treatment is immediate cardioversion or defibrillation. Because of the availability of treatment, the expected mortality is extremely low (1/1000).

EQUIPMENT

The basic equipment[27] required for EPS is described below.

• *Fluoroscopy unit:* Adequate imaging can be obtained with catheterization laboratory equipment or portable units.

• *Programmable stimulator:* The stimulator must be electrically isolated and allow introduction of one to three precisely timed premature stimuli, during both paced and spontaneous rhythm. It should allow selection of the pacing output, interval between stimuli, interval between premature stimuli, and length of pause after each stimulation sequence. It must allow a rapid changeover from pacing modes used to induce arrhythmias to pacing modes used to terminate arrhythmias. Several commercial units satisfy these requirements.

• *Multichannel physiologic recorder:* The physiologic recorder should allow the simultaneous filtering, amplification, and recording of a minimum of three surface ECG leads and four intracardiac signals. The recorder should be connected to a switch box that allows selection of intracardiac signals. Recording must be possible at paper speeds ranging from 50 mm/second to 200 mm/second. The recorder should generate time lines to allow accurate measurement. Recording systems using photographic paper are used in many laboratories. However, ink-jet recorders have the advantages of performing direct recording without any time delay and of using much less expensive paper.

• *Multichannel tape recorder:* A tape recorder allows the retrieval of any information not recorded during the study and allows replay of intracardiac events to display these for illustrative purposes. While a tape recorder is desirable, it is not essential for clinical studies.

• *Resuscitation equipment:* All standard resuscitation equipment should be available in the electrophysiology laboratory. During studies of ventricular arrhythmias I routinely have two functioning defibrillators present in the laboratory to allow for a backup unit. We apply defibrillator pads to the patient's chest at the beginning of the procedures so that defibrillation without skin burns can be achieved without delay. In some laboratories, the defibrillator is attached to the patient by means of cables to allow for more immediate defibrillation.

• *Intracardiac electrode catheters* (Fig. 9-1): A catheter with a curved tip with three electrodes spaced 1 cm apart is commonly used for recording the His potential. For atrial and ventricular recording and stimulation, the standard catheter is a quadripolar catheter, with four electrodes spaced 1 cm apart. The distal pair of electrodes can be used for stimulation while the proximal pair is simultaneously used for recording.

• *Introducer kits and cutdown tray:* These are necessary for venous or arterial access (see Chapters 2 and 3).

PERSONNEL

Personnel[27-28] required for the performance of EPS include the following specialists.

• *Clinical electrophysiologist:* EPS should be performed under the direction of a physician who is experienced in the techniques of cardiac catheterization and intracardiac recording and stimulation. This physician must be able to interpret the intracardiac electric events on line as they occur. One year of specialized training in an electrophysiology laboratory is generally accepted as a minimal requirement.

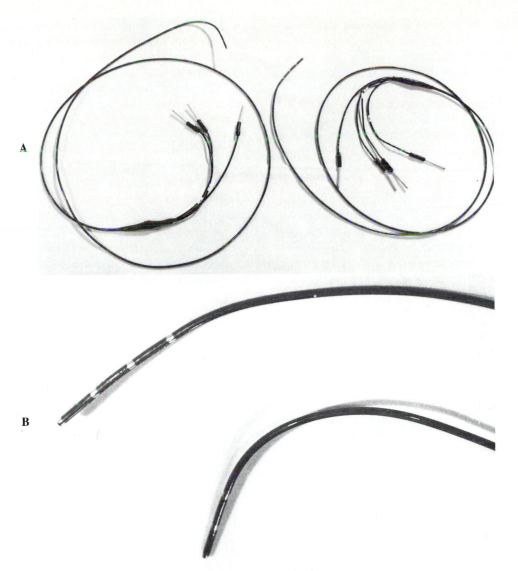

Fig. 9-1. Electrode catheters most commonly used during EPS. **A,** 6 Fr tripolar and quadripolar catheters. Note that the catheters end in electric terminals that are inserted into the switch box. **B,** Close-up of the electrode configuration on the tripolar and quadripolar catheters. On the tripolar catheter, electrograms can be recorded between the distal and middle electrodes and between the middle and proximal electrodes. On the quadripolar catheter frequently the distal and second electrodes are used for pacing, and the third and fourth electrodes are used for recording a bipolar electrogram.

• *Assistant physician:* For complex studies, a second physician who may be less experienced in electrophysiology but is experienced in the placement of cardiac catheters should be responsible for positioning and maintaining the position of the catheters. This physician should be experienced in cardiopulmonary resuscitation (CPR).

• *Nurse:* A nurse who is fully familiar with the operation of the equipment, the administration of medications, and CPR should be present in the laboratory. In some laboratories this person assumes additional duties for preoperative and postoperative teaching and may even assist in interpretation of tracings.

• *Bioengineering specialist:* A biomedical engineer or technician should be available to the laboratory for necessary maintenance of equipment function.

PATIENT PREPARATION

1. Obtain informed consent. Explain to the patient the nature of the procedure and the risks involved. If the patient has ventricular arrhythmias, explain the possibility of inducing VF in the laboratory. We explain to

patients that the occurrence of a ventricular arrhythmia in the laboratory is much preferable to its occurrence at home, and that in the laboratory we are prepared to treat this arrhythmia immediately. Most patients undergoing these studies are aware of the serious nature of their arrhythmias and are able to accept this risk without undue anxiety.

2. Discontinue all antiarrhythmic drugs at least 4 half-lives before the study. Patients with life-threatening arrhythmias should be on a monitored unit when antiarrhythmic drugs are discontinued.

3. Avoid premedication if possible because the electrophysiologic effects may influence the study. For the anxious patient or the patient at risk for emergency cardioversion, oral diazepam (5 to 10 mg 1 hour before the procedure) may be administered; diazepam produces no significant electrophysiologic effects.[29] Additional small doses of IV diazepam may be administered during the procedure. Opiates, antihistamines, and major tranquilizers should be avoided because of their anticholinergic effects.

4. The patient may take nothing by mouth for 6 hours before the procedure in case emergency cardioversion is necessary.

PROCEDURE
Catheter placement (Fig. 9-2)

1. For local anesthesia use lidocaine 0.5% or 1% without epinephrine. To avoid systemic levels of lidocaine with its attendant electrophysiologic effects, use the minimal necessary dose. When using more than 3 mg of lidocaine/kg, check blood levels of lidocaine.[30] In some laboratories mepivacaine 1% (Carbocaine) has been substituted for lidocaine.

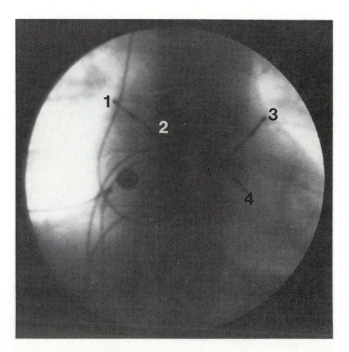

Fig. 9-2. Radiograph of typical catheter positions. Catheter *1* is a quadripolar catheter in the high right atrium. Catheter *2* is a tripolar catheter across the tricuspid valve in the approximate position to record the His bundle electrogram. Note that the catheter traverses the upper portion of the tricuspid anulus. Catheter *3* illustrates the coronary sinus position in the AP view. Note the sharp upward angulation of the coronary sinus. It is often helpful to confirm coronary sinus position in the lateral view. Catheter *4* is a quadripolar catheter in the area of the right ventricle.

2. Most electrophysiologic catheters are placed via the femoral vein. Enter the vein using the Seldinger technique with a multiple guidewire approach (see Chapter 2). After the catheters are in the inferior vena cava, pull back the sheaths to the base of the catheter. A total of 14 to 18 French sizes (i.e., three 6 Fr catheters) may be safely inserted in a single femoral vein.

3. For recording the His potential, advance the preshaped curved tripolar catheter across the tricuspid valve into the right ventricle. Pull back the catheter slowly while recording electrograms until a large His deflection is obtained. To expedite the process, it is helpful to record simultaneously from the proximal and distal electrode pairs. In the PA projection the appropriate position for recording the His potential is high in the right ventricle abutting the septum and often along the left border of the spine. If difficulty is encountered in recording a good His potential, gently rotate the catheter clockwise to provide greater proximity to the interventricular septum. When the His potential cannot be recorded with a tripolar catheter with 1 cm of distance between electrodes, a catheter with more closely spaced electrodes may be successful.

4. The most common approach to the high right atrium is from the femoral vein. It is important to obtain good contact between the distal electrode and the atrial wall. In my experience this is most often achieved by forming an arc against the lateral wall of the right atrium. In some patients the right atrial appendage, which is seen at the medial border of the right atrium overlapping the spine in the PA view, may be entered directly.

5. The common approach to the right ventricle is via the right femoral vein, with the catheter forming a loop across the tricuspid valve and anchoring in the right ventricular apex. For placement in the right ventricular outflow tract, pull the catheter back, rotate it clockwise, and advance it toward the right ventricular outflow tract.

6. The coronary sinus allows the most stable approach to left atrial recording and stimulation and is often necessary during studies of SVT. The coronary sinus may be approached from the left basilic vein (percutaneously or via cutdown) or from the femoral vein. *From the basilic vein,* pass the catheter to the lower junction of the right atrium and right ventricle where the os of the coronary sinus is found. Then rotate the catheter counterclockwise so that it points in a progressively more posterior direction. The catheter angled downward will engage the os of the coronary sinus, enter it, and form a more superior loop. Coronary sinus engagement is recognized by a characteristic angulation of the catheter in the PA view, by the posterior orientation toward the spine in the left anterior oblique and lateral views, and by the recording of a characteristic coronary sinus electrogram. The characteristic coronary sinus electrogram has atrial and ventricular components with the atrial component occurring at the end of the P wave (Fig. 9-3). After the coronary sinus has been entered, it is important to advance the catheter gently through the full length of the coronary sinus. This allows accurate localization of accessory pathways.

A *femoral approach* to the coronary sinus has been described.[28] A large loop is formed in the right atrium with the tip of the catheter pointed downward. The catheter is rotated posteriorly, engaging the coronary sinus. From the femoral approach it is often not possible to map the entire coronary sinus.

7. Left ventricular stimulation may be necessary to induce sustained VT in a small percentage of patients. In some patients left ventricular catheter mapping during induced VT may provide information about the earliest site of ventricular activation during VT. The approach is similar to that used for retrograde catheterization of the left ventricle by the femoral sheath technique (see Chapters 3 and 5). We have had good results using a standard 6 Fr quadripolar catheter. Newer catheters allowing direct manipulation of the end of the catheter are being developed.

Role of anticoagulation

The use of anticoagulation for EPS with catheters limited to the right side of the heart is controversial. Because of the appreciable risk of thromboembolism following EPS, in my laboratory all patients in whom catheters are left in place for more than 45 minutes receive full-dose heparin. The first dose (5000 units intravenously) is administered after all catheters are in place. It is not reversed when catheters are removed and a second dose (5000 units intravenously or subcutaneously) is administered 4 to 6 hours later. If left ventricular stimulation or mapping is performed, full-dose anticoagulation is mandatory.

Recording electrograms

Fig. 9-3 demonstrates typical baseline recordings.

Surface leads

Surface leads are important for determining the morphologic characteristics of induced arrhythmias, for detecting evidence of preexcitation, and for finding earliest ventricular activation. Intracardiac electrograms are

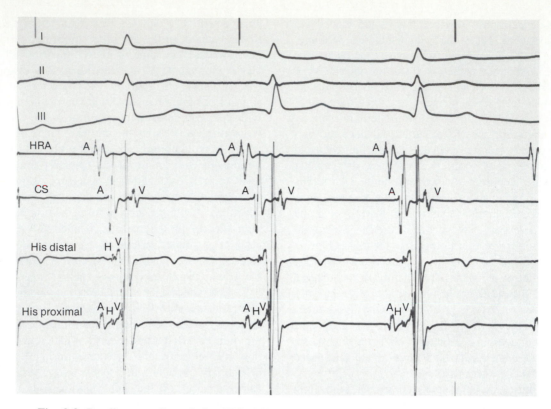

Fig. 9-3. Baseline recordings during EPS. This recording was performed on photographic paper at 100 mm/second. The first three leads are surface leads I, II, and III; the next four represent intracardiac electrograms; the high right atrial *(HRA)* electrogram demonstrates a discrete atrial *(A)* potential; the coronary sinus *(CS)* electrogram demonstrates both atrial and ventricular *(V)* potentials; and the distal and proximal His electrograms demonstrate atrial, His bundle, and ventricular potentials.

recorded simultaneously with at least three surface leads. We routinely record leads I, aVF, and V$_1$. Other laboratories use leads X, Y, and Z of the Frank vectorcardiogram.

Intracardiac electrograms

Recording bipolar electrograms. Bipolar electrograms record the potential difference between two closely spaced intracardiac electrograms and are most commonly utilized during EPS. In this manner a representation of local electric activation is obtained, and the point where the rapid deflection of the electrogram crosses the baseline is taken as the timing of local activation. To record bipolar electrograms, the ends of the electrode catheter corresponding to the appropriate intracardiac electrodes are inserted into the numbered sockets on the switch box. The dial on the switch box is set to record the difference between these two inputs, and the cable on the switch box corresponding to this dial is inserted into the amplifier.

Filtering, amplitude, and paper speed. The standard filtering for intracardiac electrograms is from 40 to 500 Hz, which removes low-frequency noise. In some instances (i.e., atrial fibrillation) change in filter settings may allow a clearer His potential.[30a]

The amplitude of the electrograms is adjusted for ease of visualization. Electrograms that are too large may overlap each other, and electrograms that are too small may be difficult to measure.

The standard paper speed for EPS is 100 mm/second. For precise mapping of the spread of electric activation, faster paper speeds may be necessary. During repeated trials of stimulation in an attempt to induce tachycardia, slower speeds may be utilized to save paper.

Validation of His potential. It is particularly important to validate that the His bundle recording represents activation of the His bundle and not right bundle branch activation or a part of atrial or ventricular activation. The most widely used method of His bundle validation

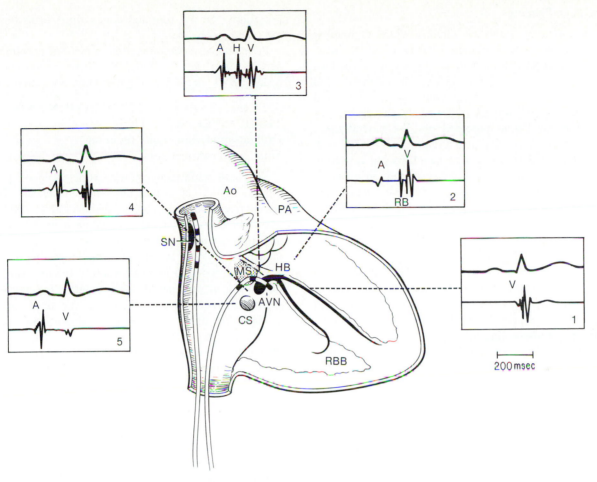

Fig. 9-4. Validation of the His bundle electrogram. The His bundle electrogram can be confirmed by slowly pulling the electrode catheter from the right ventricular cavity. This diagram illustrates the position of the catheter and the electrograms obtained with different catheter positions during withdrawal. Position *2* presents a right bundle potential; position *3*, which is further back than position *2*, documents a clear-cut His potential. (*CS,* Coronary sinus; *MS,* membranous septum; *AVN,* atrioventricular node; *HB,* His bundle; *RBB,* right bundle branch; *SN,* sinus node; *Ao,* aorta; *PA,* pulmonary artery.) (Adapted from Gallagher, J.J., and Damato, A.N.: Technique of recording His bundle activity in man. In Grossman, W., editor: Cardiac catheterization and angiography, ed. 2, Philadelphia, 1980, Lea & Febiger.)

consists of carefully recording the electrograms during a pull-back of the His catheter. The characteristic sequence of electrograms is illustrated in Fig. 9-4. Documenting the entire sequence provides strong evidence that the potential recorded simultaneous to the PR interval and between atrial and ventricular potentials represents the His bundle activation. Some workers have attempted to validate the His bundle potential by pacing the His bundle. This is a difficult technique that I have not found useful.

Technique of programmed stimulation
Type of stimuli

Standard EPS uses bipolar, cathodal, square wave stimuli of 1.5 to 2 msec duration and twice the diastolic threshold. The threshold is determined by pacing at a high output (approximately 5mA), gradually decreasing the output during pacing, and noting the output at which capture becomes inconsistent. If the threshold is greater than 1 to 2 mA, one should consider repositioning the catheter.

Incremental pacing

The stimulator allows the administration of stimuli at any fixed rate (in beats/minute) desired or at any interval (milliseconds) desired. The stimulator is synchronized to the native QRS complex, set for the desired interval, and activated. Continuous pacing at a fixed rate occurs until pacing is terminated. The pacing can then be resumed at an increased rate. We generally perform incremental pacing at intervals of 600, 500, 400, 350, 300, and 250 msec. Incremental pacing is used in evaluating sinus node function, evaluating atrioventricular (AV) conduction, inducing supraventricular and ventricular arrhythmias, and terminating supraventricular and ventricular arrhythmias.

Premature stimulation

Basic drive versus native rhythm. The stimulator allows the introduction of precisely timed premature stimuli during sinus rhythm, during paced rhythms, and during tachycardias. Paced rhythms ensure less variability and allow testing at a variety of rates; however, extrastimuli during the patient's native rhythm may provide more physiologic information. Because many electrophysiologic properties vary with heart rate, it is important to perform premature stimulation at multiple cycle lengths to maximize the induction of tachycardia. We perform premature stimulation during normal sinus rhythm, during paced rhythm at a cycle length of 600 msec, and during paced rhythm at a cycle length of 450 msec. In addition, premature stimuli are induced during any sustained tachycardia observed in the electrophysiology laboratory.

Single premature stimuli measuring the refractory period. In general, extrastimuli are administered after every eight beats of basic drive. The extrastimulus is administered late in the cycle and progressively brought closer and closer to the last beat of the basic drive. We utilize 20 msec decrements until a coupling interval of 400 msec and 10 msec decrements thereafter. A pause of 2 to 3 seconds is allowed between each sequence of basic drive and extrastimulus. The extrastimulus is moved toward the preceding beat until capture does not occur. The interval at which capture does not occur defines the *effective refractory period.* The beats of the basic drive are often called S1 and the premature stimulus is often referred to as S2.

Double and multiple stimuli. The extrastimulus technique has been expanded to include more than one premature stimulus. In administering a second premature stimulus (S3), the first premature stimulus (S2) is set at 10 msec beyond the refractory period. S3 is administered late in the cycle and gradually moved toward S2 in 10 msec decrements until it no longer captures. This procedure can be repeated for a third extrastimulus (S4), and so on.

Premature stimulation is used in measuring refractory periods, initiating SVT and VT, defining the mechanism of SVT and VT, and terminating SVT and VT.

SPECIFIC TYPES OF STIMULATION AND THEIR INTERPRETATION
Evaluation of sinus node function
Sinus node recovery time

The sinus node recovery time is determined by pacing the high right atrium near the sinus node. Three pacing rates, from just above the sinus rate to 200 bpm, should be utilized. Pacing is maintained for 60 seconds and then abruptly discontinued. The maximal sinus node recovery time is defined as the longest pause from the last paced atrial depolarization to the first sinus return cycle at any paced cycle length. The corrected sinus node recovery time is equal to the sinus node recovery time minus the patient's intrinsic sinus cycle length, and should be less than 550 msec. The presence of junctional escape beats and the presence of any pauses during the first 10 beats after cessation of pacing should be noted.

Sinoatrial conduction time

Sinoatrial (SA) conduction time can be determined by the extrastimulus method.[3] Narula[30b] has introduced a greatly simplified approach to estimating SA conduction time. For the method of Narula, the atria should be paced for eight beats at a fixed rate that is only slightly higher than the sinus rate. The return cycle following the eight beats of the Narula method is assumed to represent the intrinsic automaticity of the sinus node plus conduction time into and out of the sinus node. SA conduction time is determined by subtracting the basic cycle length from this cycle. The difference is divided by 2 and is considered normal when it is between 50 and 125 msec. A major limitation in determining the accuracy of the SA conduction time is the inevitable presence of some sinus arrhythmia. The SA conduction time requires further validation, and its clinical role is unclear. I do not routinely perform this test.

Evaluation of AV conduction
Conduction intervals

AH interval. The AH interval represents conduction time from the low right atrium through the AV node to the His bundle. The AH interval is measured from the earliest onset of the atrial electrogram and the His bundle recording to the earliest deflection of the His bundle potential from the baseline. Normal AH interval is 60 to 125 msec. The AH interval is very sensitive to autonomic influences.

HV interval. The HV interval represents conduction time from the proximal His bundle to the ventricular myocardium. The HV interval is measured from the earliest deflection of the His bundle potential from baseline to the earliest onset of ventricular activation recorded from multiple surface ECG leads or from the ventricular electrogram in the His bundle recording. The normal HV interval is 35 to 55 msec. Unlike the AH interval, the HV interval is not affected by variations in autonomic tone and is relatively constant.

Refractory periods

Refractory periods of the AV conduction system are measured by the extrastimulus technique. The relevant refractory periods include the following:

- *The effective refractory period of atrium:* The longest S1-S2 interval that fails to capture the atrium
- *The effective refractory period of the AV node:* The longest A_1-A_2 (atrial electrogram to atrial electrogram in the His bundle lead) interval that fails to result in His bundle depolarization (in some patients at some cycle lengths, atrial refractoriness will occur before AV refractoriness, and AV refractoriness cannot be determined with accuracy)
- *The functional refractory period of the AV node:* The shortest H1-H2 interval in response to any A1-A2 interval

Response to incremental atrial pacing

Pacing the atria at gradually increasing rates is used as a method for evaluating the functional properties of the AV conduction system. The normal response to atrial pacing is for the AH interval to gradually lengthen as atrial rate is increased until Wenckebach block between the A and H develops at a paced atrial cycle length of 500 to 350 msec. The rate at which AV Wenckebach block develops is very sensitive to autonomic tone. In normal persons, conduction between H and V is not affected by incremental pacing. Any prolongation of HV interval or any block between the H and V should be noted.

Evaluation of supraventricular tachycardia

Electrophysiologic testing of SVT is among the most complex of electrophysiologic studies. Performance and interpretation of these studies require a high degree of sophistication. While certain principles apply, the individual tachycardias are quite variable, and one must be prepared to encounter tachycardias with unusual features.[3,16,31]

Components of the electrophysiologic study

We perform EPS for patients with SVT in the following order.

1. Catheters are placed in the coronary sinus as well as right ventricle, His bundle position, and high right atrium.

2. The His potential is recorded during the sinus rhythm and its relationship to atrial and ventricular potentials is observed.

3. We start with ventricular stimulation in patients with SVT because the induction of troublesome arrhythmias (i.e., atrial fibrillation) is less common than with atrial stimulation. The protocol for ventricular stimulation should include incremental pacing as well as induction of a single premature stimulus during cycle lengths of 600 and 450 msec. During ventricular stimulation, particular attention is paid to the pattern of ventriculoatrial conduction (i.e., presence or absence), rate at which conduction becomes variable, and atrial activation sequence during retrograde conduction.

4. Following ventricular stimulation, atrial stimulation is performed. This includes atrial incremental pacing as well as atrial premature stimulation during sinus rhythm and during basic cycle lengths of 600 and 450 msec. If tachycardia is not induced by single extrastimuli, a second premature stimulus is added. Atrial stimulation is performed from both the high right atrium and the coronary sinus.

5. If tachycardia has not been initiated by these techniques, 1 mg of atropine is administered intravenously and stimulation repeated. Atropine often facilitates the induction of AV nodal reentry tachycardias (Fig. 9-5).

6. If tachycardia is initiated, the tachycardia can almost always be terminated by pacing techniques. Pacing may be performed from the high right atrium or coronary sinus. Single atrial extrastimulation, synchronized to the tachycardia QRS complex, can be administered throughout diastole. If single extrastimulation is ineffective, the first stimulus is set just above the refractory period and a second stimulus is added. Termination by single and double extrastimuli may provide useful information about the tachycardia. If premature stimuli are ineffective, rapid pacing will generally be effective. Pacing should be a minimum of 30 bpm faster than the tachycardia rate and should be maintained for 10 to 20 seconds before abrupt discontinuation.

Special considerations

Mapping. Mapping refers to tracing the path of a circulating reentrant impulse. Identifying the course of the impulse becomes crucial before consideration of surgical interruption of part of the circuit. The most common

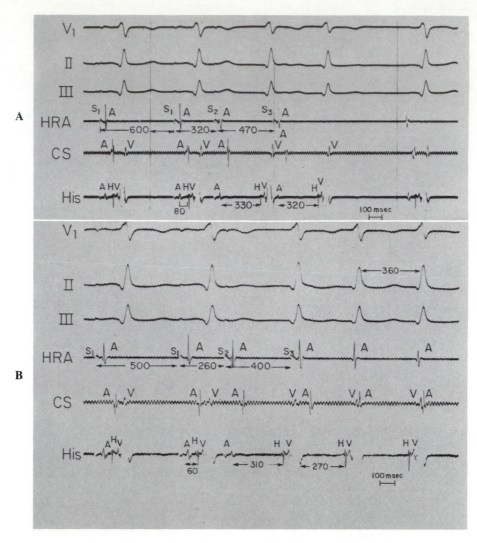

Fig. 9-5. Facilitation of induction of AV node tachycardia by atropine administration: stimulation before **(A)** and after **(B)** atropine administration. In both panels there are surface leads V_1, II, and III and intracardiac electrograms from the high right atrium *(HRA)*, coronary sinus *(CS)*, and His position. Pacing is performed in the high right atrium. **A,** Pacing is performed at a basic cycle length of 600 msec. Double premature stimuli, S_2 and S_3, are administered. Note that in the conducted beats following S_2 and S_3 a markedly prolonged AH interval is seen in the His bundle lead. This corresponds with antegrade conduction via the slow AV nodal pathway. **B,** Following administration of atropine, pacing is again done at the high right atrium, this time at a cycle length of 500 msec (because of increase in sinus rate caused by atropine). After S_3 the beat is conducted again with a prolonged AH interval, but at this time retrograde conduction via the AV node fast pathway has been facilitated by atropine, and an AV nodal reentrant tachycardia is induced. Note that atrial activation during tachycardia is simultaneous to ventricular activation. (From Wiener, I., et al.: Use of electrophysiological studies to select therapy for patients with AV nodal re-entrant tachycardia, PACE **5:**173-180, 1982.)

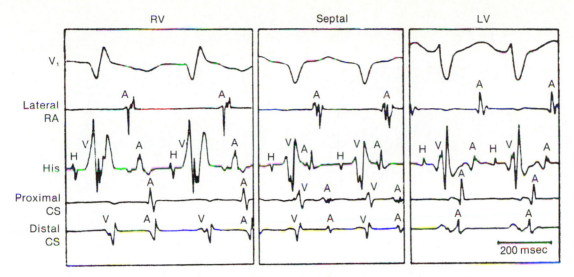

Fig. 9-6. Retrograde atrial activation during reciprocating tachycardia in patients with right ventricular, septal, and left ventricular preexcitation. With a right ventricular free wall accessory pathway, retrograde atrial activity is initiated in the right atrium and is followed by the atrial septum and left atrium, while a left ventricular free wall accessory pathway results in retrograde activation of the left atrium first, as seen in the coronary sinus *(CS)*, followed by the atrial septum and right atrium. When the accessory pathway is located in the septum itself, retrograde atrial activation is earliest in the His bundle lead, similar to the tachycardia caused by reentry in the AV node. (From Gallagher, J.J., et al.: The preexcitation syndromes, Prog. Cardiovasc. Dis. **20:**285-327, 1978.)

type of mapping is illustrated in Fig. 9-6, which shows the sequence of atrial activation during AV junctional reentrant tachycardia. Simultaneous recordings identify the portion of the atrium that is activated earliest and indicate that the tachycardia utilizes an accessory pathway that inserts in that portion of the atrium. Thus, if the tachycardia is utilizing a right-sided accessory pathway in its course from ventricle to atrium, earliest atrial activation will be in the right atrium. If the tachycardia is utilizing a left-sided accessory pathway in its course from ventricle to atrium, earliest atrial activation will be in the coronary sinus.

Evaluation of components of the tachycardia circuit. In this portion of the study, the electrophysiologist attempts to prove which cardiac structures are involved in the reentrant circuit.

If bundle branch block occurs during tachycardia or is induced by ventricular premature beats during tachycardia, increase of the tachycardia cycle length implies that an accessory pathway on the same side of the heart as the bundle branch block is used in the circuit (Fig. 9-7).

Other techniques for evaluating components of the tachycardia circuit involve the insertion of timed atrial and ventricular stimuli during tachycardia. If activation

of a certain structure results in shortening of the tachycardia cycle length, and if the configuration of the intracardiac electrograms remains unchanged, this is taken as evidence that the impulse has entered the tachycardia circuit and advanced it. Fig. 9-8 illustrates a ventricular premature beat advancing atrial activation during SVT. The fact that atrial activation is advanced without advancing His bundle activity documents the existence and utilization of another connection between ventricle and atrium (i.e., accessory pathway).

Evaluation of accessory pathways. Determining the characteristics of accessory pathways is an important aspect of electrophysiologic evaluation of SVT. Electrophysiologic testing is necessary to establish the presence or absence of an accessory pathway in cases with doubtful ECGs. In addition, EPS evaluates the potential of an accessory pathway to conduct rapidly and the participation of the pathway in the arrhythmia. We will restrict ourselves to a discussion of Kent bypass tracts.

A Kent fiber demonstrating ventricular preexcitation is considered to be present if during an atrial rhythm or atrial pacing the ventricle can be shown to be activated earlier (preexcited) than the His bundle (Fig. 9-9). During sinus rhythm the degree of preexcitation is determined by many factors (intra-atrial conduction, distance

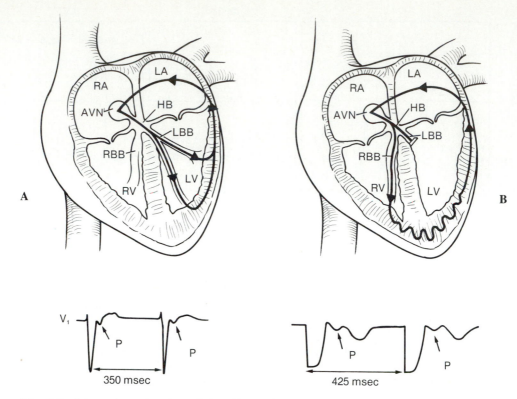

Fig. 9-7. Schematic explanation of the effects of bundle branch block during tachycardia. **A,** Tachycardia utilizing the AV node *(AVN)* from atrium to ventricle and a left-sided accessory pathway from ventricle to atrium. **B,** When left bundle branch block develops, the tachycardia circuit becomes longer. This results in a slowing of the tachycardia.

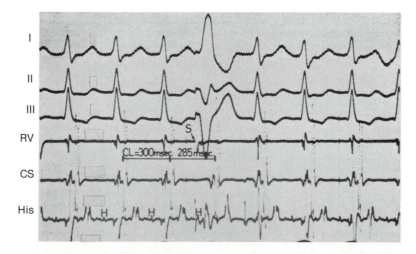

Fig. 9-8. Documentation of the participation of an accessory pathway in AV reciprocating tachycardia by administration of ventricular premature stimuli during the tachycardia. Illustrated are surface leads I, II, and III and intracardiac electrograms from the high right atrium *(HRA)*, coronary sinus *(CS)*, distal His bundle, and proximal coronary sinus *(CS)*. Note that when a premature stimulus is introduced into the right ventricular apex, the next atrial potential in the coronary sinus electrogram is advanced. This occurs without affecting the preceeding His bundle potential and indicates that ventricular premature beat enters the tachycardia circuit and advances it.

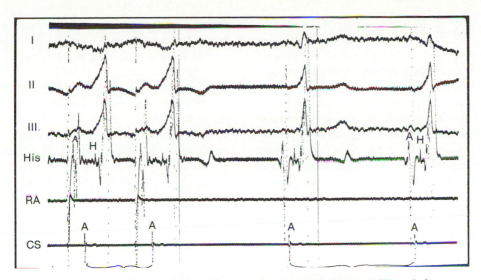

Fig. 9-9. Demonstration of preexcitation. Shown are surface leads I, II, and III, and electrograms from the His position *(His)*, right atrium *(RA)*, and coronary sinus *(CS)*. The two beats on the left are during right atrial pacing, and the two beats on the right are sinus beats. During sinus rhythm, the His deflection and the onset of ventricular activation in the surface leads are simultaneous, documenting that the ventricle is "preexcited" by a pathway other than the AV node–His axis. During the paced beats, the faster rate causes prolongation of the A-H interval, but accessory pathway conduction is unaffected. Thus, preexcitation is is accentuated and ventricular activation begins before His activation.

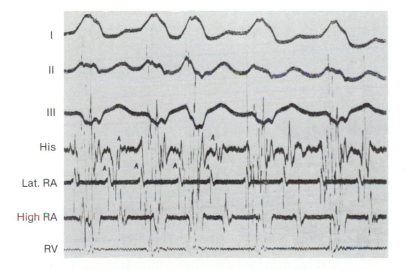

Fig. 9-10. Accessory pathway conduction during atrial fibrillation/flutter induced in the electrophysiology laboratory. Note that the atrial electrograms document a rapid atrial rhythm. Surface leads demonstrate maximal preexcitation with an irregular, rapid rate.

of the accessory pathway from the sinus node, length of the accessory pathway, and conduction time across it). Preexcitation may be minimal and even undetected during sinus rhythm despite the ability of the pathway to conduct antegradely. Demonstration of preexcitation may depend on pacing the atrium near the insertion of the accessory pathway to maximize the contribution of the accessory pathway to ventricular activation.

The functional properties of the accessory pathway may be evaluated by determining its refractory period. This is done by the extrastimulus method at multiple cycle lengths. Stimulation should be done adjacent to the atrial insertion of the accessory pathway. The refractory period of the accessory pathway is reached when a premature stimulus that captures the atrium no longer results in preexcitation. This may be manifest with preserved AV conduction over the AV node (the accessory pathway refractory period is longer than the AV node refractory period) or by complete failure of conduction to the ventricle (both accessory pathway and AV node are refractory). In some patients the atrium may become refractory before the accessory pathway, precluding accurate assessment of accessory pathway refractoriness. The effective refractory period of the accessory pathway correlates with the ability of the pathway to conduct rapidly during atrial fibrillation. However, because of other factors, such as type of atrial input and presence or absence of concealed conduction, the correlation is not precise. For this reason many laboratories advocate the induction of atrial flutter or fibrillation (by atrial pacing at a cycle length of 150 to 200 msec) so that the patient's ventricular response during atrial fibrillation can be measured directly (Fig. 9-10). If this is attempted, one must be vigilant for the possibility of very rapid rates leading to hemodynamic deterioration and requiring cardioversion.

Drug testing

One of the goals of electrophysiologic evaluation of SVT is to define a clinical drug regimen. It has been demonstrated that drugs that prevent induction of tachycardia in the electrophysiologic laboratory are effective clinically in preventing recurrences of tachycardia.

Before drug testing, it is important to document that the tachycardia can be reproducibly initiated by programmed stimulation. We have found that the most efficient means for drug testing in patients with SVT is to leave the coronary sinus catheter, which extends from the left antecubital vein to the coronary sinus, in place and perform sequential testing on multiple days.

Before any drug testing, previously administered drugs should be allowed to wash out. We prefer to repeat a control induction before each drug administration and to test only one drug or one drug and a combination on each day. The drugs should be administered slowly, with close observation for any adverse effects. A full stimulation protocol should be repeated after administration. Documentation of plasma level is critical.

The drugs for testing are selected based on the nature of the tachycardia, with close attention paid to any history of drug allergy or contraindication in the individual patient. The number of drugs and combinations to be studied in each patient have not been standardized. We prefer to test at least one AV node–blocking agent and at least one local anesthetic drug (Table 9-2).

A drug is considered effective if it prevents initiation

Table 9-2. Drugs used during EPS

Drug	Dosage	Hazards
Drugs that increase ability to induce tachycardia		
Atropine	1 mg IV	Angina, urinary retention, glaucoma
Isoproterenol	0.5-4 mg/min IV	Tachycardia, angina, hypotension
Drugs used most commonly in SVT studies		
Digoxin	0.75 mg IV	Nausea, ventricular arrhythmias
	1-1.5 mg p.o.	
Propranolol	0.15 mg/kg IV at 1 mg/min	Hypotension, congestive heart failure,
	80 mg p.o./6 hr	bronchospasm
Verapamil	0.15 mg/kg IV over 2 min followed	Hypotension
	by 0.005 mg/kg/min	
	80 mg p.o./6 hr	
Drugs used commonly in both VT and SVT studies		
Procainamide	1000-2000 mg at 50 mg/min	Hypotension, QRS widening
	750 to 2000 mg p.o./6 hr	
Quinidine gluconate	15 mg/kg at 20 mg/min IV	Hypotension, QRS widening, gastrointestinal intolerance
Quinidine sulfate	300-600 mg p.o./6 hr	Hypotension, QRS widening, gastrointestinal intolerance
Disopyramide	200-400 mg p.o. loading dose	Congestive heart failure, urinary retention
	100-300 mg p.o./6 hr	
Drugs used commonly in VT studies		
Lidocaine	5 mg/kg IV over 15 min followed	Paresthesias, seizures
	by 4 mg/min	
Mexiletine	400 mg p.o. loading	Paresthesias, seizures, gastrointestinal intolerance
	200-400 mg p.o./8 hr	
Flecainide	200-300 mg p.o./12 hr	Congestive heart failure, bradycardia, visual disturbances
Amiodarone	800-1600 mg p.o./day × 2 wk,	Pulmonary reactions, gastrointestinal intolerance, and others
	then 400 mg p.o./day	

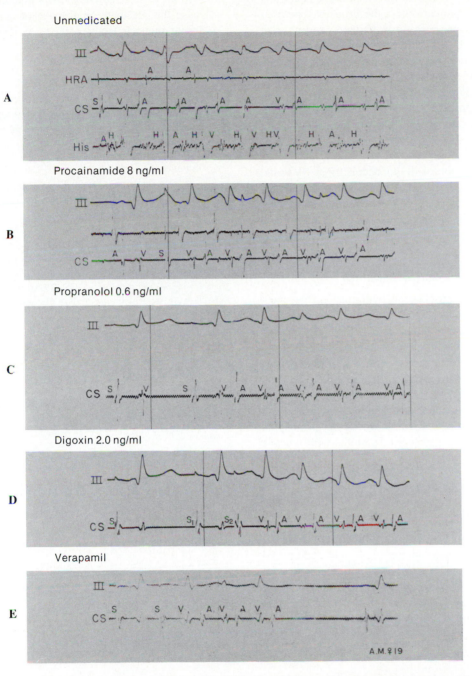

Fig. 9-11. Drug testing in a patient with SVT. **A,** Induction of tachycardia by coronary sinus pacing in the unmedicated state. This patient has a concealed accessory pathway with SVT involving the AV node and His bundle in the antegrade direction and a left-sided accessory pathway in the retrograde direction. **B to E,** Programmed stimulation on subsequent days following drug administration. This was performed by means of a coronary sinus catheter left in place. Only verapamil prevented induction of tachycardia in this patient.

of a sustained SVT. If stimulation following drug administration results in two to three reentrant beats that always terminate spontaneously, the drug may be considered effective. In occasional patients a drug that markedly slows the tachycardia rate may be acceptable for long-term therapy. However, if following drug administration more aggressive stimulation is required to induce the tachycardia but the tachycardia itself is unchanged, this is probably not an acceptable response.

Fig. 9-11 shows an example of drug testing for SVT.

Summary of types of SVT and diagnostic criteria

Complete discussion of the mechanisms of SVT and their diagnosis during EPS is beyond the scope of this chapter. A brief summary of these parameters is provided in the box on this page. The reader is referred to the studies cited in the references for more detailed discussion.

Evaluation of ventricular arrhythmias

Evaluation of ventricular arrhythmias is the most common indication for diagnostic EPS. The ability to induce ventricular arrhythmias in the electrophysiologic laboratory will vary with the arrhythmia. Table 9-3 indicates the approximate results with the most common types of ventricular arrhythmias. As the table indicates, recurrent sustained VT can be reproduced in 90% to 95% of patients. Sustained ventricular arrhythmias can be induced in up to 65% of survivors of out-of-hospital cardiac arrest. The inducibility of patients with nonsustained VT is more variable.

Components of the electrophysiologic study and drug testing

We employ the following sequence of recording and stimulation in patients undergoing evaluation for VT.[30a]

1. Catheters are placed in the high right atrium and His bundle position. After completion of atrial stimulation, the atrial catheter is repositioned in the ventricle. Many laboratories utilize three catheters so that catheter movement is not necessary (see p. 208).

2. The His potential is recorded during normal sinus rhythm. Obtaining a stable His potential is vital because the presence or absence of a His deflection during induced tachycardia is of major diagnostic importance.

SUPRAVENTRICULAR TACHYCARDIAS: TYPES, FREQUENCY, AND ELECTROPHYSIOLOGICAL FEATURES

AV nodal reentrant SVT (58%)
  Initiation and termination by APDs, VPDs, or atrial pacing during AV nodal Wenckebach block
  Dual AV nodal refractory curves and tachycardia initiation dependent on critical AH interval
  Retrograde P wave buried in QRS complex with earliest activation in His bundle lead
  Atrium and ventricle not required for tachycardia

SVT caused by AV bypass tracts (30%)
  Initiation and termination by APDs or VPDs
  Retrograde P wave with short RP interval
  Atrium and ventricle required to initiate and sustain SVT
  Eccentric retrograde atrial activation
  SVT slows with bundle branch block ipsilateral to accessory pathway
  Ability to preexcite atrium with VPD during SVT

SA nodal and atrial reentrant tachycardia (8%)
  Initiation and termination by APDs
  AV node block may exist without affecting tachycardia
  SA nodal reentrant–atrial activation sequence identical to sinus rhythm
  Atrial reentrant–atrial activation sequence different from sinus rhythm

Automatic atrial tachycardia (4%)
  Cannot initiate or terminate with APDs
  P wave differs from sinus rhythm
  AV block may exist without affecting tachycardia

Adapted from Josephson, M.E., and Seides, S.: Clinical cardiac electrophysiology: techniques and interpretation, Philadelphia, 1979, Lea & Febiger.
APD, Atrial premature depolarization; *VPD*, ventricular premature depolarization.

Table 9-3. EPS-induced arrhythmias in patients with ventricular tachycardia

Clinical arrhythmia	Induced arrhythmia			
	Sustained VT	*VF*	*NSVT*	*No arrhythmia*
Sustained VT	90%	2%	2%	6%
VF	55%	10%	15%	20%
NSVT	20%	2%	50%	28%

VT, Ventricular tachycardia; *VF*, ventricular fibrillation; *NSVT*, nonsustained ventricular tachycardia.

3. Atrial incremental pacing and atrial premature stimulation are performed. If AV Wenckebach block occurs at low rates, this will effectively exclude the diagnosis of SVT with aberrancy. Moreover, some VTs may be induced by atrial pacing.

4. Premature ventricular stimulation from the right ventricular apex is performed using single and double premature stimuli. Stimulation is performed during sinus rhythm and during two paced basic cycle lengths (generally 600 and 450 msec) (see p. 212).

5. If double extrastimuli from the right ventricular apex do not induce tachycardia, most laboratories will proceed to triple extrastimuli (discussed below). Fig. 9-12 illustrates induction of sustained VT by triple premature stimuli.

6. Rapid pacing at the right ventricular apex (starting synchronized to the native QRS) at cycle lengths of 400, 350, 300, and 250 msec is performed.

7. If right ventricular apical stimulation does not induce VT, the entire sequence of ventricular stimulation is repeated from the right ventricular outflow tract.

8. For patients in whom VT cannot be induced from the right ventricle, some laboratories repeat the entire stimulation protocol from left ventricular sites (usually one septal site and one lateral site). Because of the increased yield of arrhythmia induction with triple stimuli and because of the difficulty in performing serial drug testing from the left ventricle, I believe left ventricular stimulation has a relatively limited role in clinical EPS.

9. When VT is not induced by the standard protocol, some laboratories administer isoproterenol (initially 0.5 μg/minute, adjusted to increase sinus rate by 25% to 50%, with a maximal dose of 4 μg/minute). Isoproterenol is likely to be helpful in patients with exercise-induced sustained VT.[32] I do not believe adequate data are available to support the use of isoproterenol in other patients.

10. If tachycardia is induced, one should note the rate and configuration of the tachycardia and determine if this correlates with the patient's clinical tachycardia. If possible a 12-lead ECG should be obtained. Moreover, the diagnosis of ventricular

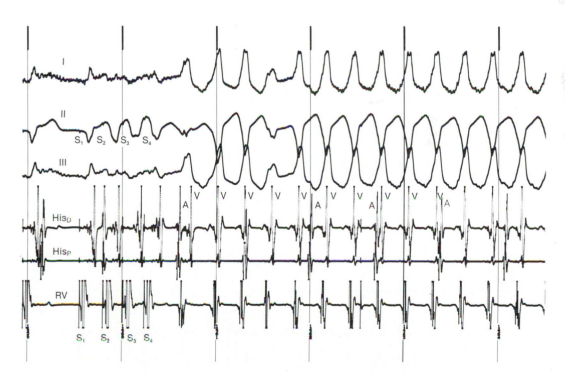

Fig. 9-12. Induction of VT in the electrophysiology laboratory. Illustrated are surface leads I, II, and III and electrograms from the distal *(D)* and proximal *(P)* His bundles and the right ventricle. Basic pacing is performed at a cycle length of 600 msec (S_1 to S_1 interval). Premature stimuli (S_2, S_3, and S_4) are administered. After several unstable polymorphic beats, a sustained monomorphic VT is induced.

tachycardia versus SVT with aberrancy must be established.

a. Ventriculoatrial dissociation is present in 50% of cases of VT, and when noted it establishes a diagnosis of VT (Fig. 9-12).

b. If ventriculoatrial correspondence is present, the absence of a His potential before each QRS, when a His potential was clearly seen during sinus rhythm, indicates the diagnosis of VT.

c. The presence of a His potential before each QRS, but with an HV interval of less than the HV interval in normal sinus rhythm, suggests that the ventricle is not activated through the AV node His axis and that the tachycardia is ventricular. Some unusual tachycardias utilizing accessory pathways may mimic this finding.

d. If a His potential is seen before each QRS and the HV interval is equal to or longer than the HV interval in sinus rhythm, the diagnosis of SVT with aberrancy is established.

11. If sustained tachycardia is induced, the next step depends on how well the tachycardia is tolerated. If the tachycardia is hemodynamically poorly tolerated, immediate cardioversion or defibrillation should be applied. If the tachycardia is well tolerated, there is time for additional maneuvers such as catheter mapping, and a less traumatic approach to termination can be employed. The following sequence is proposed.

a. Attempt termination by synchronizing the stimulator to the patient's QRS complex and administering single premature stimulation throughout diastole.

b. If single stimulation is not effective, double stimulation should be tried. Fig. 9-13 illustrates termination of the VT by double stimulation. We prefer to attempt to terminate tachycardias in this fashion because the risk of accelerating the tachycardia is less than with rapid pacing.

c. If the tachycardia does not respond to single or double stimulation, attempt to terminate the tachycardia by synchronized rapid pacing (Fig. 9-14). This requires a rate of 20 to 50 bpm faster than the tachycardia rate maintained for 6 to 15 captured beats and then abrupt discontinuation of pacing. If the initial attempt is unsuccessful, the process can be repeated with faster rates, up to a maximum cycle length of 250 to 200 msec.

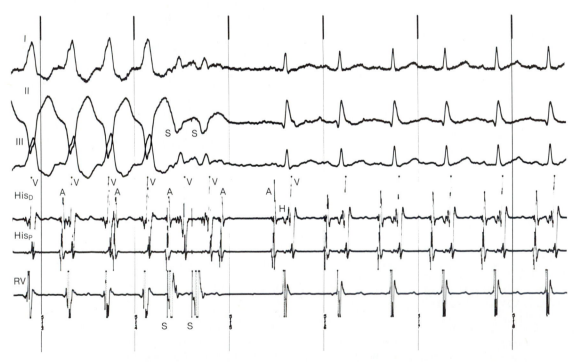

Fig. 9-13. Termination of sustained VT by double stimuli. The lead configurations are the same as in Fig. 9-12. Note that following two timed extrastimuli (*S*) administered in the right ventricle, the tachycardia is terminated.

d. If rapid pacing is ineffective in terminating the tachycardia, pace the ventricle at a rate slightly faster than the tachycardia and introduce single and double premature stimuli at the end of the pacing train.

e. If the tachycardia degenerates to VF or a hemodynamically poorly tolerated VT as a result of any of the maneuvers, perform defibrillation or cardioversion.

12. Determination of drug effects on the patient's tachycardia provides useful clinical information. The number of drugs to be tested will vary from patient to patient. Our procedure is to test more drugs in patients for whom tachycardia can be easily terminated than in patients for whom tachycardia termination requires defibrillation. During the initial study, we usually test IV procainamide. Procainamide is administered intravenously (50 mg/minute up to 1 to 2 gm) with close observation of blood pressure, heart rate, and QT interval. Following the infusion, a complete stimulation protocol is repeated. Procainamide blood levels should be determined.

On subsequent days, drug testing can be performed by means of a catheter from the antecubital or subclavian site left in place in the right ventricle apex. Principles of drug testing for VT are very similar to those discussed for SVT. To allow for washout of previous drugs I usually test only one drug or one drug and a combination on a given day. When possible a control induction should be performed before each test. Drugs to be tested are selected based on the patient's history, with particular attention to drug allergies. Drugs that are commonly tested are indicated in Table 9-2. All drugs should be administered slowly with close observation for side effects. When oral drugs are tested, they should be titrated to the maximal tolerated dose before stimulation is performed. Drug levels should be documented for both IV and oral testing. After drug administration is complete, a full stimulation protocol should be performed (see below). Fig. 9-15 illustrates drug testing in a patient with sustained VT.

Specific problems relating to drug testing are discussed below.

Special considerations

The field of induction of ventricular arrhythmias is rapidly evolving. There are several important areas of controversy at the current time which should be mentioned.

Use of triple stimuli, effects on sensitivity, and specificity of stimulation. When EPS was restricted to patients with recurrent sustained VT, and when the stimulation protocol was restricted to double extrastimuli, Vandepol et al.[33] demonstrated excellent specificity and sensitivity of the technique—that is, arrhythmias that were induced were also manifested clinically, whereas patients without clinical arrhythmias did not have inducible arrhythmias. Because the technique has been expanded to the study of patients whose clinical arrhythmias are not well characterized, (i.e., those with syncope or cardiac arrest) and because stimulation has become more aggressive (i.e., use of three and four extrastimuli), there has been increasing concern about the specificity of the results of stimulation testing. Brugada et al.[34] demonstrated that with three and four extrastimuli, malignant ventricular arrhythmias could be induced in patients who had no clinical indi-

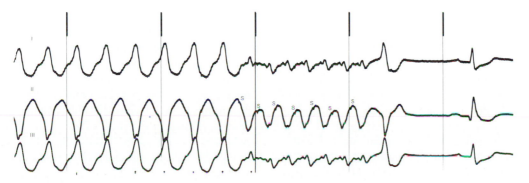

Fig. 9-14. Termination of VT with rapid pacing. Shown are three surface leads. A burst of rapid pacing at a rate of 300/minute for 7 beats (*S*) terminates the tachycardia.

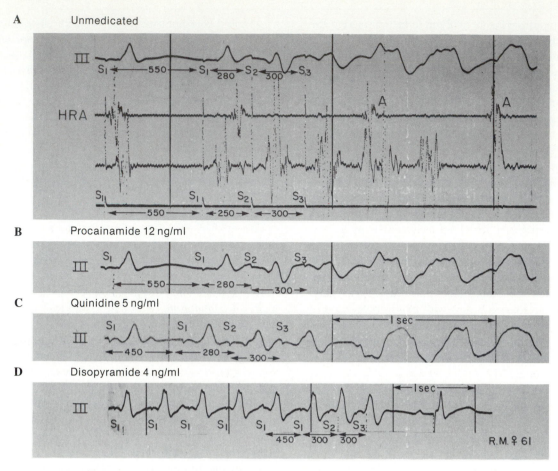

Fig. 9-15. Drug testing in a patient with VT. **A,** Tachycardia induction in the unmedicated state. **B to D,** Drug testing on sequential days using an indwelling catheter in the right ventricle. Similar stimulation protocols were used. Prevention of tachycardia occurred only with administration of disopyramide.

cations of these arrhythmias. However, Morady et al.[35] and Buxton et al.[36] have demonstrated that triple stimuli are necessary to induce certain clinical arrhythmias.

There has been no easy resolution to this problem.[37] The optimal stimulation protocol for maximal specificity and sensitivity has not yet been defined. In the interim, the results of stimulation must be interpreted in the clinical context for each patient. If stimulation induces monomorphic sustained VT in a patient who has had the same arrhythmia clinically, the induced arrhythmia will, in all likelihood, be significant regardless of how aggressive the stimulation was. However, in patients whose clinical arrhythmia is not documented, the induction of polymorphic nonsustained VT with triple extrastimuli should not be considered a positive response. The significance of

induced VF with aggressive stimulation remains controversial, but I consider this a positive finding in most patients.

End points of stimulation before and after drug administration. In most laboratories, the only end point for the stimulation protocol is the induction of a sustained ventricular arrhythmia (VT or VF), and the stimulation protocol is not discontinued for induction of nonsustained (<30 seconds) arrhythmias. Early investigators considered a drug effective in the laboratory only if it suppressed the inducibility of all VT. Swerdlow et al.[38] demonstrated that conversion of sustained ventricular arrhythmia before drug testing to less than 15 repetitive ventricular responses following drug administration is associated with a favorable outcome. A drug that markedly slows the VT so that it is well tolerated may be acceptable for long-term therapy. Drugs that make the arrhythmia more difficult to induce are probably not acceptable. Further studies are necessary on these important questions.

Significance of noninducibility. As indicated in Table 9-3, approximately 20% to 35% of survivors of out-of-hospital cardiac arrest will not have inducible sustained arrhythmias. Some laboratories have reported that this group has a favorable outcome without specific antiarrhythmic therapy and with therapy directed only at the underlying heart disease. However, this finding has been disputed by other researchers.[20-22]

Techniques of drug testing

PROCAINAMIDE: Testing of multiple drugs during EPS can be quite difficult for the patient. A method to predict the effective and ineffective drugs would be extremely helpful. Waxman et al.[39] reported that the results of stimulation following administration of IV procainamide predicted the results of stimulation during treatment with other type 1 agents. Based on this study, many laboratories restrict short-term drug testing to IV procainamide, and if procainamide proves ineffective, they proceed directly to investigational drugs. However, recent studies have suggested that even when IV procainamide is ineffective, quinidine and disopyramide may be successful in up to 20% of cases.[40] I proceed directly from procainamide to investigational drugs in patients whose induced arrhythmias are difficult to terminate. However, in patients who tolerate drug testing well, I prefer to test other type 1 drugs before proceeding to investigational drugs.

AMIODARONE: Several laboratories have reported that patients treated with amiodarone may have a good clinical response despite the drug's failure to prevent arrhythmia induction in the laboratory.[41] A possible explanation for this phenomenon is that amiodarone abolishes ventricular premature beats, removing the cause of the VT without affecting inducibility. Moreover, studies done after only 2 to 3 weeks of amiodarone therapy may not predict the effect of the drug when its steady state is reached. It should be noted that other laboratories dispute these findings and claim that EPS is a good predictor of response to amiodarone.[42]

The final answer to this question is not available at the current time. My policy is to repeat the EPS in the patient treated with amiodarone. My interpretation of these results depends on the patient's clinical arrhythmia. If well-tolerated sustained VT is reproduced with amiodarone therapy, I continue the amiodarone. However, for patients who have suffered out-of-hospital cardiac arrest, if after 6 weeks of amiodarone therapy an arrhythmia that is poorly tolerated hemodynamically remains inducible, I do not accept this as an adequate end point of therapy.

Evaluation of syncope

The electrophysiologic evaluation of syncope includes maneuvers to elicit occult bradycardias and tachycardias. I employ the following EPS protocol in patients with recurrent unexplained syncope:

1. Catheters are placed in the high right atrium and His position. After atrial stimulation the atrial catheter is moved to the RV.
2. Basic conduction intervals are recorded.
3. Sinus node recovery time is evaluated.
4. Atrial incremental pacing is used to evaluate the AV conduction system.
5. Premature atrial stimulation is administered, limited to the high right atrium, using two cycle lengths and single or double premature stimulation.
6. Ventricular stimulation from the right ventricular apex includes single and double premature stimulation during sinus rhythm, during basic cycle lengths of 600 and 450 msec, and then rapid pacing is employed to a cycle length of 250 msec.
7. A similar protocol of ventricular stimulation from the right ventricular outflow tract is followed.

We do not routinely employ triple extrastimuli, left ventricular stimulation, or isoproterenol infusion in patients with unexplained syncope.

Interpretation of findings

The true sensitivity and specificity of EPS in patients with syncope are difficult to determine. Markedly abnormal findings (i.e., markedly prolonged sinus node recovery time, infranodal block with atrial pacing, induction of rapid SVT, and induction of sustained VT) can generally be accepted as diagnostic of the cause of the patient's syncope. Other findings are less helpful. Induction of nonsustained VT should not be considered a positive response.

FUTURE DEVELOPMENTS
Diagnostic and prognostic use of ventricular stimulation

During the next several years, investigation will be directed at several very difficult questions. Whether EPS-guided therapy in survivors of out-of-hospital cardiac arrest is superior to conventional treatment based on Holter monitoring requires further exploration. The role of EPS in patients with high-grade ventricular arrhythmias and nonsustained VT requires further study.[43,44] The use of EPS to prognosticate high risk following myocardial infarction is extremely controversial and requires further study.[22,23] Studies are underway to provide information on the appropriate role of EPS in these settings.

Pacemaker therapy and the implanted defibrillator

Increasingly sophisticated antitachycardia pacemakers are being developed. A full discussion is beyond the scope of this chapter. The automatic implanted defibrillator is discussed in Chapter 14.

Surgical therapy for arrhythmias

One of the major developments has been increasing sophistication in the use of surgical techniques for both ventricular and supraventricular arrhythmias. Full discussion of this complex topic is beyond the range of this chapter, and the reader is referred to selected studies.[45-47]

Ablative therapy

There has been great interest in the use of electric charges administered through electrode catheters to treat certain arrhythmic conditions.[48] This technique was first applied for His bundle ablation in patients with intractable atrial arrhythmias. Unfortunately the technique does render the patient dependent on the pacemaker. In a registry report of 127 patients, the technique was found to be successful in 90% of patients. Complications did include VF, pericardial tamponade, and a small incidence of sudden cardiac death in the months following ablation.[49] Although this technique remains investigational, it currently appears to be the technique of choice for those rare patients in whom His bundle ablation is deemed necessary.

A similar technique has been attempted in patients with accessory pathways. While preliminary reports are encouraging for posterior septal accessory pathways,[50] cardiac perforation and tamponade have been reported in patients with left-sided accessory pathways approached through the coronary sinus.

A very small number of patients have undergone attempted electric catheter ablation of ventricular arrhythmias.[51] The technique is limited by the difficulties of catheter mapping to identify the site of origin of the arrhythmia, and further studies are awaited.

REFERENCES

1. Scherlag, B.J., et al.: Catheter technique for recording His bundle activity in man, Circulation **39:**13, 1964.
2. Wellens, H.J.J.: Electrical stimulation of the heart in the study and treatment of tachycardias, Baltimore, 1971, University Park Press.
3. Josephson, M.E., and Seides, S.: Clinical cardiac electrophysiology: techniques and interpretation, Philadelphia, 1979, Lea & Febiger.
4. Wiener, I.: Current applications of clinical electrophysiologic study in the diagnosis and treatment of cardiac arrhythmias, Am. J. Cardiol. **49:**1287-1292, 1982.
5. Scheinman, M., and Morady, F.: Invasive cardiac electrophysiologic testing: the current state of the art, Circulation **67:**1169-1172, 1983.
6. Health and Public Policy Committee: Diagnostic endocardial electrical recording and stimulation, Ann. Intern. Med. **106:**452-454, 1984.
7. Akhtar, M., et al.: NASPE Ad Hoc Committee on Guidelines for Cardiac Electrophysiologic Studies, Pace **8:**611-618, 1985.
8. Gann, D., Tolentino, A., and Samet, P.: Electrophysiologic evaluation of elderly patients with sinus bradycardias: a long term follow-up study, Ann. Intern. Med. **90:**24-29, 1979.
9. Kastor, J.: Atrioventricular block, N. Engl. J. Med. **292:**462-464 and 572-574, 1975.
10. Rosen K.M., Rahimtoola, S.H., and Gunnary, R.M.: Pseudo A-V block secondary to premature non-propagated His bundle depolarization documentation by His bundle electrocardiography, Circulation **42:**367-373, 1973.
11. Dhingra, R.C., et al.: Significance of the HV interval in 517 patients with chronic bifascicular block, Circulation **64:**1265-1271, 1981.
12. McAnulty, J., et al.: Natural history of high-risk bundle branch block, final report of a prospective study, N. Engl. J. Med. **307:**138, 1982.
13. Dhingra, R.C., et al.: Significance of block distal to the His bundle induced by atrial pacing in patients with chronic bifascicular block, Circulation **60:**1455-1464, 1979.
14. Altschuler, H., Fisher, J., and Furman, S.: Significance of isolated HV interval in symptomatic patients without documented heart block, Am. Heart J. **97:**18-26, 1979.
15. Josephson, M.E., and Kastor, J.A.:Supraventricular tachycardia mechanisms and management, Ann. Intern. Med. **87:**346-358, 1977.
16. Gallagher, J.J., et al.: The preexcitation syndromes, Prog. Cardiovasc. Dis. **20:**285-327, 1978.
17. Horowitz, L.N., Josephson, M.E., and Kastor, J.A.: Intracardiac electrophysiologic studies as a method for the optimization of drug therapy in chronic ventricular arrhythmia, Prog. Cardiovasc. Dis. **23:**81, 1980.
18. Kastor, J.A., et al.: Clinical electrophysiology of ventricular tachycardia, N. Engl. J. Med. **304:**1004-1020, 1981.
19. Swerdlow, C., Winkle, R., and Mason, J.: Determinants of survival in patients with ventricular tachyarrhythmias, N. Engl. J. Med. **305:**1436-1442, 1983.
20. Ruskin, J.N., DiMarco, J.P., and Garan, H.: Out-of-hospital cardiac arrest: electrophysiologic observations and selection of long-term anti-arrhythmic therapy, N. Engl. J. Med. **303:**607-613, 1980.
21. Morady, F., et al.: Electrophysiologic testing in the management of survivors of out-of-hospital cardiac arrest, Am. J. Cardiol. **51:**85-89, 1983.
22. Richards, D.A., et al.: Ventricular electrical instability predictors of death after myocardial infarction, Am. J. Cardiol. **51:**75-80, 1983.
23. Roy, D., et al.: Programmed ventricular stimulation in survivors of an acute myocardial infarction, Circulation **72:**487-494, 1985.
24. DiMarco, J.P., Garan, H., Hawthorne, J.W., and Ruskin, J.N.: Intracardiac electrophysiologic techniques in recurrent syncope of unknown cause, Ann. Intern. Med. **95:**542-548, 1981.
25. Gulamhusein, S., Naccareli, G.V., and Ko, P.T.: Value and limitations of clinical electrophysiologic study in the assessment of patients with unexplained syncope, Am. J. Med. **73:**700-705, 1982.
26. DiMarco, J.P., Garan, H., and Ruskin, J.: Complications in pa-

tients undergoing cardiac electrophysiological procedures, Ann. Intern. Med. **97:**490-493, 1980.

27. Gettes, L.S., et al.: Personnel and equipment required for electrophysiologic testing. Report of the Committee on Electrocardiography and Cardiac Electrophysiology, Council on Clinical Cardiology, the American Heart Association, Circulation **69:**1219H-1221H, 1984.

28. Ross, D.L., et al.: Comprehensive clinical electrophysiologic studies in the investigation of documented or suspected tachycardias: time, staff, problems and costs, Circulation **61:**1010-1016, 1980.

29. Ruskin, J.N., et al.: Electrophysiologic effects of diazepam in man, Clin. Res. **22:**302A, 1974.

30. Nattel, S., Rinkenkergen, R., Leheim, L., and Zipes D.: Therapeutic blood lidocaine concentration after local anesthesia for cardiac electrophysiologic studies, N. Engl. J. Med. **301:**418-420, 1979.

30a. Waldo, A.L., et al.: The minimally appropriate electrophysiologic study for the initial assessment of patients with documented sustained monomorphic ventricular tachycardia, J. Am. Coll. Cardiol. **6:**1174-1177, 1985.

30b. Narula, O.S., et al.: A new measurement of sinoatrial conduction time, Circulation **58:**706, 1978.

31. Ross, D., Denniss, A.R., and Uther, J.B.: Electrophysiologic study in supraventricular arrhythmias in invasive cardiology, Cardiovasc. Clin., 1985.

32. Freedman, R., et al.: Facilitation of ventricular tachyarrhythmia induction by isoproterenol, Am. J. Cardiol. **54:**765-770, 1984.

33. Vandepol, C.J., et al.: Incidence and clinical significance of induced ventricular tachycardia, Am. J. Cardiol. **45:**725-731, 1980.

34. Brugada, P., Green, M., Abdollah, H., and Wellens, H.J.J.: Significance of ventricular arrhythmias initiated by programmed ventricular stimulation: the importance of the type of ventricular arrhythmia induced and the number of premature stimuli required, Circulation **69:**87-92, 1984.

35. Morady, F., et al.: A prospective comparison of triple extrastimuli and left ventricular stimulation in studies of ventricular tachycardia induction, Circulation **70:**52-57, 1984.

36. Buxton, A.E., et al.: Role of triple extrastimuli during electrophysiologic study of patients with documented sustained ventricular tachycardia, Circulation, **69:**537-540, 1984.

37. Wellens, H., Brugada, P., and Stevenson, W.: Programmed electrical stimulation of the heart in patients with life-threatening ventricular arrhythmias: What is the significance of induced arrhythmias and what is the correct stimulation protocol? Circulation **72:**1-7, 1985.

38. Swerdlow, C., Winkle, R., and Mason, J.: Prognostic significance of the number of induced ventricular tachyarrhythmias, Circulation **68:**400-405, 1983.

39. Waxman, H.L., Buxton, A.E., Sadowski, L.M., and Josephson, M.E.: The response to procainamide during electrophysiologic study for sustained ventricular tachyarrhythmias predicts the response to other medications, Circulation **67:**30, 1983.

40. Rae, A.P., et al.: Limitations of failure of procainamide during electrophysiologic testing to predict response to other medical therapy, J. Am. Coll. Cardiol. **6:**410-416, 1985.

41. Waxman, H.L.: The efficacy of amiodarone for ventricular arrhythmias cannot be predicted with clinical electrophysiologic studies, Int. J. Cardiol. **3:**76, 1983.

42. Horowitz, L.N., et al.: Usefulness of electrophysiologic testing in evaluation of amiodarone therapy for sustained ventricular arrhythmias associated with coronary heart disease, Am. J. Cardiol. **55:**346, 1985.

43. Buxton, A.E., Waxman, H.L., Marchlinski, F., and Josephson, M.E.: Electrophysiologic studies in non-sustained ventricular tachycardia: relation to underlying heart disease, Am. J. Cardiol. **52:**985, 1983.

44. Gomes, J.A.C., et al.-Programmed electrical stimulation in patients with high grade ventricular ectopy: electrophysiologic findings and prognosis for survival, Circulation **709:**43-51, 1984.

45. Gallagher, J.J., et al.: Wolff-Parkinson-White syndrome: the problem, evaluation and surgical correction, Circulation **51:**767, 1975.

46. Horowitz, L.N., Harken, A.H., Josephson, M.E., and Kastor, J.A.: Surgical treatment of ventricular arrhythmias in coronary artery disease, Ann. Intern. Med. **95:**88-97, 1981.

47. Wiener, I., Mindich, B., and Pitchon, R.: Determinants of ventricular tachycardia in patients with left ventricular aneurysms: results of intra-operative epicardial and endocardial mapping, Circulation **65:**856, 1982.

48. Josephson, M.E.: Catheter ablation of arrhythmias, Ann. Intern. Med. **101:**234, 1984.

49. Scheinman, M., and Evans-Bell, T.: Catheter ablation of the atrioventricular junction. A report of the percutaneous mapping and ablation registry, Circulation **70:**1024-1029, 1984.

50. Morady, F., et al.: Efficacy and safety of transcatheter ablation of posteroseptal accessory pathways, Circulation **72:**170, 1985.

51. Hartzler, G.O.: Electrode catheter ablation of refractory focal ventricular tachycardia, J. Am. Coll. Cardiol. **2:**1107-1113, 1983.

Part II

THERAPEUTIC PROCEDURES

Chapter Ten

Pericardiocentesis and drainage

ARA G. TILKIAN
ELAINE K. DAILY

Pericardiocentesis is a procedure in which the pericardial space is entered with a needle or cannula and fluid is aspirated. Pericardial drainage generally involves the insertion of a catheter into the pericardial space over a needle, through a needle, or preferably over a guidewire, using a modified Seldinger technique for immediate removal of fluid or for continued drainage over hours and days.

Pericardiocentesis was first performed in 1840.[1] The widely used xiphocostal percutaneous technique was described in 1911.[2] Considerable debate still exists as to its indications and risks. Series reported from 1950 to 1980 emphasized the potential risk of the procedure and tended to discourage its use.[3-5] However, with the widespread use of echocardiography for the diagnosis of pericardial effusion, and with continued improvements in the technique of pericardiocentesis, the procedure has become increasingly more reliable and safe, stimulating renewed clinical interest.[6-10] Pericardiocentesis is now being used with increasing frequency in the management of patients with pericardial disease.

NORMAL ANATOMY

The pericardium is a strong serous sac lined by mesothelial cells. It envelops the heart and the origin of great vessels in its two layers, the visceral and the parietal pericardium. Fig. 10-1 shows the visceral layer intimately attached to the epicardium and reflected back on itself near the origin of the great vessels to form the parietal pericardium. These two layers of pericardium are separated by a potential space that normally contains approximately 20 ml of clear serous fluid.

PATHOPHYSIOLOGY

Disease, inflammation, or injury of the pericardium frequently causes accumulation of fluid in the pericardial space and the development of diffuse pericarditis, pericardial tamponade, subacute effusive-constrictive pericarditis, or chronic pericardial constriction.[11-17] Determining factors in the development of these conditions are the type of disease or injury, extent of the reaction of the pericardium (and the epimyocardium) to this injury, volume of accumulated fluid, distensibility of the pericardium, and most importantly, the rate at which this fluid accumulates in the pericardial space.

Pericardiocentesis and drainage are valuable in the diagnosis and treatment of pericarditis with pericardial effusion, pericardial effusion with cardiac tamponade, and subacute effusive-constrictive pericarditis, but they have no role in the diagnosis or treatment of pericardial constriction. It may be helpful to consider these four categories of pericardial disease as a continuum or spec-

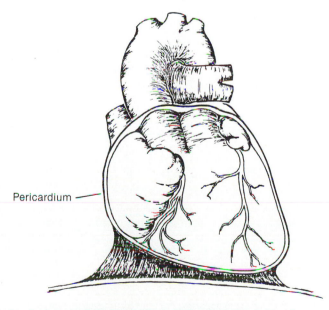

Fig. 10-1. Normal pericardium.

Table 10-1. Clinical, diagnostic, and hemodynamic features of four types of pericardial disease

Parameters	Acute pericarditis	Pericardial tamponade	Subacute effusive-constrictive pericarditis (fibroelastic)	Chronic constriction (rigid shell)
Symptoms	Chest pain; non-specific systemic symptoms	Dyspnea; fullness in chest; anxiety; agitation	Dyspnea	Dyspnea
Physical findings				
Pericardial rub	Frequent, triphasic	Frequent; may disappear as fluid increases	Often present	Usually absent
Heart sounds	Usually normal; may be muffled	May be normal; muffled if fluid is increased	Usually normal	Pericardial knock often present (early diastolic sound)
Rhythm	Usually sinus, sinus tachycardia; occasionally atrial fibrillation or flutter	Usually sinus, sinus tachycardia	Sinus; occasionally atrial fibrillation	Atrial fibrillation frequent
Venous pressure	Normal	Elevated	Elevated	Elevated
Pulsus paradoxus	Absent	Usually present and prominent	Usually present, less prominent	Occasionally present
Systemic arterial pressure	Normal	Hypotension in later stages	Normal	Normal
Ascites/edema	Absent	Generally absent	Sometimes present	Frequent
Kussmaul's sign	Absent	Absent	Usually absent	Occasionally present
ECG findings				
ST elevation, PR segment depression	Frequent, transient	May be present	Usually absent	Absent
Low voltage	Generally absent	Present with increased volume of effusion	Usually present	Usually present
Electric alternans	Generally absent	Sometimes present	Rarely present	Absent
Diffuse T wave lowering	In later stages	In later stages	Usually present	Usually present
Radiographic findings	Normal to increased heart shadow	Increased heart shadow	Increased heart shadow	Often pericardial calcification; often left pleural effusion; heart shadow usually normal
Echocardiographic findings				
Pericardial fluid	Frequently present	Always present, or almost always demonstrable	Often present	Absent
Other	Pericardial thickening (rarely seen)	RA/RV diastolic compression, inspiratory increase in RV & decrease in LV volume	Pericardial thickening (frequent)	Pericardial thickening (better seen by CT or MRI), calcification and abnormal septal motion

CT, Computerized tomography; *MRI,* magnetic resonance imaging.

Table 10-1. Clinical, diagnostic, and hemodynamic features of four types of pericardial disease—cont'd

Parameters	Acute pericarditis	Pericardial tamponade	Subacute effusive-constrictive pericarditis (fibroelastic)	Chronic constriction (rigid shell)
Hemodynamic findings				
RA pressure and waveform (see Fig. 10-7)	Normal	Elevated, with predominant systolic (X) descent, or X > Y	Elevated, X > Y or X = Y	Elevated, X = Y or X < Y
RV diastolic pressure	Normal	Elevated & equal to RA, PA diastolic, & PA wedge. No dip-plateau pattern	Elevated, equal to RA, moderate dip-plateau pattern	Elevated, equal to RA, prominent dip-plateau pattern
Intrapericardial pressure	Normal	Elevated	Elevated	Not measured
Treatment	Based on etiology	Relief of intrapericardial pressure	Relief of intrapericardial pressure & pericardiectomy	Pericardiectomy
Pericardiocentesis	Sometimes used for diagnosis	Effective treatment in most cases	Useful for diagnosis when combined with hemodynamic monitoring; palliative treatment of itself	Not used

trum, without implying a necessary progression from one form to the other (Table 10-1).

Pericarditis with effusion (without cardiac compression)

Numerous conditions can involve the pericardium and cause a reactive inflammatory change of the serous membranes and the underlying epimyocardium, with accumulation of fluid (Fig. 10-2). Some of the more common etiologic entities are listed in the box on p. 234.

The physician is aided in the clinical diagnosis of pericarditis with effusion by the combination of the presenting symptoms, findings on physical examination, ECG, chest radiograph, laboratory studies, and most importantly, the echocardiogram. In this clinical setting, pericardiocentesis and drainage are indicated only if analysis of the fluid will help make a more precise or specific diagnosis, which will alter the course of therapy.

Presenting symptoms may include systemic complaints, "pleuritic" type of chest pain, fever, sinus tachycardia or supraventricular arrhythmias, and other symptoms associated with the underlying disease process; or there may be no symptoms at all.

Physical examination may reveal a triphasic pericar-

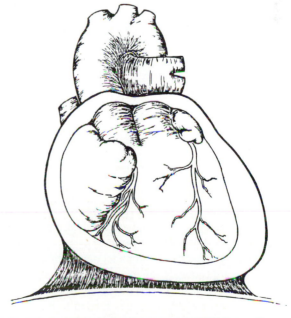

Fig. 10-2. Pericardial effusion.

COMMON CAUSES OF PERICARDITIS

Infection
    Viral pericarditis (coxsackie, influenza, and others)
    Bacterial pericarditis
    Tuberculous pericarditis
    Mycotic (fungus) pericarditis
    Parasitic pericarditis
Neoplasms
    Primary pericardial tumor (mesothelioma—rare)
    Metastatic (hematogenous or direct extension)
Chronic renal failure
Connective tissue disorders
    Rheumatoid arthritis
    Systemic lupus erythematosus
    Scleroderma
    Rheumatic fever
    Vasculitis
Myocardial infarction
    Acute myocardial infarction
    Post myocardial infarction syndrome
Trauma
    Penetrating and nonpenetrating injury
    Rupture of pseudoaneurysm
    Catheter or pacemaker perforation of the heart
    Aortic aneurysm with dissection
    Cardiac surgery
    Post-cardiopulmonary resuscitation
Radiation
Drug reactions
    Procainamide
    Hydralazine
    Minoxidil
    Isoniazid
    Penicillin
    Methysergide
    Daunorubicin
Other causes
    Myxedema
    Cholesterol pericarditis
    Sarcoidosis
    Gout
    Chylopericardium
Idiopathic causes

dial rub (not always), heart sounds that are distant (if amount of fluid is large), and other abnormalities related to the underlying disease process.

Laboratory findings may include nonspecific abnormalities of cardiomegaly on chest radiographs, ST-T wave changes on the ECG, elevated sedimentation rate, and other laboratory abnormalities related to the underlying disease process.

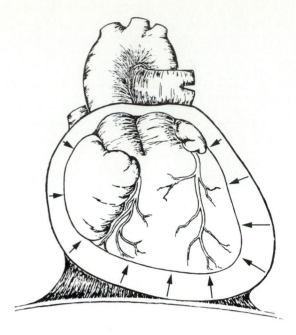

Fig. 10-3. Pericardial effusion with tamponade.

The echocardiogram is of great value in confirming the presence of pericardial effusion. It is also helpful in semiquantitating the volume of fluid, determining its relative distribution, and indicating the presence or absence of pericardial bands and fibrin strands. It may also reveal the presence of pericardial thickening.

Pericardial effusion with tamponade

In pericardial effusion with tamponade, some or all of the findings noted in pericarditis with effusion may be present. Hemodynamic effects of cardiac compression resulting from elevation of pressure within the pericardial space are also present (Fig. 10-3).

Understanding the pathophysiology of pericardial effusion with cardiac compression permits a clearer appreciation of the different clinical presentations of cardiac tamponade and the proper role and timing of pericardiocentesis and drainage in this syndrome.[14-17]

The pressure in the potential space in the normal pericardium is similar to that in the pleural space (-2 to 4 mm Hg). Fluid accumulation in the pericardial space may increase intrapericardial pressure. When fluid accumulates rapidly, as in traumatic intrapericardial hemorrhage, 150 to 200 ml of blood may cause the intrapericardial pressure to reach the steep portion of the pericardial pressure volume curve, causing a rapid rise in intrapericardial pressure and impairing ventricular filling in diastole (Fig. 10-4).

As intrapericardial pressure begins to rise, central ve-

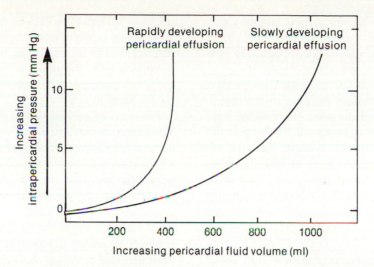

Fig. 10-4. Effects of increasing amounts of pericardial effusion on intrapericardial pressure. In rapidly developing effusions, pericardium has little opportunity to stretch and pressure/volume curve is steep. In slowly developing effusions, pericardium stretches and large effusion may develop before a steep rise in pressure occurs. (From Hancock, E.W.: Cardiac tamponade. In Scheinman, M.M.: Cardiac emergencies, Philadelphia, 1984, W.B. Saunders Co.)

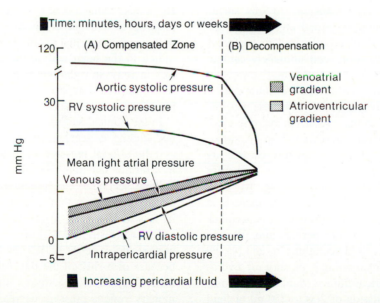

Fig. 10-5. Progressing circulatory events during cardiac tamponade. **A,** Period of effective compensation. Increasing pericardial fluid may cause increasing intrapericardial pressure, but the fluid has not accumulated rapidly enough to overcome adjustments of circulation; venoatrial gradients are maintained at some level, permitting adequate stroke volume. **B,** Period of decompensation. Either intrapericardial pressure rises too rapidly to permit compensation or compensatory mechanisms have been exhausted; pressure gradients—transvalvular and venoatrial—are rapidly liquidated, with rapidly dropping cardiac output and systemic arterial pressure. (Adapted from Spodick, D.H.: Acute cardiac tamponade, In Chung, E.K.: Cardiac Emergency Care, Philadelphia, 1980, Lea & Febiger; and from Hancock, E.W.: Cardiac tamponade. In Scheinman, M.M.: Cardiac emergencies, Philadelphia, 1984, W.B. Saunders Co.)

nous pressure rises simultaneously, maintaining a gradient between the right atrium and right ventricle during disastole and thus permitting adequate filling of the ventricle.

However, as intrapericardial pressure rises further, central venous pressure cannot increase sufficiently to maintain this gradient, and diastolic filling of the right atrium and right ventricle is impaired. This causes decreased right ventricular stroke volume, which is reflected as a decreased stroke volume by the left ventricle. Echocardiography, if done at this stage, will show right atrial collapse or compression. Cardiac output may be temporarily maintained by increased heart rate and increased ejection fraction resulting from adrenergic stimulation.

As intrapericardial pressure continues to rise, stroke volume further diminishes. Defense mechanisms of increased heart rate and increased ejection fraction may not be able to maintain adequate cardiac output. As cardiac output falls, systemic vascular resistance increases in an attempt to maintain adequate blood pressure.

As stroke volume further falls, all of these defense mechanisms are unable to compensate; this preshock (or early shock) state decompensates into frank shock, with hypotension and organ hypoperfusion. At this stage, any further increase in intrapericardial pressure and decrease in stroke volume will rapidly lead to profound shock, coronary hypoperfusion, and ultimately cardiac arrest.

The key effect of progressive increase of intrapericardial pressure is progressive reduction of ventricular volume, to a point at which compensatory increase in ejection fraction cannot prevent a severe drop in stroke volume. Cardiogenic shock and ultimately cardiac arrest ensue when compensatory increase in heart rate cannot maintain adequate cardiac output (Fig. 10-5).

The rate of development of pericardial tamponade is a function of (1) the rate at which this fluid is accumulated, (2) the compliance of the pericardium, (3) the volume of the pericardial fluid accumulated, and (4) the patient's total intravascular volume or state of hydration. Thus when the pericardium is rigid and noncompliant, the rapid accumulation of 200 to 250 ml of fluid can cause lethal tamponade in a relatively hypovolemic patient, whereas when the pericardium is compliant, slowly accumulating fluid may exceed 1 to 2 L before significant cardiac compression is produced.

Bedside observations

Cardiac tamponade is characterized by elevated and abnormal central venous or right atrial pressure; pulsus paradoxus; sinus tachycardia or an increased ventricular response to atrial fibrillation resulting from increased sympathetic output; narrowing pulse pressure; increased peripheral vascular resistance, with cold and poorly perfused skin and extremities reflecting increased adrenergic tone; progressive hypotension (late finding); and finally, cardiac arrest.

Elevation of central venous or right atrial pressure. The central venous or right atrial pressure is elevated early in cardiac tamponade and is the first compensatory mechanism that occurs in response to increased intrapericardial pressure. In the presence of hypovolemia this elevation may not be immediately evident, but fluid challenge will clearly bring it out. In addition, the early rapid filling phase of the right ventricle is inhibited because of increased intrapericardial pressure throughout diastole. This results in a decreased and finally absent diastolic Y descent in the venous pulse or right atrial pressure. This is more easily seen in the right atrial pressure waveform, which shows an elevation of the right atrial pressure with a prominent systolic X descent and a diminished Y descent (Fig. 10-6).

Pulsus paradoxus. Pulsus paradoxus is an exaggeration of the normal inspiratory decrease in systolic arterial blood pressure. In the normal state there is a 10 mm Hg or less reduction in systolic arterial pressure during inspiration. This occurs because the decrease in intrathoracic pressure that occurs during inspiration is transmitted to the heart and aorta, and because the inspiratory increase in right ventricular stroke volume does not reach the left ventricle until it has traveled through the pulmonary arteries and veins.

In the clinical setting of cardiac tamponade, this normal finding is accentuated with an inspiratory drop in systolic arterial pressure of over 10 mm Hg as a result of a further selective reduction in left ventricular stroke volume secondary to impaired left ventricular filling. During inspiration the right ventricular filling normally increases. However, in the presence of cardiac tamponade and a restricted pericardial space this increase occurs at the expense of left ventricular filling, possibly because of a shift of the intraventricular septum toward the left ventricle. In addition, during inspiration the pulmonary venous pressure decreases more than the intrapericardial pressure, causing increased pulmonary venous capacitance and further reduced left ventricular filling in diastole. These factors translate into a more pronounced reduction in left ventricular stroke volume during inspiration, causing a decrease in systolic pressure of greater than 10 mm Hg. This phenomenon—the exaggeration of a normal physiologic observation—is called *pulsus paradoxus* and can be difficult to detect at the bedside using cuff measurements, because rapid and

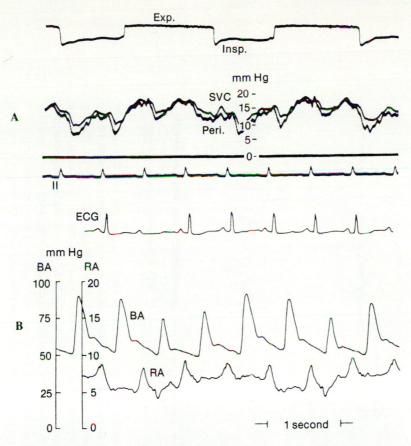

Fig. 10-6. A, Pressure recorded from superior vena cava and the pericardial space of patient with cardiac tamponade. Note there is no *Y* descent in venous pressure pulse, only descent being *X*. Note also that pressure, although elevated, falls in normal fashion during inspiration. Venous and pericardial pressures are almost identical. **B,** Brachial and right atrial pressures in patient with tamponade. Severe pulsus paradoxus is seen. No *Y* descent is seen in atrial pressure record. (From Shabetai, R.: The pericardium, New York, 1981, p. 242. Reprinted by permission from Grune & Stratton, Inc.)

abnormal respiratory patterns and arrhythmias may mask it. Intra-arterial pressure measurements more clearly elucidate this phenomenon (Fig. 10-6).

Pulsus paradoxus may be absent in advanced left ventricular hypertrophy, severe failure of the left side of the heart, atrial septal defect, severe aortic insufficiency, and extreme hypotension. Although it is frequently present in cardiac tamponade, it is not pathognomonic of this condition and can also be seen in chronic obstructive pulmonary disease, restrictive cardiomyopathy, pulmonary embolism with acute cor pulmonale, and severe hypovolemia as well as during positive pressure mechanical ventilation.

Progressive hypotension. Progressive hypotension is a late finding in cardiac tamponade. As the body's

defense mechanisms are overcome and stroke volume and cardiac output continue to drop, pulse pressure narrows and systemic blood pressure further drops. *Thus in cardiac tamponade, hypotension heralds impending cardiac arrest and signals the need for emergency relief.*

Treatment

In all cases of pericardial tamponade, definitive treatment consists of the removal of pericardial fluid by prompt pericardiocentesis and drainage (p. 241) or surgical drainage (p. 254). Volume expansion and inotropic and chronotropic agents may help in varying degrees, depending on the patient's state of hydration and ability to generate an intrinsic adrenergic response (see

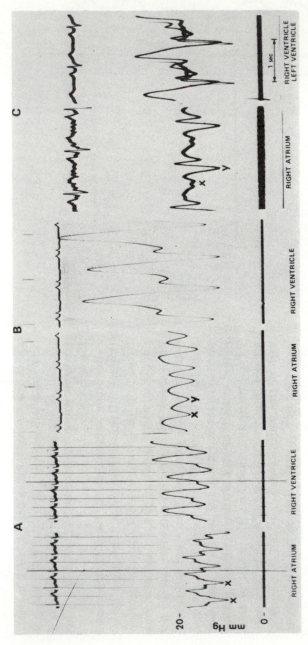

Fig. 10-7. Contrasting waveforms are seen in pressure records from right atrium and right ventricle in patients with three types of compressive pericardial disease. **A,** In record from patient with pericardial tamponade, atrial waveform shows prominent systolic (*X*) descent and absence of early diastolic (*Y*) descent, whereas ventricular waveform shows elevated early and late diastolic pressure levels and inconspicuous dip-plateau pattern. **B,** In record from patient with subacute constrictive pericarditis without effusion, atrial pressure waveform shows approximately equal *X* and *Y* descents, giving M or W contour, whereas ventricular pressure waveform shows prominent dip-plateau pattern. **C,** In record from a patient with chronic calcific constrictive pericarditis, atrial pressure waveform shows predominant early diastolic descent (*XY* pattern), whereas ventricular pressure waveform shows prominent dip-plateau pattern. All records are at same paper speed and sensitivity. (From Hancock, E.W.: On the elastic and rigid forms of pericarditis, Am. Heart J. **100:**921, 1980.)

p. 250). However, these measures are not substitutes for definitive treatment.

Subacute effusive-constrictive pericarditis

Subacute effusive-constrictive pericarditis[12,13] is characterized by constriction of the heart by the visceral pericardium in combination with free pericardial effusion, frequently under increased pressure. Thus features of pericardial tamponade and pericardial constriction may coexist (Table 10-1). In this setting, pericardiocentesis and drainage are helpful for both diagnosis and palliative treatment. Fig. 10-7 displays the contrasting waveforms in pressure records from the right atrium and right ventricle in patients with three types of compressive pericardial disease.

Diagnosis

Diagnosis is confirmed by documentation and analysis of pericardial fluid, elevation of intrapericardial pressure at the onset of the procedure with normalization after removal of pericardial fluid, and the persistence of abnormal hemodynamics in the right side of the heart. Before pericardial drainage, right atrial and right ventricular pressure are similar to those in pericardial tamponade. These pressures do not normalize after removal of fluid; instead they assume characteristics of pressures seen in the right side of the heart during pericardial constriction.

Definitive treatment

Definitive treatment requires pericardiectomy, although patients may experience improvement after the removal of pericardial fluid. This important clinical fact emphasizes the value of obtaining hemodynamic data before and after pericardial drainage (p. 252). Limited surgery (pericardial window) is generally not satisfactory.

Chronic pericardial constriction

Chronic pericardial constriction is the result of chronic, fibrotic (and later calcific) fusion of the visceral and parietal pericardial layers, causing a rigid compression of the heart. Pericardiocentesis has no role in the diagnosis or treatment of pericardial constriction (see Table 10-1 and Fig. 10-7).

INDICATIONS

Pericardiocentesis and drainage are generally indicated in those conditions in which removal and analysis of fluid will directly benefit the patient. These include the following conditions.[7,10,14]

• *Cardiac tamponade of any cause:* Essentially any condition that can cause pericardial effusion can cause pericardial tamponade. Common causes are metastatic tumor (commonly bronchogenic or breast carcinoma or lymphoma), idiopathic pericarditis, and chronic renal failure. Other causes are acute myocardial infarction (especially if anticoagulation is used), iatrogenic (cardiac catheterization, pacemakers), infection, mediastinal radiation, cardiac surgery, cardiac rupture, aortic dissection, and trauma.

Pericardiocentesis and drainage may be life-saving procedures in cases of cardiac rupture, aortic dissection, or traumatic pericardial tamponade with penetrating wounds of the heart, but definitive treatment will require surgical exploration. Blunt chest trauma may cause pneumopericardium and, if under tension (tension pneumopericardium), may precipitate pericardial tamponade. Pericardiocentesis and evacuation of the air are effective treatments.[18]

• *Infective pericarditis:* This can result from bacterial, fungal, or other rare agents (see Table 10–1).

• *Suspected cases of subacute effusive-constrictive pericarditis:* Pericardiocentesis should be performed in conjunction with right heart catheterization and hemodynamic monitoring.

• *Neoplastic pericardial disease:* Pericardiocentesis is performed for confirmation of diagnosis or instillation of local chemotherapeutic agent.

• *Pericardial effusion of unknown etiology:* Pericardiocentesis may be performed for definitive diagnosis (rarely needed).

The presence of pericardial fluid in itself is not an indication for pericardiocentesis. This procedure is generally not indicated in uncomplicated acute idiopathic pericarditis, postcardiotomy syndrome without tamponade, postmyocardial infarction syndrome without tamponade, uncomplicated pericardial effusion in patients with chronic renal failure, pericarditis with various systemic diseases without tamponade, or simple radiation pericarditis.

CONTRAINDICATIONS

Elective pericardiocentesis is contraindicated in patients who are restless and uncooperative, are receiving anticoagulation therapy, or have a bleeding disorder or thrombocytopenia (<50,000/cu mm). It is contraindicated when the presence of pericardial fluid is not definitely confirmed or is thought to be very small or posteriorly loculated, as can occur frequently after cardiac surgery. The inexperienced physician without adequate supervision or thoracic surgical back-up also constitutes a contraindication.

RISKS

The risks of pericardiocentesis include cardiac puncture (right atrium or right ventricle) with hemopericardium and pericardial tamponade, air embolism, laceration of a coronary artery (rare), pneumothorax, puncture of the peritoneal cavity or abdominal viscera, arrhythmias (usually vasovagal bradycardia), acute pulmonary edema (if pericardial tamponade is decompressed too rapidly), delayed definitive surgical treatment (where early surgical repair of the injury is needed), and missed diagnosis of neoplastic disease or tuberculosis because a pericardial biopsy was not obtained.

Most series[4,7] report a procedure-related mortality of 2% to 4%. Most of these data were accumulated before the widespread use of two-dimensional echocardiography for the definitive diagnosis and localization of pericardial effusion and before the use of fluoroscopy, hemodynamic monitoring, and the modified Seldinger technique for catheter drainage of the pericardial space (p. 241). Each of these methods improves the safety and success of the procedure. A more current series of pericardiocentesis and drainage using some of these techniques has already reported a much lower rate of morbidity and no deaths in 132 consecutive cases.[9]

The technique described in this chapter, which we have used for more than 7 years, is a synthesis of the numerous refinements that have been introduced into the procedure over the past 30 years by many investigators.[19-26] The technique is an adaptation of the basic Seldinger approach to percutaneous catheter insertion (p. 35). The safety and the efficacy of this technique have been demonstrated in children[8] as well as in patients who have undergone cardiac surgery.[25] In patients who have undergone cardiac surgery and develop cardiac tamponade secondary to loculated posterior pericardial fluid, surgical drainage is preferred.[27]

EQUIPMENT

Except for life-threatening conditions, pericardiocentesis should be performed in a controlled environment with optimal conditions and expert help. The procedure is best performed in a cardiac catheterization laboratory or a special care area (coronary or intensive care unit, operating room, emergency room) with the use of portable fluoroscopy and monitoring equipment. Necessary equipment includes:

- Full resuscitative equipment with crash-cart and defibrillator
- Fluoroscopic equipment
- ECG and hemodynamic monitoring capability
- Sterile gown and gloves
- Pericardiocentesis tray (Fig. 10-8) containing:
  Antiseptic solution, gauze sponges, towels, and drapes
  Syringes (6 and 12 ml) and #25 and #21 needles, 1 and 2 inches long
  1% lidocaine without epinephrine
  #11 scalpel
  Hemostat or needle holder
  18-gauge, thin-wall, 8 cm long, short-bevel percutaneous entry needle (10 or 12 cm needle may rarely be needed)
  Teflon-coated, flexible-tip, J-curved guidewire— 0.038 inch (1 mm), 70 cm long
  Dilators, 6 to 8 Fr, 20 cm long
  Pigtail catheter, 8.3 Fr, 40 cm long
  Connecting tube with three-way stopcock and universal connector to attach to a drainage bag
  Suture material and needle
  Test tubes for culture and laboratory analysis of fluid
  Alligator clip cable (see p. 247)
  Three-way stopcock

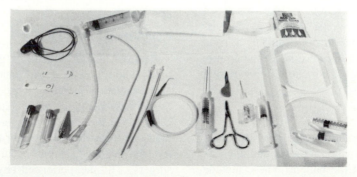

Fig. 10-8. Materials required for pericardiocentesis and drainage. Contents of pericardiocentesis tray *(right* to *left)* are listed above (see text).

Choice of drainage catheter is a personal preference; the ideal pericardial catheter has not yet been designed. Use of catheters with only an end hole is discouraged. Straight catheters with end holes and multiple side holes are satisfactory. Lock[8] has designed a pigtail catheter for use in children. The pigtail design seems to reduce the risk of trauma from the catheter tip and may improve patency of the catheter drainage sites. We have used a special-order tray made by Cook, Inc. (C-PCSY-820-AT092884) that contains the materials needed for pericardiocentesis listed above (with the exception of sterile gown and gloves). The drainage catheter used in this set is an 8.3 Fr, 40 cm pigtail catheter made of radiopaque polyurethane with six 0.05-inch (1.3 mm) side holes 3 cm from its distal tip.

PERSONNEL

The personnel listed below are required to perform pericardiocentesis with drainage.

• A physician experienced in the procedure (usually a cardiologist, cardiothoracic surgeon, or specialist in critical care medicine)

• Specialty nurses (optimally two) to monitor the patient and assist in medications and emergencies and to assist the physician in set-up, procedure, and hemodynamic monitoring

• A radiology technician for control of fluoroscopy equipment

• A cardiology technician to help with hemodynamic and ECG monitoring

• A cardiothoracic surgeon, who should be available in case of an emergency (a rare occurrence)

• A laboratory technician to process pericardial fluid

PATIENT PREPARATION

1. Explain the procedure to the patient.

2. Obtain informed consent for the complete procedure, which may include pericardiocentesis, drainage, and hemodynamic monitoring.

3. Check for confirmation of the presence of pericardial fluid on a current echocardiogram.

4. Review the indications and possible contraindications as they apply to the specific patient.

5. Check for the use of heparin or warfarin or the presence of a bleeding tendency.

6. Obtain blood count and coagulation studies if needed.

7. For an elective procedure, keep the patient fasting for 4 to 6 hours.

8. Obtain a 12-lead ECG.

9. Secure an IV route and keep it open with 5% dextrose in water.

10. Administer premedication if necessary; Sedation may be used in an apprehensive patient. *Atropine 0.6 to 1.0 mg intramuscularly or intravenously is recommended in all cases unless specifically contraindicated* (e.g., patients with glaucoma or tachycardia) to prevent vasovagal reflex of bradycardia and hypotension, which may occur at the time of puncture of the pericardium.

11. Position the patient for the left xiphosternal approach (for alternative sites see Fig. 10-11). Elevate the torso and the head at a 30° to 45° angle.

12. Shave and clean the skin before applying a liberal amount of antiseptic solution to the lower chest and upper abdominal area.

13. Drape around the xiphoid process without masking the key anatomic landmarks adjacent to it. Extend the drapes to the lower abdomen and upper thorax to permit free motion without risk of contaminating needles, catheters, or guidewires.

14. The operator should wear sterile gown and gloves; face mask and hair cover are advisable.

PROCEDURE (Fig. 10-9)
Administration of local anesthetic

The procedure is done with adequate local infiltration of 1% lidocaine without epinephrine and should be performed with little or no pain.

1. Using a 25-gauge needle on a 5 to 6 ml syringe, raise a 1 cm skin wheal 0.5 cm inferior and to the left of the xiphoid process, into the angle between the xiphoid process and the left costal margin.

2. Extend the 1% lidocaine infiltration with a 20- or 21-gauge, 2-inch needle to the left costal margin in the anticipated route of the pericardiocentesis needle to a depth of 4 to 5 cm.

Pericardial puncture

1. Make a 2 to 3 mm skin cut over the initial wheal, using a #11 blade.

2. Separate the subcutaneous tissue to a depth of 1 cm by blunt dissection with a straight hemostat.

3. Use a 10 ml syringe with 5 ml of 1% lidocaine attached to the 18-gauge, thin-wall, *short-bevel* needle. In most patients an 8 cm needle is enough, but a 10 to 12 cm needle may be necessary in very large patients. The short bevel improves the operator's sensitivity to structures and permits the safe entry of the entire needle lumen into the pericardial sac. An alternate type of needle involves use of a trochar and cannula. This requires detection of pericardial puncture by tactile sensation. We find the simple needle with its tip kept clear by injection of saline or lidocaine an easier and safer instrument to use.

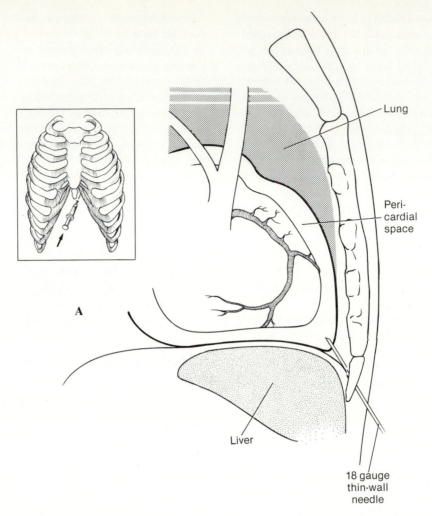

Lung

Peri-
cardial
space

A

Liver

18 gauge
thin-wall
needle

Fig. 10-9. A, Sagittal section showing subxiphoid route of pericardial aspiration and *(inset)* initial placement of thin-wall 18-gauge needle. Pericardiocentesis needle is introduced at 30° to 40° angle to frontal plane. When there is free aspiration of pericardial fluid, pericardium has been entered. Needle is not advanced further.

4. Introduce the needle/syringe assembly at 30° to 40° angle to the frontal plane and advance it, aiming the needle toward the left shoulder (Fig. 10-9, *A*) until it contacts the left costal margin. An angle greater than 45° will be directed toward the liver or stomach. Aiming toward the right shoulder or anywhere between the two shoulders is suitable if fluid volume, as seen on echocardiography, is large in this area.

5. At this point, tradition would dictate attaching an ECG lead to the needle to monitor the needle tip as it approaches the heart. For advantages and disadvantages of this, and also the actual technique, see p. 247.

6. After reaching the costal margin, tilt the needle slightly inferiorly to clear the costal margin and permit advancement toward the pericardium. Do not direct the needle more posteriorly than 30° to 40°. The only structure now between the needle and the pericardium is the membranous portion of the diaphragm. Keep the needle tip aimed anteriorly toward the left shoulder. This may require pressing the hub of the needle into the abdominal wall if the patient is obese or has a distended abdomen.

7. Advance the needle 3 to 5 mm at a time, clearing the needle tip with 0.3 to 0.5 ml injection of lidocaine and then attempting aspiration. This ensures proper anesthesia along the needle track and keeps the needle tip free of tissue or thrombus during aspiration.

8. The pericardium is entered approximately 6 to 7

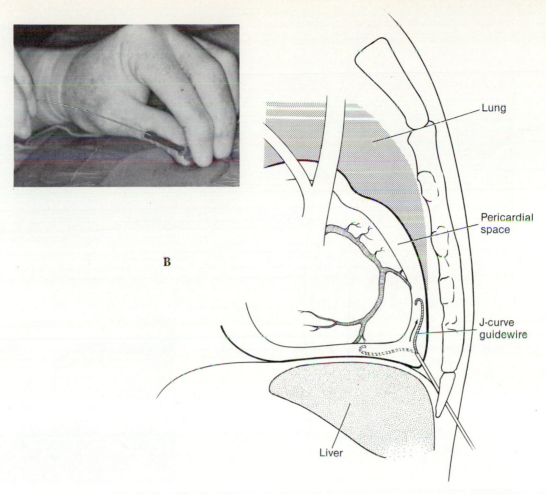

B

Lung

Pericardial
space

J-curve
guidewire

Liver

Fig. 10-9, cont'd. B, Flexible J tip of guidewire is advanced through needle into pericardial
space.   *Continued.*

cm from the skin puncture site in most adults (Fig. 10-9, *A*). The operator feels this as a distinct "giving" or "popping" sensation. We advocate not using a stopcock between the needle and the syringe to increase the "feel" and sensitivity of the operator's hand for the needle tip. The patient may experience sharp pain at the time of pericardial puncture. Infiltrate additional lidocaine at this time, if necessary.

9. If pericardial entry is achieved—as confirmed by the free aspiration of pericardial fluid—do not advance the needle any farther. (For bloody fluid see p. 250.) Do not use the hemostat as a needle stop because this may damage the thin-wall needle.

10. Remove 20 ml of fluid in a sterile syringe for basic diagnostic study.

Needle withdrawal

1. Disconnect the syringe from the needle, and under fluoroscopic guidance and confirmation, advance the flexible J tip of the guidewire well into the pericardial space (Fig. 10-9, *B*).

2. Promptly withdraw the needle, leaving the guidewire in place (Fig. 10-9, *C* and *D*). *Only at this step of the procedure is speed recommended.* The safety of the procedure is greatly enhanced by (a) minimizing the time the needle tip spends in proximity to the heart (in experienced hands this time can be reduced to 10 seconds or less), (b) substituting a flexible guidewire for the needle before any significant volume of fluid is removed and therefore before the pericardial space is reduced in volume, and (c) providing controlled atraumatic access to the pericardial space with a larger catheter.

The presence of a guidewire in the pericardial space does not provoke any arrhythmias, although its manipulation may be associated with some chest or shoulder pain.

Caution: Never withdraw the guidewire abruptly

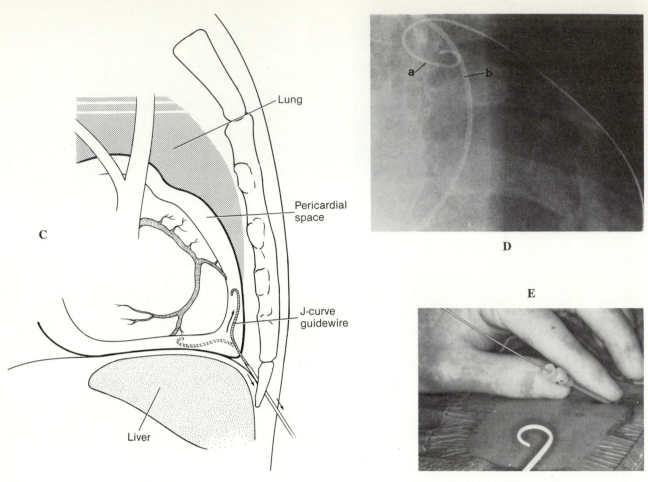

Fig. 10-9, cont'd. C, Needle is withdrawn while guidewire is left in pericardial space. **D,** AP fluoroscopic view of guidewire in pericardial sac *(a)*. Right heart catheter *(b)* is seen in RV outflow tract directed toward right pulmonary artery. **E,** Tract is dilated with use of 6 and 8 Fr dilators, advanced serially over the guidewire.

through the needle. This will risk shearing and cutting off the tip of the guidewire in the pericardial space.

Catheter insertion

1. Proceed without undue haste because the risk of damage to the heart is essentially eliminated. Before advancing the 8.3 Fr catheter over the guidewire, dilate the tract progressively with the use of 6 and 8 Fr dilators advanced serially over the guidewire (Fig. 10-9, *E*).

2. Intermittently check the wire position with the fluoroscope.

3. Next, advance the catheter over the guidewire and through the chest, using a rotating motion. As the catheter is advanced well into the pericardial space, gradually withdraw the guidewire (Fig. 10-9, *F* and *G*).

4. Attach a three-way stopcock to the catheter hub.

5. If hemodynamic data are to be obtained, attach a transducer system to the stopcock on the pericardial catheter and record intrapericardial pressure. Also obtain right heart, and systemic pressures before removal of any additional fluid. Take care that additional fluid is not infused into the pericardial space via the fluid-filled transducer system.

6. Using a 50 ml syringe, remove 50 to 100 ml of fluid and save it for various cultures and chemistry studies (see p. 254).

7. In the presence of pericardial tamponade, continue aspirating fluid until there is a clear improvement in the patient's systemic blood pressure, heart rate, and right heart pressures. Do not try to rapidly empty the entire pericardial fluid or try to promptly normalize pressure

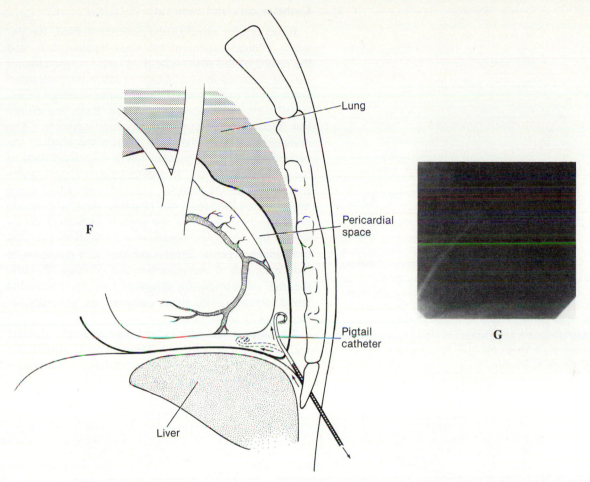

Fig. 10-9, cont'd. F, Catheter is advanced into pericardial space after proper dilatation of its path, and guidewire is withdrawn. **G,** AP fluoroscopic view of catheter in pericardial space.

in the right side of the heart because this may lead to markedly increased venous return and expose the patient to the risk of pulmonary edema.[28,29] Acute right ventricular volume overload with hemodynamic evidence of right heart failure can also be precipitated.[30] These complications of pericardiocentesis have been observed only in the presence of pericardial tamponade. Fig. 10-10 illustrates the pressure/volume relationship of pericardial fluid during pericardiocentesis in chronic pericardial effusion with tamponade.

8. After removal of several hundred milliliters of fluid, the catheter may be repositioned and advanced anteriorly or posteriorly, using fluoroscopic guidance to ensure complete emptying. The drainage procedure usually is done over 15 to 30 minutes.

9. At the end of the drainage procedure, repeat intra-

pericardial, right heart, and systemic pressure measurements. Successful treatment is confirmed by near normalization of pressures on the right side of the heart and normalization of intrapericardial pressures.

10. The pigtail catheter may be left in the pericardial space for continued drainage.

11. Secure the catheter to the skin with 3-0 silk sutures.

12. Apply sterile dressing.

13. Connect the catheter to a sterile drainage bag for continuous drainage. Secure the bag 20 to 30 cm below the midchest level. Suction is not required.

14. Cap the three-way stopcock for sterility.

15. Obtain a chest radiograph to exclude pneumothorax and confirm catheter position.

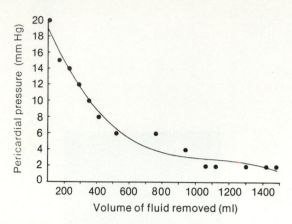

Fig. 10-10. Data obtained during pericardiocentesis of patient with cardiac tamponade owing to idiopathic pericarditis. After insertion of catheter into pericardial space, pericardial pressure was measured as increments of pericardial fluid were aspirated. Note that left-hand side of curve is steep, whereas right-hand side of curve is quite shallow. (From Shabetai, R.: The pericardium, New York, 1981, p. 239. Reprinted by permission from Grune & Stratton, Inc.)

Catheter care and removal

Based on the cause of the pericardial fluid, the patient's clinical condition, the hemodynamic data, and the results of the pericardial fluid analysis, the catheter may be removed in 1 to 2 hours or left in the pericardial space for 48 to 72 hours for continuous drainage or administration of therapeutic agents (p. 252). We do not use suction or intermittent manual aspiration. The drainage bag is secured safely below the level of the patient's midchest to prevent return of drained fluid to the pericardial space. Reaccumulation of fluid under pressure while the catheter is in the pericardial space must be rare (we have not observed this), and we do not flush the catheter or use heparin to prevent occlusion of the side holes. Injection of medications (steroids or chemotherapeutic agents) are kept at a minimum to reduce the risk of contamination and infection. Because the risk of introducing infection into the pericardial space increases with time, catheters are generally removed in 24 to 48 hours.

1. Remove the sutures and withdraw the catheter with a firm continuous pull. The catheter is usually soft and will come out easily without the need to straighten

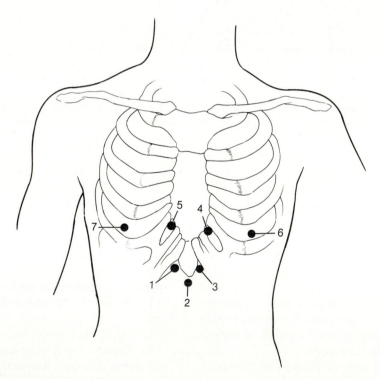

Fig. 10-11. "Standard" locations for pericardiocentesis (see text). *1* to *3,* Xiphoid approaches. *4,* Fifth left intercostal space at sternal margin. *5,* Fifth right intercostal space at the sternal margin. *6,* Apical approach. *7,* Approach for major fluid accumulation on the right side. (Adapted from Spodick, D.H.: Acute pericarditis, New York, 1959, Grune & Stratton, Inc.)

the pigtail with a guidewire. Use of a guidewire is not advisable because this would run the risk of contamination.

2. Apply a sterile dressing to the puncture site.

ALTERNATIVE APPROACHES

The described left xiphocostal approach for pericardiocentesis with the needle directed to the left shoulder is the one used most commonly and is generally considered the safest route in the presence of freely moving effusion. Other approaches (Fig. 10-11) are right xiphocostal, apical, right sided, and parasternal. It is helpful to be familiar with alternate approaches and use them when individual circumstances make such approaches desirable.

The xiphocostal approach described above with the needle directed to the *right* shoulder (Fig. 10-11, positions 1 to 3) is not routinely used unless a large amount of fluid is present in this direction. This approach carries a higher risk of injury to the right atrium and inferior vena cava, where a puncture may not be well tolerated and where bleeding complications are more serious.

Apical approach

The left pleural space and the lingula of the left lung could be punctured in the apical approach (Fig. 10-11, position 6) because they are close to this area. This route is best avoided when the pericardial fluid is suspected to be purulent, to avoid the risk of spreading infection to the lungs and the pleura. Puncture of the heart in this approach is potentially less dangerous because the coronary arteries at the left ventricular apex are smaller, and puncture of the thick-wall left ventricle (despite some normal apical thinning) poses a smaller risk of hemopericardium and tamponade as compared with puncture of the right ventricle or, worse, the right atrium. In the presence of pulmonary hypertension this route, which avoids the right ventricle, may be preferred, especially if the fluid surrounds the cardiac apex.

For the apical approach, locate the cardiac apex using radiography, fluoroscopy, or preferably echocardiography. Insert the needle 1 cm lateral to the apex and in the intercostal space below it, within the area of cardiac dullness. Direct the needle toward the right shoulder. Avoid the inferior edge of the rib because this marks the path of the intercostal artery.

Right-sided approach

The right-sided approach (Fig. 10-11, position 7) may be used when the effusion is predominantly right sided, with the right border of the cardiac silhouette 4 cm to the right of the sternal margin. Insert the needle at the fourth or fifth intercostal space, avoiding the inferior border of the ribs and directing the needle medially. Puncture of the right pleura or right atrium is a risk.

Parasternal approach

The parasternal approach (Fig. 10-11, positions 4 and 5) carries the risk of puncture of the left anterior descending coronary artery or the internal mammary (thoracic) artery. Introduce the needle in the fifth or sixth *left* intercostal space at the left sternal margin and aim it in a posterior and medial direction. The left internal mammary artery lies 1 to 2.5 cm lateral to the sternal edge; the needle should point medially to avoid this artery.

The *right* fifth or sixth intercostal space can be used, again inserting the needle at the right sternal margin and aiming posteriorly and medially to avoid the right internal mammary artery. This approach avoids the left anterior descending coronary artery but is closer to the right pleural space and the right lung.

ECG MONITORING OF NEEDLE TIP

The technique of monitoring the needle tip with an ECG was first described in 1956.[31] Since then, most discussions of pericardiocentesis have included this as an integral part of the procedure. Recently the value of this technique has been questioned.[24,25]

Procedure

A sterile electrode with alligator-type clips at each end is used. One end is attached to the metal hub of the pericardiocentesis needle and the other to the precordial lead of a properly grounded and isolated ECG recorder. The ECG limb leads are attached to the patient in the usual way. This permits continuous ECG monitoring, with the pericardiocentesis needle tip acting as an "exploring electrode." The ECG machine is set to record the V leads. As long as the needle is in direct contact with the skin or subcutaneous tissue, an ECG signal approximating V_2 (for subcostal approach) is recorded. When the needle tip makes contact with the parietal pericardium, separated from the visceral pericardium with fluid, there is no change in the ECG signal (Fig. 10-12, *A*). However, a current of injury with marked ST segment elevation is seen when the needle tip is in contact with the visceral pericardium or when the needle punctures the ventricle wall (Fig. 10-12, *B*). A sim-

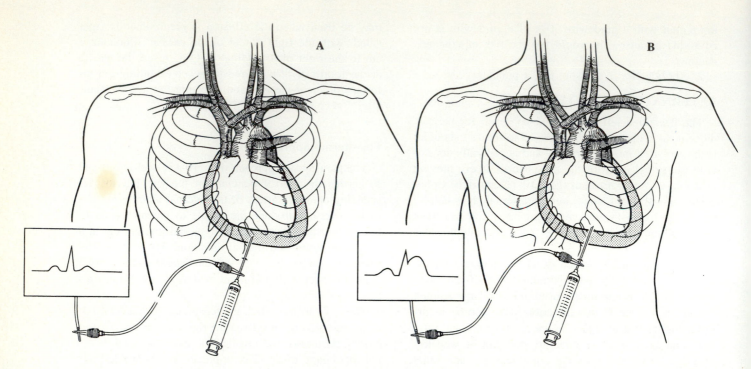

Fig. 10-12. A, ECG monitoring of needle tip. Note normal ST segment while needle tip is not touching the epicardium. **B,** When needle tip touches epicardium, current of injury ("contact" current) is reflected on ECG as elevated ST segment.

ilar type of PR segment elevation is seen if the needle punctures the atrial wall. In addition, ventricular or atrial arrhythmias or AV conduction abnormalities may be seen.

Advantages

When clear diagnostic-quality ECG tracings are obtained, cardiac puncture is avoided or immediately recognized, and the needle tip withdrawn to avoid myocardial laceration. This safety feature may be helpful if the presence of pericardial fluid is in doubt or if a Seldinger-type needle with a stylet or obturator is used, in which case it is not possible to continuously aspirate the needle tip while the pericardium is approached.

Disadvantages

Frequently, diagnostic-quality ECG tracings cannot be obtained because baseline shifts and much artifact render the technique useless.

The heart can be punctured without observing any current of injury.[23] This can occur in cases of tumor infiltration of the myocardium, myocardial infarction with fibrotic areas, and infiltrative cardiomyopathies in which the area of puncture is electrically silent. Thus the technique can give a false sense of security.

There is potential danger of ventricular fibrillation. The myocardium can receive a small but lethal shock if the operator touches both the needle and an ECG machine or other piece of electric equipment that has leakage current on its chassis and is not properly grounded; the current passes from the faulty equipment and through the operator to the needle and then to the heart.

ECG monitoring of the needle tip adds another level of complexity to pericardiocentesis and may distract the operator from paying close attention to the technique and the "feel" of the needle.

We advocate that the physician (1) be familiar with the technique and rationale of ECG monitoring of the needle tip, (2) not use this technique routinely when the diagnosis of pericardial fluid is definite and the percutaneous modified Seldinger approach for catheter drainage described here is used, and (3) use needle tip ECG monitoring—with the pitfalls and limitation in mind—when the amount of fluid is not great or when it is loculated. Surgical pericardiostomy is safer in this setting (p. 254).

TWO-DIMENSIONAL ECHOCARDIOGRAPHY

Two-dimensional (2D) echocardiography is routinely used in the diagnosis of pericardial effusion, although it is not generally used during the pericardiocentesis procedure.[9,32] It has been proposed that 2D echocardiography can enhance both the safety and the success of pericardiocentesis because it confirms the presence of pericardial fluid during pericardiocentesis, determines its location, estimates its volume, and most importantly, indicates the optimal point of needle entry and route to avoid the heart. It also confirms the location of the needle and catheter in the pericardial space with or without the use of contrast study.[9,32,32a]

If further experience confirms the value of echocardiographically directed pericardiocentesis, this may be the standard approach in the near future.

COMPLICATIONS, MANAGEMENT, AND PATIENT AFTERCARE

No special care is required following an uncomplicated pericardiocentesis and drainage over and above the care required for the underlying condition. If pericardiocentesis was done to relieve pericardial tamponade, the patient should be watched for signs of recurring tamponade. This is a real danger when a drainage catheter is not left in place or in the event that the catheter becomes occluded.

Complications of pericardiocentesis may include puncture or laceration of a cardiac chamber, laceration of a coronary artery, ventricular fibrillation, pneumothorax, peritoneal puncture, or infection.

• *Puncture or laceration of a cardiac chamber:* This is always a concern and is more likely to occur in cases involving a small amount of pericardial fluid or when the fluid is loculated. The risk of this complication cannot be completely eliminated. Simple puncture of the myocardium, especially of the left ventricle, is generally well tolerated. Right atrium or right ventricle puncture, especially if there is pulmonary hypertension, may require surgical correction. *Never advance a dilator or a catheter over the guidewire unless you are absolutely assured that the guidewire is in the pericardial space.* Otherwise, a relatively benign puncture hole could be turned into a life-threatening tear of a cardiac chamber.

If cardiac puncture occurs:
1. Recognize it immediately (see p. 250).
2. Withdraw the needle and guidewire promptly.
3. Monitor the patient for development or worsening of pericardial tamponade.
4. Summon a cardiothoracic surgeon.
5. Be prepared to repeat the pericardiocentesis if rapidly progressive pericardial tamponade develops or to proceed with surgical drainage if this becomes necessary.

• *Laceration of a coronary artery:* Coronary artery rupture is always considered a potential risk but is extremely rare. It may precipitate acute pericardial tamponade or ventricular fibrillation.

• *Ventricular fibrillation:* This may result from coronary artery laceration or needle contact with the right or left ventricle if the operator touches the chassis of an ungrounded ECG machine while also touching the hub of the needle. The leakage current on the case of the equipment travels through the operator and the needle and then to the heart. If ventricular fibrillation occurs, withdraw the needle immediately and defibrillate the heart promptly.

• *Pneumothorax:* This indicates entry into the pleural cavity, with injury to the lungs. The risk is higher in patients with chronic obstructive lung disease and when using parasternal or apical routes. Pleural tube drainage is rarely needed.

• *Peritoneal puncture:* This may occur if there is significant ascites or if the needle is not first advanced to the costal margin and then gently deflected from its surface. In the presence of ascites the operator may aspirate straw-colored fluid and may thus be convinced that the pericardial space has been entered. This will lead to inadvertent catheterization of the peritoneal space! Use of fluoroscopy will eliminate this risk. Peritoneal puncture is generally benign unless a hollow viscus is penetrated.

SPECIAL CONSIDERATIONS
Emergency treatment of life-threatening pericardial tamponade

The pericardiocentesis and drainage technique described above is suited for most cases of elective and urgent pericardiocentesis and is aimed at performing the procedure in as safe a manner as possible and obtaining as much information about the disease process as possible. However, this may not be the best approach in a setting of acute pericardial tamponade with life-threatening, rapidly progressing hypotension and shock. In such a case, the following procedures are recommended.

1. Institute immediate rapid-volume colloid or crystalloid infusion. Use 500 to 1000 ml or more over 10 to 20 minutes *while the patient is being prepared for emergency pericardiocentesis or surgical drainage.* This may increase the stroke volume and improve cardiac output by increasing the ventricular filling pressure. In a hypovolemic patient with tamponade (e.g., acute traumatic hemopericardium) the benefits may be substantial, whereas in euvolemic or hypervolemic pa-

tients with subacute tamponade the benefits are marginal.[14,33,33a]

2. Avoid positive pressure ventilation because this will further reduce venous return, stroke volume, and cardiac output. Pulmonary edema will not occur as long as pericardial tamponade, with reduced right ventricular output, is present. The risk of pulmonary edema exists after relief of pericardial tamponade when ventricular return and cardiac filling improve and cardiac output may rapidly increase. For this reason, especially if acute volume infusion has been used, the rate of pericardial decompression should be slow.

3. Administer isoproterenol (Isuprel) by IV infusion. This will increase myocardial contractility (and therefore stroke volume) and heart rate and will reduce peripheral vascular resistance; as a result cardiac output will improve. A pressor drug with dominant alpha receptor action, e.g., norepinephrine (Levophed) or metaraminol (Aramine) may also be used in patients with life-threatening hypotension.

4. Proceed to emergency needle pericardiocentesis *as soon as possible,* using a short-bevel 18-gauge thin-wall needle. In such a setting, pericardial drainage may be carried out via a simple needle pericardiocentesis without the use of a catheter. Echocardiographic guidance may be of value.

Fluoroscopy is desirable if a catheter will be introduced in the pericardial space. The procedure can be done in the cardiac catheterization laboratory or at the bedside utilizing a portable fluoroscopy unit. If emergency pericardiocentesis is done without fluoroscopy and bloody fluid is encountered, the intrapericardial location of the needle may be difficult to confirm.

5. On noting bloody fluid, immediately aspirate 50 to 100 ml and note the effect on heart rate, blood pressure, and degree of respiratory distress. If improvement is noted, then the operator is assured that the fluid is coming from the pericardial space. Further aspiration may be continued, and a catheter may be introduced for continued drainage. On the other hand, in the setting of pericardial tamponade, removing of 50 to 100 ml of blood from a cardiac chamber will cause further hemodynamic deterioration.

If a response is not clear-cut, the needle may be withdrawn and the fluid analyzed.

Theoretically, this emergency needle pericardiocentesis approach is sound. Its clinical application has not been tested or adequately reported. ECG monitoring of the needle tip in this setting has some merit, however the emergency nature of the procedure may not permit ECG monitoring.

Various other methods have been proposed for differentiating the bloody pericardial tap from cardiac puncture. However, none have had widespread use, and their application in an emergency situation is not practical. Some of these methods are:

- Checking the patient's taste response following injection of sodium dehydrocholate, saccharin, or magnesium sulfate (similar to determination of a circulation time); if the patient can taste these agents, the needle or catheter is in the cardiac chamber or a vessel
- Injecting fluorescein and using ultraviolet light to detect its circulation in unresponsive patients
- Utilizing radioisotope techniques

Hemodynamic monitoring is valuable, but pericardiocentesis should not be delayed for this. Intrapericardial pressure measurements can be dispensed with for expediency. After control of the emergency situation, definitive treatment may involve repeat pericardiocentesis under better conditions or operative surgical pericardiostomy.

Traumatic pericardial tamponade, in contradistinction to other medical conditions causing tamponade, is best treated surgically with adequate exploration. Emergency pericardiocentesis is used only as a temporizing measure and only if immediate surgery cannot be performed.

Bloody tap during elective pericardiocentesis

Pericardiocentesis may yield grossly bloody fluid. This could be an alarming experience and may lead the operator to a premature and inappropriate withdrawal of the needle. This problem should be anticipated, and a methodic approach of dealing with it should be prepared in advance. Neoplastic or uremic pericardial fluid is frequently bloody, as is the pericardial fluid of patients taking anticoagulants or those who have experienced myocardial trauma, aortic dissection, or cardiac rupture. The fluid is also frequently bloody in idiopathic or radiation-induced pericarditis. Puncture of a cardiac chamber with a pericardiocentesis needle will yield blood, which may appear indistinguishable from bloody pericardial fluid.

If bloody fluid is encountered during elective pericardiocentesis using the modified Seldinger technique with fluoroscopy, the following steps are suggested.

1. Withdraw 5 ml of the bloody fluid and send it for analysis (see Table 10-2), but do not wait for the results.

2. Advance the flexible guidewire with fluoroscopic guidance and follow its path. If there are no ectopic beats and the wire follows the well-recognized path of the pericardial sac (Fig. 10-9, *D*), then proper pericar-

Table 10-2. Comparison of characteristics of patient's blood and bloody pericardial fluid

Features	Patient's blood	Bloody pericardial fluid
Clotting	Usually (use activated clotting time tube)	No
Hematocrit	Same as hematocrit before pericardiocentesis	Usually lower
pH	Same as above	Usually lower than venous pH[34]
Po_2	Same as above	Lower than venous Po_2
Pco_2	Same as above	Higher than venous Pco_2
Drop on a gauze pad	Spreads out as a homogeneous deep red spot	Spreads with a central deep red spot with a pale peripheral halo

dial entry is confirmed, and the catheter is advanced after proper dilatation.

3. If ectopic beats occur or the wire does not freely advance in the pericardial sac, the needle may be in the right ventricle or right atrium. Withdraw the needle and guidewire without waiting for the results of fluid analysis, which may take several minutes. Proper use of this maneuver implies a working knowledge of the anticipated wire or catheter path in the pericardial space as opposed to the right ventricle or right atrium, as seen in anteroposterior fluoroscopy (Fig. 10-9, *D*).

4. Pressure recordings through the needle may yield information concerning the location of the needle tip—if this is in the right ventricle. Right atrial and intrapericardial pressures may be indistinguishable.

5. Injecting 5 ml of contrast medium under fluoroscopic observation may yield more information. Layering of the contrast material inferiorly indicates that it is in the pericardial space or at least that it is not in a cardiac chamber. On the other hand, if the contrast medium swirls and instantly disappears, a cardiac chamber has been entered.

6. The results of fluid analysis may now be checked (Table 10-2). If the analysis of the bloody fluid clearly indicates that this is blood, implying cardiac puncture, watch the patient carefully and request the help of a cardiothoracic surgeon. On the other hand, if the analysis of the bloody fluid clearly indicates that this is pericardial fluid, then a repeat attempt of pericardiocentesis is indicated, with removal of more fluid and repeated attempts to introduce the guidewire and catheter under fluoroscopic guidance.

Injection of material into pericardial space

Except for cases of uremic pericarditis or neoplastic pericardial effusion there is little need to inject material into the pericardial space. Local instillation of antibiotics for septic pericarditis has little to offer because systemic antibiotics, in addition to pericardial drainage, are required and antibiotic levels achieved in the pericardial fluid are equivalent to those in the blood.

Before the advent of echocardiography, injection of air into the pericardial space was advocated to improve radiographic visualization by contrast, permitting the diagnosis of pericardial thickening or pericardial tumor. Its routine use is discouraged because air in the pericardial space will interfere with the satisfactory performance of echocardiograms for 24 to 48 hours and because if entry into the pericardial space is not ensured, air may be injected in a cardiac chamber, with catastrophic results. This technique may have a role in some circumstances, as in cases of loculated pericardial effusions.

Neoplastic pericardial effusion

Neoplastic pericardial effusion is a common cause of pericardial effusion with tamponade. Cardiac tamponade may be the initial presentation of the malignancy. Frequently the fluid is bloody. Primary tumors of the pericardium and the heart are very rare and thus the presence of neoplastic pericardial effusion usually indicates metastatic disease, frequently breast, lung, or lymphoma-leukemia. This generally indicates poor long-term prognosis, especially for lung carcinoma, less so for breast carcinoma or lymphoma. Pericardiocentesis and pericardial drainage are frequently sufficient as palliative measures.[35-38]

For recurrent neoplastic pericardial effusion, the agents listed in Table 10-3 have been applied intrapericardially in combination with pericardial drainage.[35-37,38a] Such techniques appear to be successful in approximately 50% of cases.

Other agents used include quinacrine and thiotepa. Alternatives include anterolateral parietal pericardiectomy, radioactive gold used intrapericardially, external beam radiation, and systemic chemotherapy. The choice of treatment for the individual patient depends on a host of considerations, which are beyond the scope of this discussion.

Chronic renal failure

With increasing use of chronic dialysis, chronic renal failure is one of the more common causes of pericardial effusion and pericardial tamponade.[39,40] The following comments apply.

The presence of pericardial fluid without signs or symptoms of active pericarditis or pericardial tamponade is not an indication for pericardiocentesis or drainage. More intensive dialysis, use of regional heparin, and follow-up are required.

Actively symptomatic pericarditis with pericardial effusion frequently requires pericardial drainage, especially if attempts at medical treatment have failed. Hypotension during dialysis sessions is frequently an indication for pericardiocentesis.

Pericardial tamponade always requires pericardial drainage.

Pericardial fluid is frequently bloody and its hematocrit may approach the hematocrit of the patient.

Subacute effusive-constrictive pericarditis may be present. Hemodynamic monitoring before and after the tap is important to distinguish this from left ventricular dysfunction, which is much more frequent than constriction in dialysis patients.

Most patients with pericardial tamponade or symptomatic pericarditis will respond well to pericardiocentesis with 24 to 48 hours of continuous catheter drainage. Instillation of locally absorbable steroids (triamcinolone 50 to 100 mg/4 to 6 hours) has been used in conjunction with pericardial drainage.[40] A controlled study comparing pericardial drainage with and without use of nonabsorbable steroids has not been reported.

Pericardiectomy is reserved for patients with recurrent pericardial tamponade or patients with progressive pericardial constriction.

Definitive diagnosis of pericardial fluid: two-dimensional echocardiography and computerized tomography

Echocardiography is the method of choice for the diagnosis of pericardial effusion and for the evaluation of distribution and semiquantitation of the amount of fluid. Except in cases of life-threatening tamponade in which emergency pericardiocentesis is a life-saving procedure, 2D echocardiography should be performed before pericardiocentesis to confirm the diagnosis.

Warning: On rare occasion, a false positive diagnosis of pericardial effusion on good-quality 2D echocardiography, interpreted expertly, can occur and lead to therapeutic misadventure with the performance of an inappropriate pericardiocentesis or even thoracotomy.[41]

Table 10-3. Agents used intrapericardially for neoplastic pericardial effusion

Agent	Dosage
Tetracycline	500 mg in 20 ml normal saline (may be repeated until sclerosis occurs)
Nitrogen mustard	0.4 mg/kg
5-Fluorouracil	500-1000 mg
Bleomycin	5 mg in 20 ml sterile water

This is more likely to occur in patients who are obese or elderly or are taking corticosteroids, when anterior and posterior pericardial fat pads can mimic pericardial effusion.

The distinction is made with the help of CT scanning, which shows fluid as a highly concentrated shadow around the heart, whereas the epicardial fat line has a low concentration and is on the periphery (Fig. 10-13).

Hemodynamic monitoring

Hemodynamic monitoring during pericardiocentesis may involve right cardiac pressures, pulmonary artery wedge pressures, systemic pressures, and intrapericardial pressure. The information gained enhances the safety of the procedure and provides a more complete diagnosis.

Pressure monitoring of the right side of the heart supports the diagnosis of tamponade or constriction. In cardiac tamponade, right atrial, right ventricular diastolic, pulmonary artery diastolic, and pulmonary artery wedge pressures are equal and may range from 10 to 30 mm Hg.

Intrapericardial pressure monitoring confirms the diagnosis of pericardial tamponade, even if pressures in the right side of the heart are relatively low (low-pressure tamponade). Intrapericardial pressure will be nearly equal to the pressures in the right atrium and pulmonary artery wedge position. Postdrainage pressures confirm successful relief of pericardial tamponade when intrapericardial pressure is zero, slightly net positive, or subatmospheric, and may unmask a diagnosis of effusive constrictive pericardial disease when right cardiac pressures resemble those of pericardial constriction. After pericardial decompression, pressures on the right side of the heart may not normalize immediately but will gradually reach normal levels over several hours.

Acute right ventricular dilatation with echocardiographic features of right ventricular volume overload

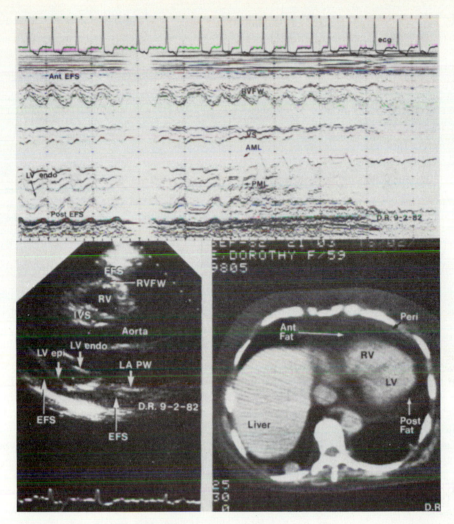

Fig. 10-13. Anterior *(Ant)* and posterior *(Post)* echo-free spaces *(EFS)* are seen by both M-mode *(top)* and 2D echocardiography *(left)*. Computed tomographic chest scan *(right)* disclosed that posterior as well as anterior echo-free spaces were caused exclusively by fat. *AML,* Anterior mitral leaflet; *Peri,* pericardium; *PML,* posterior mitral leaflet; *PW,* posterior wall; *RVFW,* right ventricular free wall; *VS,* ventricular septum. (From Rifkin, R.D., et al.: Combined posteroanterior subepicardial fat simulating the echocardiographic diagnosis of pericardial effusion. Reprinted with permission of the American College of Cardiology, J. Am. Coll. Cardiol. **3:**1335, 1984.)

has been reported immediately after pericardiocentesis for tamponade.[30] Hemodynamic measurements have suggested acute right ventricular failure. This probably reflects the temporary volume overload that follows relief of pericardial tamponade and is present in varying degrees in most patients with subacute or chronic tamponade. The hemodynamics of this temporary right ventricular overload need to be distinguished from those of effusive constrictive pericardial disease. Hemodynamic monitoring during pericardiocentesis also permits

the documentation of coexisting left ventricular dysfunction.

However, because of economic, logistic, and personnel limitations, hemodynamic monitoring is not always done. Complete hemodynamic data are essential in clinical practice only in cases of suspected subacute effusive-constrictive pericarditis. In these cases, simple removal of the fluid constitutes incomplete treatment, and documentation of persistent hemodynamic abnormality generally leads to surgical pericardiectomy. Hemody-

Table 10-4. Advantages and disadvantages of needle-catheter pericardiocentesis (as opposed to surgical subcostal pericardial drainage)

Advantages	*Disadvantages*
Effective and prompt resolution of pericardial tamponade in most patients	Safe only in experienced hands (cardiologists or cardiovascular surgeons, skilled in invasive techniques); if such expertise is not available, surgical pericardiostomy is generally safer
Easily available with fewer tools; no need for operating room personnel and surgical instruments	
Less traumatic and less involved for patient	Potential risk of cardiac puncture if amount of fluid is small, posterior, or loculated
Uses local and minor infiltration anesthetic (surgical pericardiostomy usually requires general anesthesia, although it can be done with liberal use of local anesthesia)	Requires fluoroscopy and hemodynamic monitoring for safety and optimal results
	Does not yield pericardial biopsy and thus may miss diagnosis of tuberculosis or lymphoma
Permits accurate hemodynamic measurements, including intrapericardial pressure measurement (although these measurements can be obtained in operating room when surgical approach is used, this is generally not done)	May not achieve complete drainage in the presence of extensive pericardial adhesions; in purulent pericarditis this limitation may prevent control of the infection, whereas adequate drainage with a large-bore tube after lysis of adhesions is usually effective treatment with use of systemic antibiotics
Less risk of infection than in cutdown surgical methods	Not satisfactory for treatment of traumatic hemopericardium with pericardial tamponade

namic monitoring is desirable but not essential during pericardiocentesis for pericardial effusion or pericardial tamponade when subacute constriction is not a serious consideration. At a minimum, central venous pressure should be monitored. For interpretation of hemodynamic data see Table 10-1 and Fig. 10-7.

Percutaneous pericardiocentesis versus surgical subcostal pericardiocentesis and pericardial biopsy and drainage

Surgical subcostal pericardiostomy is an excellent alternative to percutaneous pericardiocentesis and drainage.[42-45] Controversy exists as to the relative merits and safety of these two approaches. The experience of the physician and the available facilities usually determine the approach in the individual patient. More extensive surgery involving thoracotomy is generally reserved for cases requiring pericardiectomy for either recurrent pericarditis or pericardial constriction.

The advantages and disadvantages of percutaneous catheter pericardiocentesis as compared to surgical pericardiostomy are listed in Table 10-4.

Analysis of pericardial fluid

Review of the composition of pericardial fluid in different disease states is beyond the scope of this discussion. The fluid may be handled in the following manner.

1. The laboratory technician should be available at the time of the procedure to directly receive and process the specimen. If this is not possible, a responsible member of the team—the patient's attending physician or nurse—should personally carry the specimen to the laboratory and ensure proper handling and that the correct tests are performed. The aggravation of losing a specimen is difficult to overcome!

2. All specimens should be analyzed for the following:

Volume, color, character of fluid

Hematology: hemoglobin and hematocrit, white blood cells and differential count

Chemistry: protein and glucose

Microbiology: Gram stains and aerobic and anaerobic cultures, acid-fast stain and culture, fungal stains and culture

Cytology/pathology (heparinized container)

3. Additional studies listed below may be done as indicated in the individual case (See Table 10-2 for a comprehensive list of pericardial diseases)

Viral studies (rarely of clinical value)

Studies for parasites: amoeba, hydatid cyst, spirochetes, toxoplasma

Immunology/serology: fluorescent antinuclear antibody, complement CH50, C3, fungal serology (precipitin and complement fixation antibodies), quantitative latex fixation titer for rheumatoid factor, and quantitative immunoglobins

Lipoelectrophoresis for chylopericardium

Cholesterol level and microscopy for cholesterol pericardium

The specimen is saved in the laboratory for 2 weeks. Attention to details of specimen handling will be rewarding.

FUTURE DEVELOPMENTS

No major breakthroughs or discoveries are expected in pericardiocentesis or pericardial drainage in the near future, although techniques of pericardiocentesis are continually evolving. Improved pericardial drainage catheter design is anticipated. The technique of echocardiographically guided pericardiocentesis may be further validated and possibly receive wider acceptance. As the prevalence of uremic and neoplastic pericardial effusion increases, better understanding of the pathophysiology and more effective treatment may be forthcoming.

Techniques of pericardioscopy and visually guided percutaneous pericardial biopsy are in their infancy.[46-48] When fully developed, these techniques may reduce the need for surgical subcostal pericardiostomy.

PROCEDURE CHECKLIST

- ✔ Review the indications and contraindications of the procedure in relation to the specific patient.
- ✔ Note special circumstances that may apply (need for chemotherapeutic agent or steroids; need for hemodynamic monitoring).
- ✔ Obtain informed consent.
- ✔ Check equipment.
- ✔ Notify appropriate departments for a scheduled procedure (radiology, cardiology, laboratory).
- ✔ Obtain and review laboratory results: coagulation studies, echocardiogram.
- ✔ Prepare the patient: IV route, premedication, appropriate instructions, and reassurance.
- ✔ Perform pericardiocentesis and drainage.
- ✔ Process the fluid obtained.
- ✔ Obtain a chest radiograph at completion of the procedure.
- ✔ Watch for possible complications or recurrent tamponade.
- ✔ Document procedure and the outcome in medical record.

REFERENCES

1. Schuh, R.: Erfahrungen uber die Paracentese der Brust und des Herzbeutels, Med. Jahrb. d. K.K. osterr. Staates Wien. (neuste Folge 24), **33**:388, 1841.
2. Marfan, A.B.: Ponction du péricarde par l'epigastre, Ann. Med. Chir. Infect. **15**:529, 1911.
3. Fowler, N.O.: Pericardial disease. In Fowler, N.O., editor: Cardiac diagnosis and treatment, ed. 3, Cambridge, 1985, Harper & Row, Publishers, Inc.
4. Guberman, B.A., et al.: Cardiac tamponade in medical patients, Circulation **64**:633-640, 1981.
5. Kilpatrick, Z.M., and Chapman, C.B.: On pericardiocentesis, Am. J. Cardiol. **16**:722-728, 1965.
6. Wong, B., et al.: The risk of pericardiocentesis, Am. J. Cardiol. **44**:1110-1114, 1979.
7. Krikorian, J.G., and Hancock, E.W.: Pericardiocentesis, Am. J. Med. **65**:808-814, 1978.
8. Lock, J.E., Bass, J.L., Kulik, T.J., and Fuhrman, B.P.: Chronic percutaneous pericardial drainage with modified pigtail catheters in children, Am. J. Cardiol. **53**:1179-1182, 1984.
9. Callahan, J.A., et al.: Two-dimensional echocardiographically guided pericardiocentesis: experience in 117 consecutive patients, Am. J. Cardiol. **55**:476-484, 1985.
10. Callaham, M.L.: Pericardiocentesis in traumatic and nontraumatic cardiac tamponade, Ann. Emerg. Med. **13**:924-945, 1984.
11. Hancock, E.W.: Management of pericardial disease, Mod. Concepts Cardiovasc. Dis. **48**:1-6, 1979.
12. Hancock, E.W.: Subacute effusive-constrictive pericarditis, Circulation **43**:183-192, 1971.
13. Hancock, E.W.: On the elastic and rigid forms of constrictive pericarditis, Am. Heart J. **100**:917-923, 1980.
14. Hancock, E.W.: Cardiac tamponade. In Scheinman, M.M.: Cardiac emergencies, Philadelphia, 1984, W.B. Saunders Co.
15. Spodick, D.H.: The normal and diseased pericardium: current concepts of pericardial physiology, diagnosis and treatment, J. Am. Coll. Cardiol. **1**:240-251, 1983.
16. Shabetai, R.: Changing concepts of cardiac tamponade, Mod. Concepts Cardiovasc. Dis. **52**:19-23, 1983.
17. Fowler, N.O., and Gabel, M.: The hemodynamic effects of cardiac tamponade: mainly the result of atrial, not ventricular, compression, Circulation **71**:154-157, 1985.
18. Cummings, R.G., Wesly, R.L.R., Adams, D.H., and Lowe, J.E.: Pneumopericardium resulting in cardiac tamponade, Ann. Thorac. Surg. **37**:511-518, 1984.
19. Spodick, D.H.: Acute pericarditis, New York, 1959, Grune & Stratton, Inc., pp. 78–173.
20. Massumi, R.A., Rios, J.C., Ross, A.M., and Ewy, G.A.: Technique for insertion of an indwelling intrapericardial catheter, Br. Heart J. **30**:333-335, 1968.
21. MacAlpin, R.N.: Percutaneous catheter pericardiocentesis, Eur. Heart J. **1**:287–291, 1980.
22. Fallows, J.A., and Testor, B.H.: The use of a polyethelyne catheter in pericardial paracentesis, N. Engl. J. Med. **253**:872-873, 1955.
23. Sobol, S.M., Thomas, H.M., and Evans, R.W.: Myocardial laceration not demonstrated by continuous electrocardiographic monitoring occurring during pericardiocentesis, N. Engl. J. Med. **292**:1222-1223, 1975.
24. Spodick, D.H.: Pericardial aspiration (letter), Br. Med. J. **42**:64, 1980.
25. Erikson, U., Aberg, T., and Klingen, G.: Catheter pericardiocentesis in the postoperative period, Acta Radiol. Diagn. **24**:33-36, 1983.
26. Shabetai, R.: Pericardiocentesis. In Shabetai, R.: The pericardium, New York, 1981, Grune & Stratton, Inc., pp. 325-347.
27. D'Cruz, I.A., et al.: Two-dimensional echocardiography in cardiac tamponade occurring after cardiac surgery, J. Am. Coll. Cardiol. **5**:1250-1252, 1985.
28. Vandyke, W.H., Cure, J., Chakko, C.S., and Gheorghiade, M.: Pulmonary edema after pericardiocentesis for cardiac tamponade, N. Engl. J. Med. **309**(10):595–596, 1983.
29. Shenoy, M.M., et al.: Pulmonary edema following pericardiotomy for cardiac tamponade, Chest **86**:647-648, 1984.
30. Armstrong, W.F.: Acute right ventricular dilatation and echocardiographic volume overload following pericardiocentesis for relief of pericardial tamponade, Am. Heart J. **107**:1266-1270, 1984.
31. Bishop, L.H., et al.: The ECG as a safeguard in pericardiocentesis, J.A.M.A. **162**:264, 1956.

32. Chandraratna, P.A.N., et al.: Application of 2-dimensional contrast studies during pericardiocentesis, Am. J. Cardiol. **52:**1120-1122, 1983.
32a. Goldman, M., et al.: Pericardiocentesis guided by two-dimensional contrast echocardiography: a new foolproof technique (abstract), J. Am. Coll. Cardiol. **7:**95A, 1986.
33. Kerber, R.E., et al.: Hemodynamic effects of volume expansion and nitroprusside compared with pericardiocentesis in patients with acute cardiac tamponade, N. Engl. J. Med. **307:**929, 1982.
33a. Klopfenstein, H.S., et al.: Alterations in intravascular volume affect the relation between right ventricular diastolic collapse and the hemodynamic severity of cardiac tamponade, J. Am. Coll. Cardiol. **6:**1057-1063, 1985.
34. Kindig, J.R.: Clinical utility of pericardial fluid pH determination, Am. J. Med. **75:**1077-1079, 1983.
35. DeVita, V.T. Jr., Hellman, S., and Rosenberg, S.A.: Cancer: principles and practice of oncology, Philadelphia, 1982, J.B. Lippincott Co.
36. Davis, S., Rambotti, P., and Grignani, F.: Intrapericardial tetracycline sclerosis in the treatment of malignant pericardial effusion: an analysis of thirty-three cases, J. Clin. Oncol. **2:**631-636, 1984.
37. McKenna,, R.J. Jr., Ali, M.K., Ewer, M.S., and Frazier, O.H.: Pleural and pericardial effusions in cancer patients, Year Book Medical Publishers **9:**24-44, 1985.
38. Haskell, R.J., and French, W.J.: Cardiac tamponade as the initial presentation of malignancy, Chest **88:**70-73, 1985.
38a. Maher, E.R., and Buckman, R.: Intrapericardial installation of bleomycin in malignant pericardial effusion, Am. Heart J. **111:**613-614, 1986.
39. Thompson, M.E., Rault, R.M., and Reddy, P.S.: Uremic pericarditis, Cardiovasc. Rev. Report **2:**755-761, 1981.
40. Buselmeier, T.J., et al.: Uremic pericardial effusion. Treatment by catheter drainage and local nonabsorbable steroid administration, Nephron **16:**371-80, 1976.
41. Rifkin, R.D., Isner, J.M., Carter, B.L., and Bankoff, M.S.: Combined posteroanterior subepicardial fat simulating the echocardiographic diagnosis of pericardial effusion, J. Am. Coll. Cardiol. **3:**1335, 1984.
42. Prager, R.L., Wilson, C.H., and Bender, H.W.: The subxiphoid approach to pericardial disease, Ann. Thorac. Surg. **34:**6, 1982.
43. Alcan, K.E., et al.: Management of acute cardiac tamponade by subxiphoid pericardiotomy, J.A.M.A. **247:**1143-1148, 1982.
44. Little, A.G., et al.: Operation for diagnosis and treatment of pericardial effusions, Surgery **96:**738-744, 1984.
45. Permanyer-Miralda, G., Sagrista-Sauleda, J., and Soler-Soler, J.: Primary acute pericardial disease: a prospective series of 231 consecutive patients, Am. J. Cardiol. **56:**623-630, 1985.
46. Westaby, S.: Pericardioscopy—a new approach in the management of pericardial effusions of unknown aetiology, Br. Heart J. **53:**114-115, 1985.
47. Little, A.G., and Ferguson, M.K.: Pericardioscopy as adjunct to pericardial window, Chest **89:**53-55, 1986.
48. Kondos, G.T., Rich, S., and Levitsky, S.: Flexible fiberoptic pericardioscopy for the diagnosis of pericardial disease, J. Am. Coll. Cardiol. **7:**432-434, 1986.

ADDITIONAL READINGS

Fowler, N.O.: The pericardium in health and disease, Mount Kisco, NY, 1985, Futura Publishing Co., Inc.
Reddy, P.S., Leon, D.F., and Shaver, J.A., editors: Pericardial disease, New York, 1982, Raven Press.
Shabetai, R.: The pericardium, New York, 1981, Grune & Stratton, Inc.

Chapter Eleven

Intra-aortic balloon pumping

ELAINE K. DAILY
ARA G. TILKIAN

Augmentation of the diastolic pressure wave was initially studied in 1953, when Kantrowitz[1] noted the resultant increased coronary blood flow during diastole. This discovery was the basis for the development of the intra-aortic balloon (IAB) catheter by Moulopoulos and Kolff[2] in 1962. "Phase-shift-pumping," with the use of the IAB and pump, was clinically used by Kantrowitz in 1967 on patients with irreversible shock secondary to myocardial infarction. Since then, numerous investigators have studied other physiologic aspects of IAB pumping and have expanded its application to a larger number of clinical situations.[3-9]

RATIONALE

A polyurethane balloon (40 to 60 cc adult size) is mounted on a vascular catheter, inserted into the femoral artery, and positioned in the descending aorta just distal to the left subclavian artery. The balloon catheter is connected to a pump console that shuttles helium or carbon dioxide into the balloon during diastole to inflate it. During isovolumetric contraction, the gas is rapidly withdrawn to deflate the balloon (counterpulsation) (Fig. 11-1).

Inflation during diastole augments the diastolic pressure and displaces the blood in the aorta distally and proximally toward the heart and into the coronary arteries and may increase coronary blood flow, although clinical documentations of increased flow have been inconsistent.[10-13] The major advantage seems to be systolic deflation, which lowers the intra-aortic volume and pressure and reduces both afterload and myocardial oxygen consumption (MVo_2). These physiologic responses improve the patient's cardiac output and coronary circulation and temporarily improve hemodynamics. In general, counterpulsation can augment cardiac output by about 15%. Frequently, this is sufficient to stabilize the patient's hemodynamic status, which might otherwise rapidly deteriorate.

Until 1979, all IAB catheters were inserted via a surgical cutdown, generally of the femoral artery. Since then, the development of a percutaneous IAB catheter has allowed quicker, and perhaps safer, insertion and has resulted in more expeditious institution of therapy and expansion of clinical applications.

MEDICAL INDICATIONS

Medical indications for counterpulsation include:
- Unstable angina refractory to aggressive medical therapy
- Acute myocardial infarction with cardiogenic shock
- Postinfarction recurrent angina
- Papillary muscle dysfunction with acute mitral regurgitation or postinfarction ventricular septal rupture
- Recurrent intractable ventricular arrhythmias secondary to myocardial ischemia
- In conjunction with PTCA and angiography in unstable patients
- Terminal cardiomyopathy in patients awaiting cardiac transplant or implantation of an artificial heart
- Cardiac arrest, in selected cases

SURGICAL INDICATIONS

Surgical indications for counterpulsation include:
- Unsuccessful discontinuation of cardiopulmonary bypass
- Postcardiopulmonary bypass left ventricular failure, and some instances of right ventricular failure
- Major noncardiac surgery in patients with advanced LV dysfunction

Probably the most successful use of counterpulsation is as an adjunct to preoperative and postoperative management of cardiovascular surgical patients with im-

257

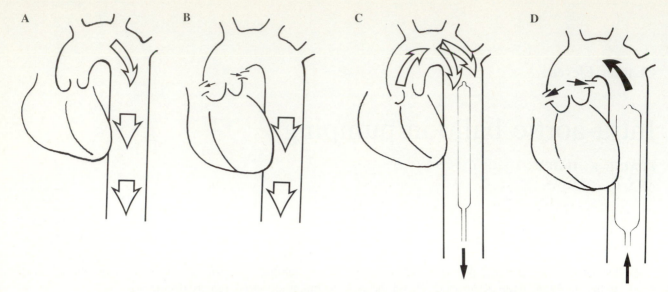

Fig. 11-1. Physiology of counterpulsation. Diagram of normal cardiac cycle pressure flow sequence as compared with the counterpulsed pressure flow sequence. **A,** Normal systole characterized by antegrade volume flow and peak intra-aortic pressures. **B,** Normal diastole showing continued antegrade volume flow and adequate intra-aortic pressure for coronary perfusion. **C,** Balloon deflation before systole, allowing antegrade volume flow from the aortic arch (systolic unloading). **D,** Counterpulsed diastole mechanically boosting volume flow retrograde to the aortic arch, heightening diastolic pressure and possible coronary perfusion. (From Daily, E.K., and Schroeder, J.S.: Techniques in bedside hemodynamic monitoring, St. Louis, 1985, The C.V. Mosby Co.)

paired left ventricular function. Elective intraoperative augmentation in high-risk patients has been shown to diminish mortality.[14]

CONTRAINDICATIONS

Absolute contraindications to counterpulsation include:
- Aortic dissecting aneurysm
- Severe aortic insufficiency
- Major coagulopathies, systemic thrombolytic therapy (unless arterial access has been secured before therapy)
- Underlying brain death, advanced or terminal neoplastic disease, or a case in which aggressive, life-prolonging treatment is not indicated

Relative contraindications to the conventional method of IAB catheter insertion include severe aortoiliac and peripheral vascular atherosclerosis. If necessary, an open-chest approach or transaortic balloon insertion through the ascending aorta can be undertaken in patients in whom femoral artery insertion is not feasible. At the time of cardiac catheterization of patients whose conditions forewarn of possible need for balloon insertion, it is prudent to secure an abdominal aortogram to aid future selection of the more appropriate femoral artery for balloon insertion.[15]

The percutaneous method of catheter insertion, along with the use of a longer sheath (16 inches), improves the chances of successful catheter placement, even in patients with moderate degrees of tortuosity. Recent surgical exposure of the femoral artery in the groin of the proposed puncture site would be a contraindication to *percutaneous* IAB insertion. If the contralateral groin cannot be used, insertion must be done via surgical cutdown.

RISKS

IAB catheterization carries the following risk[16-19b]:
- Ischemic extremities (5% to 47%)
- Thrombosis or emboli (1% to 7%)
- Arterial perforation (2% to 6%)
- Bleeding (3% to 5%)
- Infection (2% to 4%)
- Aortic dissection (1% to 3%)
- Thrombocytopenia (rare)

Table 11-1. Types, sizes, and balloon volumes of various adult IABs

Manufacturer	Catheter size	Insertion mode	Balloon volume (ml)
Datascope	12 Fr adult, 117 cm	Surgical	30-40
	8.5, 9.5 & 10.5 Fr Percor and Percor STAT-DL, 117 cm	Percutaneous or surgical	40-50
Kontron	12 Fr adult, 110 cm	Surgical	20-40
	10.5 & 12 Fr adult, 110 cm	Percutaneous	40
SMEC	12 Fr adult, 79 cm	Surgical	30-60
	10.5, 11, & 11.5 Fr adult, 79 cm	Percutaneous	30-60

LOCATION

Insertion of an IAB for counterpulsation should ideally be done in a controlled environment such as the operating room, a cardiac catheterization laboratory, a special procedures room, or an emergency room having fluoroscopic capability. However, with the advent of the percutaneous balloon catheter, insertions commonly are performed at the bedside in an intensive care or coronary care unit. Under emergency situations the IAB can be inserted percutaneously without the use of fluoroscopy. Radiologic verification of accurate catheter location should be obtained as soon as possible after insertion in these situations.

GENERAL EQUIPMENT

The following equipment is needed to perform IAB catheterization:
• Supplies for skin preparation
• Full resuscitative equipment with crash-cart and defibrillator
• ECG and pressure monitoring equipment
• Fluoroscopy equipment
• IAB catheter for percutaneous or surgical insertion (single or double chamber; 30 or 40 ml)
• Gas-driving console with emergency power source and eight electric outlets

Table 11-1 lists the types, sizes, and insertion modes of various IAB catheters.

Recommended equipment for surgical insertion

For surgical insertion, the following equipment is recommended:
• An expanded arterial cutdown tray including the following:
   #11, #15 and #20 scalpels
   Hemostats
   Two 10 cc and one 50 cc syringe
   Assorted needles (20, 22, and 25 gauge; 1½ inches and 3½ inches)
   Self-retaining retractors
   Right-angle clamps
   Scissors (Potts and suture)
   Mosquito clamps
   Cushing forceps
   Vein retractor
   Rommel hook
   Angled-jaw minimal trauma vascular clamp
   Medium hemoclips and appliers
   Vascular and bull-dog needle holders
   Bowl and cups
   Umbilical tape or Silastic snares
• Silk suture and polypropylene (Prolene) suture (4-0 or 5-0)
• Medications: lidocaine 1% without epinephrine, heparin, antibiotic for irrigation, povidone-iodine (Betadine) ointment
• Catheters
   IAB catheter (single or double chamber; 30 ml or 40 ml)
   Fogarty embolectomy catheter (3, 4, 5, and 6 Fr)
• Suction tubing
• Cautery and cautery handles

Recommended equipment for percutaneous insertion

The following equipment is recommended for percutaneous insertion:
• A percutaneous insertion tray containing:
   Drapes and towels
   Assorted syringes (50, 10, and 3 cc)
   Assorted needles (25, 22, and 20 gauge; 1½ and 3½ inches long)
   Three-way stopcocks
   Sponges

#11 scalpel
Bowls, sterile heparinized saline
Umbilical tapes (two, 18 inches long)
Male Luer plug
• Percutaneous catheter
• Percutaneous needle set, 18 gauge
• Teflon dilator (8 Fr)
• Teflon dilator/sheath assembly, 12 Fr 11 or 16 inches long
• J-tipped guidewire, 0.035 inch (0.9 mm), 120 cm long
• Medications: lidocaine 1% without epinephrine, heparin, povidone-iodine ointment

Preassemble insertion kits are available from the IAB manufacturers which supply most of the listed equipment.

PERSONNEL

The following personnel should be present for any IAB catheterization procedure.
• For surgical insertion, a cardiovascular surgeon and an assistant are needed.
• For percutaneous insertion, a cardiologist, cardiovascular surgeon, or cardiovascular radiologist experienced in the procedure should be on hand.
• A critical care nurse should be present to provide primary nursing care, hemodynamic monitoring of the patient, and administration of medications.
• A cardiovascular specialist or balloon pump nurse specialist is needed to set up and monitor IABP for counterpulsation.
• Radiology technologist should be on hand to assist with fluoroscopy.

PATIENT PREPARATION

Prepare the patient in the manner described below.
1. Explain the procedure to the patient and/or to the family.
2. Obtain informed consent.
3. Keep the patient fasting for 4 to 6 hours for an elective procedure.
4. Obtain current laboratory values, including hemogram, platelets, prothrombin time (PT), partial thromboplastin time (PTT), and bleeding time.
5. Secure and maintain an IV line. A pulmonary artery catheter for hemodynamic monitoring is highly desirable.
6. Secure and maintain an intra-arterial line. (This may not be necessary if intra-aortic pressure is monitored through the central lumen of the percutaneous IAB catheter.)

7. Check the adequacy of the ECG signal and electrode placement.
8. Connect the ECG cable and intra-arterial cable to the pump console.
9. Place patient in a supine position, restraining arms and legs if necessary.
10. Shave and prepare the patient's groin with a povidone-iodine preparation (to avoid delay if difficulty is encountered, shave and prepare both groins).
11. Apply sterile drapes to the area surrounding the prepared site.
12. Infiltrate the skin and subcutaneous tissue of the selected groin with 1% lidocaine without epinephrine.

PROCEDURES
Surgical insertion

Caps, masks, and sterile gown and gloves should be worn by the physician and assistant performing a cutdown. Caps and masks are also recommended for all personnel in the operating room at the time of the procedure. All steps described below should be done under sterile conditions.
1. Perform a routine arterial cutdown procedure (see p. 78).
2. Approximate the required length of catheter insertion by placing the catheter over sterile drapes on the patient, with the catheter tip at the junction of the first rib and the clavicle and the distal catheter extended down to the umbilicus and obliquely over to the femoral artery insertion site (Fig. 11-2). Note this distance as indicated by the black markings on the catheter, or slide the sheath seal down the catheter to the estimated exit point.
3. Test the IAB for leaks by inflating it with a volume of air equal to its capacity and submerging it in sterile saline to check for bubbles.
4. Prepare the arterial graft by beveling one end at a 45° angle to facilitate end-to-side anastamosis. *Note:* Use of an arterial graft is optional. Alternatively, the percutaneous IAB catheter can be inserted directly into the exposed artery. Placement of a 6-0 polypropylene purse string suture may be necessary to reduce arteriotomy bleeding.
5. Administer heparin IV peripherally (approximately 5000 units).
6. Attach the prepared graft to the femoral artery arteriotomy using polypropylene sutures.
7. Momentarily release the vascular clamps above the arteriotomy site.
8. Insert the completely deflated moistened balloon catheter through the graft into the femoral artery.

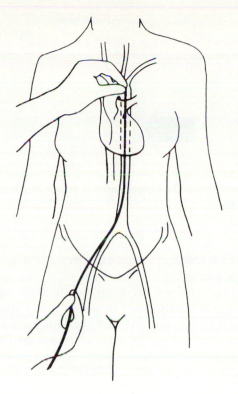

Fig. 11-2. When fluoroscopy is not used, measure the distance from below the subclavian artery extending down to the umbilicus and then obliquely over to the femoral insertion site. Note this distance as indicated by the catheter markings or by sliding the sheath seal down the catheter.

9. Advance the catheter with a slight twisting motion into the aorta until the previously determined marker reaches the skin level and the catheter tip is located just distal to the left subclavian artery.

10. Using a 50 cc syringe, forcefully inflate the balloon of the catheter with air to eliminate twists and assure proper inflation.

11. Aspirate the air and connect the balloon catheter to the pump console.

12. Begin counterpulsation.

13. Obtain a chest radiograph to determine accurate catheter position. Because the fully inflated balloon does not occlude the aorta, many clinicians obtain the chest film with the balloon kept inflated. This is very helpful in determining both proper catheter orientation and adequate inflation of the balloon.

14. Secure the graft to the catheter with heavy silk or umbilical tape. Placing a piece of Teflon felt between the catheter and the graft will provide a better seal.

15. Remove the distal clamp from the femoral artery to remove clots or air.

16. Close the subcutaneous tissue with absorbable suture (Vicryl).

17. Close the skin incision with monofilament sutures.

18. Secure the catheter to the skin with heavy silk sutures.

19. Palpate the femoral artery distal to the insertion site to verify adequacy of distal blood flow. Check pedal pulses using Doppler scanning if necessary.

Percutaneous insertion

Introduction of the percutaneous IAB catheter in 1979 greatly increased the overall use of counterpulsation.[17,20,21] Because the percutaneous route can be performed more rapidly than the surgical approach and is not dependent on the availability of a cardiac or vascular surgeon, therapy can be initiated sooner with better long-term results.

The percutaneous balloon catheter with a central lumen permits insertion of a guidewire through the lumen and facilitates passage of the balloon through atherosclerotic and tortuous vessels. In addition, contrast medium can be injected through the lumen, and intra-aortic pressure monitoring can be performed.

Caps, masks, and sterile gown and gloves should be worn by the physician and assistant performing the insertion.

Balloon preparation

1. Remove the percutaneous double-lumen catheter together with its protective tray from the sterile package. *Do not remove* the IAB catheter from its protective tray.

2. Follow the manufacturer's specific instructions for wrapping and unwrapping the balloon.

3. Attach a 50 cc syringe via the one-way valve or a stopcock to the Luer end of the IAB. Slowly aspirate a full 50 cc with the syringe to create a vacuum within the balloon. Remove the syringe, leaving the one-way valve or closed stopcock in place.

4. Approximate the required length of catheter insertion by placing the catheter over sterile drapes on the patient, with the catheter tip at the junction of the first rib and the clavicle and the distal catheter extended down to the umbilicus and obliquely over to the groin exit. Note this distance as indicated by the black markings on the catheter or slide the sheath seal down the catheter to the estimated exit point.

The newest model IAB catheter is prefolded and requires no wrapping before insertion or unwrapping after insertion.

Balloon insertion

1. Infiltrate the skin and subcutaneous tissue with lidocaine 1% without epinephrine.

2. Make a small skin incision at the insertion site with a #11 blade to facilitate insertion of the dilator.

3. Puncture the wall of the femoral artery just below the inguinal ligament with the 18-gauge percutaneous needle set (see p. 71 for complete discussion of percutaneous arterial access).

4. Insert a 0.035-inch (0.9 mm) J-tipped guidewire through the needle into the abdominal aorta. Confirm the position radiographically.

5. Remove the needle from the femoral artery, leaving the guidewire in place.

6. Insert an 8 Fr tapered dilator over the guidewire, through the skin incision, and into the femoral artery to predilate the vessel. The length of dilator inserted into the femoral artery need only be enough to dilate the puncture site. (Insertion is easier if the dilator is held close to the skin incision at a very low angle and a twisting or rotating motion is applied.)

7. Remove the 8 Fr dilator over the guidewire while applying pressure to the puncture site to control bleeding.

8. Wipe the guidewire with a sterile sponge, moistened in normal saline.

9. Insert the dilator/sheath as a unit over the guidewire into the femoral artery, using the same technique employed for insertion of the 8 Fr dilator, and advance the dilator/sheath unit into the vessel. *Note:* At least 1 inch of the 6-inch sheath (or 6 inches of the 11-inch sheath) should remain outside the skin.

10. Administer heparin (approximately 5000 units) followed by a continuous IV heparin infusion to maintain a systemic effect (usually 800 to 1200 units/hour, monitored by PTTs).

Procedures without and with the use of a guidewire follow.

Insertion without use of guidewire

1. Remove the inner dilator, leaving the sheath in place in the femoral artery (place the thumb over sheath hub to minimize bleeding from the sheath and apply pressure just above the puncture site). *Note:* The sheath should not be in the artery without the dilator or the catheter to support it for more than a few minutes.

2. While holding the hub of the sheath in the fingers of one hand, insert the tip of the IAB catheter into the sheath with the other hand (counterclockwise rotation of the IAB catheter during insertion may facilitate passage).

3. Advance the IAB catheter into the aorta, with its tip located just distal to the left subclavian artery and

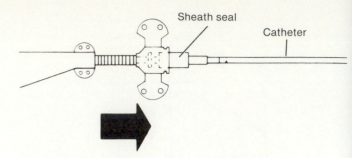

Fig. 11-3. Pushing the sheath seal down over the junction of the sheath hub and the catheter helps to reduce bleeding from the junction.

its proximal end above the renal artery; verify its location with fluoroscopy.

4. If necessary, pull the sheath back from the catheter so that approximately 1 inch (when the 6-inch sheath is used) or 6 inches (if the 11-inch sheath is used) of the sheath remains outside the skin; otherwise the balloon may not unwrap or inflate properly.

5. Push the sheath seal down over the sheath hub to control bleeding (Fig. 11-3).

6. Remove the one-way valve or the stopcock from the hub of the catheter to relieve the vacuum.

7. Follow the manufacturer's specific instructions for unwrapping the balloon.

8. Remove the inner stylet of the IAB by releasing the Luer-Lok fitting with a counterclockwise rotation of the small-end knob, allowing it to spin freely, and pull the stylet straight back.

9. Aspirate 3 ml of blood from the central lumen. If the central lumen is not to be used for intra-arterial pressure monitoring, the end should be capped with a male Luer plug.

10. Begin counterpulsation.

11. If fluoroscopy is unavailable, obtain a chest radiograph, preferably with the balloon inflated, to determine accurate position and adequate inflation of the balloon.

12. Suture or tape the sheath seal and Y fitting to the skin.

13. Palpate the femoral artery distal to the insertion site to verify adequacy of distal blood flow. Check pedal pulses, using Doppler scanning if necessary.

14. Institute IV heparin therapy (800 to 1200 units/hour) with PTT monitoring.

Insertion with use of guidewire

1. Remove the inner stylet of the IAB by rotating the stylet knob counterclockwise until it spins freely; then pull the stylet straight back.

2. Remove the inner dilator, leaving the sheath and guidewire in place in the femoral artery. Pinch the sheath around the guidewire to reduce bleeding.

3. Advance the central lumen of the IAB catheter tip over the guidewire until approximately 20 cm of wire exits the female Luer hub of the IAB.

4. Advance the IAB into the sheath, using a counterclockwise rotation of the catheter to facilitate insertion. Take care to maintain control of the guidewire as it exits the hub of the catheter. *Note:* Never insert the IAB into the sheath without the support of a guidewire or the inner stylet.

5. Advance the IAB catheter into the descending aorta, with the tip located just distal to the left subclavian artery; verify its location with fluoroscopy.

6. Pull the sheath back from the catheter to expose approximately 1 inch (if the 6-inch sheath is used) or 6 inches (if the 11-inch sheath is used) outside the skin.

7. Remove the guidewire from the central lumen of the IAB.

8. Aspirate 3 ml of blood from the central lumen and flush with 3 ml of sterile saline. If the central lumen is not to be used for intra-arterial pressure monitoring, the end should be capped with a male Luer plug. A hand injection of 10 to 20 ml of contrast medium into the central lumen of the IAB can assist in verifying appropriate intra-luminal position of the catheter.

9. Push the sheath seal over the hub of the sheath to control bleeding (Fig. 11-3).

10. Remove the one-way valve or stopcock from the hub of the catheter to relieve the vacuum.

11. Unwrap the balloon according to the manufacturer's directions. To ensure unwrapping, attach a 50 cc syringe via a three-way stopcock to the male fitting of the balloon connector. Inflate the balloon with 50 cc of air or inflating gas and *immediately aspirate*. Remove the stopcock and syringe. Meticulous attention is required to prevent inadvertent injection of air into the central lumen of the IAB.

12. Connect the balloon catheter to the pump console.

13. Begin counterpulsation.

14. Suture or tape the sheath seal and Y fitting securely to the skin to prevent accidental catheter removal.

15. Palpate the femoral artery distal to the insertion site to verify adequacy of distal blood flow. Check pedal pulses, using Doppler scanning if necessary.

16. Institute IV heparin therapy (800 to 1200 units/hour) with PTT monitoring.

Insertion via surgical cutdown

The percutaneous IAB catheter can be inserted directly into an exposed femoral artery. This may be performed after cardiopulmonary bypass or if difficulty is encountered with percutaneous insertion. The balloon catheter is prepared in the routine fashion and inserted through the arteriotomy or with the optional use of a Dacron graft. Use of a guidewire through the central lumen of the IAB can aid in passage through tortuous vessels. Removal of the IAB requires opening the incision, exposing the artery, and removing the catheter in the routine surgical manner (p. 265).

Counterpulsation

Several different types of IAB pumps are available for use in counterpulsation. It is recommended that all personnel involved in the care of a patient undergoing counterpulsation receive detailed instruction and carefully follow the specific manufacturer's recommendations and procedures for proper usage. Basic pump set-up consists of establishing power, establishing gas pressure, setting controls, and establishing ECG and arterial pressure signals.

Display the patient's arterial pressure and observe the appearance of the waveform with a distinct dicrotic notch.

To obtain an accurate arterial pressure waveform without "fling" or overdamping, avoid the use of long connecting tubing and multiple stopcocks, maintain a continuous heparinized infusion, gently flush the arterial catheter with 2 to 3 ml of heparinized solution hourly, and carefully avoid any bends or kinks in the catheter.

Obtain a reliable, artifact-free ECG with a tall (≥ 0.2 mV) positive R wave. This is essential for safe, effective intra-aortic balloon pumping. Obtaining such a signal depends on properly preparing the skin (shave the electrode site if necessary, rub the site briskly with a dry gauze pad); avoiding electrode placement on bony prominences, joints, or skin folds, and securely attaching prejelled electrodes to the skin. If 60-cycle electric interference is present in the ECG, isolate and remove the interference. Antiarrhythmic therapy may be necessary to reduce or eliminate premature beats (atrial or ventricular) that would prevent proper timing of counterpulsation.

Initiating counterpulsation

1. Connect the properly positioned balloon catheter to the pump console, tightly securing all fittings.

2. Turn on the power switch on the pump control unit.

3. Set the pump frequency switch on the control unit to *every other beat*.

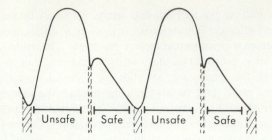

Fig. 11-4. Functional range of safe timing for counterpulsation. (From Quaal, S.J.: Comprehensive intra-aortic balloon pumping, St. Louis, 1984, The C.V. Mosby Co.)

4. Observe the augmented arterial waveform and compare it to the nonaugmented arterial waveform.

5. Adjust the inflation control so inflation occurs at the dicrotic notch of the arterial waveform; adjust the deflation control bar to achieve a 5 to 15 mm Hg diastolic unloading in the assisted arterial pressure.

Timing

Timing of inflation and deflation should not be set solely according to the ECG. Effective timing of counterpulsation is achieved through utilization of the arterial pressure waveform. Although the R wave of the ECG serves as the reference point for inflation and deflation, the normal physiologic electric/mechanical delay necessitates use of the intra-arterial waveform for more accurate timing of inflation and deflation. Inflation of the balloon can safely occur immediately after closure and before opening of the aortic valve (Fig. 11-4).[22]

Balloon deflation should occur just before the aortic valve opens. Optimal augmentation occurs when (1) the assisted diastolic arterial pressure exceeds the patients' unassisted systolic arterial pressure and (2) the assisted aortic end-diastolic pressure is 5 to 15 mm Hg lower than the patient's unassisted end-diastolic pressure (Fig. 11-5).

Proper timing can best be achieved when inflation occurs with every other beat (1:2 frequency) so as to compare the augmented with the nonaugmented arterial waveform. Fine adjustments in inflation control should be made to time the occurrence of inflation with the dicrotic notch of arterial waveform, creating a V configuration of the dicrotic notch.[22] Adjustments in the deflation control should result in a balloon-assisted systolic pressure that is lower than the patient's unassisted systolic pressure. In addition, the balloon-assisted aortic end-diastolic pressure should be 10 to 15 mm Hg lower than the patient's unassisted aortic end-diastolic pressure. Inflation should be set and adjusted first, then deflation should be optimized.

Additional timing adjustments may be necessary if the heart rate changes more than 10 beats/minute. The newest computerized IAB pump automatically and instantaneously adjusts timing for changes in heart rate

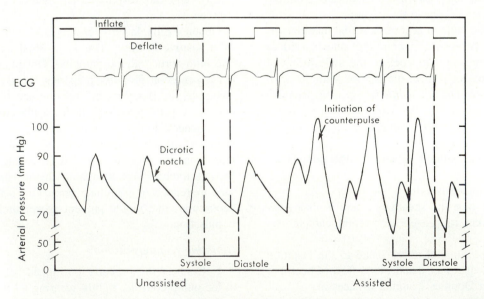

Fig. 11-5. Timing and effect of the counterpulsation sequence by the ECG and arterial pressure waveform. With initiation of counterpulsation, diastolic pressure is heightened and systolic and end-diastolic pressures are lowered. (From Daily, E.K., and Schroeder, J.S.: Techniques in bedside hemodynamic monitoring, St. Louis, 1985, The C.V. Mosby Co.)

and rhythm. Balloon pumping is most effective if the heart rate is greater than 80 beats/minute and less than 110 beats/minute in normal sinus rhythm.

Tachycardia. Heart rates above 120 beats/minute compromise the duration of diastole and therefore diastolic augmentation. Tachycardia may also pose mechanical problems in the pump's ability to track higher heart rates resulting in reduced carbon dioxide gas flow and volume. Use of helium, rather than carbon dioxide, as a driving gas is suggested for patients with higher heart rates. For heart rates greater than 120 beats/minute, decrease the pumping frequency rate to 1:2 and institute appropriate therapy to lower the heart rate.

Atrial fibrillation. Irregularity of the R-R interval poses a severe timing problem, particularly if the R wave appears early. Overall effects of augmentation are best achieved by adjusting the augmentation sequence to the shortest R-R interval. It is also prudent to adjust the deflation control bar, causing the balloon to deflate on the peak of the R wave. This prevents inflation during any systolic event, regardless of timing. Digoxin may be used to slow the heart rate; verapamil may also be used unless there is severe left ventricular dysfunction. Antiarrhythmic therapy or cardioversion may be used to achieve a sinus rhythm and improve augmentation.

Ventricular tachycardia. Ventricular tachycardia can usually trigger the balloon pump if the timing frequency is decreased to 1:3. Balloon fill time can be reduced so that balloon inflation and deflation require less time. Antiarrhythmic therapy or cardioversion is used to correct the arrhythmia.

Ventricular fibrillation. Defibrillation can be carried out in the usual manner, with discontinuation of counterpulsation for a few seconds during delivery of the current. Because the system is not completely isolated from the patient, there is the danger of damaging the unit during defibrillation.

Cardiac arrest. The IAB does not interfere with cardiopulmonary resuscitation (CPR); in fact, balloon inflation during the diastolic phase of CPR would be beneficial. If chest compressions are regular, the balloon pump will be triggered with each compression (or systole). If compressions are not regular, the balloon will automatically deflate. Balloon fill time should be reduced. The IAB catheter can be inserted percutaneously during resuscitation to provide immediate circulatory assistance.[16,17]

Intra-arterial pressure monitoring via percutaneous IAB catheter

Monitoring of the aortic pressure, rather than a peripheral artery pressure, provides a more accurate basis for timing of counterpulsation. Direct aortic pressure monitoring can be performed through the central lumen of the IAB catheter. To accomplish this, follow the steps described below.

1. Follow steps for percutaneous insertion of the IAB catheter (p. 262).
2. After removing the stylet or guidewire from the central lumen of the catheter, aspirate 3 ml of blood from the inner lumen of the IAB catheter and flush with 3 ml sterile heparinized saline.
3. Attach a three-way stopcock with a continuous flush device, transducer, tubing, and heparinized IV solution to the hub of the inner lumen of the IAB catheter (Fig. 11-6). Maintain a continuous infusion of heparinized solution.
4. Carefully ensure that all air bubbles are removed from any of the attached equipment.
5. An hourly "fast flush" of the interlumen is recommended to maintain catheter patency. Always discontinue balloon pulsation before fast flushing or blood sampling to reduce the risk of retrograde embolus.

Surgical removal of the IAB

Under sterile conditions, including the use of cap, mask, gown, and gloves, perform the following procedure to remove a surgically placed IAB.

1. Prepare and drape the operative site.
2. Infiltrate the skin and subcutaneous tissue with 1% lidocaine without epinephrine.
3. Discontinue counterpulsation.
4. Remove the skin sutures and open the wound, exposing the graft.
5. Place occluding tapes around the femoral artery distal and proximal to the balloon insertion sites.
6. Administer heparin intravenously (approximately 5000 units).
7. Cut the graft approximately 1 cm above the suture line.
8. Disconnect the pump console from the hub of the IAB catheter and attach a 50 cc syringe to the hub. Withdraw the plunger of the syringe to aspirate the balloon and assure maximal deflation.
9. Relax the proximal occluding tape while temporarily occluding the femoral artery distal to the graft site with the distal occluding tape. Remove the IAB catheter through the graft.
10. Advance a 6 Fr Fogarty arterial embolectomy catheter proximally and distally (with relaxation of the distal occluding tape) to remove any remaining clots.
11. Flush the artery with a heparinized saline solution (10 μ/ml saline).

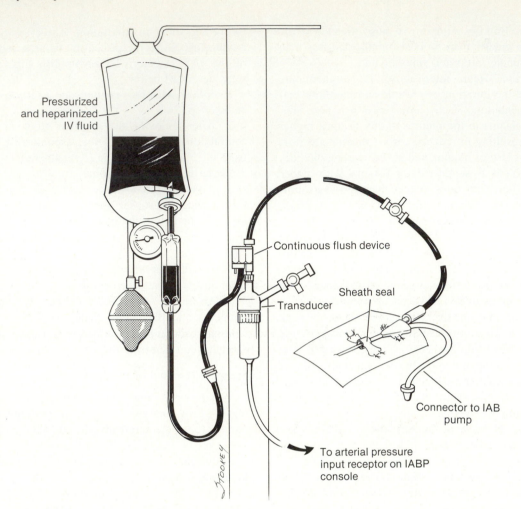

Pressurized and heparinized IV fluid

Continuous flush device

Sheath seal

Transducer

Connector to IAB pump

To arterial pressure input receptor on IABP console

Fig. 11-6. Central lumen of the IAB catheter connected to continuous flush device with heparinized solution and a transducer for monitoring of the intra-aortic pressure.

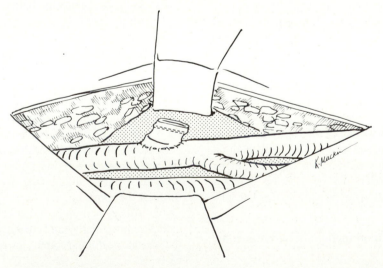

Fig. 11-7. Excess graft material is resected and the wound is ready to be closed. (From Quaal, S.J.: Comprehensive intra-aortic balloon pumping, St. Louis, 1984, The C.V. Mosby Co.)

12. Oversew the graft and leave it in place (Fig. 11-7).

13. Remove the occluding tapes.

14. Assess the quality of the distal pulse by direct palpation or Doppler scanning of the femoral artery distal to the insertion site and by palpation of the dorsalis pedis and posterior tibialis.

15. Irrigate the wound with an antibiotic solution.

16. Close the subcutaneous tissue with absorbable sutures and the skin with monofilament nonabsorbable or subcuticular absorbable sutures.

Percutaneous removal

Tapering or discontinuation of heparin 3 to 4 hours before removal of a percutaneous IAB catheter is recommended. Alternatively, heparinization may be reversed with protamine sulfate just before catheter removal.

Under sterile conditions, including the use of gloves, perform the procedure described below.

1. Prepare the insertion site with an antiseptic solution.

2. Discontinue counterpulsation.

3. Disconnect the extension tubing from the hub of the IAB catheter and attach a three-way stopcock or one-way valve and a 50 cc syringe.

4. Withdraw the plunger of the syringe to 50 cc and close the stopcock to the catheter to create a vacuum in the IAB. *Note:* do not rewrap the balloon.

5. Remove all ties and sutures from the sheath and the catheter.

6. Withdraw the IAB catheter through the sheath until the proximal end of the balloon is felt to just enter the sheath.

7. Remove both the IAB catheter and the sheath as a unit while applying digital pressure just below the puncture site.

8. Allow the wound to bleed vigourously for 2 to 3 seconds after catheter removal while still applying pressure distally.

9. Apply pressure to the proximal femoral artery and release pressure from the distal femoral artery to allow back bleeding for 3 to 5 seconds.

10. Apply firm manual pressure to both the proximal and distal portions of the femoral artery for a minimum of 30 minutes. A clamp may be used only after hemostasis is established.

11. After hemostasis is assured, apply a compression bandage. A 5- to 10-pound sandbag or a mechanical clamp may be used for an additional 1 to 2 hours.

12. Carefully examine the leg distal to the insertion site for adequate perfusion or check distal pulses with a Doppler stethoscope and check every 15 minutes for groin hematoma.

PATIENT MANAGEMENT
Monitoring the patient on IABP

Management of the patient on IABP is based on data obtained from careful noninvasive and invasive monitoring. A balloon flotation thermodilution pulmonary artery catheter should be inserted before initiation of counterpulsation to allow indirect assessment of left ventricular end-diastolic pressure via the pulmonary artery end-diastolic pressure or pulmonary artery wedge pressure, indirect assessment of right ventricular end-diastolic pressure via the right atrial pressure, and cardiac output determinations. Ideally a fiberoptic pulmonary artery catheter is used, which also permits continuous monitoring of mixed venous oxygen saturation, reflecting the adequacy of tissue oxygenation. Continuous intra-arterial pressure monitoring, usually performed via the central lumen of the IAB catheter, is necessary to appropriately time inflation and deflation and to directly assess the adequacy of perfusion pressure. Chapter 4 discusses the principles and technical aspects of performing continuous hemodynamic monitoring.

Special attention must be directed to the patient's comfort while he or she is on strict bedrest, with the head of the bed elevated no more than 30° and the insertion leg kept straight. The insertion site should be kept openly visible, at least during the first 2 to 4 hours after insertion, to assess for bleeding.

Table 11-2 lists the parameters and their monitoring frequency for patients on IABP. Table 11-3 lists the technical functions that require periodic monitoring for safe use of IABP. Abrasion of the IAB may result in perforations not detected by the system's leak detection device. Because this complication is usually associated with the appearance of blood in the IAB connecting tubing, the tubing should be examined frequently.[24a]

Cardiac catheterization of the patient on IABP

Cardiac catheterization is frequently necessary for patients on IABP to define surgically correctable lesions responsible for hemodynamic deterioration. Left ventricular angiography and selective coronary arteriography can be performed in these patients via a brachial artery cutdown (Sones technique), or percutaneously via the contralateral femoral artery (Judkins technique). Although the Sones technique avoids any mechanical interference with the IAB catheter, the Judkins technique can also be used, with special precautions. These include using a J-curve guidewire. Advance it only as

Table 11-2. Suggested monitoring schedule of hemodynamic, laboratory, and clinical parameters in patients on IABP

Parameters	*Monitoring frequency*
Hemodynamics	
RA, PA, PAW or LA pressures	Every 30 minutes until stable (& during
Intra-arterial pressure (systolic, diastolic, & augmented diastolic)	weaning), every 2 hours thereafter
CI, SVR, SWI	Every 1 hour until stable, every 4 hours thereafter
Peripheral circulation	
Quality of dorsalis pedis, posterior tibial pulses	Every 15 minutes the first hour, every 30 minutes the next 2 hours, every 2
Color, temperature, movement, & sensation of legs	hours & as needed thereafter
Doppler flowmeter	
Renal circulation	
Urine output	Every 1 hour
Cerebral circulation	
Mental status	Every 1 hour & as needed
Hematologic assessment	
Hemogram	Daily & as needed
Platelet count, PTT	Every 8 to 12 hours & as needed after therapeutic anticoagulation is obtained
Oxygenation	
Arterial blood gases	Every 8 hours & as needed
Mixed venous oxygen saturation	Continuously (via fiberoptic catheter) or every 8 hours & as needed
Vital signs	
Heart rate, respiratory rate, temperature	Every hour until stable, then every 2 to 4 hours & as needed
Auscultatory examination	
Heart sounds	Every 4 hours & as needed
Breath sounds	

CI, Cardiac index; *SVR*, systemic vascular resistance; *SWI*, stroke work index.

far as 5 cm *below* the IAB, and stopping counterpulsation while advancing the catheter (without a guidewire) past the IAB, and resuming pumping during selective positioning and angiography. After catheterization is completed, the catheter is withdrawn as far as the tip of the IAB; pumping is then discontinued while the catheter is withdrawn past the balloon; pumping is resumed and the catheter is completely withdrawn and pressure applied.

Weaning the patient from IABP

Counterpulsation can be discontinued when there is clinical and hemodynamic evidence of continued im-

proved ventricular performance, with satisfactory perfusion, and the patient has moved to a class I hemodynamic subset (Fig. 11-8). This most commonly occurs within a day or two but may take up to a week.[23]

Table 11-4 lists the hemodynamic and clinical criteria for cessation of IABP. Discontinuation of counterpulsation is always preceded by a period of gradual weaning, during which time the patient is carefully monitored for evidence of clinical or hemodynamic deterioration. Traditionally, weaning is carried out in the manner described below.

1. Reduce pumping frequency to 1:2.
2. Monitor and measure hemodynamic parameters

Table 11-3. Monitoring schedule of technical functions of the IABP

Technical function	Monitoring frequency
Record console settings	Every 2 hours or with any changes
Purge balloon	Every 2 hours & as needed
Adjust timing	Every 1 hour & as needed
Check gas gauge	Every 8 hours & as needed
Inspect tubing for presence of blood	Every 2 hours & as needed

Table 11-4. Clinical and hemodynamic criteria for discontinuation of IABP

Clinical criteria	Hemodynamic criteria
Evidence of adequate perfusion Urine output >30 ml/hour	Cardiac index >2.0 L/minute/m²
Improved mental status Skin temperature warm	MAP >70 mm Hg with minimal or no pressors
No evidence of congestive heart failure Rales absent S3 absent	PAEDP/PAWP or LAP <18 mm Hg
No life-threatening dysrhythmias	Heart rate <110 beats/minute without complex ventricular arrhythmias

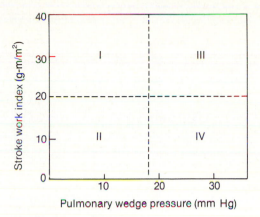

Fig. 11-8. "Shock box." Hemodynamic subsets of pump failure, which provide the rationale for therapeutic interventions, including weaning from IAB pumping. Class I: Adequate perfusion, normal filling pressures; class III: adequate perfusion, elevated filling pressures; class II: hypoperfusion, normal filling pressures; class IV: hypoperfusion, elevated filling pressures.

(CI, PAP, PAWP, RAP, SVR, heart rate), urine output, sensorium, skin temperature, Svo_2, and the presence or absence of angina every 30 minutes over the next 1 to 3 hours.

3. If the patient is hemodynamically stable, further reduce pump frequency to 1:3 for 10 to 15 minutes.

4. Repeat monitoring as in step 2.

5. If the patient is hemodynamically and clinically stable and remains in hemodynamic subset class I, the IABP is no longer needed and may be removed.

Alternative method

Alternatively, weaning may be carried out successively by decreasing the amount (balloon volume) of diastolic augmentation in addition to reducing pumping frequency. Because augmentation may depend on balloon volume more than pumping ratio, this technique may be useful in patients in whom small changes in

hemodynamic status may be critical.[12,24] Reducing the volume of gas entering the balloon is carried out in the manner described below.

Phase I

1. Reduce the balloon volume by 50% (to reduce diastolic augmentation by 25%) while maintaining a 1:1 pumping frequency.

2. Monitor and measure hemodynamic parameters, heart rate, urine output, sensorium, skin temperature, and the presence or absence of angina over the next 1 to 3 hours.

3. If patient remains stable in class I, reduce balloon volume approximately 25% more, or enough to decrease augmentation by 50% (Fig. 11-9).

4. Repeat monitoring as in step 2.

Phase II

5. If the patient remains hemodynamically stable, increase the balloon volume to its original setting (resulting in full augmentation) and reduce the pumping frequency to 1:2.

6. Repeat monitoring as in step 2 of phase I.

7. If the patient remains hemodynamically stable, reduce the balloon volume by 50% (to reduce diastolic augmentation by 25%) while maintaining a 1:2 pumping frequency.

8. Repeat monitoring as in step 2 of phase I.

Phase III

9. If the patient remains stable, reduce pumping frequency to 1:3 *or* decrease balloon volume approximately 25% to 30% more at a 1:1 frequency rate.

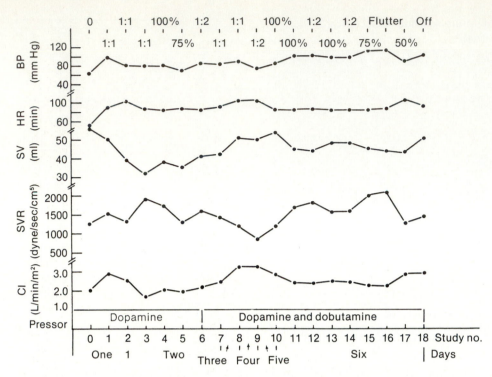

Fig. 11-9. This chart indicates changes in blood pressure (BP) as well as other cardiac function indices in the course of balloon assist at 100% augmentation with balloon assist rate of 1:1. Decrease in augmentation from 75% to 50% was done with the assist rate at 1:1, whereas decrease in the assist rate from 1:1 to 1:2 was with augmentation at 100%. This patient had multiple coronary artery bypass graft (CABG) procedures and had had a previous myocardial infarction (S/P MI). Note study no. 5 was done when augmentation was decreased to 75% and resulted in a slight decrease in cardiac index (C.I.), blood pressure, and stroke volume (SV). During study no. 14 on day 6, decrease in augmentation to 75% resulted in no significant changes except for increase in systemic vascular resistance (SVR). Compare these values with those in study nos. 5, 6, 12, and 14. *HR,* Heart rate. (From Bolooki, H.: Clinical application of intra-aortic balloon pump, Mount Kisco, N.Y., 1984, Futura Publishing Co., Inc.)

10. If the patient remains stable, discontinue counterpulsation and remove the IAB.

The flutter mode, or 1:3 pumping frequency, permits a very small amount of gas to enter the balloon, causing more movement within the aorta, but provides no augmentation. This prevents clot formation around a static balloon, which could be sheared off during catheter removal. The flutter mode should be used only briefly (10 to 15 minutes), and the balloon should never remain inactive for longer than 20 minutes.

The time required for successful weaning can vary from hours to days, depending on the hemodynamic response to counterpulsation and the length of time the patient was on IABP. Some institutions base the length of weaning time on the length of counterpulsation time. Bolooki[23] recommends 6 hours of weaning for every 24 hours of balloon pumping. This, of course, must be directed by the patient's clinical and hemodynamic status. Deterioration to class II or III during the weaning pe-

riod can often be reversed by appropriate pharmacologic intervention (volume, diuretics, afterload reducers, etc.). If the patient reverts to class I, the weaning process is continued. If, however, the change persists or further deterioration occurs, the patient is placed back on full diastolic augmentation at a 1:1 frequency.

Discontinuation of IABP after cardiac surgery depends on the patient's condition and the reason for initiating counterpulsation. A very brief weaning period (1 hour) may suffice for patients in whom preoperative IABP was electively begun for acute left ventricular dysfunction, with complete discontinuation of IABP at the close of surgery. However, in patients who receive IABP to permit discontinuation of bypass, counterpulsation should be continued for 4 to 6 hours, despite apparent hemodynamic stability. Slow weaning should then be carried out as described above.

Discontinuation of IABP should also be considered

for patients in whom no clinical or hemodynamic improvement occurs after several days of counterpulsation or patients with angiographic evidence of advanced myocardial failure with no surgically correctable lesions.

COMPLICATIONS

The complications of IABP are associated with balloon insertion, balloon pumping, and balloon removal.

During balloon insertion

Ischemic extremities (5% to 47%). Reduction of blood flow to the catheterized extremity is evidenced by poor or absent distal pulses and a cool, pale leg. Limb ischemia occurs more frequently in older patients (>70 years) and female patients.[24b] Increased incidence of ischemia related to the percutaneous or surgical insertion is associated with conflicting data.[24b,25] Preventive measures include anticoagulation with heparin, maintenance of high arterial pressure, and changing balloon insertion sites at the earliest sign of ischemia.

Management consists of catheter removal and continuous IV heparin infusion for 24 hours. Distal and proximal thrombectomy and embolectomy with the use of a Fogarty catheter may also be required. Emergency surgical revascularization may be necessary.

Inability to advance the IAB catheter (2% to 13.5%). This complication results from vessel tortuosity or severe occlusive disease and occurs more frequently in elderly patients. It may be diminished by use of a percutaneous balloon catheter with a J-tip guidewire and the use of a longer (15-inch) sheath.

Inability or difficulty in unwrapping the balloon (5% to 7%). Difficulty in unwrapping the balloon is usually evidenced by an extremely small or even absent augmentation wave. This may be caused by properties of the balloon itself or inadequate withdrawal of the longer sheath, which causes the balloon to be partially positioned inside of the sheath itself. The longer sheath should be withdrawn sufficiently, with approximately 6 inches remaining outside the skin. External rotation and torquing of the entire balloon catheter within the arterial system may facilitate balloon unwrapping. Balloon unwrapping can be ensured after correct positioning by manually inflating the balloon with a 50 cc syringe of air or inflating gas. The injected air should be immediately aspirated. The new, prefolded percutaneous IAB catheter may reduce this complication.

Arterial damage or perforation (2% to 6%). Arterial damage or perforation may not be clinically manifested. This occurrence may be discovered only at autopsy, when perforated common iliac arteries and massive retroperitoneal hematomas are noted. This complication occurs more frequently with the percutaneous method of IAB catheter insertion. If arterial damage or perforation is suspected, the vessel should be exposed and operative repair undertaken.

Aortic dissection (1% to 23%). Aortic dissection is not always clinically detected because signs and symptoms may be diffuse. Signs and symptoms of aortic dissection include back pain, inequality of pulses and blood pressure between right and left extremities, decreased renal function, increased chest pain, and neurologic deficits. Maintain a high index of suspicion when any, even momentary, resistance is encountered during passage of the IAB catheter. Intimal tears can be initiated at various sites in the arterial system, with progressive dissection occurring as the catheter is further advanced. If placement of the catheter in the subintimal layer of the femoral artery is suspected, based on tactile sensations or radiologic findings, pumping should be immediately stopped, the balloon catheter removed, and if necessary, surgical repair of the aorta undertaken.

During balloon pumping

Thrombosis or emboli
Renal (approximately 3%)
Cerebral (<1%)
Mesenteric (approximately 1%)
Peripheral (3% to 7%)
Thrombosis or emboli can occur as a direct result of propagation of clots from the catheter. Adequate heparinization may minimize or prevent this complication. Treatment depends on the site and clinical manifestations of the complications. In some instances it may be necessary to remove the IAB catheter.

Infection (local and systemic) (2% to 4%). Development of local or systemic infection can be controlled by meticulous attention to aseptic technique during insertion and daily care and dressing change at the insertion site. Prophylactic antibiotics are commonly used but their value remains debatable.

If bacteremia or septicemia develops, remove the balloon catheter and institute appropriate antibiotic therapy based on blood cultures and sensitivity results. Also remove other vascular lines because any of them may be the source of the bacteremia.

Bleeding/hematomas (1%). Bleeding around the catheter insertion site and hematoma formation can occur as a result of heparin therapy and thrombocytopenia. Persistent bleeding can sometimes be managed by direct compression but may require removal of the balloon and direct repair of the artery.

Thrombocytopenia. Reductions in platelet count are directly related to the duration of counterpulsation. Platelet counts usually return to normal quickly after discontinuation of IAB catheterization, and platelet transfusions are unnecessary unless bleeding becomes a problem. Red blood cell transfusions may be necessary if there is hemolysis and significant anemia.

During and after balloon removal

Bleeding. Bleeding from the site of catheter insertion occurs more frequently with the percutaneous method of catheter insertion, in which a large hole is made in the femoral artery and systemic heparinization is mandatory.[25] Management consists of firm manual pressure until hemostasis is established. Thereafter, tape a 10-pound sandbag over the puncture site, or use a mechanical clamp for prolonged pressure and instruct the patient to remain supine in bed for the next 12 hours. Continued bleeding or hematoma formation after full reversal of heparinization requires surgical exploration and repair of the artery.

Thromboembolus. Thrombosis or emboli can occur as a result of shearing of clots during catheter removal. Observe the patient carefully for signs and symptoms of this complication for 24 hours after catheter removal. Treatment depends on the site and clinical manifestations.

Table 11-5 lists some of the advantages and disadvantages of percutaneous IAB.

Table 11-5. Advantages and disadvantages of percutaneous intraaortic balloon catheter

Advantages	Disadvantages
More expedient insertion and initiation of therapy	Reduced control of bleeding after removal of percutaneous catheter
No surgical cutdown and repair required	Thromboembolus may occur secondary to shearing of clots during catheter removal
Can be inserted promptly and removed by nonsurgical physician	Increased incidence of leg ischemia if catheter is placed in superficial femoral artery
Can be inserted during cardiac catheterization or coronary angioplasty if patient becomes unstable	Higher incidence of complications in diabetics, women, and elderly
Cost effective, with utilization of fewer resources	Less effective at higher heart rates (>120 beats/minute) because of smaller lumen size for gas shuttle
Adaptable to all pump consoles	Possible difficulty in unwrapping of balloon catheter

FUTURE DEVELOPMENTS

Improved instrumentation, with smaller catheters and sheaths, has recently permitted the successful use of IAB pumping in children.[26,27]

Pulmonary artery balloon pumping in patients with acute right ventricular failure has been used on a limited basis with hemodynamic improvement.[28,29] Percutaneous insertion of the balloon catheter into the pulmonary artery has been used successfully in animals to ameliorate right ventricular failure secondary to increased peripheral vascular resistance. The use of pulmonary artery counterpulsation may become clinically applicable with the advent of monitoring catheters that measure right ventricular ejection fraction and thereby delineate right ventricular failure.

The use of a portable transport IABP permitting prompt initiation of hemodynamic support and safe transfer of unstable critically ill patients from community hospitals has expanded the role of counterpulsation.[29a]

Computer technology will continue to be successfully incorporated into counterpulsation technique, resulting in improved computerized monitoring and automatic fine tuning of the timing of IABP. The latest model IABP also automatically purges and refills every 2 hours, alerts the operator to changes in the patient or pump conditions, and provides 4 hours of trend information on the patient's status. The use of ocular plethysmography holds promise for noninvasively and more precisely evaluating the timing of counterpulsation.

Suitable clinical applications of counterpulsation may be better defined. Further controlled trials are needed to determine the proper indications for IABP, particularly its use as a prophylactic measure in high-risk acute myocardial infarction patients.[30]

PROCEDURE CHECKLIST

✔ Obtain consent from the patient or family.

✔ Secure a peripheral IV line.

✔ Set ECG electrodes in place with good ECG signal and tall upright R waves.

✔ Obtain a good arterial waveform via a peripheral arterial line unless the central lumen of the IAB will be used for this.

✔ Properly position a balloon flotation pulmonary artery catheter in the pulmonary artery with good pulmonary artery and pulmonary artery wedge pressures.

✔ Prepare the balloon pump console:
    Unit plugged in and power on
    Proper gas pressure and connection

ECG and arterial pressure cables connected to control system

Transducer zeroed and calibrated

Timing set

✔ Place the IAB catheter in the proper position and verify it by fluoroscopy or radiography.

✔ Aspirate, flush, and connect the central lumen of the IAB catheter to the transducer for arterial pressure monitoring (optional if a peripheral arterial line is in place).

✔ Secure IAB connection to the pump console.

✔ Begin counterpulsation.

✔ Optimize inflation and deflation on arterial waveform.

REFERENCES

1. Kantrowitz, A., et al.: Initial clinical experience with intraaortic balloon pumping in cardiogenic shock, J.A.M.A. **203:**135-140, 1960.
2. Moulopoulos, S.E., et al.: Diastolic balloon pumping (with carbon dioxide) in the aorta—a mechanical assistance to the failing circulation, Am. Heart J. **63:**699, 1962.
3. Brundage, B.H., et al.: The role of aortic balloon pumping in post-infarction angina—a different perspective, Circulation **62**(suppl. I):I-119, 1980.
4. Gerwitz, H., et al.: Effect of intra-aortic balloon pumping on myocardial blood flow distal to a severe coronary artery stenosis, Am. J. Cardiol. **49:**969, 1982.
5. Goldberg, S.: Combination therapy for acute myocardial infarction: intracoronary thrombolysis and percutaneous intra-aortic balloon counterpulsation, Cardiac Assist. **1:**1, 1982.
6. Harris, P.L., et al.: The management of impending myocardial infarction using coronary artery bypass grafting and intra-aortic balloon pump, J. Cardiovasc. Surg. **21:**405, 1980.
7. Alcan, K.E., et al.: The expanding role of intra-aortic balloon counterpulsation in critical care cardiology in a community-based hospital. Cardiovasc. Rev. Report **3:**61-69, 1982.
8. Singh, J.B., et al.: Intraaortic balloon counterpulsation in a community hospital, Chest **79:**58-63, 1981.
9. Hanson, E.C., et al.: Control of postinfarction ventricular irritability with the intraaortic balloon pump. Circulation **62**(suppl. I):I-130-137, 1980.
10. Leinbach, R.C., et al.: Effects of intra-aortic balloon pumping on coronary flow and metabolism in man, Circulation **43**(suppl. I):I-77, 1971.
11. Williams, D.O., Korr, K.S., Gewirtz, H., and Most, A.S.: The effect of intraaortic balloon counterpulsation on regional myocardial blood flow and oxygen consumption in the presence of coronary artery stenosis in patients with unstable angina, Circulation **66:**593, 1982.
12. Fuchs, R.M., et al.: Augmentation of regional coronary blood flow by intra-aortic balloon counterpulsation in patients with unstable angina, Circulation **68:**117-123, 1983.
13. Port, S.C., Patel, S., and Schmidt, D.H.: Effects of intraaortic balloon counterpulsation on myocardial blood flow in patients with severe coronary artery disease, J. Am. Coll. Cardiol. **3:**136-174, 1984.
14. Alcan, K.E., et al.: Current status of intra-aortic balloon counterpulsation in critical care cardiology, Crit. Care Med. **12:**489-495, 1984.
15. Vignola, P.A., Swaye, P.S., and Gosselin, A.J.: Guidelines for effective and safe percutaneous intraaortic balloon pump insertion and removal, Am. J. Cardiol. **48:**660-664, 1981.
16. Grayzel, J.: Clinical evaluation of the Percor percutaneous intraaortic balloon: cooperative study of 722 cases, Circulation **66**(suppl. I):233, 1982.
17. Subramanian, V.A., et al.: Preliminary clinical experience with percutaneous intraaortic balloon pumping, Circulation **62**(suppl. I):123-129, 1980.
18. Harvey, J.C.: Complications of percutaneous intraaortic balloon pumping. Circulation **64**(suppl. II):116, 1981.
19. Isner, J.M.: Complications of the intraaortic balloon counterpulsation device: clinical and morphologic observations in 45 necropsy patients, Am. J. Cardiol. **45:**260-268, 1980.
19a. Alderman, J.D., et al.: Incidence and management of limb ischemia during the use of current wire-guided intra-aortic balloon pumps, Circulation **7:**152A, 1986.
19b. Goldberger, M., Tabak, S.W., and Shah, P.K.: Clinical experience with intra-aortic balloon counterpulsation in 112 consecutive patients, Am. Heart J. **111:**497-502, 1986.
20. Subramanian, V.A.: Percutaneous intraaortic balloon pumping. Ann. Thorac. Surg. **29:**102, 1980.
21. Bregman, D.A.: Clinical experience with percutaneous intraaortic balloon pumping, Cardiovasc. Dis. Bull. Texas Heart Inst. **7:**318-324, 1980.
22. Quaal, S.J.: Comprehensive intraaortic balloon pumping, St. Louis, 1984, The C.V. Mosby Co.
23. Bolooki, H.: Clinical application of intraaortic balloon pump, New York, 1984, Futura Publishing Co., Inc.
24. Weber, K.T., Janicki, J.S., and Walker, A.A.: Intra-aortic balloon pumping: an analysis of several variables affecting balloon performance, Trans. Am. Soc. Artif. Intern. Organ **18:**486, 1972.
24a. Kayser, K.L.: Abrasion perforation of intra-aortic balloons (letter), Am. Heart J., 1985, p. 1311.
24b. Goldberger, M., Tabak, S.W., and Shah, P.K.: Clinical experience with intra-aortic balloon counterpulsation in 112 consecutive patients. Am. Heart J. **111:**497-502, 1986.
25. Bregman, D.A., et al.: Percutaneous intraaortic balloon insertion, Am. J. Cardiol. **46:**261-264, 1980.
26. Veasy, L.G., Blaylock, R.C., Orth, J.L., and Boucek, M.: Intra-aortic balloon pumping in infants and children, Circulation **68:**1095, 1983.
27. Veasy, L.G., and Webster, H.: Intra-aortic balloon pumping in infants and children, Cardiac Assist. **2:**1-6, 1985.
28. Miller, D.C.: Pulmonary artery balloon counterpulsation for acute right ventricular failure, J. Thorac. Cardiovasc. Surg. **80:**760-763, 1980.
29. Flege, J.B. Jr., Wright, C.B., and Reisinger, T.J.: Successful balloon counterpulsation for right ventricular failure, Ann. Thorac. Surg. **37:**167-168, 1984.
29a. Gottlieb, S.O., et al.: Portable intraaortic balloon counterpulsation: clinical experience and guidelines for use, Cathet. Cardiovasc. Diagn. **12:**18-22, 1986.
30. Flaherty, J.T., et al.: Results of a randomized prospective trial of intraaortic balloon counterpulsation and intravenous nitroglycerin in patients with acute myocardial infarction, J. Am. Coll. Cardiol. **6:**434-446, 1985.

Chapter Twelve

Direct current cardioversion and defibrillation

ARA G. TILKIAN
MARY B. CONOVER

Cardioversion is the procedure by which direct current (DC) that has been *synchronized* to discharge with the QRS complex of the ECG is delivered across the heart for the purpose of converting an atrial or ventricular arrhythmia to a normal sinus rhythm. This procedure, introduced in 1962, was a major breakthrough in the treatment of cardiac arrhythmias and has been in clinical use since then.[1]

Defibrillation is *nonsynchronized* cardioversion and is used when QRS complexes and T waves are not distinguishable or present, as in ventricular flutter or ventricular fibrillation. This procedure was first used in humans in 1947, using electrodes applied directly to the heart.[2] It was not until 1956 that transthoracic defibrillation was first used in humans.[3]

RATIONALE

The currents that rhythmically flow through the normal heart do so in an orderly and uniform fashion. When this order and uniformity are disturbed, supraventricular or ventricular arrhythmias result. These arrhythmias may be the result of enhanced automaticity, reentry circuits, or afterdepolarizations and may cause supraventricular and ventricular arrhythmias. It is possible to restore the heart to a normal sinus rhythm by the delivery of DC to the myocardium, either directly or through the chest wall. The electric current depolarizes a variable mass of myocardial fibers. This may interrupt a reentry circuit—one mechanism by which a ventricular or supraventricular arrhythmia may be terminated. A critical myocardial mass is required to maintain ventricular fibrillation.[4] The depolarization of a variable mass of myocardium may reduce the amount of excitable myocardium to that which is insufficient to perpetuate the fibrillation. Thus when the excitable myocardial mass is reduced to an amount less than the

critical myocardial mass required for maintenance of ventricular fibrillation, defibrillation is successful and the arrhythmia is terminated, giving the sinus node the opportunity to resume control as the dominant pacemaker.

THE VULNERABLE PERIOD

The heart is particularly susceptible to ventricular fibrillation during the so-called vulnerable period, an interval that begins and ends with the T wave but that is at its peak for about 30 msec just before the apex of the T wave of the ECG[5] (Fig. 12-1). At this point the current required to elicit ventricular fibrillation is at its lowest. In the ischemic heart the stimulus required to cause fibrillation is much less than it is in the normal heart.

To avoid precipitating ventricular fibrillation, the cardioverter is programmed so that the electric current discharges during or slightly after the QRS wave, eliminating the possibility of stimulation during the ventricular vulnerable period. This assumes that the R and T waves are clearly discernible on the ECG.

ENERGY USED FOR CARDIOVERSION AND DEFIBRILLATION

The electric output of all cardioverter/defibrillators is expressed in terms of energy. Joules (J) or watt-seconds (Ws) describe the power (watts) and the length of time it is applied (seconds). Thus energy (joules) = power (watts) × duration (seconds).

TYPES OF CURRENT WAVEFORMS

The first defibrillating current to be used was a 60 Hz alternating current (AC) (Fig. 12-2, *A*). It was first used to defibrillate a canine heart in 1933,[6] using electrodes directly applied to the heart. The use of this type of

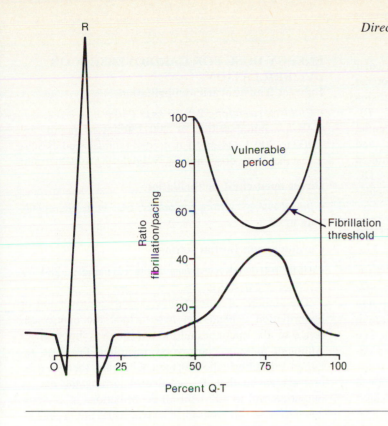

Fig. 12-1. Location of the vulnerable period in the ventricular cycle. Stimulus strength required to evoke ventricular fibrillation is minimal near the peak of the T wave. (Adapted from Geddes, L.A.: Cardiovascular devices and their applications, New York, 1984, © John Wiley & Sons, Inc.)

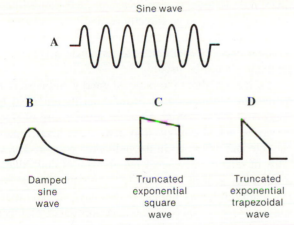

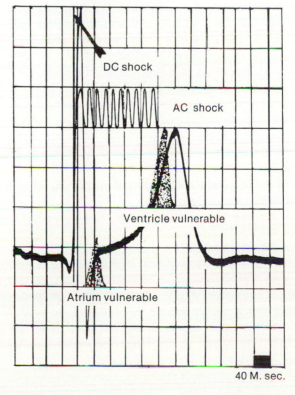

Fig. 12-2. Waveforms of currents used for defibrillation. Sine wave is an alternating current and is no longer used. Damped sine waves and the truncated exponential waves are direct current.

Fig. 12-3. Time frame for DC and AC shock compared and related to the atrial and ventricular vulnerable periods (shaded areas). Note that the AC shock of ⅕ second may end at the T wave, even when synchronized with the R wave. (From Resnekov, L. and McDonald: Complications in 220 patients with cardiac dysrhythmias treated by phase direct current shock and indications for electroconversion, Br. Heart J. **29**:926, 1967.)

current is now obsolete as it can itself cause ventricular fibrillation. The type of current in general use for the last 15 years has been DC in the form of a damped sine wave (overdamped or underdamped) (Fig. 12-2, *B*). Another type of current uses the truncated exponential waves, either square or trapezoidal (Fig. 12-2, *C* and *D*), but clinical data regarding their efficacy are limited at present. Fig. 12-3 compares the time frames of DC and AC shock and relates them to atrial and ventricular vulnerability.

TYPES OF CARDIOVERTER/DEFIBRILLATORS
Damped sine wave

The damped sine wave defibrillator consists of a capacitor, inductor, and electrodes. The energy (e.g., 400 J) is stored in the capacitor and is discharged through the inductor to the electrodes and then directly through the heart or across the thorax and through the heart. The energy delivered to the heart is less than the stored energy because of the resistance in the inductor, the internal resistance of the defibrillator, and the transthoracic impedance, which varies considerably among humans.[7] Thus the energy stored in a defibrillator can be accurately measured, as can the energy delivered into a test load (delivered energy), but the actual energy current delivered to the heart remains variable and not directly measurable.

Damped sine wave defibrillators often carry the name of one of the pioneer investigators (Gurvich, Lown, or Edmark) and have slightly different waveforms, depending on the sizes of the inductors and capacitors. For example, the Lown defibrillator has a sine wave current that reverses direction slightly (underdamped) and is 5 msec in duration; the Edmark defibrillator has a sine wave current that flows in the same direction during the pulse (overdamped) and is about 10 msec in duration (Fig. 12-2, *B*). The duration of current most commonly used to defibrillate an adult heart is 5 to 10 msec. The current intensity is variable and related to the setting of the energy control (stored energy) on the defibrillator.

Trapezoidal wave

Cardioverter/defibrillators using the trapezoidal wave (Fig. 12-2, *C* and *D*) have been available for more than 10 years. Definitive data regarding their advantages and disadvantages are lacking. Maximal output from this defibrillator is 400 J, and the threshold current needed for defibrillation is approximately the same as for the damped sine wave.[8] It has larger electrodes than do other defibrillators.

ENERGY DOSE FOR CARDIOVERSION OR DEFIBRILLATION[9-17]
Indirect transthoracic defibrillation

- *Children (weighing 2.5-50 kg):* 2 J/kg
- *Adults:* Initial setting of 200 J followed rapidly by 200 to 300 J and 360 J if needed (animal studies suggest that these doses are also valid during hypothermia)

Direct open-chest defibrillation

- *Initial energy setting for adults:* 5 J, with increments up to 20 J

Cardioversion (initial setting)

- 10 to 100 J delivered (see Table 12-1 and p. 284 for further discussion)

The amount of current flow during cardioversion or defibrillation depends on two factors: the energy selected by the operator and the transthoracic impedance. Although there is controversy regarding the dose required for defibrillation of the adult heart, there is general agreement that the practice of turning the energy output control to 400 J for all defibrillations in adults is dangerous and ill advised.[9,11] Myocardial injury and arrhythmias following cardioversion and defibrillation have been found to be directly related to the amount of energy delivered in a single shock. Thus ideally the minimal energy requirement to terminate a specific arrhythmia should be used.

Information about the minimal energy and current required for termination of different arrhythmias in humans is mostly empiric. Also, the relationship of stored energy to actual energy delivered to the heart remains variable and unknown in the individual patient. The validity of relating the energy requirement of defibrillation to the body size of the adult has been questioned. Animal and preliminary human studies have shown the feasibility of measuring transthoracic impedance and using this information to adjust the energy for defibrillation.[10,13] This may permit the operator to individualize the energy used for defibrillation and use low-energy shocks in most patients while avoiding the use of inappropriately low settings in patients with high transthoracic impedance. This approach will need further validation before it is generally accepted.

INDICATIONS

Synchronized cardioversion is used for:
- Atrial flutter or fibrillation of recent onset that cannot be converted to a sinus rhythm after the elimination or control of initiating or predisposing factors and after the use of antiarrhythmic medications

- Supraventricular tachycardia that does not respond to vagal maneuvers or antiarrhythmic therapy (a rare occurrence) and is not caused by digitalis intoxication
- Ventricular tachycardia that is refractory to antiarrhythmic drug therapy or is associated with hemodynamic instability

Defibrillation is used for:
- Rapid ventricular tachycardia with hemodynamic instability in which the QRS is wide and not clearly distinguishable from the T wave
- Ventricular flutter
- Ventricular fibrillation

CONTRAINDICATIONS FOR SYNCHRONIZED ELECTIVE CARDIOVERSION
Absolute contraindication

Supraventricular tachycardia *caused* by digitalis toxicity is an absolute contraindication for synchronized cardioversion. In this setting, cardioversion may precipitate intractable ventricular fibrillation and ultimately prove fatal.

Relative contraindications

Cardioversion is relatively contraindicated in conditions in which there is (1) either a low chance of success or a high chance of recurrence of the arrhythmia, (2) appreciable risk of precipitating a potentially more dangerous tachyarrhythmia, or (3) a risk of precipitating or unmasking a bradycardia or asystole. The chance of success, potential risk, and benefit need to be carefully evaluated in each case.

Conditions involving a low chance of success or high chance of recurrence

- Chronic atrial fibrillation of longer than 1 year, particularly in the presence of rheumatic heart disease with mitral stenosis or mitral insufficiency
- Large left atrium (>50 mm) as determined by echocardiography
- Atrial fibrillation associated with left ventricular enlargement and congestive heart failure
- Atrial fibrillation in a patient due for cardiac surgery or in a patient soon after cardiac surgery
- Active pericardial disease
- Uncompensated lung disease
- Thyrotoxicosis
- Intolerance to antiarrhythmic medications that help maintain sinus rhythm post cardioversion
- When the procedure has previously failed twice

Conditions involving a high risk of precipitating a potentially more dangerous tachyarrhythmia

- Major metabolic or electrolyte abnormalities (hypokalemia, hypomagnesemia): In these cases there is increased risk of arrhythmias following cardioversion.
- High blood levels of digitalis (subtoxic or toxic), especially in the presence of electrolyte disorder: Under these conditions, ventricular arrhythmias, including ventricular tachycardia and fibrillation, may occur in the immediate postcardioversion period. However, the presence of *therapeutic levels of digitalis* is not a contraindication to elective cardioversion.[18,19] If uncertainty exists, then careful synchronized cardioversion using energy titration will permit safe cardioversion.[20,21] The initial setting may be 10 J, with subsequent attempts at 25, 50, and 100 J or more. If the attempt at low-energy settings precipitates an acceleration of the arrhythmia or appearance of complex ventricular ectopic beats or ventricular tachycardia, then the presumptive diagnosis of digitalis toxicity is made and the procedure is best terminated. In the absence of these warning arrhythmias, progressively higher energy settings may be used until the supraventricular tachycardia is terminated.

Conditions involving a high risk of precipitating or unmasking a bradycardia or asystole

- Underlying sick sinus syndrome or concomitant atrioventricular (AV) nodal disease with abnormal AV conduction, as evidenced by a spontaneously slow ventricular response (<60/minute) to atrial fibrillation or atrial flutter
- Atrial fibrillation or atrial flutter with complete AV block, unless a pacemaker is in place or available; in these conditions cardioversion may result in profound bradycardias or asystole, requiring pacemaker therapy

In such circumstances, emergency pacing can be initiated using an external transcutaneous pacemaker, which is well tolerated as long as the patient remains under the anesthetic effect.[22] For prolonged pacing, transvenous pacing is generally needed.

RISKS OF CARDIOVERSION AND DEFIBRILLATION

Cardioversion is a standard and controlled procedure with small but definite risks that include postcardioversion tachyarrhythmias (ventricular tachycardia or fibrillation), postcardioversion bradycardias or asystole, embolization (systemic or pulmonary), myocardial injury and ventricular dysfunction, pulmonary edema, hypotension, and complications related to the use of premedication or anesthetics.

EQUIPMENT

The equipment described below is necessary to perform cardioversion/defibrillation.

- Cardioverter/defibrillator with a functioning synchronizer
- Fully equipped resuscitation cart with standard drugs used in advanced cardiac life support
- Airway: oral airway, Ambubag, Elder valve mask, and suction equipment
- Electrocardiograph
- Premedication and anesthetic

PERSONNEL

The following personnel should be on hand for an elective cardioversion.

- A physician experienced in cardioversion
- Cardiac nurse
- ECG technician
- Experienced respiratory therapist or anesthesiologist (as needed)

In elective cardioversion of high-risk patients who have underlying severe cardiopulmonary disease or when there is concern about airway management, the active participation of an anesthesiologist is required for safe cardioversion.

In elective cardioversion of low-risk patients who do not have underlying serious cardiopulmonary disease, cardioversion could safely be performed by a physician who is experienced in the use of premedication and management of airways. During such a procedure, the respiratory therapist assists in maintenance of the airway.

In an emergency, with deteriorating hemodynamic status, cardioversion should be performed without any delay and with the use of minimal (if any) premedication.

LOCATION

The procedure may be performed in any areas in which ECG monitoring and full resuscitation equipment are available, such as the critical care pavilion, monitored cardiac or medical unit, cardiac catheterization laboratory, emergency room or adequately equipped ambulatory care unit, operating room, or recovery room.

PATIENT PREPARATION

1. Explain the procedure to the patient and obtain informed consent. Try to reduce the patient's anxiety.

Avoid using the term *shock* or *electroshock*. *Electric current* or *electric energy* are suitable alternate terms. Explain the simplicity and overall safety of the procedure and the low levels of energy to be used initially.

2. Obtain the patient's current electrolyte levels, the ECG, and digoxin level and prothrombin time if applicable. Digoxin need not be withheld if there is no evidence of digitalis excess or toxicity. Administration of other antiarrhythmic agents (quinidine, procainamide, verapamil, etc.) is individualized.

3. Keep the patient fasting overnight for a morning procedure and at least 6 hours before an afternoon procedure.

4. Correct as many adverse pathophysiologic conditions as possible, such as congestive heart failure, thyrotoxicosis, respiratory blood gas abnormalities, and acid-base or electrolyte imbalance.

5. Secure an IV line and keep it open with 5% dextrose in water.

6. Record the blood pressure and continue to monitor it frequently just before and for at least 1 hour after the procedure.

7. Run an ECG rhythm strip and continue to monitor the heart rhythm during and for at least 1 hour after the procedure.

8. Acquaint the patient with the use of the Ambubag and Elder valve mask.

9. Remove the patient's dentures if these are present.

10. Secure the patient's arms and legs under soft covers.

11. Recheck the patient's ECG rhythm strip before proceeding with the administration of the anesthetic and the actual cardioversion.

ANESTHESIA

The objectives of premedication and anesthesia are to achieve sedation and amnesia to a degree that the patient will experience no discomfort and will have no recollection of an unpleasant event. The ideal agent should be safe, producing effective anesthesia with total amnesia of the electric discharges. Its onset of action should be prompt and duration of action short, with minimal respiratory depression that does not require mechanical ventilation. It should not have cardiotoxic action, either arrhythmogenic or myocardial depressant. No one agent satisfies all of these criteria.[23-25] The two regimens in common use include diazepam and methohexital sodium.

Diazepam

Traditionally, diazepam (Valium), a commonly used benzodiazepine, has been the most frequently used anesthetic agent for elective cardioversion, especially when an anesthesiologist is not in attendance.

Usual adult dose. The usual adult dose of diazepam is 5 mg IV bolus, followed by 1 to 2 mg/minute IV until the patient is asleep or unresponsive to verbal commands. Usually a total of 15 to 20 mg is needed. In patients who show unusual resistance to the effects of diazepam, up to 50 or 60 mg may be used. Inject diazepam directly into the bloodstream using a three-way stopcock between the short IV catheter and the IV tubing. This will avoid precipitation in the IV solution.

Onset of action. The onset of action is usually 2 to 5 minutes, although longer periods may be encountered in ''resistant'' patients.

Duration of sedative effect. The sedative effect of diazepam usually lasts 1 to 2 hours. Half-life exceeds 20 hours!

Advantages. Diazepam is very safe and has no myocardial and only minimal respiratory depressant action.

Disadvantages. Diazepam has a slow onset and long duration of action. It is a less than totally satisfactory anesthetic, as some discomfort and memory of the event may be experienced by the patient. Also, variable individual resistance may be encountered, especially in patients who have been chronic users of diazepam or alcoholic beverages.

A newer, water-soluble benzodiazepine—midazolam hydrochloride (Hypnoval [Roche Pharmaceutical])—has a shorter half-life and a superior sedative and amnestic effect.[26] This may be preferred over diazepam, but its use in cardioversion has not yet been reported.

Methohexital sodium

An alternative anesthetic is methohexital sodium (Brevital sodium), a very short-acting barbiturate.

Usual adult dose. The usual adult dose of methohexital is 25 to 100 mg IV bolus (0.5 to 1.5 mg/kg).

Onset of action. Methohexital sodium is a rapid acting anesthetic, working in 30 to 60 seconds.

Duration of action. The duration of action of this barbiturate is very short, rarely over 3 to 5 minutes.

Advantages. There is total anesthesia and amnesia for a very short period. Apnea is rarely encountered and usually lasts less than 1 minute.

Disadvantages. The potential of myocardial depression and hypotension exists, although the very brief duration of action makes this a minor disadvantage.

Warnings. Methohexital is not available in individual doses. It is supplied in bottles of 500 mg, 2.5 g, and 5 g for larger dose administration in operating rooms. Therefore it is necessary to prepare a solution of 10 mg/

ml with dextrose in water or normal saline. For the cardioversion procedure, prepare only 100 mg in two separate syringes to avoid potential error and accidental administration of overdose.

Any physician using methohexital should be experienced in the maintenance of airways and should be ready to support the patient's ventilation during periods of apnea.

Narcotics

The use of narcotics, either morphine or the very short-acting synthetic opiate, fentanyl, has also been advocated.[25] The respiratory depression and the longer duration of action make these agents less desirable for cardioversion.

USE OF OXYGEN DURING CARDIOVERSION AND DEFIBRILLATION

Although there is little information available relating successful cardioversion to arterial oxygen tension, there is evidence to suggest that the probability of unsuccessful ventricular defibrillation increases with hypoxia.[27] Hence the use of supplementary oxygen for cardioversion and defibrillation in patients with recognized oxygen desaturation (hypoxemia) is routine. In contrast, the need for supplementary oxygen in patients without recognized lung disease or with normal arterial oxygen tensions is not clearly demonstrated or widely recognized.

We recommend the routine use of 100% oxygen immediately before cardioversion, regardless of the patient's pulmonary status or the arterial blood gases. The rationale for this recommendation is as follows: During apnea, the arterial pCO_2 rises only about 4 to 8 torr/minute, as a consequence of the relatively large body stores of carbon dioxide. In contrast, the body's capacity to store oxygen is much less, and with patients who are breathing room air, a 40 to 50 torr decrease in arterial oxygen tension can be expected in the first minute of apnea.[28] Thus 1 to 2 minutes of apnea in the pericardioversion period—resulting from either the premedication used or the inadvertent induction of ventricular fibrillation—will cause insignificant hypercapnia and minimal respiratory acidosis but can cause profound hypoxemia, arrhythmias, or failure of cardioversion/defibrillation.

The hypoxemia resulting from postcardioversion apnea may be further aggravated by the fact that the cardioversion current is delivered at the end of expiration, when oxygen stores are reduced. Ear oximetry shows reductions in arterial oxygen saturation to 75% to 80% (corresponding to arterial oxygen tensions of 40 to 50 torr) within 30 to 60 seconds of breath holding from the end of a normal exhalation (functional residual capacity, or FRC) in volunteers who have no lung disease and are breathing room air. However, after just 2 minutes of normal tidal breathing (without hyperventilation) with 100% oxygen using a well-fitting mask and Elder valve system, no desaturation occurred in any subject, even with breath holding times of up to 3 minutes.[29] Thus the safety factor inherent in 2 minutes of preoxygenation seems obvious.

Potential dangers of oxygen

The use of oxygen during cardioversion has been criticized as a possible fire hazard. Yet if a well-fitting mask and Elder valve system are utilized, no increase in oxygen concentration can be measured at the level of the suprasternal notch. This can easily be verified using an oxygen monitor before cardioversion. The small amount of oxygen within the mask is promptly dispersed when the mask is removed immediately before cardioversion.

We recommend that the mask be removed before electric discharge. This is based on data demonstrating that a standard polyvinylchloride oxygen cannula (fire rated to self-extinguish flame at room air oxygen concentrations) would ignite and burn in the presence of 60% or greater oxygen.[30]

Patients with chronic hypercapnia are at risk of ventilatory depression from high inspired oxygen concentrations, but significant depression is rare from acute (2 minute) oxygen exposure alone. Patients with underlying pulmonary disease and ventilation/perfusion mismatch are at particular risk of more rapid and more profound oxygen falls with apnea.

Given these considerations, we make the following recommendations:
1. Use a well-fitting mask (good seal) attached to an Elder (demand) valve.
2. Administer 100% oxygen for 2 to 3 minutes. Allow the patient to breathe normally or to assist with a demand valve. Hyperventilation is neither necessary nor desirable.
3. Remove the mask from patient just before the actual cardioversion.

CARDIOVERSION TECHNIQUE

All attending personnel must avoid contact with the patient or the bed when the cardioverter is discharged. The operator should touch only the electrode handles.

Synchronizing the cardioverter

1. Connect the ECG cable to the oscilloscope of the cardioverter.

2. Monitor the ECG in the lead with the tallest R wave configuration to ensure proper synchronization.

3. *Test the synchronous discharge of the cardioverter to be sure that discharge occurs during or slightly after the R wave of the ECG.* The risk of provoking ventricular fibrillation—the main danger in cardioversion—is 3% to 5% when the procedure is done without proper synchronization. The synchronizer should be checked before each cardioversion.

Electrocardiographic gel

Completely coat the paddles with a conductive ECG gel. This will decrease the electric resistance of the skin and minimize skin burns. Pay particular attention to coating the edges of the paddles to avoid skin burns. Self-adhesive disposable electrode pads (prejelled) may be used and are equally effective.[31,31a] Their use is convenient and may enhance operator safety. Saline-soaked gauze pads may also be used.

Skin care

Before DC shock is delivered, dry the skin between the two paddles sites. If moisture or electrolyte gel connects the two paddles, current will flow across the skin instead of through the heart. If saline-soaked gauze is used, give special attention to this.

Ointments

Nitroglycerin ointments (lanolin-petroleum based) have low electric conductivity. When paddles are applied over areas where ointment is present, the ointment acts as an insulator, producing visible and audible current arcs. This reduces peak current delivered to the heart and may prevent successful cardioversion or defibrillation. In cardiac care units, such medicated ointment should not be applied over areas where cardioversion paddles may be placed. If present, they should be cleared before cardioversion is attempted. Transdermal systems of sustained nitroglycerin infusion (Transdermnitro) pose a different problem. An electric arc may form between the defibrillating paddle and the aluminum covering of the patch, causing an explosion complete with smoke![32] Do not place the paddles in contact with any transdermal delivery system.

Paddle size

The ideal paddle size remains controversial. Studies relating paddle size to body weight or body surface area in humans have not been done. Studies in animals and humans suggest that for adults, paddle size should be 10 to 13 cm in diameter.[33] For children and infants the largest electrode that allows good chest contact over its entire area is thought to be optimal. This is generally 4 to 5 cm in diameter for infants and 8 cm in diameter for children.

Paddle pressure and position

The two paddles should not touch each other and should be pressed firmly (25 pounds/paddle) against the chest surface to reduce transthoracic resistance and improve current flow to the heart.[7]

If electrode gel is used, a slight twisting motion of the paddles will ensure even distribution of the gel.

Correct paddle electrode placement is important; improper placement reduces intracardiac current flow and is an important cause of failure to cardiovert or defibrillate. Fig. 12-4 illustrates incorrect and correct paddle placements. The paddles may be applied to the chest in one of three ways; anteroapical, anteroposterior, or apical-posterior. All three positions are probably equally effective.

Anteroapical position

The anteroapical position is illustrated in Fig. 12-5. One paddle is on the anterior right chest wall below the clavicle, adjacent to but not overlying the sternum. The second paddle covers the palpable cardiac apex.

Anteroposterior position

The anteroposterior position is illustrated in Fig. 12-6. One paddle is placed over the right anterior chest wall below the clavicle, as in the anteroapical position. The second paddle is placed on the back below the left scapula (Fig. 12-6).

Apical-posterior position

The apical-posterior position is illustrated in Fig. 12-7. One paddle is placed over the cardiac apex, and the posterior paddle goes under the patient and at the angle of the *right* scapula. This placement is advantageous for patients with permanent pacemakers in the right pectoral area (Fig. 12-8). Electrodes should avoid the sternum, vertebral column, or scapula because of the high impedance of bones.

For patients with dextrocardia, the position of electrodes should be a mirror image to reflect the change in the heart's position. In patients with heart malposition or chest wall deformity, allowances for paddle position should be made to permit positioning the heart between the paddles.

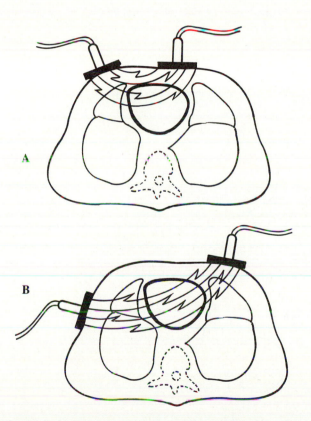

Fig. 12-4. A, When the electrode paddles are placed too close together, a substantial amount of current shunts between them and an insufficient amount reaches the heart. **B,** Wider spacing of the paddles in the anterolateral position allows a sufficient amount of current to reach the left ventricle. (Adapted from Ewy, G.A.: Defibrillating cardiac arrest victims, J. Cardiovasc. Med. **7:**44, 1982.)

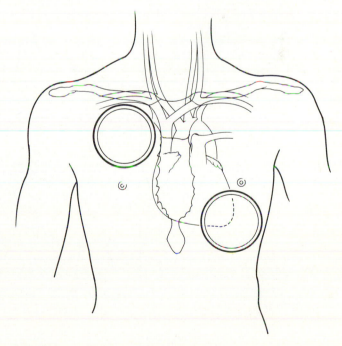

Fig. 12-5. Anteroapical position for cardioversion or defibrillation. See text.

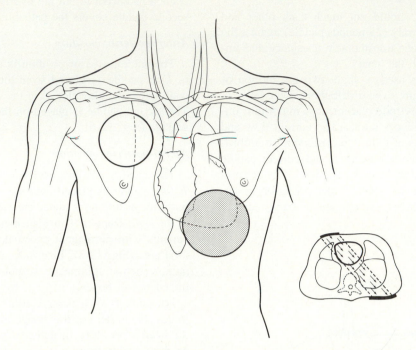

Fig. 12-6. Anteroposterior position for cardioversion or defibrillation. See text.

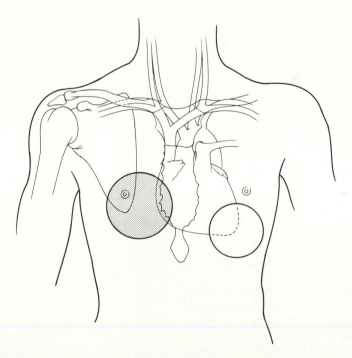

Fig. 12-7. Apical-posterior position for cardioversion or defibrillation. See text.

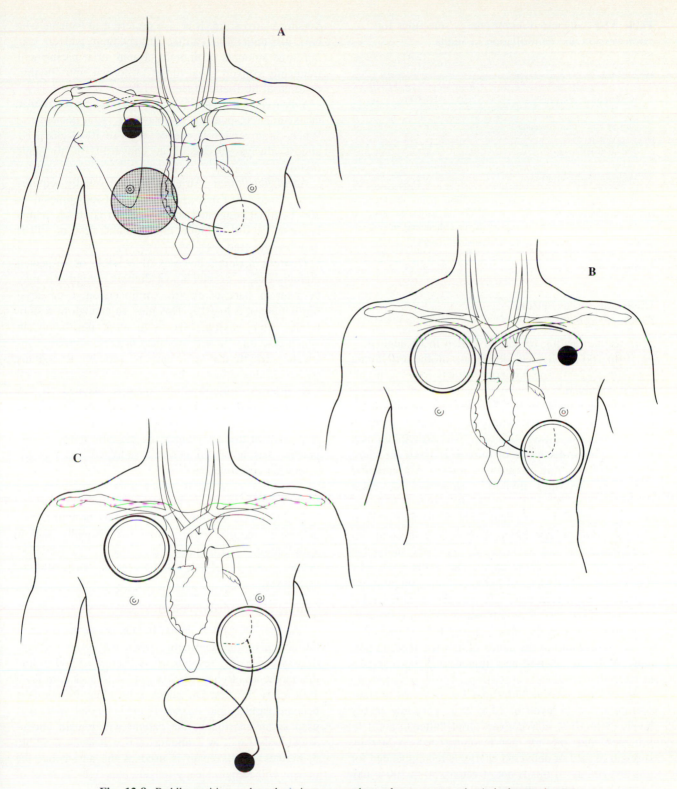

Fig. 12-8. Paddle positions when there is a pacemaker pulse generator. **A,** Apical-posterior position with the pulse generator in the upper right chest. **B,** Anteroapical position with the pulse generator in the upper left chest. **C,** Anteroapical position with the pulse generator in the lower left abdominal quadrant.

Table 12-1. Suggested *initial* energy selections for cardioversion and defibrillation in adults

Arrhythmia	Energy* (J)
	R wave synchronized
Ventricular tachycardia	10-100
Atrial flutter	20
Supraventricular tachy-cardia	50-100
Atrial fibrillation	100
	Nonsynchronized
Ventricular fibrillation	200

*If ventricular fibrillation is precipitated, turn off the synchronizer and defibrillate; otherwise the unit will not discharge. No data are available for cardioversion energy levels for arrhythmias in children and infants. For defibrillation of ventricular fibrillation in children, an initial dose of 2 J/kg is recommended.[15] If this is not effective, 4 J/kg may be used.

Choice of energy setting
Cardioversion

The initial setting for cardioversion in an adult may be 10 to 100 J delivered, depending on the arrhythmia (see Table 12-1). These energy settings have been empirically derived.

Ventricular tachycardia. Ten joules may be a large enough charge for successful cardioversion,[23] whereas 100 J is almost always effective. This arrhythmia *may* convert after a discharge of only 1 J! Even the chest thump can, on rare occasions, convert a ventricular tachycardia to sinus rhythm.[34] However, the chest thump (or very low energies) has the potential of accelerating the rate of ventricular tachycardia and precipitating ventricular fibrillation; thus its use in nonmonitored patients is not recommended. For the individual patient, the initial energy choice should be guided by the presence or absence of hemodynamic compromise, degree of anesthesia achieved, and the patient's prior response (if known). If prompt cardioversion is desired, then 100 J may be the initial energy used. In a stable patient, especially in the hands of an experienced operator, 10 J may be used and titrated to higher energies as needed.

Atrial flutter. Atrial flutter may be converted to sinus rhythm at energy levels of 20 to 25 J. Very low energy levels (5 to 10 J) may convert atrial flutter to atrial fibrillation and thus are not recommended. A starting strength of 20 J of delivered energy is recommended for this arrhythmia. If this is not effective, 50 to 100 J may be used on a repeat attempt. Rapid atrial pacing is an alternate method of treatment. It is safer than cardioversion in patients who may be predisposed to postcardio-version bradycardia. It is also preferred in patients who have just undergone cardiac surgery or in patients taking large amounts of digitalis. Rapid atrial pacing will frequently convert atrial flutter to normal sinus rhythm or to atrial fibrillation (see p. 312).

Supraventricular tachycardia. Most supraventricular tachycardias respond to verapamil or vagal maneuvers. When cardioversion is needed, a 50 to 100 J charge is almost always successful in converting it to sinus rhythm.

Atrial fibrillation. Atrial fibrillation usually requires from 100 to 150 J delivered energy and sometimes over 200 J. Initial suggested shock strength is 100 J. If this is not successful, a higher energy shock (200 or 300 J) may be delivered.

Digitalis toxicity. In cases of possible or suspected digitalis excess or subclinical digitalis toxicity, it may be safer to start all electric cardioversion, even atrial fibrillation, at 5 to 10 J. This may be enough to restore normal sinus rhythm, except in atrial fibrillation, in which case this "test dose" may disclose warning ventricular arrhythmias secondary to subclinical digitalis excess. In this situation the procedure is best terminated and alternate antiarrhythmic therapy planned. It has been suggested that the initial settings for all elective cardioversion procedures be low energy (5 to 10 J) irrespective of the arrhythmia and digitalis status.[23] This practice has not been generally adopted and remains somewhat controversial.

Defibrillation

The first defibrillatory attempt should be with 200 J delivered energy, *nonsynchronized.* Rapidly follow with 200 to 300 J and 360 J as needed. If refibrillation occurs, repeat the shock at the previously successful energy level.

Timing of the cardioversion

The first DC shock should be applied at the onset of the action of the anesthetic, when the patient is very drowsy and barely responsive. A simple method to find this moment is to have the patient count backward from 100; apply the first DC shock soon after the numbers become garbled and mixed. If methohexital sodium is used as an anesthetic, the patient will remain unconscious only for 2 to 3 minutes and will awaken within 5 minutes. If diazepam is used as the anesthetic, the patient will remain sleepy longer, although the level of consciousness will vary.

If sinus rhythm is not restored after the first DC shock, higher energy levels may be applied in titration.

Animal experiments suggest that spacing sequential energy shocks 3 minutes apart may reduce myocardial injury.[35] On the other hand, waiting 3 minutes between each electroshock application may prolong the period of anesthesia and increase the requirements for anesthetic medications. A precise risk versus benefit statement cannot be made, and we recommend proceeding with subsequent shocks without undue delay and completing the procedure as expeditiously as possible. The rhythm should be checked before each electroshock is applied; lead V_1 may be preferred because P waves may be easier to recognize in this lead. To improve current flow to the heart:

1. Remove nitroglycerin ointment on the chest where the paddles are to be applied.
2. Evenly distribute electrode gel.
3. Position the paddles correctly.
4. Maintain firm pressure on paddles.
5. Deliver the electric discharge during the expiratory phase of respiration, when transthoracic resistance is lower.

Emergency treatment of postcardioversion arrhythmias

Cardioversion may rarely precipitate bradycardia or asystole, which are more likely if there is preexisting AV block, inferior infarction, sick sinus syndrome, or use of antiarrhythmic drugs.[35a,35b] Emergency treatment may include IV atropine or isoproterenol; in very rare cases a temporary pacemaker may be required. Ventricular fibrillation may masquerade as asystole, especially if only one ECG lead is monitored.[36] Use multiple leads to avoid this pitfall. If in doubt, and if treatment of presumed asystole has not been effective, proceed to defibrillation.

A rare complication of cardioversion is ventricular fibrillation, which is frequently the result of incorrect synchronization and is treated by immediate *nonsynchronized* DC defibrillation. Lidocaine and bretylium are kept at hand for treatment of recurrent ventricular tachycardia or fibrillation. In cases in which ventricular tachycardia or fibrillation is secondary to digitalis toxicity, especially with coexisting hypokalemia or hypomagnesemia, lidocaine and bretylium may not be effective. In such circumstances, IV phenytoin (250 mg IV bolus) or IV magnesium sulfate (2 g IV over 1 to 2 minutes) may be required.[37]

Because the probability of needing these medications is very low, we recommend having them at hand but not opening or mixing them. For dosage and method of administration, see Chapter 18.

PATIENT AFTERCARE

In uncomplicated and successful cardioversion, patient aftercare is minimal.

• Maintain a patent airway and assist ventilation with an Ambubag if necessary until the patient is fully awake.
• Give nothing by mouth until the patient is awake.
• Monitor the patient's ECG and blood pressure for 2 to 4 hours.
• Record a 12-lead ECG.
• If paddle burns have occurred (indicating poor technique), use a soothing cream for symptom relief.
• If the patient is hypotensive, keep him or her supine until blood pressure is controlled; have the patient well hydrated.
• Provide medication and discharge instructions as individually needed. Most patients, after successful cardioversion, will require long-term use of antiarrhythmic medication to prevent recurrences.
• For atrial fibrillation, use quinidine beginning 24 to 48 hours before the procedure and continuing as long as necessary. Alternate medications include procainamide or disopyramide.
• For other supraventricular tachycardias, medications may include digoxin, beta blockers, or calcium blockers (verapamil or diltiazem).
• For ventricular tachycardia, antiarrhythmics that have been demonstrated to be effective by ECG monitoring or electrophysiologic studies may be prescribed. Cardiovascular surgery or implanted defibrillators are alternatives.

CARE OF THE CARDIOVERTER/ DEFIBRILLATOR

After the procedure the paddles must be carefully cleaned with soap and water. This will prevent formation of metallic oxide, which may cause pitting of the paddles and interfere with current flow. The metal surfaces of the paddles can also be cleaned with an abrasive cleaner and cold sterilized, if necessary. For regular testing of the cardioverter/defibrillator:

• Care for and store the equipment according to the manufacturer's instructions.
• Provide preventive maintenance; have the equipment checked by biomedical engineers every 3 months.
• Visually inspect the equipment and perform a charge and discharge test at 50 J into a test load once a day.

SPECIAL CONSIDERATIONS
Cardioversion and anticoagulation

Thromboembolism is a rare but serious complication of cardioversion from atrial fibrillation, be it electrically or pharmacologically achieved.[38,39] The estimates for its incidence in atrial fibrillation without prior anticoagulation range from 1.5% to 5.3%. Clinical studies suggest that the use of long-term anticoagulation before elective cardioversion reduces this risk to less than 1%. The benefit of short-term (2 to 3 weeks) anticoagulation has not been demonstrated. Controlled studies have not addressed this specific issue, and little information is available to help identify the patient who is at higher risk for thromboembolic complication.

Clinical observation has suggested that patients with rheumatic mitral valve disease, large left atria, or congestive heart failure are at a higher risk for thromboembolic complications, but these notions have not been adequately tested. Given the paucity of controlled studies, firm recommendations cannot be made. A prudent course may be to use anticoagulation in most patients with atrial fibrillation for 2 to 3 weeks before and 2 to 3 months after elective cardioversion if there is no contraindication to its use. A more selective use of anticoagulation may also be defensible.

Unless contraindicated, permanent anticoagulation should be used in patients with prior emboli, echocardiographic evidence of intracardiac thrombi, and rheumatic mitral stenosis with large left atrium.

Cardioversion during pregnancy

Atrial fibrillation during pregnancy can present a complex management problem. The rapid rate may further stress the overtaxed cardiovascular system and precipitate congestive heart failure. Thromboembolism is a concern, and anticoagulant therapy can be very hazardous to the fetus early in pregnancy or during labor. Attempts at drug (medical) cardioversion raise the possibility of maternal or fetal drug toxicity. In cases in which antiarrhythmic medications do not promptly correct the rhythm or in which there is hemodynamic deterioration, DC cardioversion *synchronized to the maternal ECG* is the treatment of choice. The safety of cardioversion in pregnancy is well documented.[40,41] The following special considerations apply.

Warfarin (Coumadin) anticoagulation is contraindicated during the first trimester or close to term, and because it passes into the milk of mothers, it should not be given to nursing mothers. If anticoagulation is considered a necessity, heparin may be used; it is a relatively large molecule and does not cross the placenta.

Most of the electric wave front passes through the chest and a small fraction reaches the maternal heart; an even smaller fraction may reach the uterus and fetus. The theoretic possibility has been raised that cardioversion synchronized to the maternal ECG is not synchronized to the fetal ECG and therefore may precipitate ventricular fibrillation in the fetal heart. Although the potential may exist, this has not been observed clinically. The ventricular fibrillatory threshold in the fetal heart has not been studied but is presumed to be high. The fact remains that no clinical case of significant fetal arrhythmia has been reported to result from synchronized or nonsynchronized electroshock therapy to the pregnant mother.

Uterine contractions and precipitation of labor secondary to electroshock have been named as potential problems but have not been observed or reported clinically.

Given these considerations, fetal ECG should be monitored during cardioversion of the pregnant woman.

Cardioversion and pacemakers

Patients with implanted pacing systems may require elective or emergency cardioversion or defibrillation and require special considerations to avoid endocardial burns, increased fibrosis at the electrode/endocardial interface, or damage to the pulse generator.[42]

Manufacturers have protected the electronic circuits in the pulse generator from the current delivered by the cardioverter; thus damage to the pulse generator is rare. However, this has produced another problem in that the energy is shunted to the myocardium via the pacing electrode and may result in endocardial burns and a loss of effective pacing, resulting from a rise in the stimulation threshold. Infrequently, the pulse generator may also be damaged, if the energy transmitted exceeds the level of protection built into the device. This may render the unit nonfunctional or change its mode and program of pacing.[42]

The following precautions should be taken when the patient has a pacemaker.

1. Position the defibrillator paddles at least 13 cm away from the pulse generator (see p. 283). This frequently necessitates the use of apical-posterior orientation (Fig. 12-8, *A*). If a posterior paddle is not available, keep the paddle as far from the pulse generator as possible and titrate the energy to permit the use of the lowest effective energy level (Fig. 12-8, *B* and *C*).

2. Have the pacemaker programmer available so that the pacemaker output can immediately be reprogrammed in case of loss of capture.

3. Within hours, and periodically for the next 2 months following the procedure, check for an expected rise in the stimulation threshold.

4. If the patient is clearly dependent on the pacemaker, consider a back-up temporary or transcutaneous pacemaker before elective cardioversion.

5. If there is a rise in the stimulation threshold, a concomitant increase in the delivered energy from the pulse generator will be necessary. This may result in a shortening of the life of the system, so careful follow-up is indicated.

6. Most *external* pacers can withstand electric shocks up to 400 J. For additional safety, turn off the pacemaker pulse generator before applying defibrillation.

MINOR COMPLICATIONS

• *Paddle burn of the skin (best prevented by meticulous attention to technique):* Treatment is symptomatic.

• *Hypotension (3% to 4%):* Keep the patient supine until the condition is controlled and have patient well hydrated.

• *Myocardial cell damage (rarely seen):* This is reflected by *persistent* ST-T segment changes and elevated cardiac enzyme levels, particularly in patients in whom higher energy levels have been used repeatedly.[43,44] Multiple low-energy shocks cause less cardiac damage than do a few high-energy shocks of similar total energy.[43,44] Transient (60- to 90-second) ST segment elevation after DC cardioversion is probably related to sustained regional myocardial depolarization in areas of highest current flow and does not reflect myocardial damage or coronary artery spasm.[45] No specific treatment is needed; monitor for arrhythmias or congestive heart failure.

• *Muscle pain:* Treatment consists of analgesics and muscle relaxants as needed.

MAJOR COMPLICATIONS

• *Systemic or pulmonary embolism (1% to 2%):* Risk is considered to be highest in the following situations: atrial fibrillation for longer than 7 days, mitral stenosis and large left atrium, prosthetic valves (especially mitral valves), cardiomyopathy, congestive heart failure, and history of embolism. Treatment includes anticoagulants. It is best to use preventive treatment in higher risk patients (see p. 285).

• *Arrhythmias:* These are usually transient. Sinus node malfunction may result in junctional or ventricular escape beats. Cardiac standstill is rarely seen and may be secondary to hypoxia, excessive premedication, the use of excessively high energy levels, or preexisting sick sinus syndrome. Ventricular tachycardia or ventricular fibrillation is rarely precipitated and may be related to improper synchronization, a high level of energy used in the clinical setting of digitalis toxicity with electrolyte imbalance, or the severity of underlying heart disease.

Most of the postcardioversion arrhythmias need no specific treatment. Symptomatic bradycardia may be treated with atropine, or isoproterenol; very rarely a temporary pacemaker may be needed. External transcutaneous pacing can be used. Ventricular arrhythmias may require lidocaine, dilantin, correction of electrolyte imbalance, and, if sustained or recurrent, repeat cardioversion or defibrillation.

• *Pulmonary edema (1% to 2%):* The exact mechanism is not clear. Contributing factors may include pulmonary embolism or depression of left ventricular function by the electric shock. Treatment is supportive.

FUTURE DEVELOPMENTS

Cardioversion has been in clinical use for almost 25 years; the procedure is well standardized and quite routine. Nevertheless, exciting research and advances in application are being made. Some of the forthcoming possibilities are described below.

• *Transvenous catheter cardioversion* for supraventricular arrhythmias (SVT or atrial flutter) or ventricular tachycardia: These newer electrophysiologic techniques may be applied in acute settings with temporary catheters or in chronic treatment in the form of implanted units[46] (see Chapters 9 and 14).

• *Automatic implanted cardioverter/defibrillator:* This is a clinical reality; 800 units have been implanted since its introduction (see Chapter 14).

• *Automatic external defibrillator:* These units are in various stages of development.[47] They distinguish ventricular fibrillation from asystole and automatically apply either defibrillating energy or external pacing impulses. When perfected, these units will add defibrillation and external pacing capabilities to basic cardiopulmonary resuscitation performed by minimally trained persons. Early application of defibrillation is expected to improve the survival rates in victims of sudden cardiac death.

• *Cardioversion and myocardial preservation:* Animal experimentation has suggested that calcium accumulation in the injured cell is a key feature of myocardial cell damage following cardioversion or defibrillation and that premedication with the calcium-blocking agent verapamil will reduce or limit such injury.[48] Human application of these observations may make cardioversion and defibrillation even safer.

• *Defibrillation energy:* The concept of choosing the proper defibrillating energy dose for each person has been proposed. Animal testing has validated the system that measures the transthoracic impedance and accordingly automatically adjusts the energy delivered.[13] Preliminary human clinical trials have showed promising results.[10] Automated impedance-based selection of defibrillation energy may replace the arbitrary levels currently used.

PROCEDURE CHECKLIST

✔ Review the indications and contraindications of the procedure in relation to the specific patient.

✔ Note any special circumstances—for example, anticoagulation, pacemaker, pregnancy, cardiac malposition, potential airway problems, and drug allergies.

✔ Obtain informed consent.

✔ Check the equipment and available medications.

✔ Notify appropriate personnel for the scheduled procedure.

✔ Obtain and review laboratory results.

✔ Review the patient's status and readiness for the procedure.

✔ Prepare the patient and give appropriate instructions and reassurance.

✔ Recheck defibrillator, synchronization, and paddle position.

✔ Recheck the ECG rhythm.

✔ Give premedication and anesthetic.

✔ Start the countdown.

✔ Warn all persons present not to touch the bed or the patient.

✔ Apply DC synchronized current in titrated energy form.

✔ If ventricular fibrillation is precipitated, apply 200 J DC nonsynchronized shock.

✔ After completing the procedure, monitor the patient for rhythm, airway patency, blood pressure, and adequacy of ventilation until the anesthetic effect is gone.

✔ Document the procedure and the outcome in appropriate medical records.

REFERENCES

1. Lown, B., Amarasingham, R., and Neuman, J.: New method for terminating cardiac arrhythmias: use of synchronized capacitor discharge. J.A.M.A. **182**:548-555, 1962.
2. Beck, C.S., Pritchard, W.H., and Feil, H.J.: Ventricular fibrillation of long duration abolished by electric shock, J.A.M.A. **135**:985-986, 1947.
3. Zoll, P.M.: Termination of ventricular fibrillation in man by externally applied electrical countershock. N. Engl. J. Med. **245**:727, 1956.
4. Zipes, D.P., et al.: Termination of ventricular fibrillation in dogs by depolarizing a critical amount of myocardium, Am. J. Cardiol. **36**:311-344, 1975.
5. Geddes, L.A.: Cardiovascular devices and their applications, New York, 1984, John Wiley & Sons, Inc.
6. Hooker, D.R., Kouwenhoven, W.B., and Langworthy, O.R.: The effect of alternating currents on the heart, Am. J. Physiol. **102**:445-454, 1933.
7. Kerber, R.E., et al.: Transthoracic resistance in human defibrillation. Influence of body weight, chest size, serial shocks, paddle size and paddle contact pressure, Circulation **63**:676-682, 1981.
8. Bourland, J.D., Tacker, W.A., and Geddes, L.A.: Strength-duration curves of trapezoidal waveforms of various tilts for transchest defibrillation animals, Med. Instrum. **12**:38-41, 1978.
9. Morgan, J.P., et al.: High-energy versus low-energy defibrillation: experience in patients (excluding those in the intensive care unit) at Mayo Clinic–affiliated hospitals, Mayo Clin. Proc. **59**:829-834, 1984.
10. Kerber, R.E., Martins, J., Olshansky, B., and Charbonnier, F.: Initial human experience with automated impedance-based energy adjustment for defibrillation and cardioversion, J. Am. Coll. Cardiol. **5**:455, 1985.
11. Weaver, W.D., Cobb, L.A., Copass, M.K., and Hallstrom, A.P.: Ventricular defibrillation—a comparative trial using 175-J and 320-J shocks, N. Engl. J. Med. **307**:1101-1106, 1982.
12. Kerber, R.E., and Sarnat, W.: Factors influencing the success of ventricular defibrillation in man, Circulation **60**:226-230, 1979.
13. Kerber, R.E., et al.: Automated impedance-based energy adjustment for defibrillation: experimental studies, Circulation **71**:136-140, 1985.
14. Gutgesell, H.P., et al.: Energy dose for ventricular defibrillation of children, Pediatrics **58**:898-901, 1976.
15. Chameides, L., et al.: Guidelines for defibrillation in infants and children, Circulation **56**:502A, 1977.
16. Tacker, W.A., Babbs, C.F., Abendschein, D.R., and Geddes, L.A.: Transchest defibrillation under conditions of hypothermia, Crit. Care Med. **9**:390-391, 1981.
17. Kerber, R.E., et al.: Open chest defibrillation during cardiac surgery: energy and current requirements, Am. J. Cardiol. **46**:393-398, 1980.
18. LeJa, F.S., Euler, D.E., and Scanlon, P.J.: Digoxin and the susceptibility of the canine heart to countershock-induced arrhythmia, Am. J. Cardiol. **55**:1070-1075, 1985.
19. Mann, D.L., et al.: Absence of cardioversion-induced ventricular arrhythmias in patients with therapeutic digoxin levels, J. Am. Coll. Cardiol. **5**:882-888, 1985.
20. Vassaux, V., and Lown, B.: Cardioversion of supraventricular tachycardia, Circulation **39**:791-780, 1969.
21. Lown, B.: Cardioversion and the digitalized patient, J. Am. Coll. Cardiol. **5**:889-890, 1985.
22. Sharkey, S.W., Chaffee, V., and Kapsner, S.: Prophylactic external pacing during cardioversion of atrial tachyarrhythmias, Am. J. Cardiol. **55**:1632-1634, 1985.
23. DeSilva, R.A., Graboys, T.B., Podrid, P.J., and Lown, B.: Cardioversion and defibrillation, Am. Heart J. **100**:881-895, 1980.
24. Coe, E.H.: Anesthesia for elective cardioversion (letter), N. Engl. J. Med. **229**:262, 1978.
25. Hagemeijer, R.V., and Smalbraak, D.W.T.: Fentanyl-etomidate anesthesia for cardioversion, Eur. Heart J. **3**:155-158, 1982.
26. Bardhan, K.D., Morris, P., Taylor, P.C., and Hinchliffe, R.F.C.: Intravenous sedation for upper gastrointestinal endoscopy: diazepam versus midazolam, Br. Med. J. **288**:1046, 1984.
27. Kerber, R.E., and Sarnat, W.: Factors influencing the success of ventricular defibrillation in man, Circulation **60**:226-230, 1979.
28. Cherniack, N.S., and Longobardo, G.S.: Oxygen and carbon-dioxide gas stores of the body, Physiol. Rev. **50**:196-243, 1970.
29. Aaronson, J.D.: Personal communication, 1985.
30. West, G.A., and Primeau, P.: Nonmedical hazards of long-term oxygen therapy, Respir. Care **28**:906-912, 1983.
31. Kerber, R.E., et al.: Self-adhesive preapplied electrode pads for

defibrillation and cardioversion, J. Am. Coll. Cardiol. **3**(3):815, 1984.

31a. Aylward, P.E., et al.: Defibrillator electrode-chest wall coupling agents: influence on transthoracic impedance and shock success, J. Am. Coll. Cardiol. **6**:682-686, 1985.

32. Babka, J.C.: Does nitroglycerin explode?, N. Engl. J. Med. **309**:379, 1983.

33. Kerber, R.E., et al.: Elective cardioversion: influence of paddle electrode location and size on success rates and energy requirements, N. Engl. J. Med. **305**:658-662, 1981.

34. Pennington, J.E., Taylor, J., and Lown, B.: Chest thump for reverting ventricular tachycardia, N. Engl. J. Med. **283**:1192-1195, 1970.

35. Dahl, C.F., Ewy, G.A., Warner, E.D., and Thomas, E.D.: Myocardial necrosis from direct current counter shock, Circulation **50**:956, 1974.

35a. Eysmann, S.B., et al.: Electrocardiographic changes after cardioversion of ventricular arrhythmias, Circulation **73**:73-81, 1986.

35b. Waldecker, B., et al.: Dysrhythmias after direct-current cardioversion, Am. J. Cardiol. **57**:120-123, 1986.

36. Ewy, G.A.: Ventricular fibrillation masquerading as asystole, Ann. Emerg. Med. **13**:910, 1984.

37. Cohen, L., and Kitzes, R.: Magnesium sulfate and digitalis-toxic arrhythmias, J.A.M.A. **249**:2808-2809, 1983.

38. Mancini, G.B.J., and Goldberger, A.L.: Cardioversion of atrial fibrillation: consideration of embolization, anticoagulation, prophylactic pacemaker, and long-term success, Am. Heart J. **104**:617-621, 1982.

39. Meyers, D.G., Gonzalez, E.R., and Nelson, W.P.: The role of prophylactic anticoagulation in cardioversion of atrial fibrillation, Cardiovasc. Rev. Report **6**:647-657, 1985.

40. Cullhed, I.: Cardioversion during pregnancy, Acta Med. Scand. **214**:169-172, 1983.

41. Finlay, A.Y., and Edmunds, V.: DC cardioversion in pregnancy, Br. J. Clin. Prac. **33**:88-94, 1979.

42. Gould, L., Patel, S., Gomes, G.I., and Chokshi, A.B.: Pacemaker failure following external defibrillation, PACE **4**:575-577, 1981.

43. Ehsani, A., Ewy, G.A., and Sobel, B.E.: Effects of electrical countershock on serum creatinine phosphokinase isoenzyme activity, Am. J. Cardiol. **37**:12-18, 1976.

44. Wilson, C.M., Allen, J.D., and Adgey, A.A.J.: Death and damage after multiple DC countershocks, Br. Heart J. **53**:99, 1985.

45. Zelinger, A.B., Falk, R.H., and Hood, W.B.: Electrical-induced sustained myocardial depolarization as a possible cause for transient ST elevation post–DC elective cardioversion, Am. Heart J. **103**:1073-1074, 1982.

46. Saksena, S., and Calvo, R.: Transvenous cardioversion and defibrillation of ventricular tachyarrhythmias: current status and future directions, PACE **8**:715-731, 1985.

47. Cummins, R.O., Eisenberg, M.S., and Stults, K.R.: Automatic external defibrillators: clinical issues for cardiology, Circulation **73**:381-385, 1986.

48. Patton, J.N., Allen, J.D., and Pantridge, J.F.: The effects of shock energy, propranolol, and verapamil on cardiac damage caused by transthoracic countershock, Circulation **69**:357-368, 1984.

Chapter Thirteen

Pacemakers

ISAAC WIENER
MARY B. CONOVER

PERMANENT PACEMAKERS

The first artificial pacemaker was implanted in Stockholm in 1958 by Elmquist and Senning.[1] The years since have seen continued progress, with pacemakers becoming increasingly compact, reliable, and sophisticated. Permanent pacemakers consist of a catheter electrode attached to a pulse generator, which is implanted subcutaneously. Over 95% of permanent pacemakers are implanted by the transvenous route.

Indications

The primary indication for a pacemaker is symptomatic bradyarrhythmias. In occasional instances, severe asymptomatic bradyarrhythmias are indications for pacemaker implantation.[2,3]

The most common indications for permanent pacemakers can be classified as follows:
- Acquired atrioventricular block
  Complete heart block, infranodal, persistent or intermittent
  Mobitz type II second-degree atrioventricular (AV) block, persistent or intermittent
  AV nodal block, Mobitz type I, only when associated with symptoms
  Atrial flutter or fibrillation with a slow ventricular response when associated with symptoms
- AV block associated with myocardial infarction
  Bundle branch block (BBB) associated with fixed or transient Mobitz type II AV block or complete block
- Sick sinus syndrome
  Sinus bradycardia and arrest when associated with symptoms
  Tachycardia-bradycardia syndrome, if drugs necessary to control the tachycardia produce symptomatic bradycardia

- Hypersensitive carotid syndrome with syncope resulting from bradycardia

Contraindications

There are very few contraindications to permanent pacemaker implantation. Implantations are contraindicated in patients with active infections; these patients should be managed with medications or a temporary pacemaker until the infection is resolved.

Risks

The risks associated with permanent pacemakers are generally small. They include:
- Catheter dislodgment, lead fracture, or other causes of pacemaker system failure
- Pacemaker syndrome and pacemaker-mediated tachycardia
- Infection or erosion of the pulse generator
- Cardiac perforation with very rare instances of tamponade
- Thrombosis of the superior vena cava or right atrium

Equipment for permanent pacemaker implantation

The following equipment is necessary for implantation of a permanent pacemaker[4]:
- Pulse generator
- Ventricular leads
- Atrial leads
- 18-gauge vascular needle
- J-tip safety guidewire, 0.035 inches (0.9 mm)
- Vein dilator with a peel-away sheath
- Well-grounded ECG
- Pacemaker systems analyzer (PSA) to measure pacing thresholds and endocardial signals
- Pacemaker programmer

- Fluoroscopy
- Standard surgical instruments and suture materials
- Back-up equipment: external pacemaker, defibrillator, emergency cart with drugs, airways, suction equipment, and emergency sets for tube thoracostomy, open thoracostomy, and pericardiocentesis

Pulse generator

The pulse generator consists of electronic circuitry, based on digital chips, and a power source for generating the electric stimuli. Lithium batteries, which last a minimum of 5 to 7 years, are used almost exclusively as the power source. The entire unit is hermetically sealed in a stainless steel or titanium housing to isolate the contents from the biologic environment.

Pacing leads

Both unipolar and bipolar pacing leads are commonly used. In the unipolar system the cathode (negative electrode) is at the distal tip of the catheter, and the body of the pacemaker is the anode (positive electrode). In bipolar systems the distal tip of the catheter is the cathode; a ring electrode, usually 1 cm proximal to the tip, is the anode. In the past unipolar leads were thinner and were thought to offer better sensing. However, more careful testing has demonstrated that sensing characteristics of unipolar and bipolar leads are quite similar.[5] Bipolar systems are less susceptible to myopotential inhibition and less prone to cause pectoral stimulation.[6,7] We prefer bipolar systems.

Ventricular leads

Ventricular leads, with silicone rubber or polyurethane insulation and removable stylets, are thin, flexible, and resilient. Lead-fixation devices such as fins and tines reduce the incidence of dislodgment and are favored by most pacemaker physicians. Fins and tines intertwine with the right ventricular trabeculae; the porous construction allows fibrous tissue growth into the pores. Active fixation devices (screw tips) may be preferable in some patients with markedly dilated right ventricles. Fig. 13-1 illustrates several of the lead configurations available.

Atrial leads

The most commonly used atrial lead has a J configuration, which allows entry into the atrial appendage. Tines help to anchor this lead (Fig. 13-1). Active fixation leads have been used to attach to the lateral atrium and are particularly useful when the atrial appendage has been removed surgically (i.e., after mitral valve surgery).

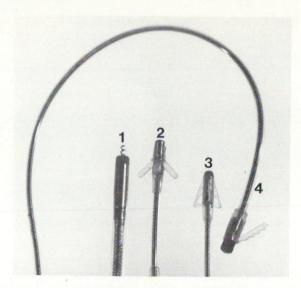

Fig. 13-1. Typical permanent pacemaker leads. *1*, Active fixation (screw-in) lead. *2*, Tined lead. *3*, Finned lead. *4*, Tined atrial J lead.

Pacemaker identification code

Pacing systems have been classified according to a universal code[8] (Table 13-1). The first letter represents the chamber paced; the second letter, the chamber sensed; the third letter, the pacing mode; the fourth letter, programmability; and the fifth letter, the antitachycardia functions. Table 13-2 defines the modes of the more commonly used three-position code, and Fig. 13-2 illustrates the basic circuitry design of the various pacing modes.

The most commonly used single-chamber pacemakers are VVI pacemakers, which have programmable output, rate, and sensitivity. Pacing and sensing occur only in the ventricle. Intrinsic ventricular activity will inhibit pulse generator output.

The most commonly used dual-chamber pacemakers are DVI and DDD pacemakers. In the DVI mode, pacing occurs in the atrium and ventricle; sensing occurs in the ventricle but not the atrium. This pacemaker is inhibited by intrinsic ventricular activity. In the DDD mode, pacing and sensing occur in the atrium and ventricle; atrial or ventricular output is inhibited by sensed atrial or ventricular activity, and ventricular output is triggered by sensed atrial activity. DDD pacemakers can be programmed to all other modes.

Selection of individualized pacing system

Selection of the proper pacing pulse generator to match the particular clinical situation is of utmost im-

Table 13-1. Five-position pacemaker code

Chamber paced (I)	Chamber sensed (II)	Mode of response (III)	Programmability (IV)	Antitachyarrhythmia functions (V)
V, Ventricle *A,* Atrium *D,* Atrium & ventricle	*V,* Ventricle *A,* Atrium *D,* Atrium & ventricle *O,* None	*I,* Inhibited (output blocked by sensed signal) *T,* Triggered (output elicited by a sensed signal) *D,* Atrial triggered & ventricular inhibited *O,* None	*P,* Programmable rate and or output *M,* Multiprogrammability (mode, AV delay, refractory period, sensitivity, hysteresis, etc.) *C,* Communicating, telemetric functions *O,* None	*B,* Burst of impulses *N,* Normal-rate competition (i.e., dual-demand pacemaker) *S,* Scanning (i.e., timed extrasystoles) *E,* External control (activated by magnet, radio, or other)

Adapted from Shively, B., and Goldschlager, N.: Progress in cardiac pacing, Arch. Intern. Med. **145:**2103, 1985. Copyright 1985, American Medical Association.

Table 13-2. Combinations of the three-position pacing code

Chamber paced	Chamber sensed	Mode	Description of function
D	D	D	Paces in either atrium or ventricle or both; senses in both chambers; mode of response can be inhibition in either chamber or atrial triggering (ventricular pacing in response to intrinsic atrial beats)
V	V	I	Paces and senses only in ventricle and is inhibited by intrinsic ventricular beats; intrinsic atrial beats do not result in paced ventricular impulses
A	A	I	Paces and senses only in atrium; output inhibited only by atrial activity (demand atrial pacing)
V	D	D	Paces in ventricle and senses in both atrium and ventricle; triggered by intrinsic atrial beats or inhibited by intrinsic ventricular beats
D	V	I	Paces in either atrium or ventricle or both; senses only in ventricle; inhibited by intrinsic ventricular beats
V	A	T	Paces in ventricle; senses only in atria; intrinsic atrial event triggers stimulus in ventricle
V	O	O	Paces in ventricle; has no sensing function
A	O	O	Paces in atria; has no sensing function
D	O	O	Paces in atria and ventricle; has no sensing function
V	V	T	Paces and senses in ventricle; sensed event triggers ventricular stimulus
A	A	T	Paces and senses in atria; a sensed event triggers atrial stimulus
O	O	O	Off

Table 13-3. Decision-making process for pacemaker selection

Condition	Associated findings	Pacemaker choice(s)
Sick sinus syndrome	Frequent atrial fibrillation or flutter	VVI
	Abnormal AV conduction	DVI, VVI*†
	Normal AV conduction	DVI, DDD, AAI, VVI*
Complete AV block	Persistent sinus bradycardia or inadequate increase in sinus rate during stress	DVI, VVI*
	Normal sinus mechanism	DDD, VVI*†
	Frequent atrial fibrillation or flutter	VVI

*Avoid use in aortic stenosis, idiopathic hypertrophic subaortic stenosis (IHSS), or pacemaker syndrome.
†For inactive patients or those with rare episodes of asystole or bradycardia.

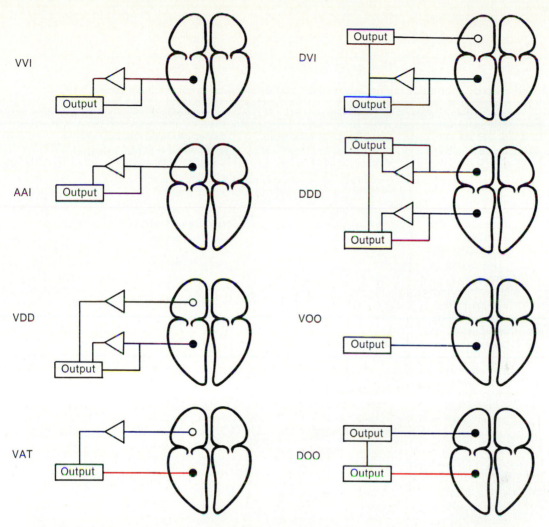

Fig. 13-2. Basic circuitry design of various pacing modes. Letters are in the order of chamber paced, chamber sensed, and mode of response. (*V,* Ventricle; *A,* atrium; *D,* both; *O,* = neither or not applicable; *I,* inhibited; *T,* triggered; ◁, sensing amplifier; □, output oscillator.) (Adapted from Ludmer, P.L., and Goldschlager, N.: Cardiac pacing in the 1980s, N. Engl. J. Med. **311:**1671-1680, 1984.)

portance.[9-11] Table 13-3 is a schematic approach to selection of the appropriate pacing system; Table 13-4 lists the indications, contraindications, advantages, and disadvantages of available pacing systems.

A few principles of pacemaker selection should be emphasized. When the patient with chronic atrial fibrillation requires a pacemaker, it generally should be a VVI pacemaker. VVI pacing is also adequate for elderly inactive patients and patients in whom the pacemaker is largely a standby device, such as those with rare sinus pauses.

Dual-chamber pacemakers should generally be used in patients with:

- Heart block with an intact sinus mechanism; these patients benefit from a pacemaker that allows the ventricular rate to increase with the sinus rate
- Sick sinus syndrome; these patients are likely to have VA conduction and a high incidence of pacemaker syndrome (p. 303)
- Noncompliant ventricles (i.e., severe hypertrophy); these patients are dependent on atrial contraction for ventricular filling
- Hypersensitive carotid syndrome; these patients often have a vasodepressor component and require maximal cardiac output

Table 13-4. Indications, contraindications, advantages, and disadvantages of available pacing systems

Mode	Indications	Contraindications	Advantages	Disadvantages
AAI	SSS with intact AV conduction	Atrial flutter or atrial fibrillation; multifocal (chaotic) atrial tachycardia Abnormal AV conduction	Preserves normal AV sequence, yet least complex system Requires single lead	Ventricle not paced if AV block should develop
VVI	Atrial flutter, atrial fibrillation, or multifocal atrial tachycardia with slow ventricular response. Infrequent episodes of bradycardia No hemodynamic benefit from AV sequential pacing Recurrent PMT	Decrease in cardiac output if AV synchrony lost (pacemaker syndrome)	Requires single lead Simple to operate Multiprogrammable Can be used with atrial arrhythmias	No change in rate in response to increased metabolic demands AV synchrony not preserved May cause VA conduction and pacemaker syndrome
VDD	Normal sinus node function with impaired AV conduction	Atrial flutter or atrial fibrillation; multifocal atrial tachycardia Sinus node dysfunction	Restores normal AV sequence if atrial rate is normal Increases ventricular paced rate when sinus rate increases	Requires two leads Does not pace atrium Requires normal atrial function Retrograde conduction may produce PMT
DVI	Atrial bradycardia with or without normal AV conduction PMT in VDD and DDD modes	Normal sinus node function Atrial flutter or atrial fibrillation; multifocal atrial tachycardia	Restores atrial rate and normal AV sequence during atrial bradycardia Does not sense in atria; thus useful in PMT	Requires two leads; is readily competitive with the atrium AV synchrony only if spontaneous atrial rate is less than automatic rate of pacemaker
DDD	Normal sinus node function with AV block	Atrial flutter or fibrillation; multifocal atrial tachycardia	May be programmed to all modes Restores normal AV sequence whether atrial rate is slow or normal	Requires two leads; can lead to PMT If sinus node dysfunction is present, paced rate is not increased to meet metabolic demands

Adapted from Ludmer, P.L., and Goldschlager N.: Cardiac pacing in the 1980s, N. Engl. J. Med. **311:**1671-1680, 1984, and from Furman, S.: Newer modes of cardiac pacing, Mod. Con. Cardiovasc. Dis **52:**9, 1983.
SSS, Sick sinus syndrome, *PMT,* pacemaker-mediated tachycardia; *VA,* ventriculoatrial conduction.

Personnel

Personnel required for a permanent pacemaker implantation procedure include the following:
- Physician (cardiologist, cardiac or thoracic surgeon) with specialized training in cardiac pacing
- Surgical scrub nurse to assist
- Circulating nurse to perform the pacemaker testing
- Radiology technician for operation of fluoroscopy
- Anesthesiologist (optional)

Location of procedure

Permanent pacemaker implantation is performed under sterile technique in a clean environment where all of the necessary equipment is available. An operating room equipped with the necessary items, a special procedure room with a fluoroscope, or the cardiac catheterization laboratory can be used.

Patient preparation

Prepare the patient for pacemaker implantation as for any other major surgery.

1. Inform the patient regarding the procedure, the risks, and what to expect.

2. Obtain informed consent from the patient and from the family, if necessary.

3. Give nothing by mouth for 6 to 8 hours before the procedure.

4. Review results of blood count, electrolytes, serum creatinine studies, coagulation studies, chest radiograph, and ECG.

5. Administer a mild sedative ½ hour before the procedure.

6. Establish an IV line before the procedure. Maintain continuous ECG monitoring.

7. Select the implant site. Both the left and right pectoral areas can be utilized. Any areas with abnormalities of the skin (i.e., abrasions) should be avoided. For patients whose occupational or recreational activities involve repetitive or detailed use of the dominant hand, the pacemaker should be placed on the contralateral side.

8. Prepare the surgical field. Strict attention to aseptic technique is mandatory for all pacemaker insertions. An area from midchest to the midaxillary line and from the jaw to the costal margin should be prepared. This includes shaving, washing with germicidal solution, and applying preparative solution the night before the procedure. Do not apply skin electrodes in the pacemaker field.

Procedure

The operation is generally done with the patient under local anesthesia. An anesthesiologist or anesthetist

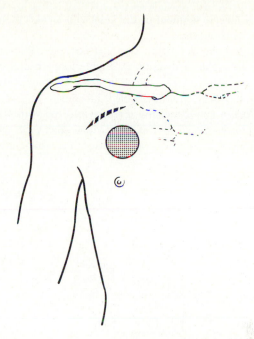

Fig. 13-3. Preferred incision. Incisions perpendicular to the deltopectoral groove are not recommended.

may be on standby. On very rare occasions (e.g., in an uncooperative patient), general anesthesia may be used.

1. Wash the intended incision site with a soap solution and apply a germicidal solution (Betadine). After a change of gloves, drape the perimeters of the field with sterile towels and cover the field with a sterile drape.

2. Administer prophylactic antibiotics, delivering the first dose just before the incision and two to three additional doses afterward.[12] Cephalosporins are commonly used. Antibiotics should be continued after the procedure for 12 to 24 hours, but no longer.

Venous access

Cephalic vein cutdown

1. Infiltrate the deltopectoral groove with 0.5% or 1% lidocaine without epinephrine. Excess lidocaine should be avoided, as lidocaine is absorbed and may suppress subsidiary pacemakers.

2. Make a transverse incision over the deltopectoral groove through the skin and subcutaneous tissues (Fig. 13-3). At this level, the fat pad in the deltopectoral groove should be easily identified. The cephalic vein courses in this fat pad.

3. Isolate the cephalic vein by blunt dissection. Often, branches of the vein are identified; ligate them with silk. Frequently, a small artery crosses the vein and must be ligated. Follow the cephalic vein sufficiently

proximal until a segment of the vein with an acceptable lumen size is exposed.

4. Secure the vein with two 2-0 nonresorbable silk sutures and ligate it distally. A double loop around the proximal portion allows the vein to be tightened after lead insertion and minimizes back bleeding.

5. Make a small incision directly into the vein with small scissors or scalpel. Gently dilate the vein with scissors or a mosquito clamp. Insert the endocardial

lead and stylet into the vein with the help of curved forceps or the introducer pick (which comes with many leads). In most cases the lead passes directly into the superior vena cava. If you encounter resistance, you may negotiate the superior vena cava by withdrawing the stylet 2 to 3 inches so that the distal catheter becomes less stiff. Rotating the catheter and asking the patient to cough or breathe deeply are often helpful. Fluoroscopy will identify instances when the catheter

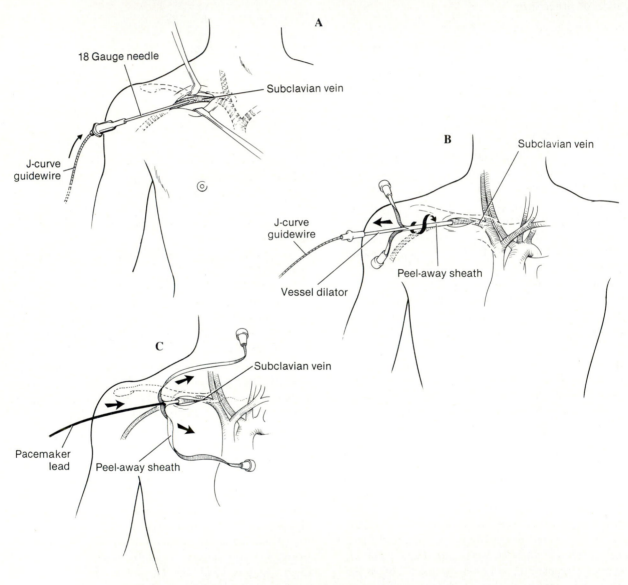

Fig. 13-4. Peel-away introducer set and the technique of pacemaker lead implantation using the subclavian vein. **A,** The **J** guidewire is introduced through the needle and the needle is then withdrawn. **B,** The vessel dilator/sheath unit is threaded over the guidewire and into the vein with a twisting motion; the vessel dilator and guidewire are then removed. **C,** The pacemaker lead is inserted through the sheath and positioned in the right ventricular apex; the sheath is then withdrawn and peeled away from the pacemaker lead. (Adapted from Miller, F.A., et al.: Permanent transvenous pacemaker implantation via the subclavian vein, Mayo Clin. Proc. **55:**309-314, 1980).

turns toward the axilla or the jugular vein. Withdrawing the catheter and rotating it will generally direct the catheter properly. In up to 50% of cases, the cephalic vein will accept both atrial and ventricular leads.

This technique is quite simple in most patients, but in approximately 20% of patients the cephalic vein is either absent or rudimentary. In these cases, deeper dissection, alternate surgical approaches (i.e., external or internal jugular vein), or placement of a subclavian introducer is necessary. The subclavian introducer can be inserted from the medial end of the incision. For dual-chamber pacing, if the cephalic vein accepts only the ventricular lead, the subclavian approach may be used for the atrial lead.

Subclavian approach[13]

1. Place the patient in the Trendelenberg position.

2. Make a 1 to 2 cm infraclavicular incision. Enter the subclavian vein through this incision with an 18-gauge needle (see Chapter 2).

3. Advance the guidewire through the needle into the central venous circulation; withdraw the needle (Fig. 13-4, *A*).

4. Pass the vein dilator, with a peel-away Teflon sheath, over the wire and into the vein, using slight pressure and a twisting motion. In some cases it is helpful to insert the dilator alone first and move this back and forth vigorously, loosening the subcutaneous tissues; then reinsert the dilator together with the sheath. Finally, remove the dilator and guidewire (Fig. 13-4, *B*).

5. Cover the end of the sheath with a finger to minimize bleeding.

6. Advance the pacemaker catheter through the sheath and position it in the right atrium. Withdraw the sheath and peel it away from the pacemaker catheter (Fig. 13-4, *C*).

Note: For dual-chamber units, both leads may be placed through a single large introducer with care to avoid tangling the two leads. We prefer a modified technique, using two wires. In this approach, when the lead is advanced into the introducer, a second guidewire is also advanced. When the first introducer is peeled back, one lead and a guidewire remain in the subclavian vein. A second introducer can be placed over the retained guidewire, the guidewire removed, and a second lead inserted through the introducer. The second introducer is then peeled away.

Lead placement, testing, and fixation

Ventricular lead

1. In placing the lead into the ventricle under fluoroscopic control, use a stylet formed into a large curve approximately 15 cm from the tip. Easy passage through the tricuspid valve can be facilitated by this U shape.

2. When the catheter is beyond the tricuspid valve, replace the curved stylet with a straight one. This allows the lead to drop into the apex of the right ventricle; the tip can then be gently advanced into the trabeculae. With tined leads, gentle traction on the lead will yield a "tugging" sensation, confirming anchoring of the lead.

3. An alternate approach uses only a single straight stylet and involves backing the lead into the apex of the right ventricle. In this approach, with the ventricular lead in the right atrium, pull the straight stylet back several inches so that a loop forms against the lateral wall of the right atrium. The body of the lead will then prolapse into the ventricle. Rotate the lead and advance the stylet to straighten the lead and allow positioning at the ventricular apex.

4. The final fluoroscopic appearance in the anteroposterior (AP) view should demonstrate stability of the distal inch of the lead, followed by a gentle bend through the right atrium (Fig. 13-5, *A*). Stability should be confirmed during deep breathing.

5. Always verify ventricular lead position in the lateral view to document anterior placement (Fig. 13-5, *B*). Posterior placement represents a lead that may be in the coronary sinus (Fig. 13-5, *C* and *D*).

6. Test the lead for both R wave amplitude and pacing threshold. An R wave of greater than 5 mV is desirable. Measure the R wave first because some patients become dependent on the pacemaker during the ventricular pacing period necessary for measuring the threshold. For unipolar measurements, a clamp in contact with the skin is used as the anode.

7. Perform threshold measurements with bipolar or unipolar configuration and the same pulse width as the pacemaker to be implanted. Both voltage and current thresholds can be tested by starting at high values and gradually decreasing the value until capture is lost. A current threshold of less than 1 mA and a voltage threshold of less than 1 V is desirable. The analyzer will also calculate the impedance from voltage and current measurements.

8. When an acceptable position is achieved, remove the stylet to minimize the risk of perforation. Gently remove the stylet under fluoroscopic monitoring to ensure that the tip does not move.

9. Pace at maximal amplitude to ensure that no diaphragmatic stimulation occurs. If diaphragmatic stimulation does occur, pull the lead back slightly and retest.

10. Anchor the lead securely with two 2-0 nonresorbable sutures, which are attached to deep muscle and tied around a suture sleeve surrounding the pacemaker lead. It is not advisable to suture directly around the pacemaker lead itself because fracture may occur.

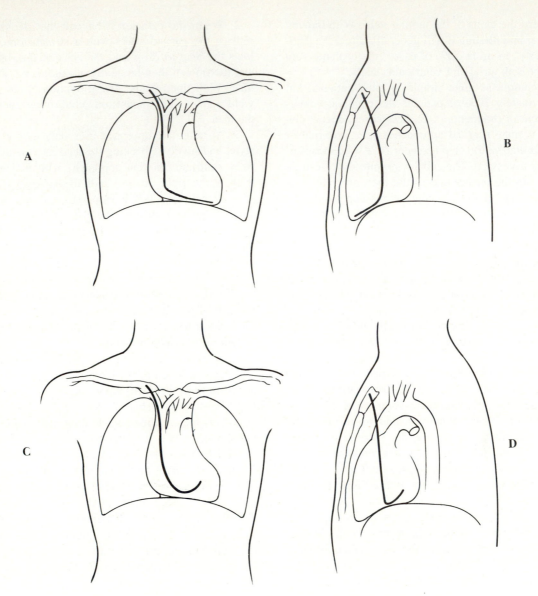

Fig. 13-5. Normal pacemaker position in the right ventricle on (**A**) anteroposterior and (**B**) lateral chest films as compared to coronary sinus position in the same views (**C** and **D**).

11. After anchoring, perform a final test of sensitivity and threshold.

12. Blood pressure should be determined during intrinsic rhythm and ventricular pacing. A significant decrease in blood pressure during ventricular pacing, especially if associated with ventriculo-atrial (VA) conduction, suggests the need for dual-chamber pacing.

13. Record all pacemaker data carefully on a standard form.

Atrial lead

1. Be sure that the ventricular lead is securely an-

chored before placing the atrial lead. The ventricular lead may be further anchored by reinserting the stylet to the level of the right atrium during atrial lead manipulation. This minimizes dislodgment of the ventricular lead during atrial manipulation.

2. Advance the atrial lead with the stylet in place so that the tip is in the low right atrium near the tricuspid valve.

3. Briskly withdraw the stylet 4 to 5 inches so that the lead can assume its preformed J configuration, engaging the atrial appendage. Slightly advance the lead,

with the stylet withdrawn, for better seating in the atrial appendage. During atrial contraction, the lead tip should be seen to move laterally and the loop to move medially. Now completely remove the stylet.

4. Use a lateral fluoroscopic view to document an anterior position of the atrial lead.

5. At this time test the atrial lead in a manner similar to the ventricular lead. In atrial leads a P wave signal greater than 2 mV is acceptable. Current threshold less than 2 mA and voltage threshold less than 2 V are desirable.

6. Anchor the atrial lead in a similar fashion to that of the ventricular lead.

7. Perform a final test of sensitivity and threshold.

Forming the pocket for the pulse generator

1. Infiltrate the subcutaneous tissue immediately superior to the pectoral muscle with 0.5% or 1% lidocaine without epinephrine.

2. Form the pocket by dissecting immediately above the plane of the pectoral muscle with the scalpel or scissors. It is important that the pocket be immediately above the muscle and not within the subcutaneous tissues. If the pocket is made within the subcutaneous tissues, blood supply to the superficial tissues may be compromised and erosion may occur. The pocket should be inferomedial to the incision, so that the pacemaker avoids both the clavicle and the anterior axillary fold. The pocket should be large enough to accommodate the pacemaker generator without undue tension on the skin above the pocket, but not so large as to permit excessive motion.

3. Strict hemostasis within the pocket is mandatory. Suture ligatures are the preferred method. Do not use electrocautery after a lead has been placed because of the danger of current leakage from the cautery through the electrode to the heart.

4. Attach the pulse generator to the lead. Covering the sleeve to the lead junction and screw cover with silicone cement is optional.

5. Coil any excess lead behind the pacemaker as the pacemaker is inserted in the pocket to minimize the possibility of cutting a lead at the time of pacemaker battery change. With some unipolar pacemakers, it is important to leave the "writing" uppermost; this directs current through a specific window and decreases pectoral stimulation. Some pacemakers allow fixation with sutures to prevent excessive migration.

6. Irrigating the pocket with triple antibiotic solution is optional.

7. Check pacemaker function again, with a magnet if necessary.

8. Close the incision with a three-layer closure using 2-0 resorbable sutures continuously for the first layer followed by interrupted 3-0 resorbable sutures and then subcuticular 4-0 resorbable sutures. There is no need for drainage tubes. Apply adhesive strips to the surface of the wound, along with antiseptic ointment and a light dressing.

Immediate postoperative care

1. Keep the patient in the postoperative recovery room until he or she is stabilized and relatively free of the effects of sedation.

2. As soon after surgery as practical, rule out pneumothorax, confirm proper electrode position, and secure a baseline for future clinical evaluations with an AP and lateral chest radiograph (Fig. 13-6). Obtain a baseline 12-lead ECG.

3. Maintain 24-hour ECG monitoring. Instruct personnel that rate alarms may not warn of loss of capture, because the monitor may interpret the pacemaker spike as a QRS complex.

Special precautions

Pacemaker insertion in the pacemaker-dependent patient requires special precautions. Whenever possible, a temporary pacemaker should be in place. After the permanent pacemaker is fully functional, the temporary pacemaker can be removed under fluoroscopic guidance so as not to dislodge the permanent pacemaker.

On occasion a temporary pacemaker is not in place, and after the first test of the pacemaker it is noted that the patient is fully dependent on the pacemaker. In these patients there is a risk of asystole when the wire is disconnected from the testing apparatus and attached to the pacemaker. In most patients this can be done without harm as long as the procedure is done expeditiously.

Pacemaker follow-up

Patients should have a thorough evaluation at 2 to 4 weeks after implantation. The history should document relief of prepacing symptoms. A physical examination should be performed, with special attention to the pacemaker pocket. Pacemaker function should be checked by a rhythm strip with magnet if necessary (see below), and accurate records should be kept of the pacemaker analysis. Any necessary adjustments can be made by programming (see below). Many physicians set the pacemaker at a high output for the first 6 weeks to avoid exit block as the lead matures. After this time period the output can be decreased to preserve battery life.

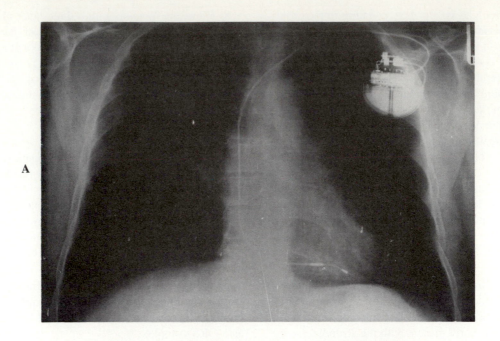

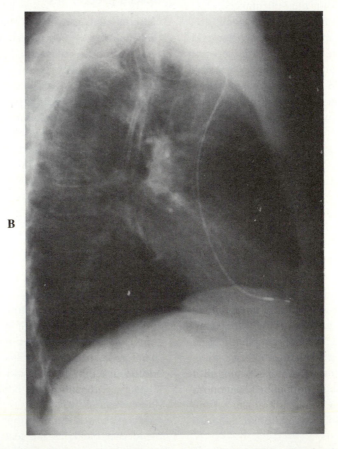

Fig. 13-6. Anteroposterior (**A**) and lateral (**B**) views of electrode configuration for dual-chamber pacing.

Later follow-up includes a combination of transtelephonic surveillance and office visits. There are no data on the necessary frequency. Most physicians check the pacemaker by one or the other modalities approximately every 2 months and increase this frequency to once monthly as the end of pacemaker life approaches.

Activation of the magnet rate is utilized clinically to evaluate the pacing function of a generator that has been suppressed by the patient's intrinsic rhythm and to evaluate battery depletion. The magnet rate results when a magnet is placed over the generator, deactivating the sensing mechanism and converting the pacemaker to a fixed-rate unit. The magnet rate is frequently different than the automatic rate. In some programmable pacemakers, end of pacemaker life is indicated only by decrease of the magnet rate, making magnet testing mandatory.

Programmability of pacemakers

Programmability is that feature by which the electronically controlled performance of a pacemaker can be noninvasively altered.[8,10,14] This alteration is permanent until the pacemaker is otherwise "reprogrammed." Almost all new pacemakers implanted in patients in the United States are multiprogrammable.

Programming is achieved by using an external programmer to transmit preselected messages in the form of a binary code, via either radiofrequency waves or a pulsed electromagnetic field, to the implanted pulse generator, which then assumes its new function. To prevent accidental reprogramming by external time-varying magnetic fields, most of the microprocessor codes require an electronic password before the code can be altered. Some models transmit a message from the pulse generator to the programmer, indicating that the instructions have been received, accepted, and acted on; otherwise, confirmation of the success of programming is obtained on the ECG tracing.

Features that can be programmed noninvasively include stimulus output (pulse duration, current, or voltage), rate, amplifier sensitivity, escape rate, hysteresis, lower and upper rate limits, AV interval, refractory periods, and mode.

Output. The voltage (V), current (mA), and pulse duration constitute the pulse generator output; each may be programmable, depending on the model.

The output may be increased to manage periods of threshold rise, such as may occur 1 to 4 weeks after implant (when fibrosis of the electrode is maximal), after cardioversion or defibrillation, during myocardial infarction, with electrolyte imbalance, or because of drug therapy.

The output may be reduced to improve battery longevity by providing the minimal level of stimulation necessary for reliable pacing. If diaphragmatic stimulation is a problem, symptoms may be alleviated by a reduction in output. Reducing the output to a subthreshold level allows the underlying rhythm to emerge and allows evaluation of conduction disorders and diagnosis of myocardial infarction. Reducing the output until capture is lost may also be used to serially evaluate the myocardial stimulation threshold.

Rate. The automatic rate is the interval between consecutive atrial- or ventricular-paced stimuli. This setting is programmable between 30 and 150 pulses/minute.

Rate may be decreased to minimize angina related to the faster paced rate, alleviate symptoms of the pacemaker syndrome by permitting the emergence of the underlying sinus rhythm, or reduce the patient's awareness of the paced rhythm.

The rate may be increased to provide a faster rate commensurate with increased metabolic needs and to suppress tachycardias.

Sensitivity. Sensitivity is the ability of the detection system of the pacemaker to recognize the intrinsic cardiac signal and to use that signal to control the output of the pacemaker. The sensing circuit recognizes the R or P wave by its amplitude and slew rate (rate of change of voltage amplitude with time). The capability to recognize slew rate allows the sensing circuit to differentiate between the QRS and the T wave.

Today's pulse generators typically have several sensitivity settings. Lower numbers (i.e., 1.0 or 1.5 mV) indicate that the unit is more sensitive to intrinsic activity, whereas higher numbers (2.5 or 3 mV) are less sensitive. The pulse generator may be made less sensitive to alleviate pacemaker inhibition resulting from oversensing of T waves or skeletal muscle electric potentials (p. 305). The pulse generator may be made more sensitive to correct failure to sense.

Escape rate and hysteresis. The escape rate is the interval between the last sensed beat and the first pacemaker beat to follow.

Hysteresis occurs when the escape interval is longer than the programmed interval (Fig. 13-7). Even though the pulse generator may be programmed to pace at 72 pulses/minute, it will not begin pacing until the rate falls below 60 beats/minute, giving the patient a greater opportunity for conducted sinus beats.

Lower and upper rate limits. Lower and upper rate limits are programmable features of the dual-chamber units that permit rate-responsive pacing. The lower (standby) rate limit is the lowest rate at which a pulse generator is programmed to track (respond to) the spon-

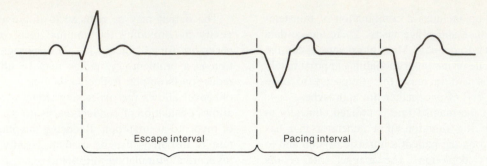

Fig. 13-7. Hysteresis. Note that the time lapse between a native beat and pacemaker escape is longer than the interval between paced beats.

taneous atrial rate. If the atrial or ventricular rate falls below the programmed lower rate limit, the generator will pace either chamber at the standby rate.

The upper rate limit is the fastest rate at which a pulse generator is programmed to track the spontaneous atrial rate on a 1:1 basis. Once this rate is exceeded, the response of the unit will vary with the manufacturer. There may be 2:1 block, Wenckebach block, or a gradual reduction to a specific "fallback" rate, which is programmable in some pacemakers. The upper rate is set to prevent any excessively rapid ventricular response to rapid supraventricular rhythms.

Refractory period. The refractory period is the period during which a pulse generator is unresponsive to an input signal. The *pacing refractory period* follows a paced complex, and the *sensing refractory period* follows a sensed spontaneous complex. The ventricular pacemaker refractory period is that time during which signals at the ventricular input are ignored. If this time is too short, oversensing of T waves may occur, delaying the next pacing impulse; if too long, there may be failure to sense closely coupled extrasystoles.

The atrial pacemaker refractory period is that time during which signals at the atrial input are ignored. The interval is initiated by the sensing of either ventricular or atrial activity and terminates at a time that may be programmed in accordance with the patient's VA conduction. The atrial refractory period may be programmed so that retrograde atrial impulses are not sensed, thus preventing pacemaker-mediated tachycardia.

Blanking period. The blanking period is a very short ventricular refractory period that is initiated in the ventricles by an atrial pacemaker pulse for the purpose of preventing the ventricular electrode from sensing the atrial pulse (crosstalk) and being inhibited by it. Fig. 13-8 illustrates the refractory periods and blanking period of a dual-chamber pacing system. If this interval is too long, it could result in delivery of the ventricular pacing pulse at the same time as an unsensed spontaneous QRS. If too short, crosstalk could result in ventricular asystole.

Mode. Pacing modes and their clinical application have already been discussed (p. 291). Several modes of function are programmable in the DDD pacemakers. For example, the DDD mode can be changed to VVI if atrial fibrillation develops.

AV interval. The AV interval should be programmed within the physiologic range (0.12 to 0.2 seconds) for maximal cardiac output. In some patients the AV interval may be programmed to allow AV conduction to occur, with the patient's native QRS inhibiting the ventricular output channel. In this way, only one output pulse is used, and battery life is preserved. In selected

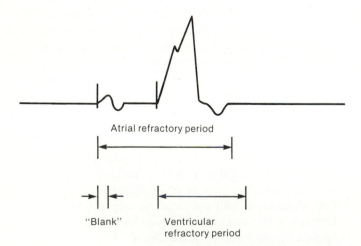

Fig. 13-8. Refractory periods and blanking period of a dual-chamber pacing system. The blanking period in the ventricular circuit disallows sensing by this circuit of the atrial output pulse (cross talk), thus avoiding inhibition of ventricular output.

patients the AV interval may be altered to prevent tachyarrhythmia.

Telemetry

Some pacemakers have a telemetry feature that allows interrogation of the pacemaker. Commonly telemetered information includes the most recent pacemaker settings. Some units provide additonal parameters such as battery status, lead impedance, marker channels for interpreting pacing or sensing, summary of percentage of paced or sensed beats, and intracardiac electrograms. These parameters may be very helpful in evaluating suspected pacemaker malfunction.

Programming procedure

Pacemakers manufactured by a given company will be programmed only by that company's programmer.[10] Each programmer comes with clear instructions for use.

Complications
Early failure to capture and sense

Early failure to capture or sense may occur in a small percentage of patients during the few days after pacemaker implantation. Catheter dislodgment is the most common cause and may or may not be seen on radiographs. Microdislodgment is more common than frank dislodgment. Instances of early failure to capture or to sense may be remedied by increasing the output amplitude or sensitivity. If programming is unsuccessful, failure to capture clearly warrants early reoperation with repositioning. Failure to sense may or may not warrant repositioning, depending on the clinical situation.

Late failure to pace

Late failure to pace may be related to change in threshold, battery depletion, or failure of the electrode or pacemaker components. In the past, reoperation was required, along with testing of the lead to determine if there was a pacemaker problem or lead problem (e.g., lead fracture). Some newer pacemakers provide information about pacemaker and lead status, allowing noninvasive diagnosis. Some late failures to pace may be corrected by programming, but others will require reoperation.

Pacemaker syndrome

The pacemaker syndrome is a group of symptoms related to adverse hemodynamic effects of ventricular pacing.[15,16] The symptoms include fatigue, dizziness, syncope, and pulmonary congestion. This syndrome is most common in patients with sick sinus syndrome who manifest with VA conduction during ventricular pacing.

Contraction of the atrium against a closed mitral valve may lead to regurgitation of blood into the pulmonary veins and may trigger atrial baro-reflexes, causing hypotension. This syndrome should be carefully checked for during any VVI pacemaker insertion (by noting the change in the blood pressure during ventricular pacing compared to spontaneous rhythm) and can be remedied by dual-chamber pacing. If pacemaker syndrome is first recognized after an implantation, programming the rate so that the majority of beats are spontaneous may ameliorate the problem. If not, reoperation for conversion to a dual-chamber unit may be indicated.

Pacemaker-mediated tachycardia

Pacemaker-mediated tachycardia occurs with VDD or DDD pacers in patients with VA conduction. The pacer synchronizes to the retrograde atrial signal, causing a tachycardia. In Fig. 13-9, note the retrograde P wave following the fourth beat. The atrial electrode senses this impulse and activates the ventricular pacemaker. There is again retrograde conduction to the atria, atrial sensing, and ventricular activation; this repetitive sequence sustains the tachycardia. A simple approach to the prevention of the problem is to program the atrial sensing refractory period of the pacer so that retrograde atrial signals beyond a certain rate are not sensed. Also, the tachycardia can immediately be terminated by switching to a DVI mode, eliminating atrial sensing.

Infection

Permanent pacemakers may be complicated by early and late infections.[17,18] *Staphylococcus aureus* is the most common offending organism in early infections, and *S. epidermis* the most common in late infections. Treatment almost always requires removal of the entire unit (see below).

Myocardial perforation and tamponade

Electrode perforation may require gentle withdrawal of the pacing catheter. Pericardial tamponade is extremely rare and requires drainage.

Thrombosis and embolism

Clinically important thrombosis of the axillary or subclavian veins and SVC syndrome[19] are rare complications with the newer leads. Anticoagulant and thrombolytic therapy are usually sufficient therapy.

Pulmonary embolism secondary to right atrial or right ventricular thrombus on a pacing wire is a very rare complication of modern pacemakers. Echocardiographic diagnosis of a large intracavity thrombus should raise the consideration of a thrombectomy.

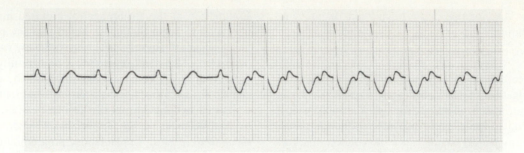

Fig. 13-9. ECG tracing of pacemaker-mediated tachycardia. A retrograde P wave follows the fourth beat and is sensed by the atrial electrode, which then activates the ventricular pacemaker. The cycle continues: each time the ventricle is activated there is a retrograde P wave, which is sensed and which activates the ventricle. (Courtesy Dan Tich, Cardiac Pacemakers, Inc.)

Erosion of the pulse generator

Rarely permanent pacemakers may erode through the skin.[20] Reoperation is required to remove the pacemaker and insert a new one in a different location.

Pacemaker reoperation

The most frequent indications for pacemaker reoperation are battery depletion, lead problems, and pacemaker erosion or infection.

Elective battery replacement is a relatively simple procedure and can be done on an outpatient basis. The technique is as described below.

1. Carefully confirm lead position with an overpenetrated chest radiograph.

2. Patient preparation, field preparation, local anesthetic, and prophylactic antibiotics are the same as for the initial implant.

3. The incision is made immediately over the old incision. The pacemaker should be gently pushed cephalad so that the body of the pacemaker, with no intervening lead, is directly under the incision. Great care must be taken not to cut the lead.

4. A fibrous sheath will have formed around the pacemaker. Identify and secure this sheath with clamps after it is incised.

5. Deliver the pacemaker through the incision and disconnect it from the lead.

6. Test the lead as at the initial implant. Thresholds less than 2 mA are acceptable for a chronic lead. If the threshold is excessively high, consider lead replacement.

7. Attach a new pulse generator to the pacemaker lead.

8. Close the pacemaker capsule and the subcutaneous layers and skin with resorbable sutures as for initial implant.

9. Postoperative management is as for the initial implant, but a period of bedrest is unnecessary.

Lead revision is similar to initial implant. When required early after initial operation, the lead can be easily repositioned. Some late cases of lead fracture can be repaired with splicing kits supplied by the manufacturer. Other cases require insertion of a new lead through alternate access on the same side or by placing an entire new unit on the other side. The old lead should be removed if possible; if not, it may be capped and anchored with suture.

Management of pacemaker infections is a difficult problem. In general, medical therapy alone has been unsatisfactory, and removal of the entire pacing system, interim use of a temporary pacemaker, and placement of a new unit on the contralateral side are recommended. In some cases without bacteremia, explantation and implantation of the new unit may be accomplished in one procedure. Removal of the long-term implanted lead is generally difficult and has been made more difficult by passive fixation leads. The basic technique applies continuous careful traction on the lead once it is dissected from all its attachments. Continuous traction by means of 1-pound weights has been employed. There is one report of multiple biopsies performed around the tip of the lead.[20] In cases of endocarditis, if these means fail, thoracotomy may be necessary.

In cases of pacemaker erosion, the lead may be saved if the erosion is detected early. It may be possible to isolate the lead relatively proximally and attach a new coupling device. The pacemaker generator is removed, the eroded pocket is closed, and the new pacemaker pack is placed in another location on the same side.[20]

Environmental hazards[21,22]

Pacemakers may occasionally sense electromagnetic interference (EMI) from other sources, both intrinsic (myopotential) and extrinsic (environmental), or they may be exposed to damaging agents.

Most pacemakers have an interference rate to which they revert if exposed to input signals above a rate determined by the manufacturer (usually 300/minute).[14] The interference rate is an asynchronous fixed-rate mode that may be the same as the automatic rate but is usually faster, so that the patient will recognize that he is in a dangerous environment and so that there will be less likelihood of competition with the native rhythm.

Intrinsic hazards (myopotentials)[6,7,23]

Oversensing of myopotentials (i.e., skeletal muscle interference with unipolar pacemaker function), may occur in as many as one third of all unipolar pacemakers implanted. Myopotentials may also cause false triggering in DDD units, as a result of pacemaker interpretation of myopotentials as P waves.

Treatment. The management of myopotential inhibition is a difficult problem. In many instances, decreasing the sensitivity of the pacemaker may be successful. Some new units allow the unipolar configuration to be programmed to a bipolar configuration. If these approaches are not successful, reoperation to place the unipolar pacemaker in a Silastic boot or to replace the entire unipolar system with a bipolar system may be necessary.

Extrinsic hazards

Improvements in pacemaker design and shielding have largely eliminated the problem of the pacemaker sensing extrinsic EMI; thus the problem is generally not of practical clinical concern. The sources of EMI that have been reported in the past, such as vacuum cleaners, electric razors, ignition systems of gasoline motors, microwave ovens with inefficient door seals, and airport weapon detectors, are not likely to present a problem for today's pacemaker. Also, the permanent pacemaker appears to be unaffected by hyperbaric chambers with up to at least 100 psi. Powerful sources of radar may inhibit pacemakers, but because of the motion of the radar beam, usually only a single beat is inhibited.

Surgical cautery. Surgical cautery has been reported as a common source of interference and may inhibit or convert the unit to an asynchronous mode. Surgical cautery may be used cautiously as long as the indifferent plate of the cautery apparatus is at a considerable distance from the heart and pacemaker and that the cutting edge of the cautery is not used near the pacemaker generator or the electrode. The patient's ECG should, of course, be monitored during the procedure.

Transcutaneous electric nerve stimulators. TENS units should be avoided in pacemaker patients, especially those with unipolar units. If the device must be used, place the electrodes as far from the pulse generator/lead system as possible.

Damaging agents

Defibrillators. Defibrillators may cause damage to pacemaker circuits. Defibrillator paddles should be placed as far as possible from the pacemaker, and the pacemaker should be fully checked after a shock is administered (see Chapter 12).

Radiation.[24-26] Studies have shown that there is no deleterious effect to the pacemaker from exposure to diagnostic x-ray radiation. However, therapeutic radiation may cause permanent malfunction of the pulse generator containing CMOS chips (the semiconductor used most commonly in modern pacemakers). Thus pacemakers should be either kept out of the field of therapeutic radiation or shielded from it. In occasional cases, it may be necessary to reposition the pacemaker to avoid the radiation field.

Magnetic resonance imaging.[27-30] Until further data are available, patients with implanted pacemakers should not be examined with magnetic resonance imaging (MRI). The static magnetic field exerts torque on the pacemaker generator and may also cause conversion to a fixed rate or false inhibition.

FUTURE DEVELOPMENTS
Automatic implantable cardioverter or defibrillator with capability for pacing

The automatic implantable cardioverter or defibrillator is a device that will allow electric treatment of tachycardias (see Chapter 14). Back-up pacing is used for any associated bradycardias.

Physiologic sensors

Currently, rate-responsive pacing is possible only in patients who have a functioning sinus mechanism. A truly physiologic pacemaker that will permit increase in rate in respone to an increase in metabolic needs is under investigation. The sensors under study include skeletal muscle activity, oxygen saturation, pH, central body temperature, and respiratory rate.[31] Further studies along this line are necessary.

Pacemaker reuse

Prospective payment systems have generated renewed interest in cost-cutting measures. In response, the North American Society of Pacing and Electrophysiology (NASPE) studied the feasibility of reusing cardiac pacemakers that are still reliable and have many years of useful life remaining. It was found that if cardiac pulse generators are properly cleaned, sterilized, tested for function and battery life, and individualized to the patient's needs, their reuse may be medically acceptable.[32] The NASPE has recommended guidelines for inhospital reconditioning of pacemakers.

The patient's perception of "second-hand" pacemakers needs to change, and legal issues must be resolved before pacemaker reuse is practiced.

TEMPORARY PACEMAKERS

A temporary pacemaker consists of a transvenous catheter electrode attached to an *external* pulse generator. Temporary pacemakers are used when the need for pacing is immediate. Temporary pacemakers may be followed by permanent pacers if the need for pacing persists or may simply be removed if the need for pacing is self-limited.

Indications

The most common indications for temporary pacing are:
- Complete heart block with slow ventricular escape
- Symptomatic sinus bradycardia, asystole, or prolonged sinus pauses
- Acute anterior myocardial infarction with complete heart block, Mobitz type II AV block, or new bifascicular block; some physicians advocate the insertion of prophylactic pacemakers for any new BBB appearing in the setting of acute anterior myocardial infarction
- Acute inferior myocardial infarction with complete heart block and poorly tolerated rates, hypotension, congestive heart failure, or ventricular arrhythmias
- Selected tachyarrhythmias such as bradycardia-induced or drug-induced torsades de pointes, atrial flutter, or recurrent sustained ventricular tachycardia
- Malfunction of implanted pacemaker
- Prophylactic use (i.e., right heart catheterization in a patient with LBBB, cardioversion of a patient with suspected sick sinus syndrome, right coronary artery angioplasty)

Contraindications

Insertion of a temporary pacemaker is generally undertaken as an emergency measure. There are no absolute contraindications. Although intravascular catheters are not desirable in patients with documented or suspected sepsis, the risk of exacerbating the infection may have to be accepted if pacing is mandatory for life support.

Risks

In a series of more than 1000 patients, complications of temporary pacemaker insertion occurred in approximately 14% of patients, without associated mortality.[33] Risks include:
- Hemothorax, pneumothorax, or thrombophlebitis, all related to complications of vascular access (see Chapter 2)
- Malignant ventricular arrhythmias induced during the period of catheter manipulation (2.3% ventricular flutter or fibrillation); the risk of arrhythmia is greater when a temporary pacemaker is introduced in the setting of acute myocardial infarction
- New pericardial friction rub (5.3%) (presumed right ventricular wall penetration or perforation)
- Right ventricular perforation (2.1%) (documented by loss of pacing)
- Cardiac tamponade necessitating pericardiocentesis (0.1%)

Equipment for temporary pacing

The following equipment is needed for temporary pacemaker insertion:
- Basic venous access tray (Chapter 2)
- Catheter introducer set (dilator, sheath, guidewire)
- Sterile sleeve
- Pacing catheter
- Fluoroscopy unit
- Electrocardiograph (well grounded)
- Pacemaker generator
- Emergency equipment as for permanent pacemaker (p. 291)

Personnel

Temporary pacemaker insertion requires the following personnel:
- Physician experienced in vascular access, catheter techniques, and pacing
- Nurse assistant and radiology technician if fluoroscopy is used

Temporary pacing catheter

The most commonly used pacing catheter is a 6 Fr bipolar catheter, which is relatively stiff and requires manipulation under fluoroscopy. Once properly positioned, it tends to be quite stable. The flow-directed, balloon-tip 4 or 5 Fr catheter is much more flexible and may be manipulated without fluoroscopy, especially if introduced via a central vein. It is reported to be associated with a shorter insertion time, lower incidence of catheter displacement, and lower incidence of serious ventricular arrhythmias during insertion.[34]

Table 13-5. Advantages and disadvantages of temporary pacing electrode insertion sites

Entry site	Advantages	Disadvantages
Basilic vein	No risk of hemothorax or pneumothorax Easily accessible by cutdown or percutaneous approach	Pacing catheter less stable Higher incidence of cardiac perforation than catheters placed via a more central location Fluoroscopy necessary
Femoral vein	Easy access to right heart using fluoroscopy Rapid insertion time Reusable access site	Increased risk of thrombophlebitis (heparin anticoagulation is frequently used) Can be dislodged by leg movement Fluoroscopy necessary
Subclavian vein	Easy accessibility Good stability, leaves the patient's extremities unencumbered Rapid insertion time Reusable access site	Small risk of hemothorax or pneumothorax during entry Risk of subclavian artery puncture
Internal jugular vein	Direct route to right side of heart, especially with right internal jugular; in emergency, better success without fluoroscopy Satisfactory stability of pacing catheter Rapid insertion time Reusable access site Complications less than via the subclavian vein	Risk of carotid artery puncture Can be dislodged with head motion Small risk of hemothorax and pneumothorax

Placement of pacing catheter using fluoroscopic guidance

1. Explain the procedure to the patient and obtain consent if possible.

2. For anatomic and technical details of venous access, see Chapter 2. The advantages and disadvantages of the different venous access routes are listed in Table 13-5.

Under fluoroscopic guidance, advance the pacing catheter to the right atrium, then through the tricuspid valve and into the right ventricle. This is easier if, before insertion, you bend the last 2 or 3 inches of the catheter at almost a 90° angle to the body of the catheter. Frequently, the catheter arcs toward the right ventricular outflow tract. If this occurs, retract the catheter slightly and rotate it gently while the patient takes a deep breath. This usually drops the pacing catheter into the right ventricular apex.

Alternatively, withdraw the catheter into the right atrium, form a loop against the lateral wall of the right atrium, rotate the catheter, and advance it through the tricuspid valve into the apex of the right ventricle (Fig. 13-10).

In some instances the catheter may enter the posteriorly located coronary sinus and simulate a right ventricular position on anteroposterior fluoroscopy. If in doubt, rotate the fluoroscope to a lateral view to ascertain if the position of the pacing catheter is anterior (right ventricle) or posterior (coronary sinus). Fig. 13-5 compares the fluoroscopic views of the two positions. Note that in the anteroposterior view both positions appear to be almost identical, whereas in the lateral view the coronary sinus position is easily distinguished from the right ventricular position.

Transvenous placement without fluoroscopic guidance

Transvenous placement without fluoroscopy has a very limited role in modern pacing. Both ECG-guided placement and blind placement have been performed in emergency situations. When these approaches are used only very flexible catheters, such as the 4 Fr balloon-

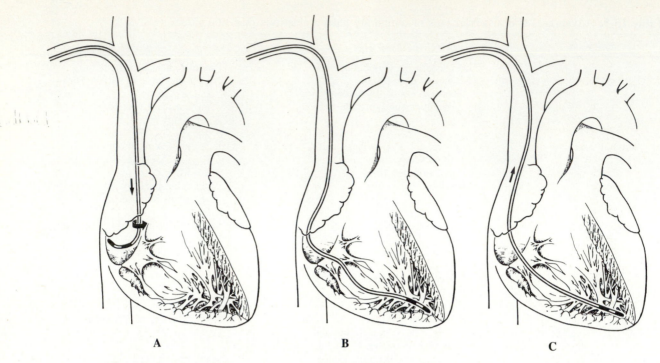

Fig. 13-10. Positioning of the pacing electrode. If the pacing catheter does not readily drop into the right ventricular apex, withdraw the catheter into the right atrium and form a loop against the lateral wall of the right atrium, rotate the catheter counterclockwise **(A),** and advance it through the tricuspid valve into the apex of the right ventricle. Next, gently advance it into the trabeculae **(B).** Gentle traction on the lead confirms anchoring **(C).**

directed catheters, should be utilized. For frank emergencies (asystole, profound bradycardia unresponsive to medication) transcutaneous or transthoracic pacing may be preferred.

ECG guidance

1. Insert the pacing catheter, preferably by the internal jugular route, and advance it to the superior vena cava.

2. Connect the distal terminal of the pacing catheter via alligator clips to the V lead of a grounded electrocardiograph.

3. Advance the catheter while monitoring the intracardiac electrogram(s), checking for the characteristic ECGs obtained from different positions in the heart.[35] The P wave, large and inverted in the superior vena cava, becomes biphasic in the mid-right atrium. As the lead enters the right ventricle, the P wave becomes small, whereas the amplitude of the QRS complex increases (Fig. 13-11). Note that contact with the ventricular wall is documented by ST segment elevation on the intracardiac electrogram (injury current). If the pacing catheter enters the pulmonary artery outflow tract, the P wave becomes negative and the QRS amplitude decreases. If this occurs, withdraw the catheter into the right ventricle and readvance it.

Blind placement of pacing catheter

If an electrocardiograph is not available, the pacing catheter may be inserted without such guidance.

1. Insert a pacing catheter preferably by the internal jugular route, as described in Chapter 2, and advance it to the superior vena cava.

2. Connect the pacing catheter to the pacemaker generator and turn the pacing rate to twice the intrinsic heart rate. Set the milliamperage at a level that is too low to capture (i.e., less than 0.2 mA).

3. Turn the pacemaker on; if the patient has an intrinsic rhythm, the pacemaker should sense but not pace.

4. Inflate the balloon and advance the pacing catheter into the right ventricle.

5. Deflate the balloon; increase output to 4 to 5 mA.

6. Advance the catheter until capture is achieved or for an additional 10 cm, whichever occurs first. If capture has not occurred at the additional 10 cm, withdraw the catheter 10 cm and begin again.

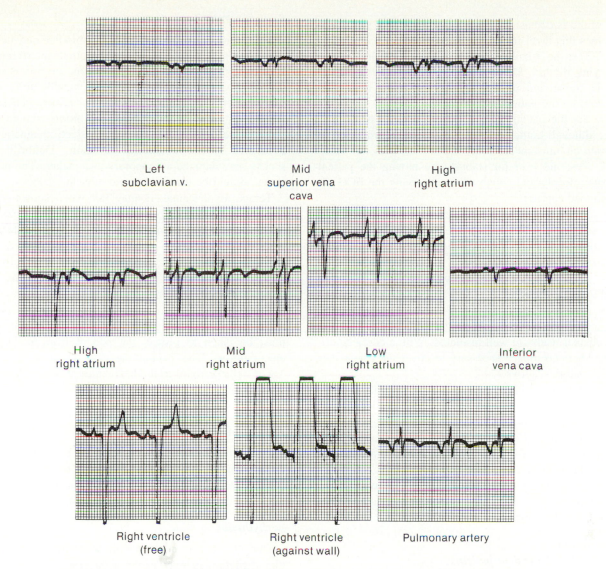

| Left | Mid | High |
| subclavian v. | superior vena cava | right atrium |

| High | Mid | Low | Inferior |
| right atrium | right atrium | right atrium | vena cava |

| Right ventricle (free) | Right ventricle (against wall) | Pulmonary artery |

Fig. 13-11. As the pacing catheter approaches the right atrium, the amplitude of the P waves progressively increases. Because atrial depolarization is inferiorly directed in this patient, P waves recorded above the atria have a negative deflection, whereas those low in the atria and in the inferior vena cava are positive. As the catheter enters the ventricle, the QRS amplitude increases markedly, and a QS complex is inscribed. When the catheter tip touches the endocardial surface, marked ST segment elevation is seen. As the electrode passes into the pulmonary artery, the QRS amplitude diminishes, and a negative P wave is inscribed because the catheter tip is again above the level of the atria. (From Bing, O.H.L., McDowell, J.W., Hantman, J., and Messer, J.V.: Pacemaker placement by electrocardiographic monitoring. Reprinted by permission of the New England Journal of Medicine **287:**651, 1972.)

Initiating pacing

1. After achieving a satisfactory right ventricular position (confirmed by fluoroscopy or intracardiac electrogram), connect the pacing catheter, using a sterile connecting cable, to the external pulse generator.

2. Test the pacing threshold by turning on the pulse generator at a moderately high output (5 mA) and at a rate higher than the patient's intrinsic rate. After satisfactory capture is achieved, gradually reduce the output until capture is lost. This milliampere level is the patient's pacing threshold (i.e., the lowest energy at which consistent capture is achieved). This is usually less than 1 mA. Repeat the step to be sure that the

threshold is consistent. The output should be set at 3 to 4 times this level for consistent capture.

3. Test the sensing function if the patient has an underlying rhythm. Do this by placing the system in demand mode and decreasing the rate until it is suppressed by the patient's rhythm.

4. Set the pacing rate—usually 70 to 80 beats/minute, although higher or lower rates may be preferred in certain circumstances.

5. Test the lead for stability by having the patient breathe deeply and cough while observing the ECG for continued capture.

6. Securely fix the pacing catheter to the skin with a 4-0 silk suture. Tension on the lead can be prevented by forming a loop in the catheter and securing it with this suture.

7. Cover the insertion site with antibiotic ointment and a sterile dressing.

8. Assess pacemaker function again.

9. The lead connection to the pacemaker and the pacemaker itself are well insulated. With modern equipment, it is no longer necessary to cover the pacemaker with a surgical glove.

10. Obtain a chest radiograph to document pacemaker position in the apex of the right ventricle and to exclude pneumothorax.

11. Obtain a 12-lead ECG. An LBBB pattern with left-axis deviation further confirms correct placement in the right ventricle. An RBBB pattern raises the suspicion of coronary sinus placement or intraventricular septal penetration but may also occur with some right ventricular locations.

Precautions
Pacemaker-dependent patients

Pacemaker insertion in pacemaker-dependent patients must be done quickly. Have the pacemaker connected to the pacing electrode and ready to pace during the insertion procedure. In patients with LBBB, special attention is required because manipulation of the pacing leads may induce RBBB, resulting in complete heart block and asystole. In these patients, use fluoroscopy whenever possible. For "blind" insertion, or insertion with ECG guidance, use the internal jugular or subclavian vein and a balloon-tip flotation catheter.

Wound care

The entry site should be kept meticulously clean. The wound should be inspected daily for evidence of infection. An antibiotic ointment and a clean dressing should be applied daily.

Environmental hazards

Most temporary pacing leads are bipolar and hence have minimal susceptibility to external interference. However, the external pulse generators are not as well shielded from interference as the implantable units. Because patients with temporary pacemakers are generally monitored, any inappropriate inhibition should be promptly recognized. On the whole, electromagnetic interference is not a clinical problem. Defibrillatory shocks may damage a temporary pacemaker. The pacemaker should be carefully tested after any shocks.

Temporary pacemakers may fail when subjected to hyperbaric conditions at 50 to 60 psi, whereas permanent pacemakers, hermetically sealed, can withstand pressures of at least up to 100 psi. Thus temporary pacing under hyperbaric conditions may be accomplished by using a permanent pacemaker attached to the patient's temporary external leads.[36]

Because the lead terminals of the temporary pacemaker are outside of the patient's body, special care must be taken to protect the patient from accidental electrocution. The pacing catheter provides a direct low-resistance route to the heart through which leakage currents may be introduced. Safeguards against leakage are discussed in Chapter 21.

Complications

For complications of vascular access and central catheterization, see Chapters 2 and 4. Complications associated with pacing include arrythmias, failure to capture, and myocardial perforation or tamponade.

Arrhythmias

During insertion of the pacing lead, atrial or ventricular arrhythmias may occur as a result of excessive catheter manipulations. Sustained arrhythmias with hemodynamic deterioration may require cardioversion or defibrillation. Recurrent arrhythmias may force reconsideration of the need for a standby pacer, but arrhythmias should not prevent insertion of a mandatory pacer.

Failure to capture or sense

Failure to capture may often be corrected by increasing the output (milliamperes) of the pacemaker. Failure to sense can often be corrected by adjusting the sensitivity of the unit. If these maneuvers are not sufficient, then the pacing catheter requires repositioning for failure to pace. Failure to sense may or may not justify repositioning, depending on the clinical situation. If a sterile sleeve has been used during the insertion, this repositioning may be accomplished without inserting a new electrode.

Myocardial perforation and tamponade

Myocardial perforation is suggested by loss of capture, intercostal or diaphragmatic stimulation, and occasionally pericardial friction rub. Interventricular septal perforation is suggested when the configuration of the paced beats changes from LBBB to RBBB. Perforation may be detected by evaluating the recording of electrograms from the pacing catheter. An electrogram with a positive R wave, mimicking a lead V_3 or V_4, suggests perforation. Perforation is treated by gently withdrawing the pacing catheter. If the patient is receiving anticoagulants, these are withheld, and the patient is closely monitored.

Pericardial tamponade is a rare complication, even in cases of documented perforation. If it does occur it must be treated with immediate pericardiocentesis and drainage (see Chapter 10).

Special considerations
External transcutaneous pacing

External cardiac pacing for asystole was introduced in 1952. It was subsequently abandoned because of the associated painful skeletal muscle stimulation. However, recently Zoll and associates[37] introduced a device for external pacing that appears to be effective and is gaining wide use. This external pacing device is capable of functioning in either the fixed-rate or demand mode. The device contains an ECG monitor, which permits sensing of the patient's intrinsic rhythm. The pacing stimulus is delivered through two large electrodes, which are moistened with tap water and applied to the patient after careful cleaning of the skin to remove salt and natural oils. The larger posterior electrode is attached in the left subscapular area, and the anterior electrode is placed in a position close to the lower left sternal edge, permitting the least pectoral muscle contraction during the stimulation. The pacemaker stimulus is a 40 msec impulse that can be delivered at any rate up to 180 stimuli/minute and at any current up to 140 mA. The operator determines the pacing rate and current with the use of dials on the pacemaker.

This device has been shown to be effective and generally well tolerated. Pacing can be maintained for more than 30 minutes. This may become the pacing method of choice during cardiopulmonary resuscitation (CPR) in asystolic cardiac arrest. In addition, the external pacemaker is likely to achieve wider use in patients considered to be at risk of developing high-degree conduction disturbances and allows insertion of an invasive pacing electrode only if bradyarrhythmias develop. The external pacing device is not suitable in patients with chest trauma or flail chest and is not well tolerated for prolonged periods.

Transthoracic pacing

Emergency pacing for asystolic cardiac arrest can be accomplished by a transthoracic technique of electrode insertion.[38] CPR is briefly suspended, and the lower sternal area is quickly swabbed with Betadine. A 10 cm cardiac needle attached to a syringe is inserted in a subxiphoid position and angled toward the left shoulder in a manner similar to pericardiocentesis. Blood return indicates entry into the right ventricle. A transthoracic pacing electrode is threaded through the needle and then gently pulled back so that the V or J at the distal end of the pacemaker makes contact with the right ventricle. The lead is then attached to the pacemaker unit. Transthoracic pacing generally has been used as a last resort and has a very poor salvage rate. It is associated with a high incidence of pneumothorax and hemopericardium. Transcutaneous pacing is likely to replace transthoracic pacing in these circumstances. The ease of applying the transcutaneous noninvasive pacemakers should lead to earlier use of pacing during asystolic arrest and may improve survival rates.

Combined temporary pacing and hemodynamic monitoring

Standard balloon flotation catheters for right-sided hemodynamic monitoring are available with ring electrodes along the body of the catheter designed to permit ventricular and atrial pacing. Ventricular pacing is usually more successful than atrial pacing. However, secure and reliable pacing capture in either chamber is neither consistently nor easily achieved. These catheters may be particularly useful in patients with LBBB who undergo catheterization in the right side of the heart. In these patients there is a small risk of catheter-induced complete heart block, and the availability of pacing electrodes may obviate the insertion of a separate temporary pacemaker. However, the combined pacing/hemodynamic catheter is not the pacemaker of choice in pacemaker-dependent patients. Newer designs may improve the reliability of these catheters

Atrioventricular sequential temporary pacing

Although most temporary pacing units use a single ventricular lead, preservation of AV synchrony may be of clinical importance.[39-41] This has been most clearly

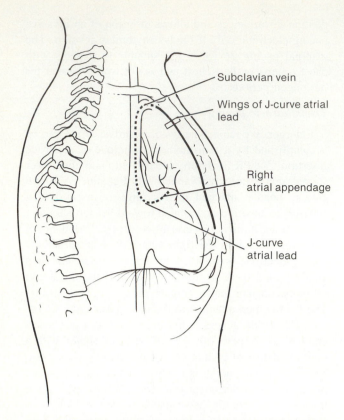

Fig. 13-12. Sagittal view showing the orientation of the wings and the distal J tip in the atrial appendage.

documented in patients with right ventricular infarction and immediately after open heart surgery but may also be important in patients with ventricular hypertrophy.

A variety of atrial pacing leads, including coronary sinus catheters and catheters that expand into a loop or spring into a Y configuration, have been used. The best-documented temporary atrial lead has a preformed J configuration similar to those used for permanent atrial pacing. J-shaped leads for temporary atrial pacing have wings perpendicular to the J-shaped portion of the lead. The lead is inserted directly into a sheath in the subclavian or internal jugular vein and positioned in the superior vena cava. The sheath is peeled back, and the lead is then pulled back under fluoroscopic guidance, or even blindly, until capture is obtained. Fig. 13-12 is a sagittal view illustrating the J tip in the atrial appendage and the wings secured with the skin side against the chest wall. This lead is successful in 95% of cases and has been shown to have excellent stability. External pulse generators for AV sequential pacing are commercially available. In addition, DDD pacemakers have been adapted for external use.

Pacing termination of atrial flutter

Rapid atrial pacing is effective treatment for termination of classical (type I) atrial flutter (atrial rate 300/ minute, saw-tooth configuration in the inferior leads).[42,43] Atypical (type II) atrial flutter (> 350 beats/ minute) or flutter/fibrillation cannot be interrupted by rapid atrial pacing. In classic atrial flutter, normal sinus rhythm is restored in a large majority of patients; however, some will be converted to atrial fibrillation.

Pacing treatment of atrial flutter is preferred to cardioversion in cases of suspected digitalis toxicity and suspected tachycardia-bradycardia syndrome. Pacing conversion does not require the sedation necessary for cardioversion and is preferred when sedation is undesirable. It is also the preferred method after cardiac surgery or during cardiac catheterization, when an avenue for atrial stimulation is readily available.

The procedure for atrial pacing to convert atrial flutter includes the steps described below.

1. Fluoroscopically confirm stable atrial position (to avoid the danger of ventricular pacing at these rapid rates).

2. Use a special rapid atrial pacemaker capable of pacing at rates approaching 400 beats/minute.

3. Establish bipolar atrial pacing at a rate faster than the flutter rate.

4. In general, it is necessary for the pacemaker to maintain a pacing rate of 115% to 125% of the atrial rate for a mean of 10 seconds.

5. When the flutter is terminated, you may see a change in configuration of the atrial-paced beats. However, with standard paper speeds this may be difficult to discern.

6. After establishing atrial pacing, abruptly terminate the pacing and see if the flutter has been converted. If the patient develops bradycardia, atrial pacing at physiologic rates may be necessary.

7. If the first attempt at atrial pacing conversion is unsuccessful, repeated attempts with more rapid rates and more prolonged pacing are warranted.

Acknowledgment: The first author is grateful to Dr. Manuel Estioko and the other members of the division of cardiothoracic surgery of the Mount Sinai Hospital, New York, N.Y., for expert instruction in the surgical aspects of pacemaker implantation.

REFERENCES

1. Elmquist, R., and Senning, A.: An implantable pacemaker for the heart, Proceedings of the Second International Conference of Medical-Electrical Engineers, London, 1959, Iliffe & Sons, Ltd.
2. Phibbs, B., et al. Indications for pacing in the treatment of brady-arrhythmias, J.A.M.A. **252:**1307, 1984.

3. Fry, R.L., et al.: Guidelines for permanent cardiac pacemaker implantation, J. Am. Coll. Cardiol. **4**:434, 1984.

4. Parsonnet, V., Furman, S., Smyth, N.P.D., and Bilitch, M.: Optimal resources for implantable cardiac pacemakers. Pacemaker study group, Circulation **68**:227A-244A, 1983.

5. Furman, S.: Electromagnetic interference, PACE **5**:1, 1982.

6. Levine, P.A., et al.: Myopotential inhibition of unipolar lithium pacemakers, Chest **82**:461-465, 1982.

7. Levine, P.A., and Klein, M.D.: Myopotential inhibition of unipolar pacemakers: a disease of technologic progress, Ann. Intern. Med. **98**:101-103, 1983.

8. Ludmer, P.L., and Goldschlager, N.: Cardiac pacing in the 1980s, N. Engl. J. Med. **311**:1671-1680, 1984.

9. Furman, S.: Newer modes of cardiac pacing, Mod. Con. Cardiovasc. Dis. **52**:9, 1983.

10. Parsonnet, V., and Rodgers, T.: The present status of programmable pacemakers, Prog. Cardiovasc. Dis. **23**:401-420, 1981.

11. Barold, S.S., Ong, L.S., Falkoff, M.D., and Heinle, R.A.: Selection of optimal pacing system for the individual patient. In Rapaport, E., editor: Cardiology update, 1981 edition, Squibb & Sons.

12. Muers, M.F., Arnold, A.G., and Sleight, P.: Prophylactic antibiotics for cardiac pacemaker implantation. A prospective trial, Br. Heart J. **46**:539-544, 1981.

13. Miller, F.A., Holmes, D.R., Gersh, B.J., and Maloney, J.D.: Permanent transvenous pacemaker implantation via the subclavian vein, Mayo Clin. Proc. **55**:309-314, 1980.

14. Duffin, E.G. Jr., and Zipes, D.P.: Artificial cardiac pacemaker. In Andreoli, K.G., Fowkes, V.K., Zipes, D.P., and Wallace, A.G., editors: Comprehensive cardiac care, St. Louis, 1983, The C.V. Mosby Co.

15. Naito, M., et al.: Reevaluation of the role of atrial systole to cardiac hemodynamics: evidence for pulmonary venous regurgitation during abnormal atrioventricular sequencing, Am. Heart J. **105**:295-302, 1983.

16. Ausubel, K., and Furman, S.: The pacemaker syndrome, Ann. Intern. Med. **103**:420-429, 1985.

17. Choo, M.H., et al.: Permanent pacemaker infections: characterization and management, Am. J. Cardiol. **48**:559, 1981.

18. Lewis, A.B., et al.: Update on infections involving permanent pacemakers: characterization and management, J. Thorac. Cardiovasc. Surg. **84**:758-763, 1985.

19. Phibbs, B., and Marriott, H.J.L.: Complications of permanent transvenous pacing, N. Engl. J. Med. **312**:1428-1432, 1985.

20. Eisenhauer, A.C.: Practical approach to pacemaker implantation, Intell. Rep. Cardiac Pacing Electrophysiol. **2**:1-7, 1984.

21. Sowton, E.: Environmental hazards for pacemaker patients, J. Roy. Coll. Phys. London **16**:159-164, 1982.

22. O'Brien, E.: Environmental dangers for the patient with a pacemaker, Br. Med. J. **285**:1677-1678, 1982.

23. Rozanski, J.J., Blankstein, R.L., and Lister, J.W.: Pacemaker arrythmias: myopotential triggering of pacemaker-mediated tachycardia, PACE **6**:795, 1983.

24. Pourhamidi, A.H.: Radiation effect on implanted pacemakers, Chest **84**:499-500, 1984.

25. Quertermous, T., Megahy, M.S., Das Gupa, D.S., and Griem, M.L.: Pacemaker failure resulting from radiation damage, Radiology **148**:257-258, 1983.

26. Katzenberg, C.A., Marcus, F.I., Heusinkveld, R.S., and Mammana, R.B.: Pacemaker failure due to radiation therapy, PACE **5**:156-159, 1982.

27. Zimmermann, B.H., and Faul, D.D.: Artifacts and hazards in NMR imaging due to metal implants and cardiac pacemakers, Diagn. Imag. Clin. Med. **53**:53-56, 1984.

28. Fetter, J., et al.: The effects of nuclear magnetic resonance imagers on external and implantable pulse generators, PACE **7**:720-727, 1984.

29. Erlebacher, J.A., Cahill, P.T., Pannizzo, F., and Knowles, R.J.R.: Effect of magnetic resonance imaging on DDD pacemakers, Am. J. Cardiol. **57**:437-440, 1986.

30. Higgins, C.: Personal communication, 1986.

31. Donaldson, R.M., and Rickards, A.F.: Toward multisensor pacing, Am. Heart J. **106**:1454-1458, 1983.

32. Furman, S.: Pacemaker re-use, PACE **8**:159-160, 1985.

33. Haynes, J.K., Holmes, D.R., and Harrison, C.E.: Five year experience with temporary pacemaker therapy in the coronary care unit, Mayo Clin. Proc. **58**:122-126, 1983.

34. Lang, R., et al.: The use of the balloon-tipped floating catheter in temporary transvenous cardiac pacing, PACE **4**:491-496, 1981.

35. Bing, O.H.L., McDowell, J.W., Hantman, J.N., and Messer, J.V.: Pacemaker placement by electrocardiographic monitoring, N. Engl. J. Med. **287**:651, 1972.

36. Kratz, J.M., Blackburn, J.G., Leman, R.B., and Crawford, F.A.: Cardiac pacing under hyperbaric conditions, Ann. Thorac. Surg. **36**:66-68, 1983.

37. Zoll, P.M., et al.: External noninvasive temporary cardiac pacing: clinical trials, Circulation **71**:937-944, 1985.

38. Roberts, J.R., et al.: Successful use of emergency transthoracic pacing in bradysystolic cardiac arrest, Ann. Emerg. Med. **13**:227-283, 1984.

39. Littleford, P.O.: Physiologic temporary pacing: techniques and indications. In Schroeder, J.S., editor: Invasive cardiology, Philadelphia, 1985, F.A. Davis Co.

40. Love, J.C., Haffajee, C.I., Gore, J.M., and Alpert, J.S.: Reversibility of hypotension and shock by atrial or atrioventricular sequential pacing in patients with right ventricular infarction, Am. Heart J. **108**:5-13, 1984.

41. Littleford, P.O., Curry, R.C., Schwartz, K.M., and Pepine, C.J.: Clinical evaluation of a new temporary atrial pacing catheter: results in 100 patients, Am. Heart J. **107**:237-240, 1984.

42. Waldo, A.L., and MacLean, W.A.H.: Diagnosis and treatment of cardiac arrhythmias following open heart surgery. Emphasis on the use of atrial and ventricular epicardial wire electrodes, Mount Kisco, N.Y., 1980, Futura Publishing Co.

43. Wiener, I.: Pacing techniques in the treatment of tachycardias, Ann. Intern. Med. **93**:326, 1980.

Chapter Fourteen

Implantation of the automatic implantable cardioverter/defibrillator

DAVID S. CANNOM

ROGER A. WINKLE

Most patients who are resuscitated from an episode of sudden cardiac death or sustained ventricular tachycardia (VT) can now be treated using serial electrophysiologic testing as a guide to drug therapy. Recurrence rates are low if an antiarrhythmic regimen can be found that prevents induction of VT. Patients failing serial drug testing have a high recurrence rate (approximately 50% per year). Most clinicians now refer such patients for either experimental antiarrhythmic therapy or electric intervention. The most promising of the electric interventions (including tachycardia converting pacemakers and intraoperative mapping) has been the automatic implantable cardioverter/defibrillator (AICD).

The development of the concept and implementation of the automatic implantable defibrillator (AID), and subsequently the AICD, has largely been the work of Dr. Michel Mirowski[1-3] and his coworkers at Sinai Hospital in Baltimore. Their work began in the late 1960s and met much initial professional skepticism. Most thought that the energy needed for successful defibrillation was more than could be stored in a miniaturized device.

However, in early canine work Mirowski showed that the actual energy requirement for direct defibrillation was only in the range of 30 to 50 joules (J).[4] He also demonstrated that to restore sinus rhythm it was only necessary to depolarize a critical cell mass, not the entire heart.[5]

Since the inception of the implantable defibrillator concept, many of its design features have successfully been addressed, including the size and location of the lead system, the way in which ventricular fibrillation is sensed, and the pulsing sequence that is used to convert ventricular fibrillation. Additionally, cardioversion capability has been added to treat VT in those patients in whom VT precedes ventricular fibrillation (VF).

In 1980 the first clinical studies were initiated, incorporating strict criteria for patient inclusion. The patient had to have survived two episodes of cardiac arrest, with at least one episode of documented VF during one of the arrests. Additionally, the documented VF had to have occurred while the patient was receiving antiarrhythmic therapy. Such stringent criteria allowed only the highest risk patients to be treated during the initial clinical trials. Nonetheless, the device functioned well, and in 1982 a second-generation cardioverter/defibrillator with an improved sensing circuit capable of sensing both VT and VF became available. Over the next 2 years, 25 centers implanted more than 400 devices with remarkably few technical malfunctions or clinical failures.[6-14] The FDA carefully monitored that activity and in 1985 then declared that the device was no longer experimental and could be implanted without agency monitoring.

The remarkable development of the AICD in the past 17 years into a highly effective clinical device comes at a time when an increasing number of patients at risk for sudden death are being identified and when the limitations of other possible therapies, including endocardial surgery and drugs such as amiodarone, are becoming more evident. Implantation of the device is a relatively simple procedure if certain guidelines are followed.[15]

AICD GENERATOR

The AICD generator consists of a sensing device, batteries, and energy storage capacitors. It is 11.2 × 7.1 × 2.5 cm, weighs 292 g, and is housed in a titanium case. The header is made of epoxy (Fig. 14-1).

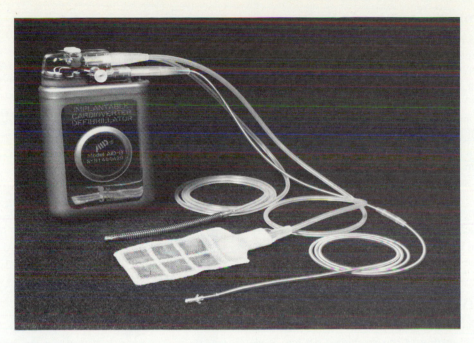

Fig. 14-1. AICD unit attached to its three leads. From top to bottom are the spring lead (right atrium), the apical patch (10 cm² small size), and the bipolar lead (right ventricular apex).

The device senses arrhythmias on the basis of two independent algorithms—heart rate and the probability density function (PDF)—both of which must be satisfied for the device to discharge.

The rate detection circuit senses an averaged heart rate, which remains above a preset value (usually 155 beats/minute), long enough to satisfy the sensing circuit. However, using rate criteria alone, the device cannot distinguish supraventricular tachycardia (SVT) from VT.

The PDF diagnoses VT or VF based on the amount of time the QRS (as sensed from right atrium to the cardiac apex or between two ventricular patch electrodes) spends away from the isoelectric baseline. The ECG waveform in sinus rhythm or SVT without aberration spends most of its time on the isoelectric baseline. Wide complex VT or coarse VF are away from the baseline a high percentage of the sense time and produce a sinusoidal waveform that easily satisfies the morphologic sensing criteria.

In the standard model AID-B (Cardiac Pacemakers, Inc.) unit both rate and PDF criteria must be met before the device is activated; nonetheless some narrow QRS rhythms, which appear sinusoidal to the device as sensed by the transcardiac leads, are still shocked. Rate-only units (model AID-BR) are also available; these units will shock any rhythm above the chosen rate cutoff. Follow-up studies comparing the AID-B and AID-BR units have shown no difference in long-term patient survival.

The AICD usually requires 5 to 20 seconds to sense VT or VF and then 5 to 15 seconds to charge its energy storage capacitors. It then delivers a 23 to 28 J shock and, if necessary, second, third, and fourth countershocks of 28 to 37 J each after additional detection and charging periods of 10 to 35 seconds. If the arrhythmia persists after the fourth shock, the unit will not recycle. This feature prevents multiple shocks in misdiagnosed rhythms. High-energy units delivering 28 to 37 J for all four shocks in the sequence are also available.

ELECTRODES

The electrodes for the AICD comprise three types of leads—a superior vena caval spring lead, a transvenous bipolar electrode, and the ventricular patch lead. The superior vena caval spring lead is 100 cm long and has a 10 cm² surface area; its lead wire is color-coded black. Rate sensing is either by a transvenous lead placed in the right ventricular apex or by a bipolar epicardial screw-in pair of leads on the left ventricle.

The ventricular patch lead is either 10 cm² (small patch) or 20 cm² (large patch) and is color-coded red. The patch is made of titanium mesh and is covered with silicone on its shiny side. Its mesh (rough) side is placed on the pericardium or myocardium during surgery.

ACTIVE MODE

In the active mode the AICD can sense arrhythmias and deliver converting shocks. The AICD is shipped in the inactive (off) mode and is turned on by placing a special donut-shaped magnet over the upper half of the generator for 30 seconds. When the generator is in the inactive mode and the magnet is applied, a continuous, somewhat shrill tone is initially heard (transmitted from the device via a piezoelectric crystal). After 30 seconds it changes from a continuous to a beeping tone, synchronous with each QRS when connected to the implanted lead system. The magnet is then removed from the unit and the device is ready for clinical use. The status of the device can be checked at any time before or after implant by placing a magnet over the generator and listening for a continuous tone (inactive) or beeping tone (active).

ELECTROPHYSIOLOGIC TEST MODE

The electrophysiologic (EP) mode of the AICD is used during final testing of the implanted device. It allows the use of lengthy (>3 seconds) ventricular induction protocols that would cause the unit to charge were its sensing circuit not blinded. The EP test mode is programmed by turning the unit off with the magnet, waiting 10 seconds, then reactivating the device by placing the magnet over the generator for 30 seconds. When the tone changes from continuous to synchronized beeping (signifying activation), the magnet is left in place on the generator and the pacing protocol is then carried out. A synchronous tone is heard with each pacing artifact. Once the arrhythmia has been induced (e.g., by 4 seconds of burst pacing at a cycle length of 250 msec; such pacing would normally initiate a charge), the magnet is removed from the generator. Only then does sensing of the arrhythmia begin. The sensing cycle takes longer in this mode, possibly up to 30 to 45 seconds or more in VT. Use of a magnet to inhibit the sensing circuit adds approximately 10 seconds to detection time (2 to 5 seconds for gain control to focus and stabilize and 5 seconds for sensing circuits to begin detection). In VF, detection time is shorter.

MAGNET TEST

During routine follow-up, use of a special external testing device (AIDCHECK-B; Fig. 14-2) and a donut magnet allows noninvasive estimation of the life of the batteries and determination of the number of shocks delivered to the patient. The small probe of the AID-CHECK is placed near the upper end of the device (over the region of the epoxy header), and the magnet is applied for 2 to 5 seconds just below the probe over

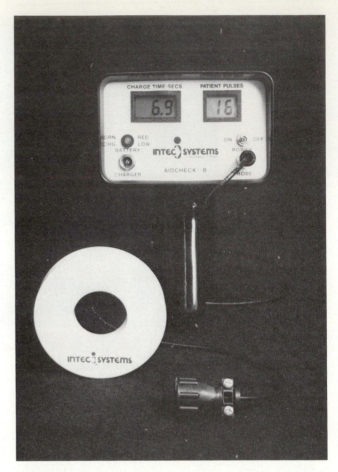

Fig. 14-2. AIDCHECK device attached to its probe, which for magnet tests is placed near the raised circular area on the front of the AICD. The digital charge time of the device (in seconds) is displayed on the left side of the AIDCHECK. Patient pulses are seen on the right side. The defibrillator magnet is in the lower left corner.

the upper half of the pulse generator. Several QRS synchronous tones indicate proper positioning of the magnet. A charging cycle is initiated when the magnet is removed, and the AIDCHECK displays the charge time and patient pulses. The magnet test charge is dumped internally, and the total number of charges stored in the battery is reduced by one. This discharge does not appear as an additional patient pulse during subsequent AIDCHECKs; therefore magnet test charges must be recorded separately in the patient's record.

TERMINOLOGY
Redirect

Redirect is the feature by which a charge can be directed away from the patient and into the device if necessary. During EP testing, ventricular rhythms often

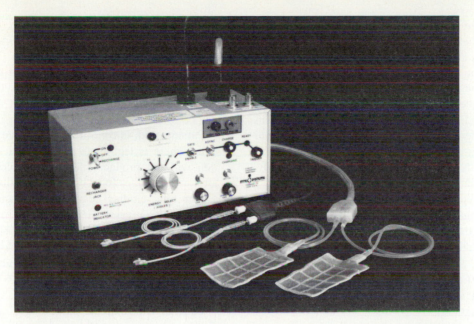

Fig. 14-3. The external cardioverter/defibrillator (ECD) box attached to a different set of leads than in Fig. 14-1. Two large patches are shown, along with two epicardial screw-on electrodes for rate sensing (rather than a right ventricular bipolar electrode). The ECD is used for determining DFTs at operation and for measuring electric signals between one spring/patch lead and the bipolar lead.

terminate after the unit has sensed the rhythm but before it discharges. Placing the magnet quickly over the upper portion of the device for only 2 to 3 seconds directs the charge internally rather than to the patient. A redirect is signaled by a rapid series of beeping tones (signifying that the device has been triggered to redirect). *Caution:* The magnet must be removed after the beeps are heard; otherwise the capacitor could be damaged by overcharging.

Defibrillation threshold

The defibrillation threshold (DFT) is the minimum amount of energy required for successful, reliable termination of an induced rhythm. It is measured at the time of implantation with the use of the external cardioverter/defibrillator (ECD) device (Fig. 14-3).

Sense time

Sense time (detect time) is the time from the onset of the arrhythmia to the initiation of the charging of the capacitors. Its duration is 2.5 to 5 seconds for VF and 5 to 20 seconds for VT.

Charge time

The charge time of the capacitor is under 10 seconds unless the battery is near its end of life. If a charge time greater than 10 seconds is detected, the magnet test should be repeated one or two times because charge times may be prolonged if the capacitor has not been charged for a long period of time. The AIDCHECK-B measures charge time during a magnet test or at implant testing.

INDICATIONS

The indications for AICD implantation have expanded in the past 2 to 3 years. In the early days of investigational use, patients were required to have survived two cardiac arrests before being eligible. The device is now recommended for the categories of patients described below.

Survivors of *sudden cardiac death* not associated with acute myocardial infarction, whose inducible arrhythmias are not controlled pharmacologically, are candidates for AICD implantation. The 1-year mortality without the AICD for this group of patients is 35% to 40% despite empiric antiarrhythmic therapy.

The AICD is also indicated for patients with more than one *cardiac arrest* whose arrhythmia cannot be induced during EP testing.

Patients with *sustained VT* who have had a clinical recurrence on conventional antiarrhythmic medications or who have failed serial EP testing but have not yet had a recurrent episode of VT while taking a drug known to be ineffective during EP studies benefit from AICD implantation. Episodes of sustained VT that would cause the unit to function should not occur more than 1 to 2 times per month for reasons of patient comfort. An example of such a case would be one in whom, after one episode of clinical VT, sustained VT remains easily inducible despite trials of procainamide, quinidine, or a beta-blocking drug. Especially important in this subgroup is the patient in whom standard type I agents have failed and long-term amiodarone therapy is being considered. Although amiodarone is more effective clinically than most other antiarrhythmic agents for recurrent VT, the incidence of serious side effects was previously underestimated. Most patients have an easier time with the AICD than with long-term, high-dose ($\geq$400 mg/day) amiodarone therapy. We generally prefer to implant an AICD rather than begin long-term amiodarone treatment.

Patients with long QT syndrome who have been resuscitated from sudden cardiac arrest are also candidates for AICD implantation.

Intraoperative mapping

Some patients for whom drug therapy has failed are candidates for intraoperative mapping and subendocardial resection of the arrhythmogenic focus rather than the AICD. Clinical criteria for selection of the operative candidates are not agreed on.

Electrically directed surgery is recommended for patients with coronary disease who have VT with one or two stable morphologic conditions and have an ejection fraction of approximately 40% or more. (Patients with polymorphic VT or with monomorphic VT and a low ejection fraction are currently referred for an AICD.)

Electrically directed surgery is also used for patients with very frequent or incessant VT for whom all drug treatments have failed. Such patients are not ideal candidates for intraoperative mapping because of high operative risk.

Patients having intraoperative mapping surgery should have two large ventricular patch leads placed without intracardiac leads at the time of their surgery. An epicardial bipolar pair should also be placed, and DFT measurements should then be performed if at all possible. Even though the precise meaning of these DFTs is uncertain, they do provide a baseline for future DFT determination if a pulse generator is later implanted.

Postoperatively, if the patient has recurrent arrhythmias or has inducible arrhythmias following EP studies, the remaining intracardiac leads and a pulse generator can be implanted.

CONTRAINDICATIONS

There are a few important contraindications to the use of the AICD.

Patients with frequent nonsustained or sustained VT that cannot be controlled with antiarrhythmic drugs may not be candidates because of frequent triggering of the device. Such cases are rare.

Patients with uncontrolled congestive heart failure, in which there is legitimate concern that AICD implantation will not produce substantial prolongation of life, are not candidates for AICD implantation. The Stanford 1-year total cardiac death rate in their VT/VF group with an AICD was 10.1%, nearly 10 times their annual rate of death from arrhythmia.[13] Most of the cardiac deaths occur in patients with a very low ejection fraction. The device should not be implanted unless the patient can be expected to have at least 6 to 12 months of productive life.

Patients with extreme psychologic uncertainty about the device are not candidates for AICD implantation.

Centers not having adequately trained personnel (electrophysiologist, cardiovascular surgeon, specially trained nurses) and operating room equipment to allow full EP studies and dedication to long-term patient follow-up should not implant the device.

EQUIPMENT

In the operating room the following equipment must be available:

- Anterior and posterior paddles for external cardioversion; the posterior paddle is placed under the left shoulder, and the anterior paddle kept sterile on the operating field (External paddles must be used when the AICD is connected to the implanted lead system!)
- A back-up pair of small, hand-held internal defibrillator paddles that may be applied directly to the heart if there are technical problems with the anteroposterior paddles; in such a case the AICD should not be connected or the electronics will be destroyed
- Two external defibrillators capable of delivering 400 J
- A programmable stimulator that can do both standard and ramp pacing
- A multichannel physiologic recorder with strip chart to display ECGs and intracardiac electrograms (Honeywell AR6); a six-channel magnetic tape interface is optional but not essential
- A device that will deliver AC or rectified AC fibrillating current for testing DFTs (e.g., operating room fibrillator box)
- The external cardioverter/defibrillator (ECD) box and accessories
- Appropriate cables to make connections between the

AICD generator, ECD box, and physiologic recorder (ECD accessories)
- AIDCHECK-B device
- Two sterile magnets
- Two sterile AIDCHECK probes for performing the magnet test after implantation but before the wound is closed.
- Two sets of bipolar sensing leads; these may be a single bipolar catheter for right ventricular apical sensing (Intec/Cardiac Pacemakers, Inc. [CPI]) or a bipolar pair of screw on leads for epicardial sensing (Intec/CPI); both should be available
- AICD pulse generator; ideally each center would have available the following units:

  Standard rate (>155 beats/minute), standard energy (AID-B)

  Rate only (>155 beats/minute), high energy (AID-BR)

  High rate (>175 beats/minute), standard energy

  Standard rate (>155 beats/minute), high energy
- Two standard SVC spring leads
- Four large ventricular patches
- Four regular-size ventricular patches
- Set of four monitoring leads with adaptor pins
- Subclavian vein puncture set
- A 14 Fr sheath and dilator set (for the spring lead) and a 9 Fr sheath and dilator set (for the bipolar transvenous lead)
- A pacing systems analyzer with appropriate sterile cable (e.g., CPI PSA) for evaluation of bipolar lead signals
- Portable fluoroscopy unit

PERSONNEL

Successful implantation of the device requires more than technical skills. The patient must be carefully prepared before operation. The team must have full working knowledge of the AICD, its indications, and techniques for implantation; and the institution must have the capability of carefully monitoring the patient during and after operation. Few centers in any metropolitan community will have this type of personnel-intensive cardiology service. Only by implanting devices frequently are skills maintained and the difficulties encountered at implantation mastered.

Members of the medical care team must include personnel with the skills described below.

• A cardiologist-electrophysiologist who has a thorough background in ventricular arrhythmia treatment and contemporary induction techniques should perform the implantation. Many implantations should be observed before the first is done.

• The cardiovascular surgeon should have a special interest in arrhythmias; this is important during DFT testing, which must be understood and cannot be rushed.

• The anesthesia team must be able to deal with hemodynamically unstable patients.

• The operating room nursing team should be familiar with ventricular arrhythmic surgery and the equipment required to perform such procedures to ensure proper instrumentation and safety to compromised cardiac patients.

• A nurse, ideally with a background in electrophysiology and EP testing, should be available to do the preoperative teaching, train nurses in the recovery area, coordinate data acquisition during the operation, and ensure the proper function of the physiologic recorder and tape system during surgery.

• Specialists in equipment performance and management from the manufacturer should be available to lend technical support during the first few cases.

• A clinical psychologist, social worker, or psychiatrist with a special interest in patients with life-threatening arrhythmias should be available.

• A cardiologist responsible for the patient's long-term follow-up is essential. A decision must be made postoperatively as to whether this physician will do the noninvasive follow-up magnet testing or whether this is the responsibility of the implanting physician.

The importance of careful preparation and teamwork cannot be overemphasized. Many technical problems can (and will!) occur at surgery; the problems can be minimized if the team is well prepared and experienced.

PATIENT PREPARATION
Before admission

Before admission for implantation of the device itself, the patient must undergo the following procedures:
- Complete hemodynamic and angiographic study so that the decision can be made about the need for either coronary artery or valvular surgery at the time of implant
- Thorough EP study, with careful notation of the induction programs and the rates and forms of the ventricular tachycardia(s) induced
- Maximal treadmill stress test to assess maximal heart rate with exercise and anticipate the postoperative need for a beta blocker to prevent the heart rate from reaching rates that may trigger the AICD
- Discontinuance of amiodarone for as long as possible before operation; amiodarone may interfere with successful defibrillation of VT/VF induced during intraoperative EP studies

Careful judgment about this last issue is crucial. If there is suspicion that the patient will be receiving amiodarone postoperatively, then the drug should be given right up to the time of surgery. By giving amiodarone, DFTs will accurately reflect any adverse impact the drug might have on DFTs. If the drug is withheld but then restarted sometime postoperatively, the patient's postoperative threshold could be altered unbeknown to the physician; the AICD might then not function appropriately.

Admission

During admission for implantation of the AICD itself the patient should undergo the following procedures.

1. Treat any congestive heart failure.
2. Test preoperative pulmonary function for the identification of underlying chronic obstructive pulmonary disease or interstitial lung disease. Optimal care of any underlying pulmonary disease is helpful in reducing postoperative complications.
3. Educate the patient and the family as to the function of the device, its potential usefulness, and problems that may arise. Alteration of body image by the device should be discussed openly with the patient. The current device is large and deforming; close-fitting clothing is not comfortable because of the generator, and bulging will be apparent when the patient is in beach attire.
4. Obtain informed consent.
5. Determine preoperative complete blood count, serum electrolytes, magnesium, blood urea nitrogen, prothrombin time, and partial thromboplastin time (PTT), and obtain chest radiograph and ECG.
6. Discuss the implantation with the patient's medical insurer and obtain preoperative authorization for an implantation, whenever this is required.
7. Check that the ECD box has been charged and will discharge appropriately.
8. Check the AIDCHECK-B for charge.
9. Check the operating room for the supplies that will be needed during the procedure.

PROCEDURE
Preparation

1. Before administering general anesthesia, connect the patient to the ECG cables, establish an intra-arterial pressure-monitoring line, and position the posterior defibrillating paddle below the left scapula.
2. Introduce a Swan-Ganz catheter from the right internal jugular vein, if needed.
3. Insert a Foley catheter.
4. Test the selected AICD with the AIDCHECK-B to ensure proper charge times and then inactivate it. (Record preimplant magnet test results.)

Insertion of leads

1. Administer general anesthesia and place the patient in a slight Trendelenburg position, with the left thorax elevated.
2. Make a limited skin incision under the left clavicle.
3. Enter the subclavian vein with a standard needle and position the guidewire in the mid-right atrium by fluoroscopy. If a transvenous sensing lead is to be used, enter the vein a second time and position a second guidewire in the mid–right atrium.
4. Place a 9 Fr sheath over either guidewire and through this advance the bipolar lead to the right ventricular apex; wedge the lead firmly in the ventricular apex. Be sure the lead is not in the coronary sinus.
5. Ensure adequate right ventricular apical monitoring capabilities by measuring pacing thresholds and R wave amplitude from the bipolar lead using a CPI PSA. The R wave amplitude should be greater than 5 mV, if possible, and the threshold less than 1 mA.
6. Pass a 14 Fr sheath over the other guidewire and pass the spring electrode through the sheath to the mid–right atrium. Half of the lead should be above and half below the junction of the superior vena cava and the right atrium. The lead usually falls easily into place. *Note:* Introduce the bipolar lead before the spring lead to prevent displacement of the spring lead.
7. Remove both sheaths and secure the spring lead with the supplied fixation device (lead anchor).
8. Tie the bipolar lead down well, using standard ties over the lead fixation sheath.

Thoracotomy

1. Return the patient to a flat position and perform a standard anterolateral thorocotomy through the fifth or sixth intercostal space. Use blunt dissection to free the cardiac apex from surrounding fatty tissue.
2. A choice must be made between beginning with a small (10 cm^2) or large (20 cm^2) patch. A spring/small patch configuration is effective in 75% of patients, but in 25% of patients it will not give adequate DFT measurements, necessitating another configuration. To save time, we favor beginning with a spring/large patch configuration because it is not possible clinically to identify the patients who will not obtain adequate DFTs with a spring/small patch configuration.
3. Sew the patch over the anterolateral left ventricle to the left ventricular side of the interventricular septum. Place the dull, rough side of the patch on the pericardium or myocardial surface and sew it on with 6 to 8 mattress sutures (2-0 Tycron suture). If epicardial sensing leads are used, sew them close together (no

more than 1 to 2 cm apart) on the anterobasal left ventricle.[16,17]

Note: Other surgical approaches can be used. A median sternotomy is used if bypass or valvular surgery is being done in conjunction with implantation of the AICD. Other centers have used a subxiphoid or subcostal approach. (Choices are based on criteria such as heart size and previous surgery.)

Initial electrophysiologic measurements

1. Tunnel the spring lead and bipolar lead into the thorax through the second intercostal space or directly subcutaneously.

2. Using the ECD box and its connections, display recordings of three ECG leads, an unfiltered spring/patch electrogram, an unfiltered bipolar electrogram, surface ECG, and the intra-arterial pressure on the physiologic recorder. Introduce 5 mV calibration signals from the ECD box. Obtain paper and magnetic tape recordings from all leads.

R wave amplitude: The R wave in the bipolar electrogram should ideally be 5 mV to ensure adequate sensing. This amplitude may be different during VT or VF. If it is less than 2 mV, a new electrode position (in the right ventricle or on the left ventricular epicardium) must be found. The spring/patch electrogram will look much like a surface ECG with a 1 to 10 mV R wave.

R wave duration: R wave duration should be less than 100 msec; if it is greater than 150 msec, improper sensing may occur.

Abdominal pocket

1. Make a horizontal or vertical skin incision approximately 10 cm long in the left abdominal wall slightly below the level of the umbilicus.

2. Use blunt dissection down to the level of the fascia. In particularly slender patients, especially male patients, make the abdominal wound as low as possible to avoid pressure from a belt and trousers.

3. Place the AICD unit in the pocket with the epoxy header in the midline. If a vertical abdominal pocket is used, place the header superiorly.

Determination of DFTs

1. Proceed with EP testing, using the ECD box and a traditional stimulator (Medtronic), which is attached to the ECD input. A set routine must be followed to keep the number of defibrillation tests as low as possible and to ensure clinically meaningful results.

2. Determine the DFTs in both VT and VF. Because the AICD itself could potentially convert VT to VF, be sure that the device can convert both VF and VT. For VT induction we try to use the same EP protocol that was successful at preoperative testing, but this often is not possible because of the effects of anesthesia. If standard techniques do not work after a few minutes' trial, quickly employ nonclinical techniques. One effective nonclinical technique is ramp pacing. The ventricle is initially paced at a cycle length corresponding to the effective refractory period (ERP) of the ventricle (approximately 270 msec); this rate is quickly increased (i.e., the pacing interval is shortened on the stimulator) over a few seconds. Invariably, coarse VT or VF is induced.

3. After VT is induced, *count accurately* from 1 to 15 seconds and then activate the ECD box, which has been precharged at 25 J. By waiting this long to initiate defibrillation, the postoperative clinical setting is more precisely duplicated than if less time elapses before cardioversion. The risks in waiting this long are no more marked than they will be clinically postoperatively. Determine the DFT beginning at no greater than 25 J and then reduce to 20, 15, 10, 5, and occasionally 1 J.

4. Now determine the DFT for VF. The usual method of inducing VF is with AC rectified current. Do not deliver AC current via the sensing leads because it may cause local tissue damage and scarring and may affect chronic sensing.

Note: If the patient is clinically unstable or has poor left ventricular function, we would determine the DFT for VF only and might elect to not evaluate all energies listed above.

Guidelines for determining DFTs

Determining DFTs is the most important part of the intraoperative testing, and great care must be taken. The following guidelines should be adhered to.[18,19]

1. Use multiple energies to determine the exact DFT and the margin of patient safety.

2. Determine the DFT for both VT and VF, even if the patient has not had clinical VF. VT can usually be induced by ramp pacing; VF can be reliably induced using bursts of AC current.

3. If lower energy levels (e.g., 10 J) fail to terminate the rhythm, then deliver rescue shocks of 25 J through the ECD box as quickly as possible. If two 25 J rescue shocks fail to terminate the rhythm, then the surgeon must deliver conventional cardioversion, using the anteroposterior paddles.

Margin of safety

A 10 J margin of safety is ideal. By this we mean the DFT should be 10 J less than the maximal energy

Table 14-1. Relationship of DFT to electrode configuration

Energy tested with ECD at implant	Result of testing	Recommended spring-patch configuration
1 to 15 J	Successful conversion	Spring/large patch
25 J	Successful, but 20 J not effective	Large patch/large patch—if this reduces DFTs, use regular unit; if not, use high-energy unit
25 J	Variable result	Implant generator unless device accelerates rate; then do not implant device
25 J	Unsuccessful	Implant leads; bring patient back in 2 weeks off medication for retesting

in the implanted AICD pulse generator. If a standard unit is used, successful conversion with 15 J during DFT testing ensures a comfortable margin of safety.

If relatively high energies do not work, many difficult judgments must be made at surgery (see Table 14-1). A typical spring/large patch configuration, in our experience, works in 80% of patients; in another 15% of patients, two patches give adequate DFTs. In the remaining 5% of patients, no configuration reliably induces conversion.

If 20 J does not induce conversion, but 25 J reliably does, a second patch is sewn on the left ventricle in a superoposterior position. The left ventricle then is almost entirely cupped between the two patches. Often, two large patches significantly reduce the DFT and thus can be used with a standard unit. If the DFT remains between 20 and 25 J with two large patches, it is safest to use a high-energy unit. Care should be taken to make sure the two patches are not too close together. This may cause "fringing effect," which can increase impedance.

When the DFTs are 25 to 40 J

Conversion to NSR is variably accomplished in some patients with stable VT with 25 J. If the device is not always successful and does not accelerate the rhythm, a high-energy unit can be implanted. In an occasional patient the DFT is between 25 and 40 J, even with two large patches, and a unit is not implanted in these patients. We have taken the following approach with these patients.

1. The leads are tunneled into the abdominal wound and capped, and the patient is brought back in 3 or 4 weeks for repeat determination of DFTs in the operating room under general anesthesia, just as at the initial implant.

2. In the interim all antiarrhythmic agents are discontinued, especially amiodarone; frequently, midrange DFTs are subsequently found at retesting.

3. Between the two procedures such patients may be sent home with family members trained in CPR. An external defibrillator is recommended for home use if appropriate instruction of the family is possible. For selected patients, continuous home ECG monitoring using telemetry and transtelephonic transmission is instituted (CELIA System, Cardiac Communication, Ltd., Northridge, Calif.).

4. Sound clinical judgment is necessary in making decisions about DFTs at surgery. We spend a great deal of time using various patch configurations in troublesome cases to give a 10 J margin of safety. We have varied the position of the second patch if the DFTs are close to being adequate, and often in a patient with a large heart, a position can be found that will bring the DFTs into the 15 to 20 J range.

5. If two patches are successful, then the superior vena caval spring lead is removed. The polarity of the two patches must be recorded (both are color-coded red), and one of the two patches must be identified by placing a tie around its end. Lead serial numbers should be carefully recorded under these circumstances.

On completion of DFT determination

1. After DFT determinations are completed, tunnel the three leads from within the thorax out through the fifth intercostal space and then subcutaneously down to the abdominal pocket. A #28 Argyle chest tube and long forceps (uterine packing forceps) are a useful means of doing this.

2. Activate the pulse generator and perform a magnet test before removing it from its sterile shipping case if this has not already been done.

3. Deactivate the pulse generator and give it to the surgeon.

4. Wipe the color-coded leads dry and insert them tightly into the generator. Use mineral oil if insertion seems difficult. Tighten the set screws just enough to prevent their being pulled out by gentle tugging.

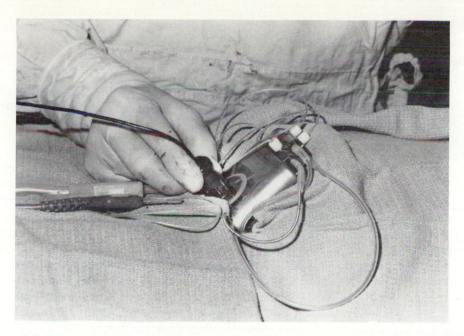

Fig. 14-4. Final testing of the AICD at surgery. The AICD rests in the abdominal wound; attached to it are the three leads from the heart and the temporary monitoring leads, which run from the header to the ECD box. The surgeon holds the AIDCHECK probe over the center of the AICD to determine charge time during the final induction. After completing this final check of the sensing and converting properties of the device, the monitoring leads are removed and replaced with set screws.

The final magnet test

If the DFT determinations have been done carefully, the final test of the AICD is usually successful.

1. Perform a final magnet test with the device resting in the abdominal pocket itself and attached to the special color-coded monitoring leads that are supplied with the device.

2. Again display the signals from the monitoring leads (bipolar pair, spring/patch) on the physiologic recorder.

3. Place a sterile AIDCHECK probe over the header and hold it in place. The AIDCHECK-B must be on and watched. The AICD must be in the pocket for testing; otherwise "noise" may prevent detection of the induced arrhythmia (Fig. 14-4).

4. Again induce VT through the ECD box, but take care to keep the pacing protocol under 2 to 3 seconds if a rapid drive rate is used. Ideally the EP test mode should be used. Alternating current (AC) is sensed by the device as noise.

5. If a pacing protocol longer than 3 seconds is necessary, place the device in EP mode.

6. Have a magnet ready, as redirection might be necessary if the tachycardia spontaneously terminates.

Recycling will occur if the first shock is not successful.

7. Back-up *external* cardioversion must be available in the event that the device is ineffective after recycling three times or if 60 seconds has elapsed.

8. Be sure that the device can both sense and cardiovert VT and VF. To ensure both sensing and converting capability, use the EP mode at final testing. If the device is not blinded (in the EP mode), the pacing sequence itself may activate the device and its sensing capability will not be evaluated at final testing.

9. Cap the pulse generator screw ports with special cap screws to prevent seepage of body fluid into the generator header and also to prevent myopotentials from causing inappropriate shocks.

10. Place the device in the abdomen, with the header toward the midline. Perform routine closure (Parsonnet pouch available if desired).

11. Deactivate the device if electrocautery is to be used; it may trigger the device.

12. Deactivate the device before leaving the operating room. Many patients have postoperative VT that will trigger the device, and these rhythms are best treated with short-term antiarrhythmic medications.

Magnet test failure

It is unusual for the implanted AICD system not to detect an induced rhythm during final testing. The reasons described below should be considered if failure occurs.

1. Power line interference can inhibit the device or extend detection time.

2. Inadequate signals from the bipolar lead may require repositioning.

3. The averaged arrhythmia rate may be below the rate cut-off value. The rate-sensing properties of the device necessitate that a polymorphic VT ideally be 30 beats/minute greater than the cut-off and a monomorphic VT be 10 beats/minute greater to prevent prolonged detection by the rate-sensing circuit.

4. Morphology (PDF) criteria may not be fulfilled. A VT that has a rapid morphology phase lasting less than 100 msec might not be detected as "sinusoidal" by the PDF sensing circuit. Solutions to this problem include use of a rate-only unit or use of two large patches with an AID-B unit.

With experience—the same team doing multiple procedures in the same manner—the time for implantation can be as little as 2½ hours. The initial cases in any institution can be very time-consuming, usually because of uncertainty about the ECD box and the electric connections. Surgical problems are few. Careful attention to the patient's hemodynamic status is mandatory, with enough time allowed between cardioversions/defibrillations for the blood pressure to return to baseline.

COMPLICATIONS
Operative death

The 30-day operative mortality is between 2% and 3%. This rather high figure is in large part attributable to the severity of underlying cardiac and pulmonary disease. In our experience two of four deaths resulted from postoperative pneumonia in patients with underlying chronic obstructive pulmonary disease (one had been treated with amiodarone), and the other two deaths resulted from congestive failure. Stricter selection criteria should reduce the operative mortality. The device should not be to used as a "last ditch" therapy in severely ill patients.

Lead migration

In 2% to 3% of patients, lead migration, usually of the spring lead, has required reoperation. In one patient the spring lead migrated to the level of the right iliac vein. In two other patients it migrated into the inferior vena cava. In one patient the spring lead migrated extravascularly. With use of the fixation device (lead anchor) at the subclavian incision site, this problem should occur less frequently.

Lead fractures

In the early experiences 2% to 3% of patients developed lead fracture that required reoperation. This has been less of a problem recently.

False positive shocks

In the initial Stanford experience with the AICD, 37 of 52 patients (71%) received a total of 463 shocks for rhythms varying from VT to sinus tachycardia.[13] It is impossible to identify the cardiac rhythm that prompted the shock unless the patient is being monitored. It is therefore imperative to obtain Holter monitoring records on patients receiving frequent shocks and to connect these patients to an arrhythmia surveillance telephone system, such as transtelephone ECGs with continuous loop memory. If, on the basis of the clinical setting (such as shocks with extreme exercise), sinus tachycardia seems the likely cause, a beta-blocking drug is given.

Infections

Infection requiring explantation of the device has occurred in less than 2% of patients. The infection usually begins early in the pocket and is often caused by a *Staphylococcus* organism. Any suspicion of pocket infection warrants a careful evaluation, and if an organism is cultured from the pocket, usually the unit and the three leads must be removed. This can be a life-threatening infection and must be treated promptly and aggressively. Late infections are rare to date, except in patients with colonization from another source.

Generator explantation

Among the patients in the Stanford experience, two had their device explanted before hospital discharge because at final EP testing the unit could not reliably cardiovert VT.

Death caused by ventricular arrhythmia

The incidence of recurrent sudden cardiac death has dropped strikingly in these high-risk patients with the use of the AICD. In this group of patients in the Stanford experiment, the annual sudden death rate was 17% using primarily EP-guided antiarrhythmic therapy and electrosurgery. With the use of AICD the sudden death rate in a comparable (nonrandomized) group of patients dropped to 1.3% in the entire study (1 of 52 patients).[13]

Concomitant drug therapy

The majority of patients are discharged on a concomitant antiarrhythmic drug treatment to control frequent episodes of VT, nonsustained VT, sinus tachycardia, and episodes of atrial fibrillation or SVT. Most are taking amiodarone (often 200 mg/day, rather than higher doses) or a beta-blocking drug, although a wide variety of agents are employed. Efficacy is judged on clinical grounds. Adding antiarrhythmic drugs can theoretically alter the DFTs; if DFTs were marginal at initial implant and an antiarrhythmic drug is added, repeat EP testing should be done to ensure that the device functions adequately in the presence of these medications.

Ventricular tachycardia induced during magnet tests

Ventricular tachycardia has occurred infrequently during routine magnet testing; the magnet triggers a nonsynchronized discharge, which in turn induces VT and VF. This experience underscores the importance of having complete external defibrillation equipment available during magnet tests. Ideally, the patient should also be monitored.

Pacemaker-AICD interaction

Temporary or permanent pacemakers can interfere with AICD arrhythmia sensing by two distinct mechanisms.

• *Detection inhibition:* If a patient develops VT or VF that the pacemaker does not sense, the pacemaker will continue to pace. In turn, the AICD might ignore the VT or VF and base its arrhythmia analysis on pacemaker artifact signals. Analysis of electrograms (from the spring/patch or bipolar pair of leads) for the presence of pacing spikes at surgery should clarify whether the pacing artifact is being sensed by the AICD. This is particularly important during VF, in which case a bipolar pacemaker might continue to fire with the patient in VF, thus inhibiting the AICD. If a patient has both a pacemaker and an AICD, he must be evaluated in VF to ensure that no unsafe interaction occurs between the two devices.

• *Double counting:* The AICD has a short refractory period (150 msec); if there is local intraventricular conduction delay, then both the pacing artifact and the evoked response will be counted by the device. If the pacemaker rate is greater than one half the AICD rate limit, both rate and morphology criteria can be met because ventricular pacing resembles VT. Also, with dual-chamber pacemaker units, one device can count both the atrial and ventricular pacer strikes and resulting depolarizations. A shock is then delivered in response to this tripled rate.

These problems can be anticipated in patients requiring a pacemaker and an AICD. The following guidelines are offered:

1. Use only bipolar pacing systems with patients who have an AICD
2. The bipolar pacing systems should be closely spaced and as far away as possible from the AICD rate-detection electrodes
3. If right ventricular endocardial bipolar pacing leads are present, sew the AICD epicardial sensing leads on the posterior left ventricle with 1 cm spacing
4. Two endocardial leads, pacing and AICD sensing, should not be placed in the same heart chamber
5. A final EP test is mandatory in patients who have a permanent pacemaker to ensure proper AICD function

Electromagnetic interference

Electromagnetic interference (EMI) may cause either inhibition of the sensing system or inappropriate discharge. Diathermy or magnetic resonance imagers may damage the components of the AICD system. Electrocautery may be used only when the pulse generator has been deactivated. (EMI from sources such as small motors will probably result only in inhibition.)

Interaction with standard defibrillators

If an external defibrillation were of sufficient magnitude AICD failure might occur, but to date this has not occurred. In emergency situations we have used defibrillation without damage to the device. If internal paddles are applied to the heart during surgery, the generator should be disconnected from the lead system or AICD damage will occur.

IMMEDIATE AFTERCARE

1. Transfer the patient from the recovery room to the surgical intensive care unit. Both the surgeon and the cardiologist should follow the patient's progress. Postsurgical progress is often slow because of splinting at the site of the thoracotomy.
2. Use antiarrhythmic drugs only as needed for acute arrhythmias; lidocaine is the preferred drug.
3. Pay careful attention to the patient's often compromised hemodynamic status; avoid myocardial depressants. Continue hemodynamic monitoring until the patient is stabilized.
4. Cardioversion or defibrillation can be performed externally without damage to the device.

5. Treat any early manifestation of pneumonia aggressively.

6. Move the patient to a telemetry-monitored ward when the chest tube is out.

7. If the patient is having nonsustained VT that may trigger the device, oral antiarrhythmic medications are needed. Administer a beta-blocking drug to younger patients who experience rapid sinus rates on the preoperative treadmill stress test.

8. Perform a final EP study before discharging the patient, usually on the fifth to seventh day, at a time when the patient's oral antiarrhythmic therapy has been initiated. The unit is activated and a magnet test performed. Either the active mode or the EP mode is chosen during the test, depending on the difficulty of induction. The patient experiences a shock during this test while awake; this indicates that the device is working properly. This testing is especially important and should be performed several times if DFTs were marginal at the time of implant (based on patient tolerance).

LONG-TERM FOLLOW-UP
Patient education

The patient should wear a medalert identification bracelet or necklace and carry an identification card with AICD information (supplied by CPI/Intec). If possible, a member of the family should be instructed in CPR, and the patient taught how to perform cough CPR.

Psychologic support of the patient and his or her family is important. Many centers have now started support-group meetings for their AICD patients.

Full activity is possible for the patient unless sinus tachycardia activates the device. In such cases beta-blocking drugs are used. Driving is usually permitted unless the patient is having unsafe neurologic symptoms. Swimming is not allowed because of the danger of aspiration during a tachyarrhythmia.

Office visits

The patient is seen every 2 months the first year and every month after that by a physician and nursing staff fully knowledgable about the device. An interval history is taken and a magnet test performed at each visit. Two magnet tests are performed at each visit if the first charge time is long. The second charge time is invariably shorter than the first and should be under 10 seconds. Specific Elective Replacement Indicators should be used to evaluate magnet test results. Full resuscitative equipment must be available when a magnet test is performed.

Battery elective replacement indicator

Manufacturers provide tables that allow accurate estimation of the battery's end of life based on the magnet test. Battery life has been 12 to 24 months, and occasionally longer than 2 years. A new generator can be implanted with only a one-night hospital stay.

Discharge of the AICD

The patient is asked to call the physician if the device discharges, and an effort is made to determine what type of rhythm triggered the device. If multiple shocks occur over a short period of time, the obvious reversible causes, such as electrolyte imbalance, new congestive heart failure, or new ischemia should be investigated. Holter monitoring and transtelephonic devices with a memory loop are helpful in monitoring these cases. New antiarrhythmic medications or changes of an old regimen are often necessary.

FUTURE DEVELOPMENTS
Improvements on the AICD

The presently available AICD unit performs effectively and with few component failures. Future refinements in the unit will allow programmability of the generator (rate, duration of VT before shock, energy of shock). A memory loop in the generator will read the ECG of the rhythm that caused the unit to discharge and allow more precise antiarrhythmic therapy.

Parallel technologies

Parallel technologies have been developed that use different electrophysiologic mechanisms to interrupt VT. The Medtronic device uses either single synchronized low-energy (1.7 J) VPDs or a programmed train of impulses by a single transvenous catheter placed in the right ventricle. The risk of accelerating the rate of a stable VT makes defibrillation back-up highly desirable clinically. This unit can also function as a pacemaker for bradycardia.

Single-catheter system

Finally, a single-catheter system for use with an AICD has recently been developed. It transmits a defibrillating current between the right atrium and right ventricle and does not necessitate a ventricular patch and thoracotomy. Initial acute evaluation results compare favorably with the traditional spring/patch configuration.

Acknowledgment: The authors gratefully acknowledge the careful review of the manuscript by Andra C. Thomas, R.N. (Intec—CPI, Inc.).

REFERENCES

1. Mirowski, M., et al.: Standby automatic debibrillator, Arch. Intern. Med. **126:**158, 1970.
2. Mirowski, M., et al.: Ventricular defibrillation through a single intravascular catheter electrode system, Clin. Res. **19:**328, 1971.
3. Mirowski, M., Mower, M.M., Gott, V.L., and Brawley, R.K.: Feasibility and effectiveness of low-energy catheter defibrillation in man, Circulation **47:**79, 1973.
4. Mirowski, M., et al.: A chronically implanted system for automatic defibrillation in active conscious dogs, Circulation **58:**90, 1978.
5. Mower, M.M., et al.: Patterns of intraventricular catheter defibrillation, Circulation **45,46**(suppl II): II-25, 1972.
6. Mirowski, M., et al.: Termination of malignant ventricular arrhythmias with an implanted automatic defibrillator in human beings, N. Engl. J. Med. **303:**22, 1980.
7. Mirowski, M., et al.: Clinical treatment of life-threatening ventricular tachyarrhythmias with the automatic implantable defibrillator, Am. Heart J. **102:**265, 1981.
8. Reid, P.R., et al.: Clinical evaluation of the internal automatic cardioverter-defibrillator in survivors of sudden cardiac death, Am. J. Cardiol. **51:**1608, 1983.
9. Winkle, R.A.: The implantable defibrillator and ventricular arrhythmias, Hosp. Pract. **18:**149, 1983.
10. Mirowski, M., et al.: Mortality in patients with implanted automatic defibrillator, Ann. Intern. Med. **98:**585, 1983.
11. Reid, P.R., et al.: Implantable cardioverter-defibrillator: patient selection and implantation protocol, PACE **7:**1338, 1984.
12. Mirowski, M., et al.: Clinical performance of implantable cardioverter-defibrillator, PACE **7:**1345, 1984.
13. Echt, D.S., et al.: Clinical experience, complications and survival in 70 patients with the automatic implantable cardioverter/defibrillator, Circulation **71:**289, 1985.
14. Mirowski, M.: The automatic implantable cardioverter-defibrillator: an overview, J. Am. Coll. Cardiol. **6:**461, 1985.
15. Winkle, R.A., et al.: Practical aspects of cardioverter/defibrillator implantation, Am. Heart J. **108:**1335, 1984.
16. Watkins, L. Jr., et al.: Surgical techniques for implanting the automatic implantable defibrillator, PACE **7:**1357, 1984.
17. Lawrie, G.M.:, Griffin, J.C., and Wyndham, C.R.C.: Epicardial implantation of the automatic implantable defibrillator by left subcostal thoracotomy, PACE **7:**1370, 1984.
18. Winkle, R.A., et al.: The automatic implantable defibrillator: local ventricular bipolar sensing to detect ventricular tachycardia and fibrillation, Am. J. Cardiol. **52:**265, 1983.
19. Winkle, R.A., et al.: Cardioversion/defibrillation thresholds in man using a truncated exponential waveform and an apical patch-SVC spring electrode configuration, Circulation **69:**766, 1984.

Chapter Fifteen

Coronary angioplasty

JACK A. PATTERSON
ARA G. TILKIAN

HISTORICAL PERSPECTIVE

Attempts of nonsurgical catheter treatment of obstructive vascular disease date back to 1964, when Charles Dotter and Melvin Judkins[1] described their techniques of peripheral vascular dilatation using progressively larger catheters and forecast applications of such techniques to the coronary arteries. This technique did not receive wide acceptance or application in the United States, and criticism focused on its causing endothelial injury with vascular occlusion and emboli. A reinforced balloon catheter dilatation method was next proposed and applied in a few patients with iliac artery narrowing.[2] This technique did not receive much attention until Andreas Gruentzig[3] designed a smaller flexible catheter with a distensible balloon at its tip and reported on his successful results of peripheral vascular dilatation in 1977. The keys to success appeared to be the use of small, flexible catheters permitting passage to small distal vessels, and the capability of inflating the balloon to a *predetermined diameter* under increasingly high inflation pressures. This permitted a controlled compression or splitting of focal atheromatous lesions without major trauma to the entire vessel wall or adjacent segments of the vessel.

Encouraged by results of peripheral angioplasty, Gruentzig promptly extended this technique to coronary arteries, initially with experiments in dogs and subsequently in humans during aortocoronary bypass surgery. Having demonstrated the efficacy of the technique and being satisfied with its safety, Gruentzig[4,5] performed the first percutaneous transluminal coronary angioplasty in a human in September 1977. This work was presented at the fiftieth annual American Heart Association Scientific Session in 1977, where a standing room only audience in a huge hall gasped in amazement as Andreas Gruentzig showed the coronary arteriograms of the first (and successful) coronary angioplasty performed in man. A new era in cardiology was being introduced.

In the subsequent 5 years, this technique received cautious acceptance,[6] then underwent several technical modifications, the most important of which was the introduction by Simpson et al.[7] of the movable and steerable guidewire technique for directing the dilatation catheter to the coronary artery branches. Improvements in design and construction of guiding and dilatation catheters, guidewires, and peripheral accessories, coupled with widespread availability of high-resolution angulated imaging equipment, have rapidly propelled this technique into common use. Within a decade, coronary angioplasty has moved from experimental treatment available in university research centers to accepted treatment applied worldwide and gradually extended to an increasingly larger subset of patients with coronary artery disease (Table 15-1).[8]

The literature and the cardiovascular community are unanimous in crediting Andreas Gruentzig for his pioneer work in coronary angioplasty. Less recognized were Gruentzig's untiring and uncompromising efforts to personally teach his techniques to his colleagues and encourage them to take those techniques to their communities. He insisted on critical scientific methods of testing and evaluating the results of the procedure, endeavoring to distinguish fact from fancy. The boundaries of the technique were extended gradually and cautiously under controlled investigation and critical evaluation of results, with patient safety always a first consideration. Thus, having fathered coronary angioplasty, Andreas Gruentzig demonstrated a loving, caring, and very responsible parenthood! With his untimely death we have all lost a great teacher and an esteemed colleague.[9]

In this chapter we will review the technique of coronary angioplasty and highlight its procedural aspects in

Table 15-1. The development of coronary angioplasty

	1977	1979	1980-1981	1982	1985-1986
Status	1st angioplasty performed	Technique introduced ($n = 200$)	Investigational ($n = 400$)	Accepted treatment ($n > 3000$)	Worldwide use ($n > 100,000$)
Indications		Single-vessel CAD	Single-vessel CAD	Single-vessel CAD	Single & multi-vessel CAD
Patients suitable for CABG who can be treated successfully with PTCA		5%	10%	Approx. 15%	25%-50% (Some claim >90%)
Multivessel angioplasty		Rare	Rare	Rare	20%+ in many centers, 50% in some centers
Primary success rate (SVA)		60%-80%	—	70%-80%	90%+
Emergency surgery (SVA)		6%-10%	—	5%-10%	<3%
Myocardial infarction (SVA)		5%	—	—	2.5%
Major complications (myocardial infarction, emerg. surg., death) (SVA)		10%	—	—	4%
Minor complications, (emerg. reangiography, VT/VF, BBB, vascular repair, tamponade)		—	—	—	9%
Restenosis		20%-30%	—	—	20%-30%
Death					
Single-vessel angioplasty		0.8%	—	—	0.1%-0.9%
Multivessel angioplasty					0.5%-2%

VT, Ventricular tachycardia; *VF*, ventricular fibrillation; *BBB*, bundle branch block; *CABG*, coronary artery bypass grafting; *SVA*, single-vessel angioplasty; *PTCA*, percutaneous transluminal coronary angioplasty; *CAD*, coronary artery disease.

the light of our experience with the procedure since early 1981.

PRELIMINARY CONSIDERATIONS AND PREPARATION
Indications

Indications for coronary angioplasty are still evolving.[8,10-15] When this procedure is being considered, four important questions must be asked: (1) Can the procedure be performed with a high probability of success? (2) Will a successful result benefit the patient? (3) Is it better than other available treatment options? (4) Can the procedure be performed safely?

A definite indication exists if the answer to all of these questions is "yes." A relative contraindication is identified if the answer to any one of these questions is "no," and careful reconsideration is in order. A strong contraindication is present if the answer is "no" (or "maybe") to two or more questions; performing coronary angioplasty in such a case would invite disaster.

The indications and contraindications of coronary angioplasty are still evolving and are determined by (1) the experience and the judgment of the person performing the procedure, (2) the technical and support facilities available, (3) the design of available equipment, (4) the capability and experience of the cardiovascular surgical back-up team, and (5) the individual, clinical, and angiographic characteristics of the patient. Ultimately, a randomized study will be necessary to compare the long-term results of coronary angioplasty with those of medical treatment or aortocoronary bypass surgery in different subsets of patients.

Classic indications (1979)

Classic indications exist for the patient who is a candidate for aortocoronary bypass surgery and has single-vessel coronary artery stenosis with the following findings:
- Recent onset angina not well controlled with medications
- Objective evidence of myocardial ischemia
- Proximal, discrete stenosis
- Concentric, noncalcified lesions
- Subtotal obstruction
- Good left ventricular function

These original indications established in 1979 remain valid today. Angioplasty in such cases can be performed safely, with a high probability of success, and with substantial benefit to the patient. It is the procedure of choice when medical treatment has not controlled the patient's angina.

Extended indications (1986)

- Proximal left anterior descending coronary artery or dominant right coronary artery stenosis with demonstrable ischemia, with or without angina
- Multiple discrete lesions in a single vessel (there are no absolute morphologic contraindications, i.e., the stenosis to be dilated may be distal, eccentric, long, partially calcified, or totally occluded and may involve points of vessel bifurcation)
- Selected cases of multivessel coronary artery stenosis with relatively refractory angina and demonstration of myocardial ischemia
- Acute evolving myocardial infarction (selected cases) with or without the use of thrombolytic therapy
- Saphenous vein bypass graft stenosis (or internal mammary graft stenosis), preferably discrete and at the distal anastomotic site
- Restenosis after a first or second successful angioplasty
- Variant angina in the presence of fixed anatomic obstruction (debatable indication; see p. 367)
- Atherosclerosis with high-grade obstruction following cardiac transplantation
- Selected patients who are not acceptable candidates for aortocoronary bypass surgery but who may benefit from palliative angioplasty, such as patients with severe obstructive lung disease, advanced age, disseminated malignancy, or prior aortocoronary bypass surgery with high risk for reoperation

Coronary angioplasty has been extended to these groups by experienced operators, who have performed the procedure with decreasing morbidity and mortality; however, the beginner is advised to adhere to the classic indications until he or she acquires the skill and judgment that come with experience.

The temptation to perform ''cosmetic angioplasty'' must be resisted. In the absence of angina or ischemia and with little risk to life, a coronary artery with a moderate stenotic lesion accessible to the balloon catheter should not be dilated. Angioplasty in this setting may precipitate acute occlusion and myocardial infarction or may predispose to accelerated atherosclerosis and restenosis at a faster rate than that of the natural history of the disease.[12]

Relative contraindications

There are few absolute contraindications to coronary angioplasty. As with indications, contraindications are still evolving and are highly subject to the experience and judgment of the operator and the support available at the facility.

Some generally accepted contraindications[10-16] for elective coronary angioplasty are discussed below.
- Left main coronary artery stenosis constitutes a relative contraindication[15,16] where morbidity and mortality of coronary angioplasty are high and restenosis may have a clinically malignant presentation and where aortocoronary bypass surgery has proven long-term benefits. Most of the exceptions to this are in the category of ''protected'' left main lesions where previous surgery has been partially successful. There are also rare emergency situations where angioplasty may be used before surgery to stabilize a patient who has acute left main artery occlusion.

Preliminary results of palliative angioplasty in patients with left main coronary artery disease are encouraging.[15] However, most centers would prefer revascularization in these cases.
- ''Left main equivalent'' (e.g., when the vessel to be dilated supplies most of the viable left ventricle and the contralateral vessel supplying an area of old myocardial infarction is obstructed) also represents a relative contraindication. It is possible to dilate such stenosis, with benefit to the patient. However, in this setting the requirement for patient safety is not met: acute occlusion during or immediately following coronary angioplasty may precipitate acute hemodynamic instability, pulmonary edema, shock, or intractable arrhythmias, and emergency revascularization surgery may not be successful. In such a case, the question must be asked: ''If the vessel I propose to dilate has a total occlusion, will the patient survive with the help of

full support including emergency aortocoronary bypass surgery?" If the answer is "probably not," a definite contraindication exists and the procedure should not be done! This also applies to patients with advanced left ventricular dysfunction who may not survive emergency surgery. To reduce the risk for such patients some centers have designed a combined catheterization, angioplasty and surgery suite to reduce the time required for emergency surgery in case of complications. Using such a facility has reduced the time to emergency cardiopulmonary bypass to approximately 10 minutes, permitting emergency revascularization without myocardial infarction.[17]

Additional relative contraindications include the following:

- Three-vessel coronary artery disease with disabling angina where long-term benefits of *surgical* revascularization are well established
- Critical valvular disease not caused by acute myocardial ischemia
- Chronic total occlusion: If patency is reestablished, the chance of reocclusion is high (see p. 369)
- Variant angina with documented coronary artery spasm: Response of these patients to angioplasty has been unpredictable with a high chance of recurrence; these patients are best treated with coronary vasodilators (see p. 367)
- Stenosis at the orifice of vessels (involving the aortic wall): Disease here may not respond well to dilatation

Risks and complications

Risks and complications[11,13,18-24] of single-vessel coronary angioplasty have gradually declined with increased operator experience and improved equipment. However, as the technique extends to multivessel angioplasty and complex (high-risk) conditions, the risks and complications are expected to increase.

The most complete information on risks and complications comes from the National Heart, Lung, and Blood Institute (NHLBI) registry data,[18-21,23] where more than 75% of patients had single-vessel angioplasty, and from the careful follow-up done at Emory University,[11,13] where until recently more than 75% of patients had single-vessel angioplasty. Thus, the risks cited in Table 15-2 apply mostly to single-vessel coronary angioplasty unless otherwise specified. In this table the risks from two time frames are compared. Those cited for 1979 to 1982 include the performance of some relatively inexperienced operators using first-generation equipment and are overestimates for today. Conversely, the reports of risks for 1984 to 1985 are from centers with extensive experience, large numbers of cases, and excellent support facilities and thus are probably underestimates when applied to the general community. With current techniques as applied in the general community, the true risk probably lies between these two extremes.

Complications have been higher in women and in patients with unstable angina or eccentric lesions. Mortality has been higher in women and in patients over age 60 years, patients with prior aortocoronary bypass surgery, and patients with left main coronary artery disease.

Personnel

The operating physician must be experienced in cardiac catheterization, coronary arteriography, and coronary angioplasty and an expert in the care of critically

Table 15-2. Risks of coronary angioplasty (single vessel)*

	1979-1982	1984-1985
Death	1%	0.1%-0.5%
Failure to dilate	15%-30%	5%-10%
Acute occlusion	4%-10%	2%
Emergency surgery	6%-10%	2%-3%
Myocardial infarction	5%-13%	1%-2%
Right ventricular puncture & pericardial tamponade	?	1%
Coronary artery aneurysm	Rare	Rare
Coronary artery rupture	Rare	Rare
Coronary artery emboli	Rare	Rare
Iatrogenic left main stenosis caused by catheter trauma	Rare	Rare
Vascular complications	Same as for diagnostic cardiac catheterization (see pp. 119 and 122)	
Arrhythmias (ventricular fibrillation, complete heart block)	Slightly more than seen in diagnostic cardiac catheterization	

*The risk in the general community probably lies within these extremes—see text.

ill patients.[25] For the safe performance of this procedure extensive experience in coronary arteriography is necessary but not sufficient; additional technical skills, maturity, and knowledge are also required for this demanding procedure. These skills may be acquired by visiting medical centers where angioplasty is performed frequently, attending courses, and participating in preceptorship programs. Formal cardiovascular training programs have started to incorporate angioplasty in the syllabus of their third and fourth years.[26]

Training guidelines have been published by the Society of Cardiac Angiography.[25]

Thus the personnel required for angioplasty include the following:

- Operating physician experienced with the procedure
- Physician to assist at the catheterization table
- Nurse to assist in the sterile field, helping with catheter exchanges, injections, balloon dilatations, etc.
- Circulating nurse, responsible for providing supplies, administering medications, monitoring the patient, and responding to emergencies.
- Radiology technologist to ensure optimal performance of the radiology equipment
- Cardiovascular technologist, responsible for hemodynamic and ECG monitoring
- Cardiovascular surgical team on standby, including cardiovascular surgeon, anesthesiologist, and cardiopulmonary perfusionist ready for immediate surgery if needed

Table 15-3. Guiding catheters

Manufacturer	Type	Design	Construction
ACS	Femoral	Judkins* Amplatz El Gamal Coronary bypass Internal mammary	Polyethylene outer layer; Aramid (epoxy-fiberbraid) midlayer; Teflon inner liner; radiopaque tip marker on tapered tip catheters
	Brachial	Similar to Stertzer (see below)	Polyethylene outer layer; Aramid midlayer; Teflon liner
USCI	Femoral (Myler)	Judkins type* Amplatz type King Multipurpose El Gamal Coronary bypass Internal mammary Arani double loop§	Polyurethane outer layer; wire braid midlayer; Teflon inner liner
	Brachial ‖ (Stertzer)	Multipurpose type I, small, medium, large (with and without side holes)	Woven Dacron with soft flexible tip, wire braid, inner layer, & Teflon inner liner
		Multipurpose type II, medium & large (no side holes)	As above
IM	Femoral Brachial	Same as above	Polyurethane outer layer; wire braid midlayer; Teflon inner liner; 1 mm radiopaque tip-marker
Angiomedics	Femoral	Softip Judkins Amplatz Multipurpose Coronary bypass	Deformable tip, polyurethane outer layer; wire braid midlayer; Teflon inner liner; Celgard coating
Schneider-Medintag	Femoral	Judkins, Amplatz, El Gamal, Burassa	Same as USCI
	Brachial	Small, medium, large	With and without side holes; same as USCI

ACS, Advanced Cardiovascular Systems, Inc.; *USCI,* United States Catheter and Instrument Corp., C.R. Bard, Inc., *IM,* Interventional Medical, Inc.

*Available with side holes for right coronary catheter.

†Tapered tip with radiopaque markers.

The angioplasty suite

The angioplasty suite[27] is a dedicated cardiac catheterization room with some special features:

- High-resolution and multimode image intensifier with x-ray tube/image intensifier configuration capable of angulated projections and rapid changing of these projections; biplane imaging capability is recommended but not essential
- High-resolution television monitor with freeze frame video capacity through a tape recorder or a hard disk for simultaneous display of guiding projections next to the real-time images
- Immediate availability of the intra-aortic balloon pump (IABP) and anesthesia equipment

The angioplasty suite should have easy access to the cardiovascular operating suite. For performance of angioplasty in high-risk patients, a combined angioplasty/cardiovascular surgery operating suite is highly desirable.[17] Given the current techniques, elective angioplasty can be performed only in hospital settings with complete cardiovascular surgical capabilities.

Angioplasty equipment

Advances in coronary angioplasty have been directly related to improvements in equipment design and construction.[13,28-30] The rapid evolution of the sophisticated angioplasty equipment available today is credited to the innovative technology of the catheter industry, guided by pioneers in the field.

Usable shaft length	Available sizes Outside diameter (Fr)	Inner diameter (inches)	Largest guidewire (inches)	Approx. price (1986)
100 cm	8.8	0.076	0.063	$75
	8.0	0.072	0.063	
	8.8/8.0†	0.076	0.063	
	8/7.5†	0.072	0.063	
	7.0‡	0.065		
90 cm	8 with 1 cm tip tapered to 7.5	0.072	0.063	$82
100 cm	9.0	0.072	0.063	$84
	8.0	0.072 (large lumen)	0.063	
		0.068 (standard)	0.063	
90 cm	8.3	0.067	0.035 with introducer	$87
90 cm	8.3	0.067	0.035 with introducer	$87
100 cm	8.0	0.074	0.063	$75
	9.0	0.082		
90 cm	8.0	0.074	0.035 with introducer	$80
100 cm	9.0	0.080	0.063	$85
	8.0	0.076		
100 cm	9.0	0.071	0.063	
	8.0	0.071	0.063	
90 cm	8.3	0.071	0.035	

‡Can be used only with Hartzler LPS dilatation catheter.
§Available with 1.5 and 2.6 cm tips and with 90 and 75 degree final curves. All have a perfusion side hole.
‖ Multipurpose type I has soft flexible distal tip, similar to Sones coronary catheter, except for its nontapered tip. Multipurpose type II has a soft preformed tip, similar to Castillo modification.

Physicians performing coronary angioplasty need to be intimately familiar with the characteristics and special features of the equipment used in the procedure. In this section we will summarize the important technical information concerning the currently used equipment. Obsolete equipment or equipment in a development or testing stage will not be discussed. Technology in this area is changing rapidly, therefore current manufacturer information should always be reviewed. Each manufacturer provides instructions and clinical inservice on the special preparation and handling of its equipment.

Guiding catheters[13,29-32] (Table 15-3)

Design. A longitudinal section of a representative guiding catheter is illustrated in Fig. 15-1. Its design has followed that of diagnostic coronary arteriography catheters. Practically all of the coronary catheters used for diagnostic angiography (both femoral and brachial approach) are available as guiding catheters, but with different construction. These catheters are made of three layers—an inner Teflon lining to reduce friction between the guiding and the dilatation catheters, a midlayer made of either epoxy and fiber braid (Advanced Cardiovascular Systems, Inc. [ACS]) or a wire braid (USCI) to permit torque control, and an outer layer of polyethylene (ACS) or polyurethane (USCI and others) providing stiffness and ability to retain preformed shape (memory).

The femoral guiding catheter is 100 cm long and has an 8 or 9 (8.8 for ACS) Fr outside diameter. The brachial catheter is 90 cm long and has an 8 or 8.3 Fr outside diameter. Traditionally, the tip of these catheters is short and not tapered, increasing their potential for causing intimal injury. There are also minor differences in their internal diameter depending on the manufacturer (Table 15-3). Tapered tip guiding catheters are also available and have a marker at their tip. This modification permits use of 9 Fr (body) catheters with their increased support and flow, with 8 Fr tips that reduce the risk of occluding flow at the coronary ostium, whereas the 8/7.5 Fr version may permit a deeper seating of the catheter tip in the coronary ostium. A longitudinal section of the tip portion of an ACS tapered tip guiding catheter is illustrated in Fig. 15-2. The tip marker facilitates fluoroscopic monitoring of the tip location. Manufacturers will accommodate requests for special configuration, size, or lengths (advance notice is required).

Choice of catheters. Various factors considered in the choice of the guiding catheter (fit of the diagnostic catheter and anatomy of the proximal coronary artery, aorta, and coronary lesion) are discussed in the section

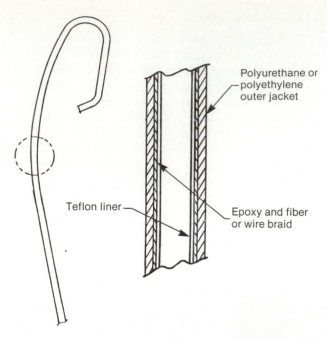

Fig. 15-1. Longitudinal section of a representative guiding catheter.

Polyurethane or polyethylene outer jacket

Teflon liner

Epoxy and fiber or wire braid

on procedure. There is no single catheter or system that is "better" for all cases. A most important requisite for successful angioplasty is a guiding catheter that (1) will provide proper coaxial seating in the coronary ostium without occluding the flow and (2) is capable of providing support and "power" for the passage of the dilatating catheter through high-grade or distal stenosis. This choice is not always easy. Careful review of the diagnostic angiogram and the seating of the catheters used in diagnostic coronary artiography provides helpful clues. Variation in the coronary anatomy must also be considered (see pp. 353 to 354). The choice of 8 Fr versus 9 Fr guiding catheters entails trade-offs.

An 8 Fr catheter provides greater flexibility and versatility, permitting selective catheterization of the left anterior descending or circumflex coronary artery with less potential of trauma to the proximal coronary artery. Occluding the right coronary artery flow is less likely. Contrast material delivery is compromised, and proximal (guiding catheter) pressures may be somewhat damped.

A 9 Fr catheter provides better torque control than does the 8 Fr as well as excellent contrast material delivery and guiding catheter pressures. It is more stable and provides better support to the dilatation catheter. However, risk of occluding flow in the right coronary artery is greater, and selective intubation of the left anterior descending or circumflex coronary artery carries

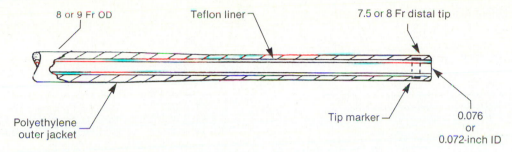

Fig. 15-2. Longitudinal section of the tip portion of an ACS tapered-tip guiding catheter. Note the tip marker, which helps to fluoroscopically locate the catheter tip.

increased risk of traumatizing the proximal left main coronary artery.

Right coronary artery guiding catheters with side holes on their secondary curve partially overcome the problem of occluding flow in a relatively small right coronary artery, where 9 Fr or even 8 Fr guiding catheters are used. A disadvantage of these catheters is inability to obtain satisfactory selective angiograms because the contrast is partially injected into the sinus of Valsalva. This may compromise the ability to precisely position the dilatation catheter or define the results of the dilatation procedure.

The introduction of high flow and the tapered tip guiding catheter is aimed at providing the advantages of both the 8 and 9 Fr catheters while reducing or eliminating the disadvantages.

Dilatation catheters[13,29-33] (Table 15-4)

The original dilatation catheter consisted of a nonsteerable balloon catheter with a fixed wire at its tip. This catheter could not be maneuvered easily and did not permit safe recrossing of a dilated segment.

The creation of dilatation catheters with steerable and movable guidewires was a key step in the development of the angioplasty technique. Basic requirements for such a catheter are that it be small, soft, and flexible to allow passage through tight stenoses. At the same time it must permit prompt expansion to a predetermined diameter, withstand high inflation pressures, and permit prompt deflation. Additional requirements are that it be radiopaque and permit the use of steerable guidewires, pressure monitoring at the tip, and injection of contrast material distally. In a short span of 5 years, industry has met the challenge of providing us with dilatation catheters that meet these requirements. Each manufacturer has added modifications to this basic design (Table 15-4).

Simpson-Robert and Simpson Ultralow Profile Catheter (ACS). Fig. 15-3, *A* illustrates the basic design of

the ACS catheter, which is constructed of two concentric polyethylene tubings. The inner tubing (inner member) is used for passage of the guidewire, injection of contrast medium, and pressure measurements. The outer tubing (balloon member) has the balloon formed at its tip. There is a vent tubing between the two tubes to allow purging of air from the catheter during filling of the balloon with contrast material. The stiffness of the shaft of the catheter can be varied by advancing or withdrawing the vent tube within the inner lumen. There is a radiopaque distal tip marker.

Delta (ACS) catheter. The Delta catheter is illustrated in Fig. 15-3, *B*. This catheter, a modification of the basic ACS design, has a larger inner diameter and tip side holes that permit more adequate contrast injections and pressure monitoring. The vent tube is eliminated.

Hartzler LPS catheter (ACS). Fig. 15-4, *A* illustrates the design of the Hartzler LPS catheter, a steerable dilatation catheter. Note that unlike the basic ACS design, there is no inner tubing. The balloon tubing is extruded directly over a small guidewire, permitting a very low profile, but does not permit the use of an inner movable guidewire. The guidewire fixed in the balloon tubing can be steered by applying torque to the central knob on the proximal end of the catheter. Because there is no inner lumen, distal pressure measurements and contrast material injections are not possible. The marked low profile of this catheter permits passage into very small, tortuous, and distal coronary artery branches.

Hartzler-Micro dilatation catheter. This is a further modification of the Hartzler LPS catheter (Fig. 15-4, *B*). It has a lower profile and no vent tube; the balloon is self-venting. There is an independently torqueable wire that can be rotated and moved to and fro for approximately 10 cm but cannot be removed. Contrast injection is not possible.

Gruentzig-Dilaca low-profile steerable (LPS) catheter (USCI). The Gruentzig low-profile steerable catheters are illustrated in Fig. 15-5. These catheters are con-

Table 15-4. Dilatation catheters

Manufacturer	Design	Balloon length (mm)	Balloon diameter (mm)	Material	Shaft outer diameter Fr (mm)
ACS	Simpson-Robert	20	2.0-4.0	PE	4.3 (1.43)*
	Delta	20	2.0-4.0	PE	4.3 (1.43)
	Simpson Ultralow profile	20	2.0-3.0	PE	4.3 (1.43)
	Hartzler-LPS	20	2.0	PE	2.9 (0.96)
			2.5		3.2 (1.06)
			3.0		3.5 (1.15)
	Hartzler-Micro	20	2.0-3.0	PE	2.9(0.96) − 3.5(1.15)
			3.5		3.6 (1.18)
			4.0		3.7 (1.22)
USCI	Gruentzig-Dilaca LPS	25	2.0	PVC	4.3 (1.43)
		25	2.5-4.0		4.3 (1.43)
	Gruentzig-Dilaca LPS II	20*	2.0	PVC	4.3 (1.43)
			2.5-4.0		4.3 (1.43)
	Gruentzig-Dilaca Profile Plus	20	2.0	PVC	4.3 (1.43)
			2.5-4.0		4.3 (1.43)
Mansfield Scientific, Inc.	Heart-Trak Heart-Trak III	20	2.0-4.0	PE	4.5 (1.50)
Scimed	Trac	20	2.0-3.5	PO	4.3 (1.43)
	Tracplus	20	2.0-3.5	PO	4.3 (1.43)
American Edwards	Hybrid catheter	20	2.0	PE	3.9 (1.3)
			2.5		3.9 (1.3)
			3.0-4.0		3.9 (1.3)
Schneider-Medintag	Gruentzig steerable (low profile)	20	2.0-4	PVC	4.3 (1.43)
	Pass Key LCX (super low profile)	20	2.0	PVC	4.3 (1.43)
		20	2.0-3.0	PVC	3.6 (1.2)

PE, polyethylene; *PVC*, polyvinylchloride; *PO*, polyolefincopolymer; *ACS*, Advanced Cardiovascular Systems, Inc; *USCI*, United States Catheter and Instrument Corp., C.R. Bard, Inc.; *LPS*, Low Profile Steerable.
*Also available in 12 mm balloon length.

structed with a double-lumen shaft made of polyvinylchloride. The larger lumen is for distal pressure measurements, contrast medium injection, and the passage of the movable guidewire. The smaller lumen is for inflation and deflation of the balloon.

Gruentzig Dilaca Profile Plus. The newest of the USCI dilatation catheters has a balloon length of 20 mm (instead of 25 mm), lower profile, and is constructed of polyethylene terepthalate (PET), which provides a low friction coefficient similar to polyethylene and can withstand inflation pressures up to 20 atmospheres without stretching. The published specifications of these and other catheters are displayed in Table 15-4.

Comparison of USCI and ACS catheters. The difference in construction and material used in these types of catheters has resulted in different performance characteristics. There are no formal comparisons of these two catheter systems. Both systems perform well and are satisfactory in most circumstances.

It appears that the USCI catheter (Gruentzig Dilaca) generally permits better distal pressure measurements and contrast material injection with the guidewire in place. This is possible because the cross-sectional area of its lumen is greater than that of the ACS, Simpson Robert, and Simpson ultra-low profile catheters (Fig. 15-6). These USCI catheters have a slightly stiffer shaft, permitting a more effective transmission of force in passing the distal balloon tip through severe stenosis, an advantage that is generally lost in distal or tortuous vessels.

Tip		Largest guidewire (inches)	Average deflated profiles (inches)		Average deflation time (seconds)	Approx. price (1986)
Outer diameter (inches)	Inner diameter		2 mm balloon	3 mm balloon		
0.035-0.05	0.02	0.018	0.045	0.055	6-10	$420
0.035-0.05	0.022	0.018	0.044	0.054	6-12	$445
0.025-0.035	0.016	0.014	0.040	0.050	6-10	$475
0.023		Fixed guidewire Tip 1 or 3 cm	0.035	0.043	6-10	$525
0.024	0.010	Movable guidewire 0.015 (not removable) 2 or 3 cm tip	0.036	0.043	6-10	
0.022	0.016	0.014	0.039		4	$400
0.026	0.020	0.016		0.050	6-12	$400
0.022	0.016	0.014	0.036		5	$445
0.026	0.020	0.018		0.050	5-10	
0.022	0.019	0.014	0.032		5	$450
0.026	0.020	0.018		0.040	5-10	
0.030	0.021	0.018	0.055	0.058	3-5	$400
0.026	0.020	0.018	0.04	0.049	3-4	
0.026	0.020	0.018	0.04	0.049	3-4	
0.025	0.021	0.018	0.04		4	$425
0.030	0.021			0.050	6	
0.035	0.021					
0.028		0.014				
		0.010	0.037			
0.024		0.012		0.053		

*Shaft diameter of 4 mm balloon in Simpson-Robert is 4.7 Fr.
All dilatation catheters have shaft length of 135 cm except Schneider, which is 130 cm long.

The ACS dilatation catheters have a slightly lower profile. The polyethylene material and catheter construction provide more flexibility and ease in negotiating tortuous vessels and permit freer motion of the guidewire through the catheter. The inflation of the balloon is more rapid. However, the Simpson-Robert and Simpson ultra-low profile catheters are suboptimal for distal contrast material injection or pressure monitoring while the guidewire is in place. To overcome this, a new catheter has been designed (Delta System) to permit satisfactory distal contrast agent injection and pressure measurements.

The balloon at the distal tip of all dilatation catheters is constructed so that it can withstand and transmit increasingly higher inflation pressures without large changes in its diameter. This prevents overstretching of the balloon and rupture of the arteries at high pressures. The balloon diameters of USCI catheters (polyvinylchloride) vary slightly based on the inflation pressure used. It appears that the preset balloon diameter is reached at approximately 6 to 8 atmospheres; at inflation pressures below this, the balloon diameter is approximately 10% less, and at pressures over this, balloon diameters can be increased by approximately 10%. Table 15-5 cites these parameters for the USCI catheter line. ACS catheters (polyethelene) do not change diameter with the inflation pressure. This information is important in matching the diameter of the balloon to the diameter of the coronary artery being dilated. The danger of overstretching the artery cannot be overempha-

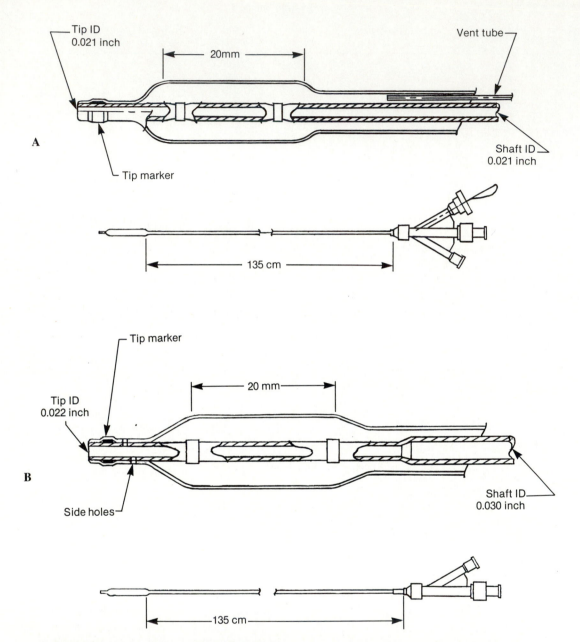

Fig. 15-3. A, Longitudinal section of the Simpson-Robert-ACS catheter. The polyethylene inner tubing is used for passage of the guidewire, injection of contrast material, and pressure measurements. The outer tubing has the balloon formed at its distal tip. Note the vent tube between the two tubings. When the balloon is filled with contrast material, air can be evacuated from the balloon. **B,** Longitudinal section of the Delta dilatation catheter. There is a slightly increased inner diameter, tip side holes, and no vent tube.

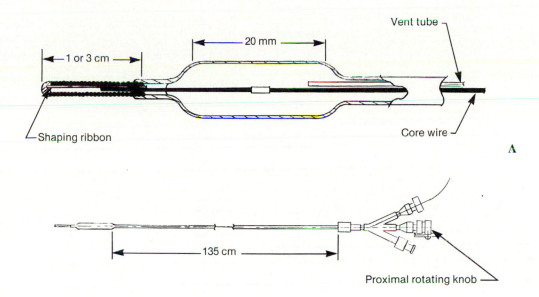

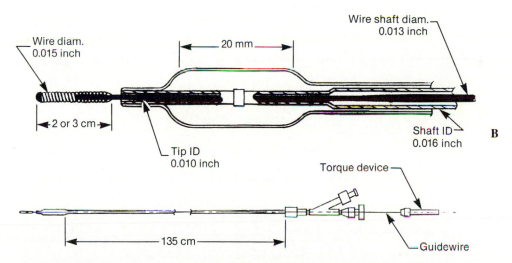

Fig. 15-4. A, Longitudinal section of the Hartzler LPS catheter (ACS). Note that there is no inner tubing, the balloon being formed over a small guidewire. One radiopaque marker is located at the center of the balloon. A rotating knob changes the direction of the tip. **B,** Longitudinal section of the Hartzler Microcatheter. There is a self-venting balloon and an independently movable and torqueable guidewire that can be moved 10 cm, but cannot be removed from the catheter. There is no vent tube.

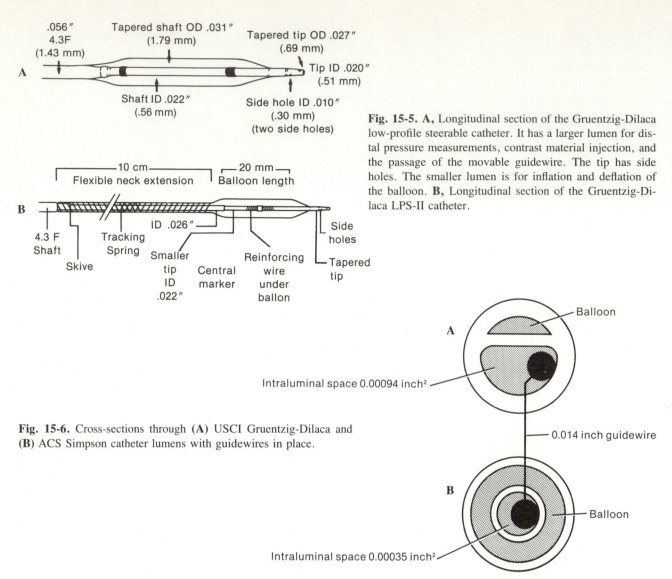

A, .056" 4.3F (1.43 mm) — Tapered shaft OD .031" (1.79 mm) — Tapered tip OD .027" (.69 mm) — Tip ID .020" (.51 mm) — Shaft ID .022" (.56 mm) — Side hole ID .010" (.30 mm) (two side holes)

B, 10 cm Flexible neck extension — 20 mm Balloon length — 4.3 F Shaft — Tracking Spring — Skive — Smaller tip ID .022" — ID .026" — Central marker — Reinforcing wire under ballon — Side holes — Tapered tip

Fig. 15-5. A, Longitudinal section of the Gruentzig-Dilaca low-profile steerable catheter. It has a larger lumen for distal pressure measurements, contrast material injection, and the passage of the movable guidewire. The tip has side holes. The smaller lumen is for inflation and deflation of the balloon. **B,** Longitudinal section of the Gruentzig-Dilaca LPS-II catheter.

A — Balloon — Intraluminal space 0.00094 inch² — 0.014 inch guidewire — B — Balloon — Intraluminal space 0.00035 inch²

Fig. 15-6. Cross-sections through **(A)** USCI Gruentzig-Dilaca and **(B)** ACS Simpson catheter lumens with guidewires in place.

Table 15-5. Inflated diameters of USCI® Gruentzig Dilaca® low-profile steerable balloon catheters

Inflation pressure (bars)	Balloon size				
	2.0 mm	2.5 mm	3.0 mm	3.5 mm	4.0 mm
4	1.85	2.25	2.70	3.22	3.66
5	1.93	2.34	2.81	3.33	3.78
6	2.02	2.42	2.90	3.42	3.92
7	2.10	2.50	2.98	3.54	4.04
8	2.18	2.59	3.07	3.63	4.17
9	2.26	2.65	3.15	3.72	4.29
10	2.35	2.73	3.28	3.80	4.41
11	2.43	2.83	3.32	3.90	4.55
12	2.53	2.89	3.40	3.97	4.66
13	2.70	3.00	3.46	4.02	
14		3.09	3.55		

Reproduced by permission of C.R. Bard, Inc.

sized. Dissection and rupture have occurred under such circumstances.

Tandem balloon catheters are now only available in Europe (Schneider-Medintag) and are designed for stepwise dilatation of severe stenoses or combined dilatation of a proximal and distal stenoses with one catheter.[29a] In the United States this is currently accomplished by sequential use of the same dilatation catheter or its exchange over a guidewire for a smaller or larger diameter dilatation catheter. Tandem balloon catheters are expected to be available in the United States in the near future.

Guidewires[13,28-32] (Table 15-6)

The development of the movable and steerable guidewires was a major step in the advancement of the angioplasty technique. The requirements of angioplasty likewise prompted the development of versatile and sophisticated guidewires. The following are desirable or necessary characteristics of an angioplasty guidewire.

Visibility. Angioplasty wires must be easily seen by means of fluoroscopy. Stainless steel wires with diameters of 0.018 inch or less are not easily seen with most fluoroscopy units. This problem was solved by using gold or platinum in the distal weld of the guidewire. Subsequently platinum was used in the distal coil, making currently used angioplasty wires easily seen with standard fluoroscopy.

Steerability (torque control). Angioplasty guidewires must be steerable to permit passage into tortuous vessels and branches. Early workers using movable guidewires were limited by lack of steerability. Now most angioplasty guidewires are constructed so that they provide satisfactory torque control (see Table 15-6). This feature has extended the application of angioplasty to tortuous vessels and side branches that otherwise could not be negotiated.

Flexibility. Angioplasty guidewires should be soft at the tip to permit nontraumatic passage through the coronary artery and reduce the chance of dissection. Tip flexibility is achieved by ending the tapered core several centimeters before the tip. On the other hand, some tip stiffness may be required to provide trackability and steerability to permit passage through a fresh thrombus or a chronic occlusion. The Teflon coating of the tip causes increased stiffness. Some guidewires have the tip free of Teflon coating, making it more flexible. These requirements for varying degrees of tip flexibility (and length of flexible tip) have prompted the production of a variety of guidewires with sometimes confusing names and designations (see Table 15-6 for details on guidewire construction). There is much need for standardization as well as some designation on the proper role of the different guidewires.

Shapability (maleability). Angioplasty guidewires should have tips that can be shaped into various size curves to suit the individual requirements, and these curves should be retained (memory). The introduction of tip-forming ribbons at flexible wire tips has made this possible. Extending the tapered core of the guidewire to its tip (full-body wires) is an alternative method that increases the stiffness of the tip as well as the potential for intimal trauma. These curves may be set in the factory or made as needed.

Trackability. Trackability refers to the ability of the wire to follow the tip when the tip has engaged a side branch. Angioplasty wires should possess a degree of trackability to permit passage to side branches with acute angles. Trackability also refers to the ability to advance the dilatation catheter over the wire. This function would require some stiffness in the wire; thus, both extreme flexibility and trackability are not possible in the same wire. The different guidewires available try to achieve varying degrees of compromise in favor of one or the other requirement. Full-body wires with their tapered core extending to the tip provide maximal trackability and steerability.

Size. Commonly used guidewires have diameters of 0.018 to 0.014 inch (0.46 to 0.36 mm). Guidewires in development have diameters 0.012 and 0.010 inch (0.30 and 0.25 mm). The larger wires (0.016 and 0.018 inch) permit better steerability and catheter tracking, especially around sharp angles. They provide more stability and support as well as axial strength in crossing tight stenosis. The smaller wire (0.014 and 0.012 inch) is superior for distal injection of contrast material and measurement of distal pressures and also allows the use of smaller profile dilatation catheters.

Table 15-6 lists the currently available guidewires. These are all 175 cm long, except the exchange guidewire, which is 300 cm long. Fig. 15-7, *A* to *C*, illustrates guidewire construction.

Guidelines for guidewire use. Proper use of the guidewire is crucial to the safe and successful performance of angioplasty.

1. Handle the guidewire carefully. Avoid bending the wire; torque control will be lost in a bent wire.

2. The guidewire should meet no resistance in the dilatation catheter. If the wire meets resistance in the coronary artery, the operator should feel this. The wire should not be forced. Independent and free motion of the guidewire in the dilatation catheter is important for providing tactile information to the operator and for safe steering and negotiating of acute angles.

Text continued on p. 346.

Table 15-6. Angioplasty guidewires

Manufacturer	Type	Diameter (inches)	Coating	Tip construction
ACS	SOF-T	0.018	Teflon for body of wire; with or without Microglide for distal 37 cm	3 cm floppy platinum coil at its tip, with shaping ribbon in distal tip
	Multipurpose (PDT)	0.014	Same	Tapered core ends 1 cm from tip; 1 cm tip has shaping ribbon
	Hi-torque standard (stiff or intermediate)	0.018 & 0.014	Same	30 cm flexible spring wire; tapered core (0.003 inch) extends to tip & is wrapped with platinum alloy coils
	High-torque floppy	0.018 & 0.014	Same	30 cm flexible spring; tapered core ends 2 cm from tip. Shaping ribbon provides tip with memory. Distal gold tip weld
	High-torque floppy exchange	0.018 & 0.014	Same	Same
	Exchange	0.018 & 0.014	Same	5 cm tapered core wrapped with platinum alloy coils
USCI†	Steerable J	0.014 & 0.016	Teflon	Tapered core extends to tip weld; 25 cm flexible radiopaque platinum tip ends with 30° bend
	Flexible straight	0.014 0.016	Teflon	Tapered core ends 2 cm short of distal tip, forming ribbon in distal 2 cm, straight tip
	Flexible J	0.014 0.016	Teflon	Same as above except tip ends with 30° bend
	Very flexible straight	0.014	Teflon	Tapered core ends 3 cm short of distal tip, forming ribbon in distal 3 cm, straight tip; 25 cm flexible radiopaque platinum tip
	Very flexible J	0.014	Teflon	Same as above with tip ending in 30° bend
	Flexible straight exchange	0.014‡	Teflon	2 cm flexible tip & 25 cm radiopaque platinum tip
Mansfield Scientific, Inc.	Heart track	0.014	Teflon up to 35 cm from tip	Tapered core extends to a straight tip
Schneider-Medintag	Straight or J	0.014 0.012 0.010		
	Exchange	0.012 0.014		
	Kaltenbach (long-wire technique) straight or J	0.012		Ball-shaped tip; straight or J

Features*				
Torque	Flexibility	Malleability	Use	Approx. price
3+	3+	2+	When there is moderate need for tip steering in tortuous vessels	$47
2+	3+	2+	With low-profile system	$47
4+(.018)	2+	3+	When exact tip movement is needed; good for side branches and total chronic occlusions; has stiff tip; potentially traumatic	$55
4+(.018) 3+(.014)	3-4+ 2+	2+ 2+	When exact tip movement is needed; nontraumatic, good for recrossing dilated lesions or acute occlusions; excellent all purpose (.018); also available in 300 cm as exchange wire	$50
2+	3+	2+	For dilatation catheter exchange	$75
1+	4+	1+	Same	$75
4+(.016) 3+(.014)	1−2+ 2+	4+(.016) 3+(.014)	When minimal wire steering and manipulation is needed; excellent for old (chronic) total occlusions; potentially traumatic	$50
3+ 4+(.016)	3+	2+	For straight vessels; for curves, tip may be bent	$50
3+ 4+(.016)	3+	2+	When good tip movement is needed, as in moderately tortuous vessel and side branches	$50
3+	4+	1+	When good tip movement is needed; nontraumatic tip, could be bent; suitable for recrossing lesions or acute occlusions	
3+	4+	1+	Same as above	$50
3+	3+	2+	Dilatation catheter exchange	$65
3+	2+	3+	When little wire manipulation is needed; good for chronic occlusions; potentially traumatic	$50
4+	2-3+	3+		
2+	2-3+	3+		

†All USCI guidewires can be attached to a USCI *extension wire*, permitting catheter exchanges.
‡Distal 125 cm is 0.014 inch, proximal 175 cm is 0.016 inch.

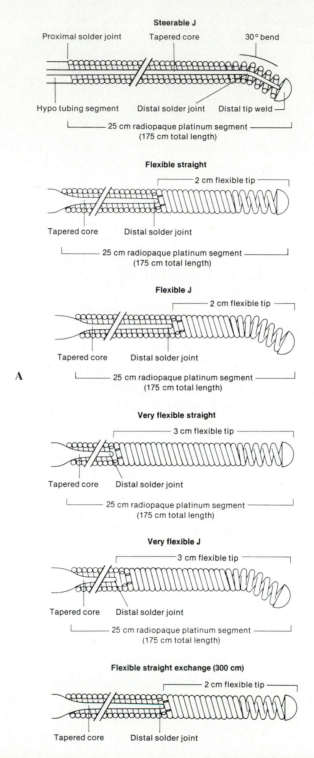

Fig. 15-7. A, USCI guidewire construction. See Table 15-6 for details.

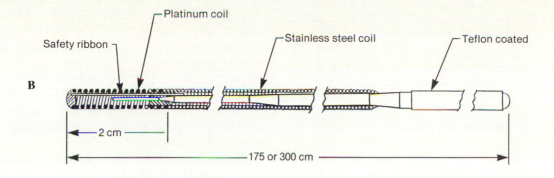

B

Safety ribbon — Platinum coil — Stainless steel coil — Teflon coated

←— 2 cm —→

←———————————— 175 or 300 cm ————————————→

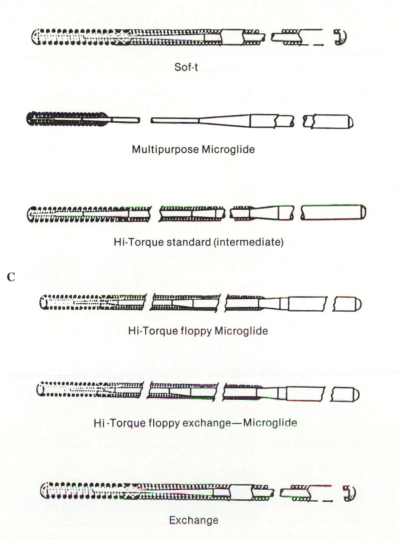

Sof-t

Multipurpose Microglide

Hi-Torque standard (intermediate)

C

Hi-Torque floppy Microglide

Hi-Torque floppy exchange—Microglide

Exchange

Fig. 15-7, cont'd. B, Details of construction of ACS-high torque floppy guidewire. **C,** ACS guidewire construction. See Table 15-6 for details.

3. Different functions are served by different guide-wires. Choose the proper guidewire as a part of the pre-planning strategy. As the procedure progresses (or stalls!) do not hesitate to change the guidewire if circumstances change. Choice of guidewire and change of guidewire should be reasoned exercises and not matters of trial and error.

4. Preshape a wire in anticipation of needs based on the coronary anatomy observed. Do not hesitate to gently reshape the wire multiple times if necessary. Discard a wire if the tip becomes damaged.

5. Always observe the wire tip by means of fluoroscopy during advancement of the catheter. Buckling indicates resistance. Do not force the guidewire.

6. Advancement or withdrawal of the guidewire should be gentle; never advance or withdraw it rapidly. If withdrawal meets resistance, pull back the whole system gently.

7. Always advance the floppy tip of the guidewire past the stenosis and distally into the vessel. This permits positioning the stiffer shaft of the guidewire across the stenosis, providing stability and ease of advancement of the dilation catheter across it.

8. When reintroducing a guidewire in the dilatation catheter within the coronary artery, make sure that the tip of the dilatation catheter is free within the arterial lumen. If doubt exists, inject a small amount of contrast material through the dilation catheter and observe the flow.

9. All efforts should be expended to confirm that the wire is intraluminal and in the correct vessel. It is very important that the tip of the guidewire is not positioned in a side branch just distal to the lesion to be dilated. Avoid introducing the guidewire tip into septal branches—ventricular arrhythmias may occur. Confirm wire position in orthogonal views.

10. Do not apply torque to a wire without observing tip movement fluoroscopically. Do not overtorque a wire in one direction if the tip of the wire is not moving.

11. Do not bore a guidewire through a stenosis or total occlusion; the guidewire may become entrapped within the stenosis.

12. Use the exchange guidewire when indicated. After initial guidewire/catheter passage to the area of stenosis, if a larger dilatation catheter is needed, use the exchange guidewire to safely recross a dilated segment or avoid negotiating a difficult proximal coronary anatomy.

Inflation devices

Inflation devices are illustrated in Fig. 15-8. ACS offers an easy-to-use disposable device (Indeflator), consisting of a 10 cc syringe bonded to a one-way stop-

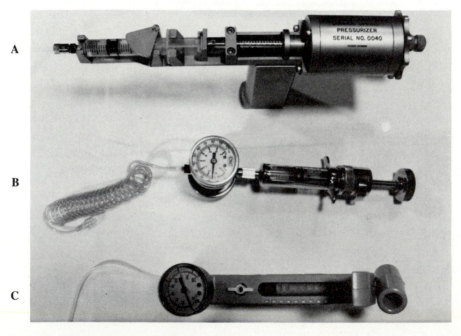

Fig. 15-8. Inflation devices: (A) The Dorros-Spring pressurizer, (B) the USCI inflation device, and (C) the ACS Indeflator.

cock, coupled to a pressure regulator. This leads through a connecting tube and a male Luer fitting to the dilatation catheter. Pressure and balloon inflation are generated by squeezing on the handle or by turning the handle clockwise. Deflation is achieved by the opposite movement.

USCI and Interventional Medical provide easy-to-use reusable inflation devices, similar in concept to the Indeflator. Their simple design consists of a metal syringe adaptor with a stainless steel gauge. The syringe barrel is screwed down and provides a calibrated balloon pressure.

The Dorros-Spring Pressurizer* is an easily sterilized, reusable, hand-held, stainless steel inflation device with a calibrated spring that produces controlled inflation (up to 16 atmospheres) and deflation. It uses a disposable 5 cc plastic syringe and standard pressure tubing.

The carbon dioxide gun was the initial device used for rapidly inflating the dilatation balloon while keeping a continuous negative pressure on it during deflation. It is now obsolete as it is expensive, burdensome, and dangerous (possible balloon rupture).

There is much personal preference as well as unsubstantiated opinion about the superiority of one manufacturer's products as compared with those of another. There are no control or comparative studies. Users of the equipment are urged to become familiar with the technical specifications of the products as well as their design and construction features and to understand the basic concepts in the proper choice of these devices. Ultimately, operators will form their own opinion based on their personal interpretation of the information and their experience.

Trouble-shooting equipment problems

Murphy's law applies to angioplasty. Even in experienced hands with careful attention to detail, things can and will go wrong. Many of the pitfalls and how to handle them are covered in the procedure section. Equipment problems may include the following.

Balloon rupture. Current dilatation catheters in common use will withstand inflation pressures of 10 to 12 atmospheres with 10% to 15% increase (stretching) of their preset diameter (polyvinylchloride catheters) at maximal pressures. Higher inflation pressures will frequently cause balloon rupture; defective balloons may rupture at lower pressures. Although frequently well tolerated, balloon rupture is always undesirable because

---

*Available from Cardiovascular Diagnostic Services, Inc., Suite 930, 811 E. Wisconsin Ave. Milwaukee, WI 53202.

(1) the overstretching before rupture of the balloon may predispose to coronary artery overstretching and possible arterial rupture, (2) balloon rupture may risk introduction of air into the coronary artery, and (3) rupture necessitates removal of the balloon and the guidewire (unless an exchange guidewire was used). Unless the dilatation was successful, recrossing with the new guidewire and balloon may be difficult and risky. A ruptured balloon may not easily be pulled back across the lesion and inside the guiding catheter.

We recommend the following:
1. Do not deliberately exceed the recommended inflation pressures.
2. If balloon rupture occurs and there is any difficulty in pulling the balloon across the stenosis, use intracoronary nitroglycerin to relieve any possible spasm and gently and continuously pull on the dilatation catheter while applying negative pressure until it is withdrawn across the stenosis.
3. If the ruptured balloon cannot easily be pulled inside the guiding catheter, withdraw the guiding catheter and the dilatation catheter as one unit.

Guidewire breakage. Angioplasty guidewires are delicate instruments with variable tip construction to meet different needs. Understanding the construction of these wires will permit safer use. The safety ribbons on the tips of these flexible guidewires have reduced the risk of tip separation and guidewire fragment embolism. If the tip of a guidewire is caught in an arterial branch, and the operator, unaware of this, applies extreme torque, the tips can break off. It is important to recognize this and take the proper action.

1. If caught in an arterial branch, the wire will meet resistance when withdrawn and its tip will not move.

2. Observe the tip by means of fluoroscopy while gently pulling the wire back.

3. If free withdrawal is not possible, advance the dilatation catheter over the guidewire to the distal tip of the wire and then try to pull them out as one unit.

Guidewire kinks or bends. If kinks or bends develop in the guidewire, use a new wire.

Guiding catheter kinks. Guiding catheters do not handle torque as well as diagnostic coronary arteriography catheters. Their larger inside diameter can cause kinks when considerable torque is applied. This is particularly a problem in the approach to the right coronary artery. The development of kinks in the coronary catheter may prevent its easy withdrawal through the introducer. The problem is recognized when torque applied at the proximal end of the catheter is not transmitted to its tip. This is usually solved by reversing the direction of the torque and gently pulling the catheter in the introducer.

Patient preparation

Patient preparation for angioplasty is similar to that for cardiac catheterization. The patient is admitted to the hospital 12 to 24 hours before the scheduled procedure, and the following preparations are made.

1. Review the patient's medical condition and confirm the need for angioplasty.

2. Instruct the patient on the procedure and what to expect, preferably with the help of pictures or slides. Obtain informed consent.

3. Make adequate preparation for emergency surgery, although the need is infrequent (approximately 2% to 5%). This should include consulting a cardiovascular surgeon, typing and cross-matching of blood, and keeping the patient fasting for at least 8 hours.

4. Review laboratory studies before coronary angioplasty: complete blood count, electrolytes, creatinine, ECG, and chest radiograph. Other laboratory studies should be performed as individually required.

5. Continue all necessary cardiac and noncardiac medications. Some physicians have recommended stopping beta blockers, but the use of beta blockers does not seem to be associated with an increased incidence of ischemic episodes after angioplasty.[34] Patients are given enteric coated aspirin (325 mg by mouth twice a day) and dipyridamole (Persantine) (75 mg three times a day), preferably 48 hours before the procedure. In some centers Persantine is administered only after the procedure or not used at all. One study suggests that the combined use of aspirin and dipyridamole before angioplasty decreases the incidence and clinical significance of acute coronary thrombus after the procedure.[35] A randomized study is in progress (Mayo Clinic) comparing the use of aspirin/Persantine and placebo.

6. Establish a secure IV line 1 to 2 hours before the procedure.

7. Use an external urinary catheter or a Foley catheter if necessary, especially when a lengthy procedure is anticipated.

8. Administer diazepam, a barbiturate, or a narcotic 30 minutes before the start of the procedure. In addition, give a calcium blocker and a long-acting nitrate preparation.

Drugs used during angioplasty

The following drugs are either routinely used or occasionally needed in emergencies during coronary angioplasty and should be immediately at hand: nitroglycerin (sublingual and injectable forms), heparin, calcium blockers (oral or sublingual nifedipine, diltiazem, IV verapamil), atropine, metaraminol (Aramine), lido-

caine, morphine, and dopamine. For details on these drugs see Chapter 18. Their use will be discussed in the section on procedures. Thrombolytic agents (streptokinase, urokinase, tissue plasminogen activator—see Chapter 16) should also be available.

Based on animal experimental data, IV dextran was used routinely during angioplasty during the early 1980s with the hope of preventing a layering of platelets and thrombus formation at the site of angioplasty. However, experiments in dogs have failed to show benefits,[36] and two studies in humans of the use of IV dextran during angioplasty have shown no benefit to either the success rate or the acute occlusion rate.[37,38] Potentially fatal anaphylactoid reactions secondary to the use of dextran 40 have been reported.[39] Based on these data, we and many others no longer use it. Other experienced operators continue to use IV dextran during angioplasty (500 ml of 10% dextran 40 started 30 minutes before and continued during the procedure at 100 ml/hour) (Gentran: 50 g dextran 40 in 500 ml 5% dextrose in water).

Review of the coronary cinearteriogram

Before starting the procedure, carefully review (rereview) the coronary cinearteriogram. This inspection will help you in making an intelligent choice of catheter and guidewire, determining what degree of curve or bend to form at the guidewire tip, and anticipating difficulties that may arise in reaching the area of the stenosis or positioning the wire tip in a suitable area past the stenosis. This review should include the following steps.

1. Pay careful attention to the aortic root and origin of the coronary artery to be dilated to determine the position and seating of the guiding catheter in the coronary ostium. Is its position stable? Does wedging appear to be a problem?

2. Decide on the best approach—femoral or transbrachial (see pp. 350 and 353).

3. Decide on the size and type of guiding and dilatation catheters to be used (see pp. 334 and 335).

4. Determine the projection and angulation most helpful in approaching the stenosis. This may not be the same projection chosen for viewing the balloon and subsequent angioplasty during the dilatation.

5. Inspect the path that the guidewire will take from the coronary artery ostium to the area of stenosis and into the distal branches. It may appear that the guidewire will naturally follow the main artery lumen and seek the area of the stenosis. This is frequently not the case! Side branches and bends, which are generally ignored during routine review of coronary arteriograms,

now need to be inspected with care. The guidewire can and will find ways of getting to side branches that you never knew existed!

Inspection of the area of stenosis

1. Is the immediate area of stenosis symmetrical, hourglass shaped (relatively easy to cross), or eccentric (difficult to cross)? The angiographic estimation of the severity of narrowing does not necessarily correlate with ease or difficulty in passing a wire or balloon catheter across the stenosis.

2. Is the stenosis discrete and focal, or long? This determination will help you choose the dilatation balloon with the correct length, place it properly, and choose the site(s) of repeat dilatations.

3. Is the lesion calcified? Densely calcified plaques may often cause resistance to balloon passage and may require higher dilatation pressures.

4. What is the diameter of the coronary artery lumen immediately before and after the area of stenosis to be dilated? This is an important estimate. To aid you in this, use the diameter of the diagnostic angiographic catheter as an internal reference marker. The outside diameter of an 8 Fr angiographic catheter is 2.6 mm; a 7 Fr catheter has an outside diameter of 2.3 mm, and both have tips (5 Fr) with outside diameters of 1.65 mm. Determine the size of dilatation balloon to be used to match the inside diameter of the artery. For a particularly narrow or calcified stenosis, one may deliberately undersize the balloon and plan on stepping up to a larger balloon with the help of an exchange guidewire. If in doubt, err on the side of undersizing the balloon.

5. Does the lesion involve any side branches? Will inflation of the balloon risk occlusion of a major branch? Does the anatomy call for use of the double wire technique (see p. 357)?

6. If multivessel angioplasty is being planned, the same stepwise approach needs to be applied to each vessel and area of stenosis to be dilated. Also, plan the sequence of dilatation; the most critical or severe stenosis is generally dilated first.

Pacing during coronary angioplasty[11,40-43]

The need for emergency pacing during angioplasty occurs in 1% to 2% of patients. A right ventricular pacemaker is routinely used in all dominant right coronary (or dominant circumflex) artery angioplasties. A pacemaker is frequently used as a standby unit in left coronary artery angioplasty as well, where in addition to its back-up pacing function, it provides an internal reference point to mark the area of the stenosis. Traditionally, stiff-wall Dacron catheters have been used

(Myler catheter, or a nonlumen 6 Fr bipolar pacing catheter). Complications of right ventricular puncture and pericardial tamponade have been reported with a frequency of 1%. Systemic heparin, combined with traumatic handling of these stiff pacing catheters, is at fault. Acute pericardial tamponade requiring emergency pericardial drainage and cessation (or reversal) of heparin is a most unwelcome complication during an otherwise successful angioplasty! The following suggestions are made:

1. If you are going to use these stiff pacing catheters, handle them very cautiously and delicately.

2. Use guidewires in manipulating these catheters through the right ventricle.

3. Consider using a nontraumatic, balloon-tip, multipurpose pacing catheter[43] (p. 17) or a 5 Fr transvenous pacing electrode.

4. In cases with low risk of major bradycardia (left anterior descending angioplasty), consider the use of a standby transcutaneous external pacer. A balloon-tip flotation right heart catheter may be used for "marking" the lesion.

Satisfactory results have been described for use of the angioplasty guidewire for emergency coronary pacing.[40] We have no experience with this technique, but we are concerned that it will risk coronary artery dissection or thrombus. Its routine use cannot be recommended.

Second review of the coronary cinearteriogram

Having chosen the type of approach, guiding catheter, dilatation catheter, guidewire, and pacing catheter, take another look at the cinearteriogram.

1. Are there collateral vessels? Collateral vessels are frequent in the presence of totally occluded or severely narrowed arteries. The presence of a rich network of collaterals is always reassuring. The patient will tolerate the period of balloon inflation well, prolonged inflations are possible, and if a total occlusion is precipitated it will be better tolerated.

2. How much viable left ventricle is being served by the coronary artery to be dilated and what is the status of the other coronary arteries? Keep the guidelines for patient selection and contraindications in mind. If the procedure cannot be carried out safely, this is your last chance to gracefully back off!

Review of the patient's medical record

Specifically check the report of the cardiac catheterization study to note if any special difficulties were encountered during the procedure in relation to vascular access, choice of catheters, contrast material reaction, and so on. Ensure that patient preparation has been carried out properly and that informed consent is documented in the medical record.

Preplanning

Review the procedure with your assistants. Discuss any questions and choice of alternatives. Even the best-laid plans will be modified and sometimes abandoned during the actual angioplasty procedure. However, starting the procedure with a set but flexible plan will ensure a smoother operation.

Ensure availability of surgical back-up and intra-aortic balloon pump. Being convinced that the angioplasty procedure is necessary, and having informed the patient, secured consent, and addressed the technical details, you are now ready to begin the procedure.

The following section will outline the steps involved in a smoothly performed, successful, uncomplicated angioplasty, using the femoral route. The following special considerations are discussed separately: transbrachial approach (p. 353); difficulty negotiating the various vessels, vein, and internal mammary grafts (p. 353); bifurcation lesions (p. 357); equipment and technical problems and how to deal with them (p. 347); and management of complications (p. 361).

THE ANGIOPLASTY PROCEDURE*
Femoral approach

1. Prepare the patient in a manner similar to that for cardiac catheterization (see Chapter 5).

2. Enter the right or left femoral artery and vein using the percutaneous Seldinger technique; position the proper-size long arterial and regular-length venous introducers (see Chatpers 2 and 3).

3. Administer heparin—10,000 units intravenously. An additional 5000 units is given if the procedure is prolonged over 2 hours. (For discussion concerning dextran see p. 348).

4. Secure both introducers to the skin with sutures so that the sheath will remain secure during catheter manipulation.

5. Introduce a multipurpose pacing catheter with a lumen through the venous sheath and with *gentle* manipulation place it in the right ventricle or pulmonary artery (see p. 349). Ensure pacing capture.

6. Obtain right heart pressures; this information will be valuable if the patient develops hemodynamic instability.

7. Introduce the guiding catheter with its 0.063-inch (1.6 mm) guidewire protruding through the arterial

*See references 11, 13, 44-58.

sheath. Advance it to the thoracic aorta and across the aortic arch to the ascending aorta.

8. Remove the guidewire and flush the catheter. Record aortic pressures. Fill the catheter with contrast medium.

9. Advance the guiding catheter gently to the coronary ostium of the artery to be dilated. This is usually done in the left anterior oblique projection.

10. Obtain stable coaxial catheter seating in the aortic root, properly aligned to the coronary ostium.

11. Check catheter tip pressures for damping.

12. Visualize the coronary artery on the cinearteriogram and record the data on videotape or disc. Determine if there has been any change in the coronary artery anatomy as compared with the prior diagnostic study.

13. Choose the projection and angulation that give the best view of the area of the stenosis and the initial approach to it; freeze guiding frames for reference during the remainder of the procedure.

14. Inject intracoronary nitroglycerin (100 to 300 μg) via the guiding catheter. Sublingual nifedipine (10 mg) may also be given.

15. Withdraw the guiding catheter to a position just proximal to the coronary ostium.

16. Introduce the properly prepared dilatation balloon catheter with its guidewire through a Y connector and into the guiding catheter. Advance 10 cm of guidewire beyond the dilatation catheter.

17. Connect the Y connector to the guiding catheter while flushing the catheter to ensure bubble-free connections. The guiding catheter, dilatation catheter, and manifold system are illustrated in Fig. 15-9.

18. Measure pressures at the guiding catheter tip and the dilatation catheter tip. This is the time to confirm that satisfactory pressures are recorded. There should be no appreciable difference between the mean pressures at this point.

19. Under fluoroscopic control, reengage the coronary ostium with the guiding catheter and gently advance the dilatation catheter with the guidewire protruding from it to the tip of the guiding catheter.

20. Independently advance the guidewire without the dilatation catheter into the coronary artery, *always visualizing the tip of the guidewire with fluoroscopy.* Inject contrast material repeatedly through the guiding catheter to help locate the correct branch and steer the guidewire into it. The "frozen" guiding frame is used for reference during advancing of the guidewire.

21. Position the guidewire well beyond the stenosis and deep into the distal lumen of the primary artery, avoiding kinks or loops. Ensure proper position by

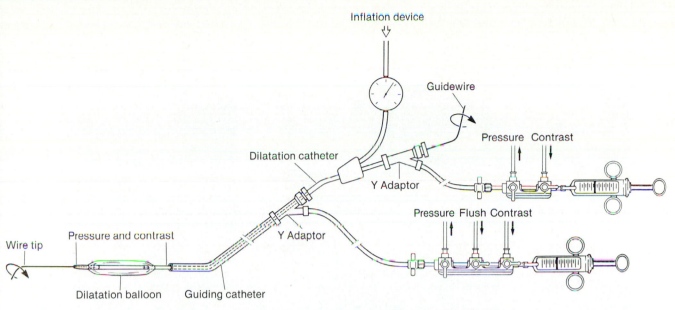

Fig. 15-9. The guiding catheter, dilatation catheter, and manifold system.

small injections of contrast material through the guiding catheter and view in multiple projections.

22. Advance the dilatation catheter toward the stenosis while holding the guidewire back.

23. Repeat intracoronary administration of nitroglycerin (100 to 200 µg).

24. With angiographic and pressure monitoring and while holding the guidewire back, advance the dilatation catheter and position it *across* the stenosis, trying to place the central area of the balloon at the area of the most severe narrowing. Apply firm forward pressure on the guiding catheter during this maneuver, because you may encounter considerable back-pressure as the dilatation catheter engages the stenosis. Having the patient cough may help advance the balloon.

25. Record the change in the mean distal pressure and the estimate of the mean pressure gradient across the stenosis.

26. Confirm optimal balloon position by injecting a small amount of contrast material proximally via the guiding catheter, or if needed, distally via the dilatation catheter, to assess distal flow and proper position of the radiopaque balloon markers in relation to the stenosis. *Do not inflate the balloon unless correct balloon position is confirmed!* Permit the contrast agent to clear.

27. Perform the dilatation (see p. 366) under fluoroscopic control (Fig. 15-10).

28. Observe balloon inflation and the deformity produced by the lesion on the balloon. This verifies correct balloon positioning. Note the pressure required to fully dilate the balloon. Record the first and subsequent dilatations briefly by means of cineangiography. Note the change in the pressure gradient with each inflation and deflation. Injecting a small amount of contrast material via the dilatation catheter will be helpful for assessing distal runoff and may also improve the distal pressure waveform, especially if high inflation pressures have been employed.

29. Completion of the procedure is determined by full balloon inflation, the number of dilatations performed, satisfactory pressures and duration of inflation, the low residual gradient across the stenosis, and the preliminary (and frequently suboptimal) cineangiographic view obtained with the dilatation catheter still across the stenosis. Long stenosis should be dilated at the outflow of the lesion, at the midportion, and finally at the inflow portion of the stenosis.

30. Ensure balloon deflation and gently withdraw the dilatation catheter proximal to the area of stenosis while advancing the guidewire so that its tip is kept safely distal to the area of stenosis to ensure ability to recross the stenosis if the need arises. Monitor pressures during this pull-back.

31. Visualize the coronary artery with combined injections in the guiding and dilatation catheters with the guidewire still across the lesion. Inspect the area of the dilated vessel segment. If the pressure and angiographic results are satisfactory (see p. 364), the procedure is essentially completed.

32. If these results are not satisfactory, readvance the

A   B   C

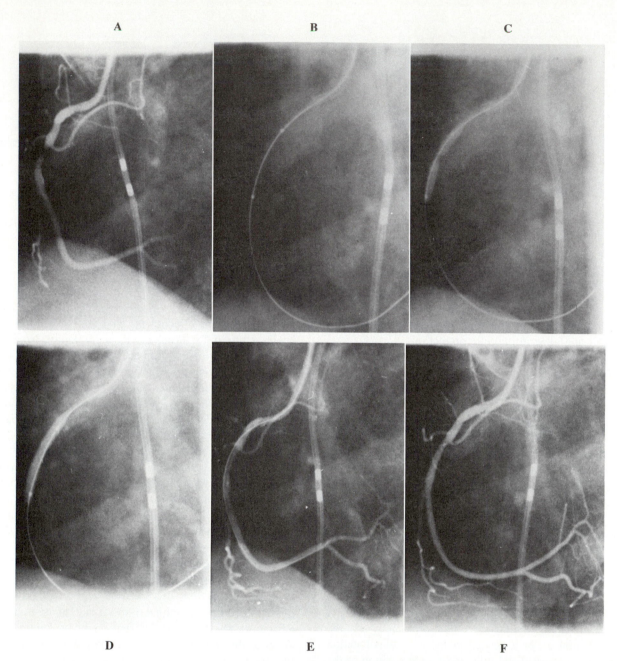

D   E   F

Fig. 15-10. Angioplasty of a high-grade stenosis in the proximal right coronary artery, left anterior oblique projection. **A,** Predilatation arteriogram showing proximal stenosis. **B,** Proper position of the guidewire and the dilatation catheter, before inflation of the balloon. **C,** Initial balloon inflation. Note the deformity produced by the lesion on the balloon. **D,** Balloon fully dilated. **E,** Postdilatation preliminary arteriogram with the guidewire still across the dilated segment, showing satisfactory result. **F,** Final postdilatation arteriogram showing good result.

dilatation catheter over the guidewire to the area of stenosis, determine any residual gradient, and repeat the dilatation, possibly using higher dilatation pressures and longer duration.

33. After successful dilatation, leave the guidewire in the coronary artery across the stenosis and withdraw the dilatation catheter within the tip of the guiding catheter. Observe the patient.

34. Administer intracoronary nitroglycerin (100 to 300 μg) through the guiding catheter.

35. If the patient has no chest pain and the ECG and hemodynamic pressures remain stable for approximately 5 to 10 minutes, remove the guidewire and dilatation catheter assembly.

36. Obtain the final selective coronary arteriogram via the guiding catheter in multiple projections. Carefully review this final coronary study before terminating the procedure.

37. Withdraw the pacing catheter under fluoroscopic control to the inferior vena cava. If a multipurpose Swan-Ganz type of catheter was used, it may be left in the pulmonary artery for monitoring purposes, especially in a high-risk patient.

38. Remove the guiding catheter. Insert and secure the arterial introducer into the sheath to prevent its kinking or buckling while permitting pressure monitoring and blood sampling. Secure all catheter and side arm tips with IV drip infusion apparatus. Heparin is not reversed.

39. Transfer the patient to the monitored cardiac care ward (see p. 360).

Brachial approach[30,47,48]

Diagnostic and interventional procedures can be performed with comparable results from brachial or femoral approaches. The angiographer should utilize the approach with which he or she is most familiar and utilize the alternate under select conditions only if thoroughly versed and comfortable with it. This caution, appropriate for diagnostic angiography, is mandatory for coronary angioplasty.

Advantages of the brachial approach include (1) vascular access when limited by disease or previous surgery; (2) improved ability to deal with some anatomic variants; (3) improved control about the orifice of the vessel (flexible soft tip of the brachial guiding catheter and easier torque control from the arm permit safer superselective intubation of a vessel, which is particularly useful in the right coronary artery); and (4) early removal of the catheter at completion of procedure and early ambulation.

It is estimated that approximately 10% of angioplasty procedures are either more easily done or can only be done via the brachial approach.

Insertion of the guiding catheter

1. Perform the brachial cutdown as for diagnostic angiography (p. 78).

2. The insertion of the guiding catheter is facilitated by a catheter introducer, which should be preloaded with a safety J guidewire. Insert the introducer into the arteriotomy 3 to 4 cm and gently advance the guidewire independently another few centimeters. Now, advance the entire system to the point where the guiding catheter reaches the arteriotomy. Introduction of the blunt-tip guide is eased by a plastic vessel lifter (Beckton-Dickinson), which is used to open and stretch the arteriotomy during catheter insertion.

3. Advance the guiding catheter to the aortic root under fluoroscopic guidance and withdraw the guidewire and catheter introducer.

We give 5000 units of heparin intravenously before performing the arteriotomy and another 5000 units intra-arterially through the guiding catheter after insertion. Instillation of heparin in the brachial artery distal to the arteriotomy has been suggested. This is mechanically more difficult and may not offer any significant advantage over adequate systemic heparinization.

Right coronary artery

The right coronary artery is catheterized in the left anterior oblique projection. A small-curve Stertzer guide is used for most patients with normal anatomy and straight origins of the right coronary artery from the aortic root. Wider aortic roots or right coronary vessels that course superiorly from their origin or have the "sheperd's crook" configuration frequently require a medium-size curve. Larger curves are rarely required in the right coronary artery. The guiding catheter can usually be slipped deep into the artery while the patient inspires deeply. A further power fulcrum can be developed by looping the catheter gently on the opposite aortic wall. If the proximal right coronary artery has a superior direction, it is usually necessary to develop a loop in the sinus of Valsalva and increase the loop size gradually with further advancement, rotation, and upward traction on the catheter until a suitable configuration is obtained.

Once the guiding catheter is suitably positioned, the guidewire can be negotiated distally in the vessel across the stenosis. The balloon catheter can often be advanced across a tight stenosis safely by further deep intubation with the guiding catheter once the balloon is beyond the guide. Side holes are not necessary as episodes of guiding catheter wedging can be kept brief and the guide withdrawn toward the orifice without losing its position in the right coronary artery. These considerations make the brachial approach generally preferable for right coronary artery angioplasty.

Left coronary artery

The left coronary artery is approached as in diagnostic arteriography. However, for coronary angioplasty, the long loop position is usually required to obtain a power position. Selective catheterization of the left anterior descending coronary artery is facilitated by clockwise rotation and upward traction of the guide while the loop size is increased.

Similar maneuvers favor circumflex artery catheterization with counterclockwise rotation. Curved, steerable guidewires are of assistance as in the femoral technique. We have found the Castillo curves (type II) and Amplatz femoral guides helpful in approaching the circumflex coronary artery.

Preformed left coronary artery Judkins-type guiding catheters can engage the left coronary artery from the left brachial artery in the same manner as from the femoral approach and can be used with minimal manipulation.

After completion of the procedure, closure of the brachial cutdown site is similar to that following diagnostic angiography (p. 78).

Special technical considerations[11,13,44-46]
Approach to the left anterior descending coronary artery

Approach left anterior descending (LAD) coronary artery lesions via the femoral route, using the Judkins catheter, or via the transbrachial route, using the Stertzer catheter. With the Judkins catheter, proper size selection will ensure a stable seating position in the coronary ostium (see p. 136). When the catheter approaches the LAD/circumflex junction, its tip may be pointing to the LAD or circumflex artery. Its direction is estimated based on the preferential flow of the contrast medium during the coronary arteriogram and is confirmed when the guidewire preceding the dilatation catheter preferentially enters one or the other vessel.

If the tip of the catheter points toward the circumflex artery and the guidewire enters this vessel (Fig. 15-11, A), withdraw the guidewire into the catheter, rotate the guiding catheter anteriorly (counterclockwise), and advance it slightly (Fig. 15-11, B). This will direct the tip of the catheter anteriorly and superiorly toward the LAD artery (Fig. 15-11, C). This repositioning is further helped if the catheter size is slightly smaller for the given aortic root (i.e., Judkins 3.5 Fr left coronary catheter in a normal aortic root or 4.0 to 4.5 Fr in a dilated aortic root). Perform such a manipulation gently, with continuous monitoring of catheter tip pressures, to reduce risk of trauma to the left main coronary

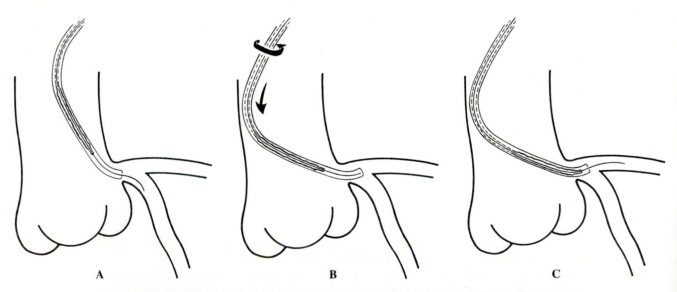

Fig. 15-11. A, The tip of the left Judkins coronary guiding catheter is resting in the left main coronary artery and pointing toward the circumflex artery (right anterior oblique view) so that the guidewire enters this vessel. **B,** The guidewire is withdrawn into the guiding catheter, which is then rotated counterclockwise and advanced slightly, with the tip directed anteriorly and superiorly toward the LAD artery. **C,** The guidewire is advanced into the LAD artery.

artery (LMCA). More aggressive manipulation of the guiding catheter may be necessary during passage of the dilatation catheter across the stenosis. This can be done with reasonable safety, but *only* if the dilatation catheter is advanced past the tip of the guiding catheter, thus partially protecting the LMCA from trauma from the guiding catheter tip. An 8 Fr catheter is safer for such maneuvers. If the LMCA is a long segment or the LAD branches off at a sharp angle, it may not be possible to direct the tip of the catheter to the LAD. Given such a circumstance, entry into the LAD is accomplished by manipulation of the steerable guidewire with a gentle curve at its tip (Fig. 15-12). Use left anterior oblique, caudal, or cranial projection, whichever gives a better visualization of the separation of the LAD and circumflex arteries. Advance the guidewire independently of the dilatation catheter. Steer its gently curved tip in an alternating anterior (counterclockwise) and posterior (clockwise) rotations, with slight withdrawal and advancement until the proper direction is achieved. Continuous rotation of the wire in one direction is not advisable. After the guidewire enters the LAD, advance it and steer it past the stenosis all the way to the cardiac apex, if possible, before advancing the dilatation catheter to the area of the stenosis. If resistance is met and difficulty encountered in crossing the stenosis with the dilatation catheter (e.g., if the guiding catheter backs out of the coronary ostium when the dilatation catheter is pushed forward), investigate the cause of the difficulty. Ensure proper wire position away from side branches and deep in the distal portion of the LAD at the apex. Be sure the wire has not kinked on an eccentric plaque. If wire position is optimal, then additional pressure (force) must be exerted on the dilatation catheter via the guiding catheter. To accomplish this, advance the guiding catheter deeper in the LMCA (now partially protected with the shaft of the dilatation catheter) while pulling back slightly on the dilatation catheter. This is sometimes referred to as the "push-pull" technique. Deeper intubation of the vessel then allows a firmer support from which the dilatation catheter may be advanced across a tight stenosis. This maneuver is generally safe with an 8 Fr guiding catheter and a widely patent left main coronary artery. It is not recommended with a 9 Fr guiding catheter, especially in a smaller or diseased left main coronary artery. The same push-pull technique can be used with distal guidewire and dilatation catheter. The guidewire can be pulled back slightly and the dilating catheter simultaneously advanced. Having the patient cough during the maneuver also can assist in crossing the tight stenosis.

Pressures should be monitored at the tip of the guiding catheter at all times. Pressures may damp for brief periods, but deep intubation should be performed with speed and extreme caution. If successful, it should bring down and position the heel of the Judkins guiding catheter against the opposite wall of the aorta. This position stabilizes the guiding catheter and permits additional pressure to be applied to the dilatation catheter and thus facilitates crossing severely narrowed or hard

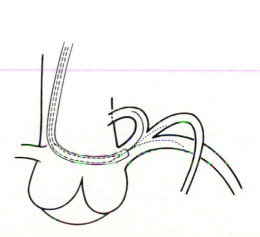

Fig. 15-12. Left anterior oblique, caudal view showing guidewire manipulation to permit entry into the LAD artery.

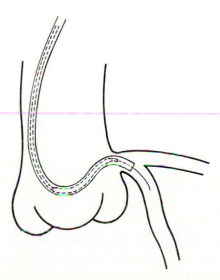

Fig. 15-13. Amplatz catheter in the left coronary artery with its tip pointing to the circumflex branch (right anterior oblique view).

lesions. If deep intubation of the guide has been necessary, withdraw the guide as soon as the balloon is properly positioned. After crossing the stenosis, gently pull back the guiding catheter until it is free in the LMCA; check the pressure at its tip. Continue to be careful regarding the guiding catheter position throughout the dilatation procedure. Withdrawal of the dilating catheter frequently causes the guiding catheter to slip deeper into the coronary vessel. If this maneuver is not successful, the use of the Amplatz or other guiding catheter may be tried. Complete the dilatation process as described on p. 351.

The King multipurpose or El Gamal catheter or using the Stertzer catheter via the transbrachial approach will rarely help when the difficulty in crossing the lesion is due to its "hardness."

Approach to the circumflex coronary artery

Amplatz catheter. The Amplatz catheter is well suited for approach to the circumflex coronary artery. Its tip points inferiorly and when seated in the LMCA, it usually points to the origin of the circumflex artery (Fig. 15-13). This permits easier passage of the guidewire and dilatation catheter. A gentle single curve at the wire tip helps this passage if the LMCA is long. Sharp curves on the steerable guidewire tip must be avoided, as this will make crossing the area of the stenosis difficult.

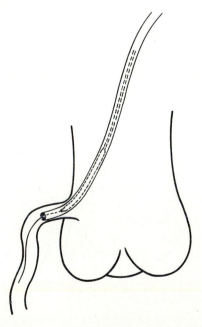

Fig. 15-14. Left anterior oblique view of the Judkins right coronary guiding catheter in the right coronary artery.

After completion of the procedure, gently remove the Amplatz guiding catheter from the LMCA. Fig. 15-13 illustrates the tip of the catheter well engaged in the left coronary orifice. *Do not pull* the catheter to free its tip; this may traumatize the LMCA. Gently advance the shaft of the catheter until the tip is freed and falls into the aortic cusp. Rotate the catheter and withdraw it.

Judkins catheter. The Judkins catheter, with its tip pointing upward, is not ideally suited for approach to the circumflex coronary artery, which is directed posteriorly and inferiorly at its bifurcation from the LMCA. If the diagnostic study was performed with a Judkins-type catheter, the films should be carefully reviewed with attention toward the direction of the catheter tip.

If a Judkins left coronary guiding catheter is used for approach of the circumflex coronary artery, the following maneuvers will help.

1. Choose a larger than usual catheter size (4.5 to 5 Fr Judkins left coronary catheter for a normal aorta). This will help direct the catheter tip more toward the circumflex coronary artery (Fig. 15-11, *A*). We have noted that the left guiding catheters (USCI) are slightly larger than comparably sized diagnostic coronary arteriography catheters.

2. In advancing the steerable guidewire with its gentle single curve, the wire will frequently enter the LAD, given the direction of the tip of the Judkins catheter. To overcome this, shape the tip of the guidewire so that it has a double curve (S form). Thus the distal tip of the guidewire can be steered inferiorly, while the guiding catheter tip may still point superiorly. This is illustrated in the lower guidewire position in Fig. 15-12.

Approach to the right coronary artery

Approach to the right coronary artery poses a different set of problems. There is a wider choice of suitable guiding catheters, including the Judkins, Amplatz, King multipurpose, Stertzer, El Gamal, and Arani catheters. For the transbrachial approach, the Stertzer catheter is preferred. For the transfemoral approach, the Judkins right coronary catheter is used most frequently and no difficulty is usually encountered in properly seating it in the right coronary artery ostium (Fig. 15-14). However, a King multipurpose or Amplatz catheter may also be suitable.

If the catheter tip wedges in the proximal right coronary artery, reposition it until satisfactory seating is established. Do not load the guiding catheter with the dilatation catheter or guidewire unless stable coaxial seating without wedging is established. If difficulty is encountered at this stage, choose an alternative guiding catheter (Amplatz, King multipurpose, Arani, or Judkins guiding catheter with side holes), or proceed via the transbrachial approach.

If the proximal right coronary artery is excessively tortuous and superiorly directed (Fig. 15-15), anticipate difficulty in crossing a tight stenosis. Most of the force applied to the dilatation catheter will be absorbed by the tortuous vessel and will cause the guiding catheter to back off. Such a tortuous right coronary artery is best approached transbrachially. If the femoral route is used, the Arani double loop catheter with a 75 degree curve at its tip—pointing the tip superiorly—may be very helpful.[49]

If the area of stenosis is distal and severe, enough force cannot be applied by the guiding catheter tip for the dilating catheter to pass across the stenosis without difficulty.

If the proximal coronary artery is large, you may pass the guiding catheter over the dilatation catheter into the body of the right coronary artery. To do this, pull back on the dilatation catheter while advancing the guiding catheter. Monitor tip pressures and use small injections of contrast medium via the guiding catheter tip to detect possible wedging. This maneuver is similar to that performed in the LMCA and will permit appreciably more force to be applied to the dilatation catheter. Performed rapidly and with caution, this technique is generally safe.

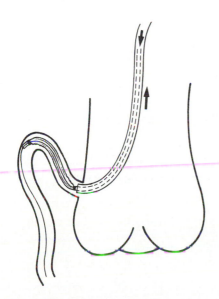

Fig. 15-15. Left anterior oblique view of a tortuous and superiorly directed proximal right coronary artery. Force applied to the dilatation catheter (*short arrow*) causes the guiding catheter (*long arrow*) to back off.

The Judkins right coronary catheter is ill-suited for this maneuver because of the near 90° angle at its tip. It is much better (and safer) to use the King multipurpose catheter or the transbrachial Stertzer approach.

In approaching distal right coronary artery or circumflex artery stenoses, especially in a tortuous vessel, it is advisable to start the procedure with a small, low-profile balloon, perform a preliminary dilatation, and then step up to the definitive balloon with the help of an exchange guidewire. For such a tortuous vessel, chose a balloon that is slightly smaller than the artery and avoid high pressure inflations to reduce the chance of vessel dissection.

Bifurcation lesions[50-56]

Bifurcation lesions most often involve the LAD and its diagonal branches or circumflex marginal vessels, but could also involve the right coronary artery system. If a side branch vessel originates at the site of the stenosis to be dilated, there is risk of side branch occlusion (Fig. 15-16). This risk is higher (10% to 15%) if the ostium of the branch vessel has a stenosis. Such occlusions may be well tolerated and may show spontaneous recanalization but may also cause myocardial infarction. They can frequently be prevented by a double guidewire technique.

In order to determine the need for this technique, carefully assess the angiogram with the following questions.

1. Does the side branch involved originate from the area of the stenosis itself?
2. Is the side branch large enough to warrant an independent bypass if the patient were to have bypass surgery?
3. Is there a stenosis at the origin of the branch vessel?

If the answers to these questions are all positive, the patient should be considered a candidate for the double wire and sequential dilatation technique. This technique requires two separate approaches with two guiding catheters, two balloons, and two guidewires via bifemoral or brachial-femoral approaches.[53] The balloon sizes and guidewire choice will be dictated by the anatomy of the vessels involved. Long duration (60 to 120 seconds) and low pressure inflations are used in these double guidewire sequential inflation methods. This technique is more appropriate for bifurcation stenosis in the LAD. The steps involved are:

1. Position the first guidewire across the stenosis that requires more manipulation. The more difficult vessel is negotiated first to minimize excessive manipulation of the second guidewire while the first guidewire is in place. Withdraw the first guiding catheter with its bal-

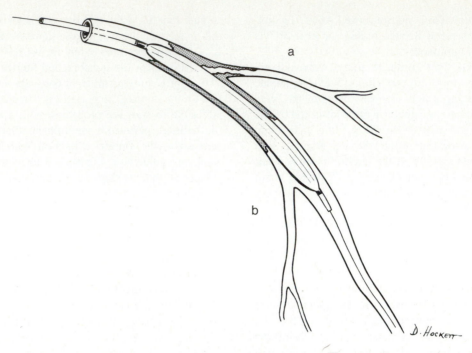

Fig. 15-16. Side branch occlusion during angioplasty may occur if *(a)* the side branch vessel originates at the site of the stenosis to be dilated and the lesion extends into the branch vessel. Branches originating from the adjacent normal artery *(b)* are generally safe, even if within the segment dilated. (Adapted from Meier, B., et al.: Risk of side branch occlusion during coronary angioplasty, Am. J. Cardiol. **53:**10-14, 1984.)

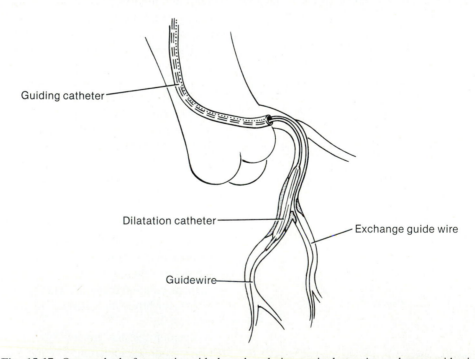

Fig. 15-17. One method of protecting side branches during angioplasty. An exchange guidewire is positioned across the bifurcation, in the vessel to be protected. The dilatation catheter, with its own guidewire, is used for the principal lesion. One guiding catheter is used. See text and Table 15-7 for details. (Adapted from Oesterle, S.N., et al.: Angioplasty at coronary bifurcations: single-guide, two-wire technique, Cathet. Cardiovasc. Diagn. **12:**57-63, 1986.)

loon within it into the aortic sinus, leaving the guidewire in a stable distal position.

2. Position the second guiding catheter in the left coronary ostium and advance its guidewire into the coronary artery, past the secondary area of stenosis, and into the distal vessel.

3. Determine the sequence of dilatations to be performed. The largest vessel supplying the largest area of myocardium is dilated first. Proceed with positioning the proper guiding catheter in the coronary ostium, advance the dilatation catheter over the guidewire and across the area of stenosis, and perform the dilatation.

4. After successful dilatation, withdraw the balloon into the guiding catheter, leave the guidewire in a stable position distal to the stenosis dilated, and withdraw the guiding catheter from the coronary ostium.

5. Perform postdilatation arteriography to determine success of angioplasty and patency of the side branch. If the result is successful and the side branch has no stenosis and has remained patent, no further dilatations are needed. If the side branch has a stenosis or is occluded following angioplasty of the main vessel, then proceed to dilate the side branch.

6. Introduce the second guiding catheter into the coronary ostium, advance the balloon over the previously positioned guidewire, and perform the angioplasty.

7. After successful dilatation of the side branch, cross the major vessel and perform the final inflation there. Document the result on arteriography.

Application of this technique to the right coronary artery or circumflex vessel is more difficult. A modification can be used where one guiding catheter is used and an exchange guidewire positioned across the side branch.[56] Dilatation of the main stenosis is performed using a separate guidewire and dilatation catheter. The side branch is approached and dilated over the exchange guidewire if it has a high-grade stenosis or if it occludes after dilatation of the main vessel. This simplified method of dealing with bifurcation lesions may also be applied to the left coronary artery (Fig. 15-17). Table 15-7 lists potential combinations of dilatation catheter, guiding catheter, and guidewire using this technique. Any combination chosen must be tested on the table, before use, to assure independent motion of the exchange wire and the dilatation catheter in the guiding catheter.

Simultaneous inflations, originally described as "kissing balloon coronary angioplasty,"[52] are cumbersome and appear to be associated with a high rate of restenosis, possibly related to overdistention and mechanical damage to the vessels. Those simultaneous inflations should probably be abandoned or reserved for unusual situations in which the side branch or major vessel closes despite sequential dilatations. In such cases the simultaneous inflations should be done with relatively low pressures.

Bypass grafts

Vein grafts. Vein grafts can be approached with the King multipurpose catheter, the El Gamal catheter, the Arani catheter, or the coronary bypass guiding catheter. The King multipurpose catheter may need to be shaped to a 70° or 80° curve to achieve a stable graft position. Proximal anastomotic areas of stenosis or stenosis within the body of the graft are not optimal for dilatation because of a high rate of recurrence. Ostial sten-

Table 15-7. Potential combinations of catheters and guidewires for side branch protection

Guiding catheter	Exchange wire	
	014 inches	*018 inches*
	Dilatation catheter	
ACS catheters		
8.8 Fr (ID0.076 inches)	2.0-4.0 mm S/R	2.0-3.0 mm S/R
	2.0-3.0 mm S/ULP	2.0-3.0 mm S/ULP
	2.0-3.0 mm H/LPS & H/M	2.0-3.0 mm H/LPS & H/M
8 Fr (ID0.072 inches)	2.0-3.0 mm S/R	2.0 mm only S/R
	2.0-3.0 mm S/ULP	—
	2.0-3.0 mm H/LPS & H/M	2.0-3.0 mm H/LPS & H/M
USCI catheters		
9 Fr, 8 Fr large lumen (ID0.072 inches)	2.0 mm LPS, LPS II, & PP	2.0 mm LPS, LPS II, & PP
	2.5-3.5 mm LPS, LPS II, & PP	
8 Fr (standard) (ID0.068 inches)	2.0 mm LPS & LPS II	
	2.5 mm LPS, LPS II, & PP	

ACS, Advanced Cardiovascular Systems, Inc; *S/R,* Simpson-Robert; *S/ULP,* Simpson Ultralow Profile; *H/LPS,* Hartzler LPS; *H/M,* Hartzler Micro; *USCI,* United States Catheter Instrument Corp., C.R. Bard Inc; *LPS,* Lo Profile Steerable; *LPS II,* Lo Profile Steerable II; *PP,* Profile Plus.

oses may require very high inflation pressures. Stenosis at the distal anastomotic site or past the graft in the native coronary artery can be dilated with good long-term results.

Internal mammary (thoracic) grafts. Internal mammary artery grafts have achieved popularity and increased use because of their superior long-term patency as compared with vein grafts. Stenoses in the body of the internal mammary artery are rare. Experience with dilatation of distal anastomotic site stenosis or stenosis in the distal coronary branches is still limited.[57,58] A specially designed internal mammary artery guiding catheter (8 Fr shaft, 7.5 Fr tapered tip with marker) (Table 15-3) is similar in shape to the internal mammary angiographic catheter (Table 5-5). With increased use of internal mammary artery grafts, experience with angioplasty in this vessel will probably grow.

Ostial lesions

Attempt of dilatation of ostial lesions is generally unrewarding. Technically they are difficult to dilate, results are not encouraging and long-term follow-up is limited.

CARE OF THE PATIENT AFTER ANGIOPLASTY
Care following successful angioplasty[11,13,59-61]

The guidelines for the care of the patient following successful angioplasty have evolved empirically and have not been tested rigorously. They are as follows.

1. Leave both venous and arterial introducers in place.

2. If the venous introducer has a pacemaker catheter, remove this catheter and position a double-lumen Swan-Ganz catheter in the pulmonary artery or insert a soft Teflon catheter in the venous sheath to maintain patency.

3. Insert the introducer back into the arterial sheath and attach a stopcock to its hub. This will prevent kinking or collapse of the sheath and permit intra-arterial pressure monitoring and blood sampling.

4. If the procedure was successful and review of the coronary arteriogram shows no evidence of intimal tear (large intimal flap), further heparin administration is not considered necessary. Do not reverse the heparin used during the procedure with protamine sulfate. If the procedure was otherwise successful, but an intimal tear is present, further administration of heparin is advisable for 24 hours (continuous IV drip, 800 to 1200 units/hour). Monitor partial thromboplastin time (PTT), maintaining it at 2 to 2½ times control level, keep the patient in the coronary care unit, continue IV nitroglyc-

erin, monitor intra-arterial pressure, and avoid hypotension. Taper dosages of heparin and IV nitroglycerin in 12 to 24 hours and discontinue them by 24 hours. Because the mechanism of angioplasty frequently involves some intimal tear (whether or not seen with angiography), many investigators use heparin routinely for 12 to 24 hours following all coronary angioplasty procedures. For all patients we continue IV heparin overnight and remove the sheath early in the morning following the procedure.

5. Move the patient from the angioplasty suite to the cardiac care unit with close nursing care and ECG and blood pressure monitoring for at least 6 hours and usually overnight. Nursing observations should include inspection of cardiac catheter site, observation of rhythm, blood pressure, peripheral pulses, and evaluation for any chest pain.

6. Resume or start the following medications:
   a. Resume nitrates and calcium antagonists and continue them throughout the hospital stay. Their long-term (3 to 6 months) use is generally recommended, empirical, and frequently individualized.
   b. Aspirin, 325 mg/day: This dose is empiric, since manufacturers happen to make aspirin tablets of 325 mg! Some physicians recommend 60 mg (one tablet of baby aspirin), and others 325 mg two times/day. Aspirin is continued for 6 months.
   c. Most centers use dipyridamole, 75 mg three times/day, for 3 months following angioplasty.

It is apparent that most of the drug treatment following angioplasty is concocted by "clinical judgment" and that this neglected area needs investigation to put it on a rational basis. It is entirely possible that rates of acute reclosure and late restenosis could be reduced if the proper use of these or other agents is identified.

7. If the patient remains stable, remove both venous and arterial sheaths after the heparin effect is cleared and apply *manual compression* until satisfactory hemostasis is established (usually 10 to 15 minutes). PTT may be checked before this step. The use of sandbags or mechanical clamps for this initial step of hemostasis is discouraged.

If the heparin effect is still present, longer manual compression may be needed. Occasionally a small amount of protamine sulfate may be used at this stage to help establish hemostasis.

8. After satisfactory hemostasis is established, keep the patient on complete bed rest for at least 6 hours.

9. The patient is advised to walk 6 to 8 hours after removal of all catheters and adequate hemostasis. At

this time, check the femoral (or brachial) pulses and review the ECG and hemoglobin levels. Check the creatine phosphokinase level if there is any suspicion of myocardial necrosis. Check the potassium and serum creatinine levels if a large amount of contrast agent was used or if there is preexisting renal disease. Patients are usually discharged 48 hours after an uncomplicated angioplasty.

10. Discuss medications, activity program, return to work plan, and follow-up plans with the patient.

11. Arrange for stress treadmill evaluation, preferably with thallium imaging within 1 to 2 weeks of the procedure.

12. Long-term follow-up generally includes treadmill (with thallium imaging if possible) evaluation 3 to 6 months following the procedure and yearly thereafter. Coronary arteriography is reserved for (a) patients with return of angina pectoris, (b) patients who have positive thallium treadmill results, or (c) situations in which it is critical to know if the procedure remains successful, and (d) experimental study protocols where the results of treadmill thallium evaluation are unreliable.

Care following unsuccessful angioplasty

When angioplasty is attempted and results are not successful, the care of the patient must be individualized. Assuming that the patient was a suitable candidate for aortocoronary bypass surgery, these guidelines are offered.

1. If the area of stenosis was manipulated by wire or balloon catheter but not crossed, or crossed by the balloon catheter and the balloon inflated without success, then the patient is potentially unstable and at risk of acute occlusion, and aortocoronary bypass surgery should be promptly performed.

2. If the lesion has not been traumatized, then the patient can be taken back to a cardiac care floor and cared for as are patients following cardiac catheterization, and then prepared for elective surgery.

3. Check the hematocrit and ECG, as well as creatinine, potassium, and cardiac enzyme levels 12 to 24 hours following the failed angioplasty as a part of preparation for surgery.

Care following development of acute coronary occlusion associated with angioplasty*

Acute coronary occlusion is the most serious complication related to coronary angioplasty; the risk is 2% to 5%. The mechanism of occlusion may involve vessel dissection, spasm, intramural hematoma, or thrombo-

*References 22, 24, 62-71.

sis. The mechanisms involved are frequently unknown. All efforts should be aimed at reopening the vessel or establishing flow past the occlusion.

Occlusion before guidewire/catheter manipulation

If acute occlusion occurs at the site of the stenosis and before any guidewire or dilatation catheter has crossed the lesion, the most likely mechanism is coronary artery spasm, coronary thrombus, or embolism. In any case, such an event suggests a break in technique in that the patient should have been fully heparinized and premedicated with nitrates and calcium antagonists, and should have received intracoronary nitroglycerin. The following guidelines are offered:

1. Visualize the vessel angiographically, and inject 200 μg of nitroglycerin into the coronary artery and repeat as needed.

2. Give sublingual nifedipine (10 mg).

3. Administer heparin.

4. If the vessel is not promptly opened, proceed to intracoronary thrombolysis with modest doses of a clot-selective thrombolytic agent, thus keeping the surgical treatment option open. An equally acceptable or possibly preferable alternative is trying to cross the obstruction with a flexible guidewire, followed by the balloon, and attempt dilatation in a manner similar to that employed for spontaneous acute myocardial infarction.

5. If the vessel cannot be opened expeditiously with the combined use of intracoronary nitroglycerin, thrombolysis, and angioplasty, the patient is usually taken to emergency surgery. IABP may help stabilize the patient during the transfer arrangement.

6. If the vessel can be opened and adequate flow is established, the angioplasty procedure may be completed.

Occlusion after guidewire/catheter manipulation

If acute occlusion of the vessel occurs after guidewire and catheter manipulation of the lesion, dissection of the vessel is another likely mechanism (in addition to spasm or thrombus). As with acute occlusion before guidewire and catheter manipulation, proceed with intent to open the vessel with intracoronary nitroglycerin, and attempt recrossing and redilating.

Ability to successfully dilate a total occlusion caused by dissection of the artery and to maintain long-term patency is not predictable, but experience has been encouraging. Approximately 50% of these vessels can be opened and kept open with the repeat angioplasty attempt. Thrombolytic treatment in this setting is controversial.

If the vessel cannot be promptly opened and kept open with satisfactory blood flow, proceed to emergency surgery.

If the vessel can be opened and successfully dilated, obtain a postdilatation arteriogram and observe the patient closely for 24 hours, while continuing IV heparin and nitroglycerin.

If the lesion and the patient appear stable, emergency surgery can be avoided. Coronary arteriography repeated in 24 hours and before the arterial sheath is removed may help in the decision-making process.

Occlusion after successful coronary angioplasty

Occlusion following successful coronary angioplasty usually occurs within 2 to 3 hours of completion of the procedure (majority within 30 minutes) or 2 to 3 hours after discontinuation of heparin and is manifested by chest pain, ST segment shifts, arrhythmias, and hemodynamic instability. The likely mechanism is coronary artery spasm (early occlusion while the patient is still receiving heparin therapy) or coronary artery thrombosis (late occlusion occurring after heparin therapy is discontinued). Rarely a late extension of a coronary artery dissection can occur.

Given current hypotheses concerning the sequence of events that culminate in spontaneous myocardial infarction[65,66] and keeping in mind the vessel pathologic processes induced by angioplasty, it is remarkable that the occurrence of acute coronary occlusion following angioplasty is the exception and not the rule!

1. Immediately administer IV nitroglycerin (100 to 200 μg) and sublingual nifedipine (10 mg).

2. Mobilize the angioplasty and the cardiovascular surgical team and transfer the patient to the angioplasty suite.

3. While the cardiovascular surgical suite is being prepared, attempt to reopen the vessel with intracoronary nitroglycerin, followed by repeat angioplasty, especially if the occlusion is total. In cases where intracoronary nitroglycerin is ineffective in establishing some flow and an angioplasty guidewire cannot be passed through the occlusion to the distal vessel, a thrombolytic agent may be infused directly into the coronary artery. This will be effective if the mechanism of occlusion was a thrombus. Such an approach will open the artery and avoid emergency surgery in approximately 50% of patients.

4. Reopening the vessel may eliminate the need for emergency surgery, or at least the patient will go to surgery with an open vessel and perfused myocardium with a limited or relatively insignificant myocardial infarction.

5. If the vessel cannot be reopened in 20 to 30 minutes, do not continue attempts. Transfer the patient to the operating room with the support of IABP, especially if he or she is hemodynamically unstable. If the occlusion has been recrossed with a guidewire, then a coronary infusion catheter with side holes (reperfusion "bail-out" catheter) can be positioned across the occlusion with the use of an exchange guidewire and to establish some flow to the myocardium while preparations for surgery are in progress. For this technique to be successful, a substantial perfusion pressure across the proximal and distal side holes of the catheter is required. Preliminary use of this coronary perfusion catheter in humans has been encouraging.[71] If this catheter is not used, then the angioplasty guidewire is best left across the obstruction, as it may help maintain some vessel patency and distal perfusion while preparations for surgery are underway.

If an intimal dissection had occurred during the initial "successful" angioplasty, or the initial angioplasty was technically difficult, it may be best to proceed directly to surgery at the time of acute occlusion, because the chance of successful repeat angioplasty may not be very high. The cardiovascular surgeon should be alerted to the likelihood of coronary artery dissection, to avoid insertion of the graft into the false lumen of the coronary artery.

If the patient develops symptoms of coronary artery occlusion following angioplasty, and yet the arteriogram shows the involved vessel to be patent with good flow, consider a differential diagnosis of (1) acute pericarditis secondary to right ventricular pacemaker perforation, with or without pericardial tamponade,[42] (2) localized pericarditis secondary to coronary artery dissection,[63] or (3) small side branch occlusion.[51,54]

Other complications

Coronary artery perforation or rupture[71-75] during angioplasty is a rare but potentially lethal complication. It is best avoided by carefully matching the dilatation balloon size to the vessel size and confirming the intraluminal position of the dilatation catheter before inflating the balloon. When perforation occurs, it may precipitate acute pericardial tamponade with a possible fatal outcome. Reported treatment measures have included reversal of heparin effect with protamine, pericardiocentesis, reocclusion of the bleeding vessel with the balloon, and emergency operation.

Other complications are arrhythmias, emboli, vascular complications, or right ventricular puncture and pericardial tamponade.

Treatment of vascular complications or arrhythmias

is similar to when these occur in association with cardiac catheterization and arteriography (see Chapter 5).

Pericardial tamponade responds well to pericardial drainage and cessation of anticoagulation (see Chapter 10).

Use of IABP

IABP has been found useful for (1) critically ill patients (usually with acute myocardial infarction or cardiogenic shock) who are candidates for angioplasty but are too unstable to have cardiac catheterization and angioplasty; and (2) patients who develop acute vascular occlusion during or following the procedure.[76,77] IABP can be used to stabilize patients in the latter group for an attempt at reopening the vessel or, if this fails, for transfer to the operating room.

Emergency aortocoronary bypass surgery

With rare exceptions, patients who undergo elective coronary angioplasty are also prepared for aortocoronary bypass surgery in case of acute vessel occlusion.[20,22,78] The rare exceptions are in cases in which an acute occlusion will not be treated surgically, such as in patients with advanced chronic obstructive pulmonary disease or malignancy.

In the National Heart, Lung, and Blood Institute registry the necessity for emergency aortocoronary bypass surgery was 6.6%.[20] In 1985 to 1986 it can be as low as 3% in patients undergoing single-vessel angioplasty. Most centers, early in their experience, report emergency surgery rates of 6% to 10%, whereas established centers have rates of 2% to 3%. Thus, need for emergency aortocoronary bypass surgery in the setting of coronary angioplasty decreases with the increased experience of the angioplasty team. With the experienced team, patient selection is improved, technical errors are fewer, and, most importantly, emergency conditions are frequently corrected in the angioplasty suite, where total acute occlusions are often successfully recrossed and redilated.

Because some patients will require emergency surgery, elective coronary angioplasty is not performed without this capability. However, in acute myocardial infarction with total (and sometimes subtotal) vessel obstruction, emergency coronary angioplasty has been performed without immediate surgical back-up to avoid delay in the procedure.

The risks associated with emergency surgery for failed angioplasty are relatively high and include increased risk of operative death, perioperative myocardial infarction, hemorrhage, infection, and sternal complications. Overall surgical mortality ranges from 3.5% to 6% and perioperative myocardial infarction from 30% to 40%. The rate of hospital death of patients having emergency surgery and who have sustained significant myocardial infarction approaches 10%.[22,78]

The mortality of emergency surgery could possibly be reduced by more regular use of IABP, use of coronary infusion catheter during preparation for cardiopulmonary bypass, and reduced time to cardiopulmonary bypass. Emergency surgery for failed multivessel angioplasty should bypass all involved vessels, even if some were successfully dilated.

SPECIAL CONSIDERATIONS
Vessel pathologic conditions caused by angioplasty (mechanism of angioplasty)

Experimental animal models, postmortem studies, and a few pathologic studies of arteries in humans who had undergone angioplasty have shown a variety of mechanical injuries to the vessel at the area of the angioplasty, although the tissue adjacent to the dilated atherosclerotic lesion or plaque does not seem to be damaged.[79-85] Among the pathologic findings are the following:

- Endothelial desquamation and intimal dissection extending into the media of the vessel: The fibrous cap overlying an atherosclerotic plaque is frequently ruptured (Fig. 15-18).

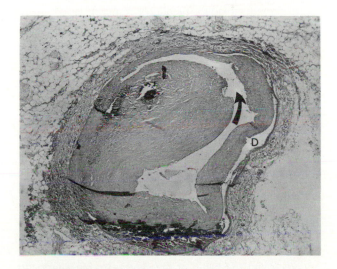

Fig. 15-18. Section of LAD artery at the site of angioplasty, revealing splitting *(arrow)* of the atherosclerotic plaque and a dissecting hematoma of the outer media *(D)*. The split has enlarged the original lumen. (From Block, P.C., et al.: Morphology after transluminal angioplasty in human beings, reprinted by permission of the New England Journal of Medicine **305:**382-384, 1981.)

- Medial stretching, especially of the uninvolved or nondiseased portion of the vessel: Overstretching of the vessel with oversized balloons can cause vessel perforation and rupture.
- Compaction (plaque compression, remolding) of the atherosclerotic plaque: This may occur with soft, noncalcific lesions; fluid extrusion may also occur.
- Distal embolization: This does not appear to cause clinical problems.

The healing phase (days to weeks) following angioplasty may be characterized by phagocytosis, fibrosis, and retraction and subsequent endothelialization, making the lumen larger. In patients with recurrent stenosis the "healing" phase seems to be characterized by excessive intimal proliferation and development of atherosclerotic lesions indistinguishable from other de novo lesions observed in the same artery. Why some vessels "heal" by further reduction of the plaque and others by restenosis remains unexplained.

Some of the "plaque fracture" and "dissecting clefts" described in patients and attributed to the angioplasty procedure can also be observed at postmortem examination in the coronary arteries of patients who have not had angioplasty.

Morphologic data concerning graft angioplasty are limited. It appears that angioplasty in saphenous vein grafts early after surgery (less than 1 year) causes stretching of the vein, whereas in older grafts the mechanism includes plaque fracture or rupture.

Pressure gradient across the stenosis[11,13,86-89]

Gruentzig and other workers have emphasized the importance of measuring pressures at both the tip of the guiding catheter (aortic and proximal coronary artery pressure) and the tip of the dilatation catheter.[11,13] Thus when the dilatation catheter crosses the area of the stenosis, a pressure gradient is obtained that may be of value in assessing the severity and functional significance of the stenosis, in addition to the anatomic or the angiographic assessment.

The quality of pressure tracings during the angioplasty procedure is directly related to the attention given to proper preparation of the guiding and dilatation catheters, Y connectors, manifolds, and transducers. The accuracy and the value of these pressure measurements have been questioned.[86,88] The following guidelines are offered.

1. Pressure measurements and the evaluation of gradients are valuable if a reliable pressure tracing can be obtained. The accuracy or the absolute value of the pressure is not important. The diastolic pressure gradient is of greater significance than the systolic gradient. One can use the *mean pressures* and *directional changes* in the mean pressures.

2. Reliable measurements of mean pressures at the tip of both catheters add to the information acquired from arteriography and help the angiographer in the following ways.

a. It is easier to recognize when the distal tip of dilatation catheter has crossed the stenosis. If the dilatation catheter occludes the vessel, the distal pressure recorded reflects the pressure of the collaterals and may not aid in determining when the stenosis is crossed.

b. Directional changes in the mean pressure gradient before inflation and after deflation of the balloon indicate whether the balloon inflation has made a difference in the size and the functional significance of the lesion.

c. There may be a correlation between a higher restenosis rate with higher residual gradient,[89] and thus provide a second index, in addition to the arteriogram, of a successful or unsuccessful angioplasty. A persistent pressure gradient, especially if the angiographic result is suboptimal, is an indication for further inflations.

3. The aim of the procedure is performing a successful angioplasty, not obtaining hemodynamic data! If, after a reasonable effort, meaningful hemodynamic measurements cannot be obtained, proceed with the study with only fluoroscopic and angiographic control. If full balloon inflation has been performed with satisfactory inflation pressures and duration and the cineangiographic result looks successful, do not continue the procedure with repeated inflations to bring the "gradient" to a predetermined level. In this setting "chasing" a possible artifactual gradient may lead to complications, including acute vessel occlusion.

4. Reliability of pressure gradients is questioned when one is dealing with small vessels, acute bends in vessels, multiple lesions in a vessel, or guiding catheters with side holes.

Immediate postangioplasty cinearteriogram

The cinearteriogram of the dilated coronary artery obtained immediately after angioplasty is an important study.[90] It can be obtained with the guidewire left in the dilated artery, with the balloon catheter pulled into the dilatation catheter, and with a simultaneous injection of contrast medium via the dilating and guiding catheters. If visualization is inadequate, the guidewire and dilatation catheter may be removed and a diagnostic-quality coronary injection obtained. An exchange

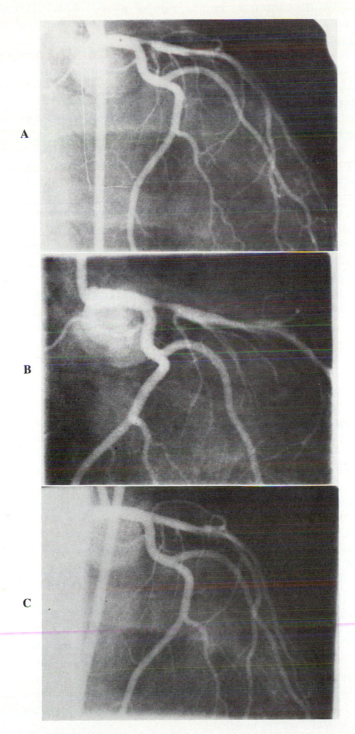

Fig. 15-19. Successful angioplasty of a lesion in the proximal LAD artery. **A,** Predilatation arteriogram. **B,** Arteriogram taken immediately after PTCA reveals pronounced haziness in the dilated lesion. **C,** Arteriogram performed 2 weeks later reveals resolution of the haziness and a smooth-wall dilatation. (From Holmes, D.R., et al.: Angiographic changes produced by percutaneous transluminal coronary angioplasty, Am. J. Cardiol. **51:**676, 1983.)

guidewire may be positioned across the stenosis before the dilatation catheter is removed, especially if the patient seems unstable. This arteriogram will tell the operator if the procedure appears successful and can be terminated, or if further dilations (longer inflation time, higher inflation pressure, or larger balloons) are needed. It is best to make this determination with a guidewire still across the lesion, especially if difficulty was encountered in crossing the stenosis. However, where the postdilatation angiogram has been disappointing, we have not hesitated to recross a dilated stenosis that appeared suboptimally dilated but without dissection using a very flexible guidewire.

Some operators rely only on the postangioplasty coronary arteriography for determination of the success of the procedure, whereas most combine this angiographic information with the information obtained from the pressure gradient. Frequently one is not dealing with a yes or no (success/failure) situation. The pressure gradient may have been reassuringly abolished while the angiographic result may look "suboptimal" with intravascular haziness (Fig. 15-19).

On the other hand, a degree of stenosis may be reduced from 90% to 50%, at which point the information from the pressure gradient may be important in declaring this a success or failure. The diverse angiographic findings following coronary angioplasty have been presented by Holmes et al.[90]; careful review of this article is rewarding.

The ultimate decision of a successful result versus the need for repeat angioplasty is made on the basis of (1) the cinearteriogram, with developing and reviewing of the films if necessary, (2) pressure gradients, (3) the patient's condition, and (4) operator experience.

In borderline cases it may be advisable to repeat coronary arteriography in 30 minutes or leave the arterial sheath in place and obtain a follow-up coronary arteriogram in 24 to 48 hours. Angiographic changes occurring within 30 minutes and again at 24 to 48 hours after angioplasty have shown improvement or worsening in approximately 20% of cases.[91-93] The decision for repeat angioplasty may be based on this information, as well as the patient's clinical course.

Balloon inflations

There are no firm data or controlled studies to determine the optimal number, pressure, or duration of inflation. High balloon dilatation pressure has been correlated with lower residual pressure gradients, but this has not been directly related to reduction in restenosis rate. These practices regarding balloon inflation have

evolved mostly from experience, anecdotal cases, "feeling," and reasoned judgment.[10,11,13,45,94] The following guidelines are offered.

1. Begin with low inflation pressures. Limit initial inflation to 3 to 4 atmospheres for 15 to 20 seconds. Use this inflation to confirm optimal balloon position and test the "hardness" of the lesion.

2. Subsequent inflation pressures with optimal balloon position should be higher to permit full inflation of the balloon and "splitting" or breaking of the plaque. This may occur with pressures of 4 to 5 atmospheres or may require 10 to 12 atmospheres (sometimes higher). Currently available balloons may burst at 12 to 13 atmospheres. Newer balloons may tolerate pressures as high as 20 atmospheres, but their safety remains untested. Generally, try to open the stenosis with the lowest pressure necessary.

3. Following splitting of the plaque, repeat the inflation at 1 to 2 atmospheres higher. This is considered a "molding inflation." Except for the first "test" inflation, continue balloon inflations for 50 to 60 seconds if tolerated by the patient. Longer duration of inflation may be necessary in selected cases. If very high–pressure inflations are required to split the plaque, molding inflations should be done at a pressure that is 1 to 2 atmospheres lower.

If after a minimum of three inflations—test inflation, splitting inflation, and molding inflation—the pressure gradient across the lesion is less than 15 mm Hg and the angiogram confirms good results, there is no need for repeated, higher pressure or longer inflations. If reliable pressures indicate a residual gradient of more than 20 mm Hg and especially if the coronary angiogram shows suboptimal results, the procedure should be repeated with inflations at a higher pressure and longer duration, until either the pressure gradient is reduced to below 20 mm Hg or angiographic results look satisfactory.

Do not insist on a perfect result. If you aim for abolishing the pressure gradient and ending with a normal- or near-normal-looking artery all of the time, you will risk a higher chance of major coronary artery dissection or a higher rate of acute occlusion. Judgment of when to stop is only acquired by experience, with the help of careful review of the cineangiogram and pressure data.

Physiologic and clinical changes during balloon inflation

The sequence of mechanical, electrocardiographic, and clinical effects during coronary angioplasty during the period of balloon occlusion have been studied.[95,96]

Clinical ECG and echocardiographic monitoring during balloon inflation have shown the following changes in the order listed:

1. There is hypokinesis of the left ventricular segment supplied by the coronary artery being occluded.
2. Dyskinesis soon follows hypokinesis (20 to 30 seconds).
3. ST segment shifts on ECG usually follow the wall motion abnormalities.
4. Chest pain may follow the appearance of ST segment shifts approximately 30 to 40 seconds after balloon inflation.

These abnormalities usually clear approximately 20 seconds after reperfusion. Abnormalities of diastolic left ventricular function may take longer to recover.[97] Currently, balloon inflation is continued for 30 to 40 seconds and, if well tolerated, up to 1 to 1½ minutes. This short duration of total occlusion in an otherwise uncomplicated angioplasty is not associated with any evidence of myocardial necrosis. It is not known if longer duration is safe or beneficial. When myocardial injury occurs, as evidenced by prolonged chest pain and elevation of creatine kinase MB isoenzyme, there is usually occlusion of a small side branch with myocardial necrosis.[98] Such events are generally well tolerated if the occluded side branch is small.

Anatomic (angiographic) characteristics of the lesion[13,99]

The initial (and ideal) angioplasty-suitable lesion described by Gruentzig and associates remains the easiest to dilate. Other types of lesions are now routinely subjected to angioplasty, and the experience shows that:

- Concentric stenosis continues to respond well, with a success rate greater than 90%.
- Eccentric lesions can be dilated, with a primary success rate of approximately 80%. Failure is usually due to inability to cross or to dilate the area of stenosis. The chance of acute closure is higher, especially if the eccentric lesion is also a long lesion.
- Calcifications in the lesion usually indicate a "hard" lesion, requiring higher inflation pressures. Totally encircling circumferential calcification may not respond to balloon dilatation.
- Obstructive lesions just at or immediately distal to acute bends are more prone to dissection and acute closure.
- Bifurcation lesions can be safely dilated if both vessels are protected (see p. 357).
- Extreme tortuosity of a vessel proximal to a lesion

(usually seen in the right coronary artery) may absorb the force applied on the dilatation catheter and prevent its passage through the stenosis.

Coronary artery spasm

The role, if any, of angioplasty in patients with variant angina and coronary artery spasm in association with obstructive anatomic disease continues to be debated.[100-102] Experience has shown that:

- In most cases treatment with combinations of nitrates and calcium antagonists is satisfactory.
- Successful dilatation is possible with primary success rates similar to those for other groups.
- Refractory coronary artery spasm during and immediately after the dilatation procedure does not appear to be a problem.
- Acute reclosure rates are the same as in patients without coronary spasm.
- Angina and coronary artery spasm are abolished in some but not all patients.
- Preliminary studies show a substantially higher recurrence rate (approximately 50%) at 2 to 3 months with symptoms of coronary artery spasm occurring in association with restenosis.
- A very high restenosis rate (80%) was observed in patients with coronary artery spasm who did not continue calcium antagonist therapy after angioplasty.

The issue remains unresolved. We manage these patients with aggressive medical treatment; failures are rare. In a patient for whom medical treatment has truly failed and who requires aortocoronary bypass grafting for control, we would consider coronary angioplasty, especially for a patient with single-vessel disease. The patient is kept on therapy with combined calcium antagonists and long-acting nitrates, as well as aspirin and dipyridamole for at least 6 months after the procedure.

Coronary artery spasm may appear for the first time after successful angioplasty. This is usually accompanied by fixed obstruction (restenosis) and can be refractory to the usual antianginal medications. This appears to be more frequent in younger patients and those with noncalcific lesions.

Coronary artery thrombus and unstable angina

Angiography in the early phase of acute myocardial infarction frequently demonstrates an intraluminal thrombus and a totally or subtotally occluded infarct-related artery. Coronary artery thrombus is a recognized common precipitating cause of acute myocardial infarction.[65,66,103]

Coronary artery thrombus also plays a significant role in the syndrome of unstable (crescendo) angina[103,104]; in such cases recurrent mural thrombus formation may alternate with intermittent thrombus fragmentation in a dynamic, cyclic manner that may culminate in total vessel occlusion and myocardial infarction. Thus, in many patients with the syndrome of unstable angina pectoris, an active coronary artery thrombus is present, although not always recognized by means of coronary arteriography. Fiberoptic coronary angioscopy is more sensitive in determining these thrombi.[105,106]

Coronary angioplasty in patients with known coronary artery thrombus has been reported.[107] In these patients there was increased risk of developing complete occlusion either during or after the attempted coronary artery dilatation. Recommendation has been made to treat such patients with 24 hours of heparin infusion following angioplasty procedure.

Results of angioplasty in patients with the clinical syndrome of unstable angina have been reported.[108-112] It appears that angioplasty in these patients carries the same risk and success rate as in patients with stable angina pectoris and is a satisfactory alternate to surgical revascularization.

Based on these observations, the following guidelines are suggested for the management of patients with unstable angina pectoris.

1. Medical treatment should be aggressive, with long-acting nitrates, IV nitroglycerin, calcium antagonists, beta blockers, and systemic heparinization. The role of thrombolytic therapy is under investigation. IABP may be of value.

2. Early coronary arteriography should be performed, preferably after the patient's condition has stabilized.

3. If angiographic or angioscopic diagnosis of coronary artery thrombus can be made and angioplasty is considered, precede elective angioplasty by 12 to 24 hours of heparin administration and use thrombolytic therapy before the angioplasty, followed by 12 to 24 hours of heparin administration after successful angioplasty. If the observations initially reported by Falk[104] on the role of coronary artery thrombus in the syndrome of unstable angina are confirmed and accepted, thrombolytic therapy may be extended to this subgroup before coronary angioplasty and independent of the angiographic diagnosis of coronary artery thrombus.

Acute myocardial infarction[113-125]

Acute myocardial infarction is almost always accompanied by angiographically demonstrated total or subtotal occlusion of the vessel supplying the affected myocardium. Frequently intracoronary thrombus is present. Opening this obstruction and reestablishing flow early in the evolution of myocardial infarction is successful in relieving the chest pain, arresting the process of infarction, and limiting the left ventricular damage. This can be achieved by coronary angioplasty, systemic or selective intracoronary thrombolysis, or surgical revascularization.[113-120] Preliminary results have shown that emergency angioplasty is a feasible method of opening the infarct-related vessel or occluded vein grafts and that emergency angioplasty may precede or follow thrombolytic treatment in this syndrome. Both thrombolytic agents and angioplasty open the artery, with residual stenosis being much less following angioplasty.[118] *The indications, timing, and effectiveness of this type of treatment in acute myocardial infarction are not firmly established by controlled studies.* Our approach to this difficult problem early in the course of evolving myocardial infarction is the following.

1. We direct initial efforts to opening the infarct-related artery medically, using IV nitroglycerin, calcium-blocking agents, systemic heparin, and frequently systemic (IV) thrombolytic treatment (see Chapter 16). We generally defer emergency arteriography or angioplasty until the patient's condition stabilizes and the process of infarction seems arrested or the process better clarified.

2. For carefully selected patients in whom large amounts of left ventricular myocardium are at risk (as judged by the clinical presentation, ECG, or emergency echocardiography), we proceed to emergency coronary arteriography followed by additional selective intracoronary thrombolytic treatment or emergency angioplasty. The sequence of these is usually directed by whichever can be performed faster.

3. The area of total or subtotal occlusion or thrombus is *gently* probed with a *flexible* angioplasty guidewire; force is not applied. The guidewire usually passes beyond the thrombus without much difficulty. Guiding catheter injections are done to document the intraluminal location of the wire. Passage of guidewire through a thrombus may help thrombolysis by increasing penetration of the thrombolytic agent. After a stable guidewire position has been secured, the dilatation balloon catheter is advanced thru the area of the occlusion. Initial inflations are done at 2 to 4 atmospheres, while the balloon is observed fluoroscopically. Angioplasty is continued until patency and good angiographic result are established.

4. During emergency angioplasty for acute myocardial infarction, only the infarct-related vessel is approached and dilated. Complete diagnostic coronary arteriography is done. Left ventriculography may be

deferred or performed with less contrast material, especially if the patient's condition is unstable. If obstruction is identified in coronary arteries not involved in the myocardial infarction, these are not dilated at the same time. Risking an acute occlusion and additional infarction in this noninvolved segment could be catastrophic. After stabilization of the infarct artery and recovery from myocardial infarction, the issue of revascularization surgery or follow-up angioplasty can be addressed.

5. During angioplasty procedure, analgesics, antiarrhythmic agents, and hemodynamic support for complication of myocardial infarction are used. We have used morphine sulfate and diazepam for relief of pain. The use of general anesthesia during angioplasty in patients with acute myocardial is being investigated.

Coronary angioplasty for acute myocardial infarction has been reported to have a low mortality. Angioplasty in patients with acute myocardial infarction complicated by cardiogenic shock has been reported with a mortality of 25% to 40%, suggesting substantial benefit.[108-111] Results of randomized studies (in progress) are not yet available to document the risk and benefit of this form of treatment of myocardial infarction as compared with currently accepted treatment methods. Until definitive data is available, primary angioplasty for treatment of acute myocardial infarction remains investigational.

Chronic coronary artery occlusion

Successful angioplasty in totally occluded coronary arteries in the absence of acute myocardial infarction has been reported by many groups.[126-136] The combined experience appears to show that:

- Totally occluded vessels can be opened with angioplasty weeks and months following the occlusion. Intracoronary thrombolytic therapy may be of help in establishing partial reperfusion and guiding the angioplasty procedure.
- The rate of primary success is generally lower than for angioplasty in the absence of total occlusion. The longer the occlusion has been present, the lower the success rate.
- The procedure is relatively safe because of the presence of collaterals. Risk of precipitating acute occlusion, myocardial infarction, or the need for emergency surgery is quite low.
- Higher reocclusion and restenosis rates are encountered.
- Totally occluded vein grafts can be opened with angioplasty.

In approaching totally occluded vessels, a soft flexible guidewire is first used. If this is not successful, a stiffer wire may next be used. The occluded segment is probed and gently explored with the guidewire tip. Force is not applied. Once the guidewire is passed, its intraluminal position should be confirmed by using multiple views before the dilatation catheter is advanced or the balloon inflated. Low-profile, small balloons are initially used. If larger balloons are needed, they may be introduced.

Multivessel angioplasty

The technique of coronary angioplasty, initially applied to patients with single-vessel coronary artery disease, has now been extened to patients with obstruction in two or more coronary arteries.[10,11,13,23,137-142] This has been a natural evolution of the technique, given the positive experience accumulated in patients with single-vessel coronary angioplasty, the expanded capability offered by the steerable guidewire, and the fact that most patients have multivessel disease. Hartzler[10,137] has been an early and aggressive proponent of applying angioplasty to patients with multivessel disease, whereas Gruentzig and colleagues[11,13,138] have advised caution and restraint in extending the angioplasty technique to this subset of patients.

This much is known. First, angioplasty is feasible in selected patients with multivessel coronary artery disease. This may involve multivessel or single-vessel coronary angioplasty. Also, multivessel coronary angioplasty can be carried out in one sitting. The vessel with the most severe stenosis and supplying the greatest amount of myocardium at risk is dilated first. Second, success rates are similar to those for patients with single-vessel coronary angioplasty. Third, risks are higher especially in patients over the age of 70 years.[139] Emergency surgery and mortality risks are increased (see Table 15-8). Fourth, the clinical recurrence rates are higher. Individual vessel recurrence rates may be similar to that after single vessel angioplasty, but cumulative clinical recurrence of angina or myocardial ischemia is probably higher than that after single vessel angioplasty.[140]

Important unknowns involve the following questions: Will multivessel angioplasty prolong life for patients with two- to three-vessel coronary artery disease? Will it decrease or increase the risk of myocardial infarction? How does it compare with medical and surgical treatments of patients with multivessel coronary artery disease? Which subset of patients with multivessel coronary artery disease are safe candidates? In which subset of patients is complete revascularization necessary and in which subset is partial revascularization adequate? In which subset of patients is angioplasty too risky?

Principles applied in the section on indications and

Table 15-8. Major complications of coronary angioplasty: single vessel disease versus multiple vessel disease

	Single vessel disease		Multiple vessel disease*	
	Emory U.† 1980-1986	French registry 1981-1985‡	Emory U. 1980-1986	French registry 1981-1985
Number of patients	4361	2385	1316	813
Success	93%	73%	87%	78%
Emergency surgery	2.6%	4.1%	3.2%	4.5%
Myocardial infarction	2.2%	5.2%	2.8%	5.8%
Death	0.1%	0.9%	0.5%	2.2%
Recurrence	Approximately 25%-30%			

*Also includes some patients with multivessel angioplasty and multilesion angioplasty.
Sources: †S.B. King, M.D., and G.S. Roubin, M.D. (personal communication).
‡Bertrand, M.E., et al.: French percutaneous transluminal coronary angioplasty (PTCA) registry: four years experience (abstract), J. Am. Coll. Cardiol. **7:**21A, 1986.

contraindications are valid in addressing these questions.

It is clear that when the technique of coronary angioplasty is standardized and is not undergoing substantial change, the results of angioplasty must be compared with results of medical and surgical treatment in a large randomized study in an effort to determine the role of angioplasty in multivessel coronary artery disease. Such a study is underway (Bypass Angioplasty Revascularization Investigation—BARI), sponsored by National Heart, Lung, and Blood Institute, but definitive results are not expected before the early 1990s.

Intraoperative angioplasty

The desirability or feasibility of intraoperative angioplasty was first discussed at the first coronary angioplasty conference sponsored by the National Heart, Lung, and Blood Institute, in Bethesda, 1979, but progress in this field has been slow.[143-144] Catheter designs are still being tested and the protocols remain experimental, with no long-term follow-up of results. Intraoperative angioplasty of inaccessible segments of the LAD artery, septal perforators, or the distal branch of this vessel may be of some value, although the overall benefits remain unproven.

In general, intraoperative angioplasty should be considered only in vessels that cannot be bypassed, because the graft occlusion rate is lower than the rate of recurrence of occlusion following angioplasty.

Angioplasty following aortocoronary bypass surgery

Angioplasty is performed following aortocoronary bypass surgery because of either graft stenosis and occlusion or development of new obstructive coronary artery disease in native vessels. Many patients with recur-

rent angina either early or late following aortocoronary bypass surgery can be spared reoperation with the use of angioplasty.[117,145-148]

Dilatation of graft stenosis is most successful when the stenosis involves the distal anastomotic site, with primary success rates of 80% and recurrence rates as low as 15%. Stenosis of the proximal anastomotic site or the midbody of the graft can be dilated with similar success but with a much higher restenosis rate (approximately 50%). Vein graft dilatation should probably be reserved for relatively new grafts. The proximal stenosis is usually mechanical and may merely require stretching; those in the body are more likely intimal hyperplasia and do not respond as well in the long term to dilatation. Older grafts are often filled with friable material, and working within these grafts may be hazardous. The angiogram should be reviewed carefully and grafts with irregular lumens avoided.

If acute occlusion is encountered and emergency surgery is required, there is higher operative risk partly as a result of the increased time required in achieving cardiopulmonary bypass. Thus, if total occlusion of the vein graft or the vessel is apt to precipitate a complicated or major infarction which the patient may not survive, reoperation may be a safer choice.

Short-term results

Coronary angioplasty is successful in increasing the luminal diameter and improving myocardial blood flow in the majority of patients.[149-151] A successful result can be claimed when (1) the mean diameter narrowing of the vessel is reduced by 20%, (2) the pressure gradient across the stenosis is abolished or substantially reduced (ideally to <15 mm Hg), (3) symptoms of myocardial ischemia are eliminated, and (4) the patient does not require surgery. Success rates of single-vessel coronary angioplasty have improved from 60% to over 90%. Clearly success rates will be directly influenced by the experience of the operator, as well as case selection. A novice may have a success rate of less than 50% in complex cases, while the master can achieve virtually 100% success rates in simple cases. Success rates achieved in the early National Heart, Lung, and Blood Institute study (60% to 70%) should be considered the minimal accepted rates, given the current technology.

When an operator achieves primary success rates of 80% to 90%, then he or she may cautiously extend the case selection to more difficult cases and hope to keep success rates at the same level.

Successful angioplasty achieves the following:
- Relieves angina
- Improves myocardial perfusion as proven by treadmill testing, thallium imaging, and arteriography
- Increases exercise tolerance
- Increases coronary blood flow as determined by coronary sinus flow measurements
- Improves left ventricular function at rest and exercise

Long-term results

Many questions remain unanswered about the long-term results of angioplasty. Most of our information is obtained from the follow-up of a subgroup of 2200 of approximately 3000 patients enrolled in the National Heart, Lung, and Blood Institute registry from March 1979 to September 1981.[18] One-year follow-up has shown sustained improvement in 72%, repeat angioplasty in 14%, bypass surgery in 12%, myocardial infarction in 3%, and death in 1.6%. In a longer follow-up of 2 to 3 years, the percentage of sustained improvement was lower and additional patients have required angioplasty or revascularization surgery.

A 5-year follow-up of the initial 50 patients reported by Gruentzig showed sustained improvement in many, with 8 of 11 patients having late arteriograms showing excellent and long-lasting effect.[152] Larger series show similar results.[153] Restenosis rates have remained at approximately 20% to 30% (see below).

Preliminary data reveal the following:
- In patients who have undergone successful angioplasty, the improvement lasts 6 months or longer in at least 70% of patients.
- For patients with no restenosis at 6 months, the rate of late restenosis is very low.
- Maintenance of functional improvement and an angina-free state correlate well with long-term vessel patency.

- The mortality in patients who have undergone single-vessel angioplasty is approximately 1%/year. This appears to be very similar to the mortality for medically and surgically treated patients in this subgroup.
- The mortality in patients who have undergone multivessel angioplasty (limited follow-up) is approximately 3%/year. Because patients were not randomly selected, this experience cannot be compared in any meaningful way with data for patients with multivessel disease treated medically or surgically.

Thus angioplasty, when successful, clearly relieves the symptoms and improves the quality of life. Its effect on the incidence of myocardial infarction or long-term survival is unknown and will remain so until a properly designed, randomized study addresses the issue.

Restenosis[18,154-165]

The true incidence of restenosis is not known because a uniform definition has not been adopted and repeat arteriography is not routinely done. The best estimates are that restenosis occurs in approximately 20% to 30% of patients.

Restenosis may occur as early as within 1 month of angioplasty, when searched by a thallium-imaged treadmill study. Clinically it is usually announced by the return of angina 2 to 6 months following successful angioplasty and is accompanied by ischemic response to treadmill testing. Rarely, restenosis may manifest by acute myocardial infarction or sudden death.

Preliminary studies suggest that restenosis may be more frequent in younger patients, patients with unstable angina, patients who have variant angina with documented coronary artery spasm (especially if calcium antagonists are not used after angioplasty), patients with uncontrolled hyperlipidemia and an increased incidence of atherosclerosis in other coronary vessels, patients with a long history of angina, patients who have undergone dilatation of totally occluded vessels, and patients with LAD artery lesions. Restenosis is also more frequent following suboptimal angioplasty where a significant gradient ($\geq$20 mm Hg) remained across the stenosis or arteriography did not show a satisfactory result. The last category is probably not restenosis but primary failure to dilate sufficiently.

The rate of restenosis may be lower in cases where the postangioplasty gradient was abolished or reduced to 15 mm Hg or less, intimal dissection was noted immediately after angioplasty, hyperlipidemia is absent, or higher balloon inflation pressures were used.

Restenosis does not appear to be related to the patient's sex, type of stenosis, or long-term use of warfarin anticoagulation. Diltiazem used 3 months after angioplasty in patients without coronary artery spasm did not reduce the restenosis rate. Effects of aspirin or dipyridamole are not known. Additional studies will be required before these preliminary findings are accepted as definitive.

Repeat angioplasty (second or third) is frequently performed following restenosis. Success rates are as good or better than rates for the primary angioplasty, and restenosis rates are similar to those for the first procedure. Given the present rates of restenosis, it is clear that (1) restenosis and the possible need for repeat angioplasty should be considered as a integral part of angioplasty (thus, patients should be informed and prepared for this development before they undergo their first angioplasty) and (2) the high rate of restenosis remains the major and unsolved limitation of angioplasty.

Economics

Assuming an 80% primary success rate in the short term, angioplasty appears to cost 40% less than aortocoronary bypass surgery. The true all inclusive cost of angioplasty over long periods of time may not compare so favorably.[166-169] Initial cost estimates did not consider the costs of standby surgeons, anesthesiologists, and operating room facilities, all necessary for the procedure. The 20% to 30% restenosis rate with subsequent repeat angiography and angioplasty is another expense that needs to be considered. When these expenses are added, the long-term cost savings of angioplasty may be less substantial.

At a time when medical payment systems are rapidly evolving from a nonrestrictive cost-based reimbursement and fee-for-service system to a prospective prepayment system, the economic impact of angioplasty will be closely monitored.

Table 15-9. Aortocoronary bypass surgery (ACBS) versus percutaneous transluminal coronary angioplasty (PTCA) (1986)

	ACBS	PTCA
Known effects	Improve myocardial blood flow Relieve angina, myocardial ischemia Effective palliative measures	
Experience	Time tested since 1967	Relatively new (1977)
Randomized studies available?	Yes; long-term effects better known	No; long-term effects not well known; randomized study started (1986)
Primary success rate	90%-95% (grafts open at time of hospital discharge)	±90%
Functional outcome	Comparable	
Recurrence rate		
1 yr	10%-15%	20%-30%
10 yr	50%	Not known
Availability	Wide	Wide
Cause of myocardial infarction	4%-5%	1%-2% for single vessel 2%-4% for multivessel*
Suitability of repeat procedure	With difficulty & increased risk	With ease
Morbidity	Substantial	Reduced
Patient acceptance	Concern & some reluctance	Generally well accepted
Mortality—1st operation	<1%-5%	0.1% for single vessel* 0.5%-2% for multivessel*
Reoperation mortality	5%-10%	Probably same as 1st operation
Hospital stay	6-10 days	2-3 days
Return to work	4-10 wk	2-4 days
Direct cost	2-3 times that of single PTCA	Will probably be further reduced
Long-term all inclusive costs	May be comparable	
Improvement in survival	Confirmed in some subgroups	Not known

*Predicated on expert immediate revascularization capability.

Coronary angioplasty versus aortocoronary bypass surgery

Coronary angioplasty and aortocoronary bypass surgery are two different and effective mechanical means of increasing coronary perfusion in patients with coronary artery disease. One or both of these palliative procedures may be used, in either order, in efforts to improve the quality and sometimes the quantity of life. Although claims for the superiority of angioplasty are sometimes made, its only *proven* advantages are its reduced morbidity, better patient acceptance, ease with which it can be repeated, and possibly its reduced cost.[10,13,169]

It is hoped that before the end of this decade controlled studies will be organized to yield information to guide the clinician in choosing the appropriate treatment. Table 15-9 summarizes some of the observations made when the technique and results of coronary angioplasty are compared with those of aortocoronary bypass surgery.

FUTURE DEVELOPMENTS

The future of coronary angioplasty appears promising.[170-181] The technique is new, and the potential for improvement and innovation is great. Efforts are aimed at clearing of atherosclerotic plaques using spark errosion, laser endarterectomy, laser assisted balloon angioplasty, and mechanical rotary catheters. All such techniques are in very preliminary stages.[170-177]

A system to permit temporary perfusion of an occluded coronary artery with oxygenated blood is being researched. Progress in these fields is anticipated in the coming years.[178-179]

Improvement in angioplasty equipment is also anticipated. Dilatation catheters with smaller shafts and lower profiles will be developed, extending the technique to peripheral coronary artery branches. Further improvements in guidewires are feasible, and guidewires with diameters of 0.010 inch will be widely available. Guiding catheters will probably undergo improvement to permit better torque control coupled with atraumatic tips.

The techniques of pressure measurements to determine gradients across coronary artery stenosis and determination of severity of stenosis will improve. It is likely that catheter systems will be available that will permit determination of flow across the stenosis before and after dilatation.[181]

Advances in our understanding of the mechanism and thus effective management of acute reclosure and early restenosis will probably be slower in coming.

A randomized study comparing coronary angioplasty with coronary bypass grafting and medical treatment is being organized. The study is expected to be completed by 1994.

Acknowledgement: The help of Carl Simpson in the preparation of this chapter is gratefully acknowledged.

REFERENCES

1. Dotter, C.T., and Judkins, M.P.: Description of a new technique and a preliminary report of its application, Circulation **30**:654-670, 1964.
2. Dotter, C.T., et al.: Transluminal iliac artery dilatation: nonsurgical catheter treatment of atheromatous narrowing. J.A.M.A. **230**:117-124, 1974.
3. Gruentzig, A.: Percutaneous transluminal recanalization of chronic arterial occlusion with a dilatation technique, Baden-Baden, Germany, 1977, G. Witzstrock-Verlag.
4. Gruentzig, A.: Transluminal dilatation of coronary artery stenosis, Lancet **1**:263, 1978.
5. Hurst, J.W.: The first coronary angioplasty as described by Andreas Gruentzig, Am. J. Cardiol. **57**:185-186, 1986.
6. Rapaport, E.: Percutaneous transluminal coronary angioplasty, Circulation **60**:969-972, 1979.
7. Simpson, J.B., Baim, D.S., Robert, E.W., and Harrison, D.C.: A new catheter system for coronary angioplasty, Am. J. Cardiol. **49**:1216-1222, 1982.
8. The expanding scope of coronary angioplasty, Lancet, June 8, 1985, pp. 1307-1308.
9. Hurst, J.W.: Tribute: Andreas Roland Gruentzig (1939-1985). A private perspective, Circulation **73**:606-610, 1986.
10. Hartzler, G.O.: Coronary angioplasty: indications and results. In Schroeder, J.S., editor: Invasive cardiology, Philadelphia, 1985, F.A. Davis Co., pp. 97-107.
11. King, S.B. III, Douglas, J.S., and Gruentzig, A.R.: Percutaneous transluminal coronary angioplasty. In King, S.B. III, and Douglas, J.S. Jr.: Coronary arteriography and angioplasty, New York, 1985, McGraw-Hill Book Co.
12. Ischinger, T., et al.: Should coronary arteries with less than 60% diameter stenosis be treated by angioplasty? Circulation **68**:148-154, 1983.
13. Libow, M.A., Gruentzig, A.R., and Greene, L.: Percutaneous transluminal coronary angioplasty, Curr. Probl. Cardiol. **10**:5-55, 1985.
14. Hastillo, A., et al.: Serial coronary angioplasty for atherosclerosis following heart transplantation, Heart Transplantation **4**:192-195, 1985.
15. Biamino, G., et al.: Left main coronary PTCA is a reasonable palliative procedure (abstract), J. Am. Coll. Cardiol. 5:520, 1985.
16. Gershony, G., et al.: Percutaneous transluminal coronary angioplasty of protected and unprotected left main coronary stenosis (abstract), J. Am. Coll. Cardiol. 7:238A, 1986.
17. McAuley, B.J., Selmon, M., Sheehan, D.J., and Simpson, J.B.: Coronary angioplasty of high risk patients in a combined catheterization laboratory–operating room setting (abstract), Circulation **72**(suppl. III-217):868, 1985.
18. Kent, K.M., et al.: Percutaneous transluminal coronary angioplasty: report from the registry of the National Heart, Lung, and Blood Institute, Am. J. Cardiol. **49**:2011-2020, 1982.
19. Cowley, M.J., et al.: Acute coronary events associated with percutaneous transluminal coronary angioplasty, Am J. Cardiol. **53**:12C-16C, 1984.

20. Cowley, M.J., et al.: Emergency coronary bypass surgery after coronary angioplasty: the National Heart, Lung, and Blood Institute's percutaneous transluminal coronary angioplasty registry experience, Am J. Cardiol. **53:**22C-26C, 1984.

21. Cowley, M.J., et al.: Sex differences in early and long-term results of coronary angioplasty in the NHLBI PTCA registry, Circulation **71:**90-97, 1985.

22. Reul, G.J., et al.: Coronary artery bypass for unsuccessful percutaneous transluminal coronary angioplasty, J. Thorac. Cardiovasc. Surg. **88:**685-694, 1984.

23. Dorros, G., et al.: In-hospital mortality rate in the National Heart, Lung, and Blood Institute percutaneous transluminal coronary angioplasty registry, Am. J. Cardiol. **53:**17C-21C, 1984.

24. Hollman, J., et al.: Acute occlusion after percutaneous transluminal coronary angioplasty—a new approach, Circulation **68:**725-732, 1983.

25. Weaver, W.F., et al., and the Laboratory Performance Standards Committee: Guidelines for physician performance of percutaneous transluminal coronary angioplasty, Cathet. Cardiovasc. Diagn. **11:**109-112, 1985.

26. Scanlon, P.J.: The training for and practice of percutaneous transluminal coronary angioplasty: results of two surveys, Cathet. Cardiovasc. Diagn. **11:**561-570, 1985.

27. Williams, D.O., et al.: Guidelines for the performance of percutaneous transluminal coronary angioplasty, Circulation **66:**693-694, 1982.

28. McAuley, B.J., Oesterle, S., and Simpson, J.B.: Advances in guidewire technology, Am. J. Cardiol. **53:**94C-96C, 1984.

29. Gruentzig, A.R., and Meier, B.: Current status of dilatation catheters and guiding systems, Am. J. Cardiol. **53:**92C-93C, 1984.

30. Topol, E.J., Myler, R.K., and Stertzer, S.H.: Selection of dilatation hardware for PTCA—1985, Cathet. Cardiovasc. Diagn. **11:**629-637, 1985.

31. Simpson, C. (Advanced Cardiovascular Systems, Inc.): Personal communication, 1986.

32. La Violette, P. (USCI): Personal communication, 1986.

33. Meier, B, et al.: Tandem balloon catheter for coronary angioplasty (abstract), J. Am. Coll. Cardiol. **7:**213A, 1986.

34. Krucoff, M.W., et al.: Safety of beta blockers with coronary angioplasty (abstract), J. Am. Coll. Cardiol. **7:**239A, 1986.

35. Barnathan E., et al.: Aspirin and dipyridamole pretreatment in the prevention of acute thrombus formation during coronary angioplasty (abstract), J. Am. Coll. Cardiol. **7:**64A, 1986.

36. O'Gara, P.T., et al.: Effect of dextran and aspirin on platelet adherence after transluminal angioplasty of normal canine coronary arteries, Am. J. Cardiol. **53:**1695-1698, 1984.

37. Swanson, K.T., et al.: Efficacy of adjunctive dextran during percutaneous transluminal coronary angioplasty, Am. J. Cardiol. **54:**447-452, 1984.

38. Bradlau, C.E., et al.: Is routine dextran infusion during coronary angioplasty (PTCA) necessary? (abstract), Circulation **72**(suppl. III-399):1595, 1985.

39. Brown, R.I.G., et al.: The use of dextran-40 during percutaneous transluminal coronary angioplasty: a report of three cases of anaphylactoid reactions—one near fatal, Cathet. Cardiovasc. Diagn. **11:**591-595, 1985.

40. Meier, B., and Rutishauser, W.: Coronary pacing during percutaneous transluminal coronary angioplasty, Circulation **71:**557-561, 1985.

41. Dorros, G., et al.: Percutaneous transluminal coronary angioplasty: report of complications from the National Heart, Lung, and Blood Institute PTCA Registry, Circulation **67:**723, 1983.

42. Goldbaum, T.S., et al.: Cardiac tamponade following percutaneous transluminal coronary angioplasty: four case reports, Cathet. Cardiovasc. Diagn. **11:**413-416, 1985.

43. Jacob, A.S., et al.: Use of pulmonary artery pressure and pacing catheter during PTCA, Cathet. Cardiovasc. Diagn. **12:**64-65, 1986.

44. Hall, D., and Gruentzig, A.: Percutaneous transluminal coronary angioplasty: current procedure and future direction, A.J.R. **142:**13-16, 1984.

45. Block, P.C.: Percutaneous transluminal coronary angioplasty. In Yu, P.N., and Goodwin, J.F., editors: Progress in cardiology, Philadelphia, 1982, Lea & Febiger, pp. 1-18.

46. Levin, D.C., Boxt, L.M., and Meyerovitz, M.F.: Percutaneous transluminal coronary angioplasty, Radiol. Clin. North Am. **23:**597-611, 1985.

47. Dorros, G.: The brachial artery method to peripheral transluminal angioplasty, Cathet. Cardiovasc. Diagn. **10:**115-127, 1984.

48. Stertzer, S.: Personal communication, 1986.

49. Arani, D.T.: A new catheter for angioplasty of the right coronary artery and aorto-coronary bypass grafts, Cathet. Cardiovasc. Diagn. **11:**647-653, 1985.

50. Pinkerton, C.A., Slack, J.D., Van Tassel, J.W., and Orr, C.M.: Angioplasty for dilatation of complex coronary artery bifurcation stenoses, Am. J. Cardiol. **55:**1626-1628, 1985.

51. Meier, B., et al.: Risk of side branch occlusion during coronary angioplasty, Am. J. Cardiol. **53:**10-14, 1984.

52. Meier, B.: Kissing balloon coronary angioplasty, Am. J. Cardiol. **54:**918-920, 1984.

53. Zack, P.M., and Ischinger, T.: Experience with a technique for coronary angioplasty of bifurcational lesions, Cathet. Cardiovasc. Diagn. **10:**433-443, 1984.

54. Vetrovec, G.W., Cowley, M.J., Wolfgang, T.C., and Ducey, K.C.: Effects of percutaneous transluminal coronary angioplasty on lesion-associated branches, Am. Heart J. **109:**921-925, 1985.

55. Shiu, M.F., and Singh, A.: Spontaneous recanalisation of side branches occluded during percutaneous transluminal coronary angioplasty, Br. Heart J. **54:**215-217, 1985.

56. Oesterle, S.N., et al.: Angioplasty at coronary bifurcations: single-guide, two-wire technique, Cathet. Cardiovasc. Diagn. **12:**57-63, 1986.

57. Kereiakes, D.J., George, B., Stertzer, S.H., and Myler, R.K.: Percutaneous transluminal angioplasty of left internal mammary artery grafts, Am. J. Cardiol. **55:**1215, 1985.

58. Giorgi, L.V., et al.: PTCA of distal coronary stenosis via patent internal mammary artery grafts—improved recent experience (abstract), J. Am. Coll. Cardiol. **7:**105A, 1986.

59. Thornton, M.A., et al.: Coumadin and aspirin in prevention of recurrence after transluminal coronary angioplasty: a randomized study, Circulation **69:**721-727, 1984.

60. Mehta, J.: Role of platelet antagonists in coronary artery disease: implications in coronary artery bypass surgery and balloon-catheter dilatation, Am. Heart J. **107:**859-869, 1984.

61. Galan, K.M., Gruentzig, A.R., and Hollman, J.: Significance of early chest pain after coronary angioplasty, Heart Lung **14:**109-112, 1985.

62. Marquis, J., et al.: Acute coronary artery occlusion during percutaneous transluminal coronary angioplasty treated by redila-

tion of the occluded segment, J. Am. Coll. Cardiol. **4**:1268-1271, 1984.

63. Slack, J.D., Pinkerton, C.A., and Nasser, W.K.: Acute pericarditis after percutaneous transluminal coronary angioplasty, Am. J. Cardiol. **55**:843-844, 1985.

64. Schofer, J., Krebber, H., Bleifeld, W., and Mathey, D.G.: Acute coronary artery occlusion during percutaneous transluminal coronary angioplasty: reopening by intracoronary streptokinase before emergency coronary artery surgery to prevent myocardial infarction, Circulation **66**:1325-1331, 1982.

65. Davies, M.J., and Thomas, A.C.: Plaque fissuring—the cause of acute myocardial infarction, sudden ischaemic death, and crescendo angina, Br. Heart J. **53**:363-373, 1985.

66. Maseri, A., Chierchia, S., and Davies, G.: Pathophysiology of coronary occlusion in acute infarction, Circulation **73**:233-239, 1986.

67. Kern, M.J., and Eilen, S.D.: Coronary vasospasm complicating PTCA, Am. Heart J. **109**(part 1):1098-1101, 1985.

68. Hollman, J.: Acute occlusion syndrome post PTCA (letter), Am. Heart J. **109**:1403, 1985.

69. Shiu, M.F., Silverton, N.P., Oakley, D., and Cumberland, D.: Acute coronary occlusion during percutaneous transluminal coronary angioplasty, Br. Heart J. **54**:129-133, 1985.

70. Bredlau, C.E., Abi-Mansour, P., Ball, E.M., and King, S.B.: Acute coronary occlusion syndrome after successful coronary angioplasty (PTCA): angiographic features, treatment strategy (abstract), Circulation **72**(suppl. III-217):866, 1985.

71. Hinohara, T., et al.: Experience with use of the reperfusion catheter prior to emergency bypass surgery (abstract), J. Am. Coll. Cardiol. **7**:153A, 1986.

72. Meier, B.: Benign coronary perforation during percutaneous transluminal coronary angioplasty, Br. Heart J. **54**:33-35, 1985.

73. Kimbiris, D., et al.: Transluminal coronary angioplasty complicated by coronary artery perforation, Cathet. Cardiovasc. Diagn. **8**:481-487, 1982.

74. Saffitz, J.E., Rose, T.E., Oaks, J.B., and Roberts, W.C.: Coronary arterial rupture during coronary angioplasty, Am. J. Cardiol. **51**:902-904, 1983.

75. Grollier, G., et al.: Coronary artery perforation during coronary angioplasty, Clin. Cardiol. **9**:27-29, 1986.

76. Alcan, K.E., et al.: The role of intra-aortic balloon counterpulsation in patients undergoing percutaneous transluminal coronary angioplasty, Am. Heart J. **105**:527-530, 1983.

77. Murphy, D.A., et al.: Surgical management of acute myocardial ischemia following percutaneous transluminal coronary angioplasty: role of the intra-aortic balloon pump, J. Thorac. Cardiovasc. Surg. **87**:332-339, 1984.

78. Golding, L.A.R., et al.: Early results of emergency surgery following coronary angioplasty (abstract), Circulation **72**(suppl. III-218):869, 1985.

79. Waller, B.F., et al.: Status of the major epicardial coronary arteries 80 to 150 days after percutaneous transluminal coronary angioplasty analysis of 3 necropsy patients, Am. J. Cardiol. **51**:81-84, 1983.

80. Mizuno, K., Kurita, A., and Imazeki, N.: Pathological findings after percutaneous transluminal coronary angioplasty, Br. Heart J. **52**:588-590, 1984.

81. Isner, J.M., and Fortin, R.V.: Frequency in nonangioplasty patients of morphologic findings reported in coronary arteries treated with transluminal angioplasty, Am. J. Cardiol. **51**:689, 1983.

82. Sanborn, T.A., et al.: The mechanism of transluminal angioplasty: evidence for formation of aneurysms in experimental atherosclerosis, Circulation **68**:1136-1140, 1983.

83. Block, P.C.: Mechanism of transluminal angioplasty, Am. J. Cardiol. **53**:69C-71C, 1984.

84. Waller, B.F., et al.: Morphologic observations after percutaneous transluminal balloon angioplasty of early and late aorto-coronary saphenous vein bypass grafts, J. Am. Coll. Cardiol. **4**:784-792, 1984.

85. Buktany, J.W., Silver, M.D., Schwartz, L., and Aldridge, H.: Morphological changes following coronary angioplasty (PTCA) and causes of restenosis (abstract), Circulation **72**(suppl. III-140):558, 1985.

86. Feldman, R.C., and Anderson, D.J.: Gradients at PTCA. Physiological or artifactual? (abstract), J. Am. Coll. Cardiol. **5**:525, 1985.

87. Sigwart, U., Grbic, M., Coy, J., and Essinger, A.: High fidelity pressure gradients across coronary artery stenosis before and after transluminal angioplasty (PTCA) (abstract), J. Am. Coll. Cardiol. **5**:521, 1985.

88. Busch, U.W., Sebening, H., Beeretz, R., and Heinze, R.: Reliability of pressure recordings via catheters used for transluminal coronary angioplasty, Texas Heart Inst. J. **11**:160-164, 1984.

89. Hodgson, J.M., and Williams, D.O.: The transstenotic pressure gradient during coronary angioplasty predicts long term clinical success (abstract), Circulation **72**(suppl. III-371):1481, 1985.

90. Holmes, D.R., et al.: Angiographic changes produced by percutaneous transluminal coronary angioplasty, Am. J. Cardiol. **51**:676-682, 1983.

91. Hinohara, T., et al.: Angiographic changes occurring within 24 hours of PTCA (abstract), Circulation **72**(suppl. III-219):873, 1985.

92. Sanders, M.: Angiographic changes thirty minutes following percutaneous transluminal coronary angioplasty, Angiology—J. Vasc. Dis. **36**:419-424, 1985.

93. Powelson, S., et al.: Incidence of early restenosis after successful percutaneous transluminal coronary angioplasty (PTCA) (abstract), J. Am. Coll. Cardiol. **7**:63A, 1986.

94. Meier, B., et al.: Higher balloon dilatation pressure in coronary angioplasty, Am. Heart J. **107**:619-622, 1984.

95. Hauser, A.M., et al.: Sequence of mechanical, electrocardiographic and clinical effects of repeated coronary artery occlusion in human beings: echocardiographic observations during coronary angioplasty, J. Am. Coll. Cardiol. **5**:193-197, 1985.

96. Alam, M., et al.: Echocardiographic evaluation of left ventricular function during coronary artery angioplasty, Am. J. Cardiol. **57**:20-25, 1986.

97. Wijns, W., et al.: Effect of coronary occlusion during percutaneous transluminal angioplasty in humans on left ventricular chamber stiffness and regional diastolic pressure-radius relations, J. Am. Coll. Cardiol. **7**:455-463, 1986.

98. Oh, J.K., Shub, C., Ilstrup, D.M., and Reeder, G.S.: Creatine kinase release after successful percutaneous transluminal coronary angioplasty, Am. Heart J. **109**:1225, 1985.

99. Meier, B., et al.: Does length or eccentricity of coronary stenoses influence the outcome of transluminal dilatation? Circulation **67**:497–499, 1983.

100. Hollman, J., et al.: Coronary artery spasm at the site of angioplasty in the first 2 months after successful percutaneous transluminal coronary angioplasty, J. Am. Coll. Cardiol. **2**:1039-1045, 1983.

101. David, P.R., et al.: Percutaneous transluminal coronary angioplasty in patients with variant angina, Circulation **66**:695-696, 1982.

102. Corcos, T., et al.: Percutaneous transluminal coronary angioplasty for the treatment of variant angina, J. Am. Coll. Cardiol. **5**:1046-1054, 1985.

103. DeWood, J.B., et al.: Intracoronary thrombus in nontransmural myocardial infarction and in unstable angina pectoris, Am. J. Caridol. **52**:1-6, 1983.

104. Falk, E.: Unstable angina with fatal outcome: dynamic coronary thrombosis leading to infarction and/or sudden death. Autopsy evidence of recurrent mural thrombosis with peripheral embolization culminating in total vascular occlusion, Circulation **71**:699-708, 1985.

105. Gotoh, K., et al.: Angiographic visualization of coronary thrombus during anginal attack in unstable angina (abstract), Circulation **72**(suppl. III-112):445, 1985.

106. Aherman, C.T., et al.: Fiberoptic coronary angioscopy identifies thrombus in all patients with unstable angina (abstract), Circulation **72**(suppl. III-112):446, 1985.

107. Mabin, T.A., et al.: Intracoronary thrombus: role in coronary occlusion complicating percutaneous transluminal coronary angioplasty, J. Am. Coll. Cardiol. **5**:198-202, 1985.

108. Williams, D.O., et al.: Evaluation of the role of coronary angioplasty in patients with unstable angina pectoris, Am. Heart J. **102**:1-9, 1981.

109. De Feyter, P.J., et al.: Emergency coronary angioplasty in refractory unstable angina, N. Engl. J. Med. **313**:342-346, 1985.

110. Haft, J.I., et al.: The coronary arteriographic lesion of acute unstable angina (abstract), Circulation **72**(suppl. III-113):451, 1985.

111. Sharma, B., et al.: Short term efficacy of coronary angioplasty in unstable angina pectoris (abstract), Circulation **72**(suppl. III-370):1477, 1985.

112. Wohlgelernter, D., et al.: Coronary angioplasty of the ''culprit lesion'': an alternative approach in the management of unstable angina with multivessel disease (abstract), J. Am. Coll. Cardiol. **7**:19A, 1986.

113. Holmes, D.R., et al.: Percutaneous transluminal coronary angioplasty, alone or in combination with streptokinase therapy, during acute myocardial infarction, Mayo Clin. Proc. **60**:449-456, 1985.

114. Pepine, C.J., et al.: Percutaneous transluminal coronary angioplasty in acute myocardial infarction, Am. Heart J. **107**:820–822, 1984.

115. Erbel, R., et al.: Combined medical and mechanical recanalization in acute myocardial infarction, Cathet. Cardiovasc. Diagn. **11**:361-377, 1985.

116. Papapietro, S.E., et al.: Percutaneous transluminal coronary angioplasty after intracoronary streptokinase in evolving acute myocardial infarction, Am. J. Cardiol. **55**:48–53, 1985.

117. Slysh, S., Goldberg, S., Dervan, J.P., and Zalewski, A.: Unstable angina and evolving myocardial infarction following coronary bypass surgery: pathogenesis and treatment with interventional catheterization, Am. Heart J. **109**:744-752, 1985.

118. O'Neill, W., et al.: A prospective randomized clinical trial of intracoronary streptokinase versus coronary angioplasty for acute myocardial infarction, N. Engl. J. Med. **314**:812-818, 1986.

119. Rothbaum, D.A., et al.: Emergency percutaneous transluminal coronary angioplasty in acute myocardial infarction (abstract), J. Am. Coll. Cardiol. **7**:149A, 1986.

120. Braunwald, E.: The aggressive treatment of acute myocardial infarction, Circulation **71**:1087-1092, 1985.

121. Topol, E.J., et al.: Sequential intravenous thrombolysis and coronary angioplasty vs. direct PTCA therapy for acute myocardial infarction (abstract), J. Am. Coll. Cardiol. **7**:18A, 1986.

122. O'Neill, W., et al.: Coronary angioplasty therapy of cardiogenic shock complicating acute myocardial infarction (abstract), Circulation **72**(suppl. III-30):1234, 1985.

123. Rutherford, B.D., Hartzler, G.O., McConahay, D.R., and Johnson, W.L. Jr.: Direct balloon angioplasty during acute myocardial infarction in patients with severely compromised hemodynamics (abstract), Circulation **72**(suppl. III-308):1232, 1985.

124. Brown, T.M. Jr., et al.: Percutaneous myocardial reperfusion (PMR) reduces mortality in acute myocardial infarction (MI) complicated by cardiogenic shock (abstract), Circulation **72**(suppl. III-309):1233, 1985.

125. Heuser, R.R., et al.: Coronary angioplasty in the treatment of cardiogenic shock: the therapy of choice (abstract), J. Am. Coll. Cardiol. **7**:219A, 1986.

126. Kereiakes, D.J., et al.: Angioplasty in total coronary artery occlusion: experience in 76 consecutive patients, J. Am. Coll. Cardiol. **6**:526-533, 1985.

127. Rickards, A.F.: Should angioplasty be attempted for occluded vessels? Proceedings of the British Cardiac Society, Br. Heart J. **52**:89, 1985.

128. Libow, M.A., Leimgruber, P.P., Roubin, G.S., and Gruentzig, A.R.: Restenosis after angioplasty (PTCA) in chronic total coronary artery occlusion (abstract), J. Am. Coll. Cardiol. **5**:445, 1985.

129. Dervan, J.P., Baim, D.S., Cherniles, J., and Grossman, W.: Transluminal angioplasty of occluded coronary arteries: use of a movable guide wire system, Circulation **68**:776-784, 1983.

130. Umans, V.A., et al.: Long term follow up after elective PTCA of totally occluded coronary arteries, not associated with acute MI (abstract), J. Am. Coll. Cardiol. **5**:521, 1985.

131. Holmes, D.R., et al.: Angioplasty in total coronary artery occlusion, J. Am. Coll. Cardiol. **3**:845-849, 1984.

132. Ferguson, D.W., et al.: Combined intracoronary streptokinase and percutaneous coronary angioplasty for reperfusion of chronic total coronary occlusion, J. Am. Coll. Cardiol. **4**:820-824, 1984.

133. Rose, G.C., and Dillon, J.C.: Variables associated with successful reopening of totally occluded coronary arteries using PTCA alone (abstract), Circulation **72**(suppl. III-369):1475, 1985.

134. Klein, M.I., et al.: Percutaneous transluminal coronary angioplasty of 100% and 99% lesions (abstract), Circulation **72**(suppl. III-370):1479, 1985.

135. Wexman, M.P., et al.: Patient selection, complications and predictors of success in PTCA of total occlusions (abstract), Circulation **72**(suppl. III-141):563, 1985.

136. Safian, R.D., et al.: Long term results and follow-up of coronary angioplasty of totally occluded coronary arteries (abstract), Circulation **72**(suppl. III-141):562, 1985.

137. Hartzler, G.O., et al.: ''Long-term'' clinical results of multiple lesion coronary angioplasty in 500 consecutive patients (abstract), Circulation **72**(suppl. II-139):556, 1985.

138. Bredlau, C.E., et al.: In-hospital morbidity; and mortality in patients undergoing elective coronary angioplasty, Circulation **72**:1044-1052, 1985.

139. Hartzler, G.O., et al.: Late results of multiple lesion coronary angioplasty in an aged population (abstract), J. Am. Coll. Cardiol. **7**:21A, 1986.

140. Hollman, J., et al.: Recurrent stenosis after coronary angioplasty (abstract), J. Am. Coll. Cardiol. **7**:20A, 1986.

141. Hernandez, J., Vandormael, M.G., Harper, J.M., and Deligonul, U.: PTCA in multivessel coronary disease: influence of degree of revascularization (abstract), Circulation **72**(suppl. III-139):554, 1985.

142. Vlietstra, R.E., et al.: Balloon angioplasty in multivessel coronary disease: importance of complete revascularization at 1-year follow-up (abstract), Circulation **72**(suppl. III-139):555, 1985.

143. Fogarty, T.J., and Kinney, T.B.: Intraoperative coronary artery balloon-catheter dilatation, Am. Heart J. **107**:845-850, 1984.

144. Wallsh, E., Adjunctive operative coronary artery balloon-catheter dilatation: review of Lenox Hill experience, Am. Heart J. **107**:856-858, 1984.

145. Douglas, J.S., et al.: Percutaneous transluminal coronary angioplasty in patients with prior coronary bypass surgery, J. Am. Coll. Cardiol. **2**:745-754, 1983.

146. Block, P.C., et al.: Percutaneous angioplasty of stenoses of bypass grafts or of bypass graft anastomotic sites, Am. J. Cardiol. **53**:666-668, 1984.

147. Corbelli, J., et al.: Percutaneous transluminal coronary angioplasty after previous coronary artery bypass surgery, Am. J. Cardiol **56**:398-403, 1985.

148. Reeder, G.S.: Angioplasty for aortocoronary bypass graft stenosis, Mayo Clin. Proc. **61**:14-19, 1986.

149. Lewis, J.F., et al.: Effects of transluminal coronary angioplasty on left ventricular systolic and diastolic function at rest and during exercise, Am. Heart J. **109**:792-798, 1985.

150. Hirzel, H.O., Nuesch, K., Gruentzig, A.R., and Luetolf, U.M.: Short- and long-term changes in myocardial perfusion and percutaneous transluminal coronary angioplasty assessed by thallium-201 exercise scintigraphy, Circulation **63**:1001-1007, 1981.

151. Hartzler, G.O., et al.: Coronary blood-flow responses during successful percutaneous transluminal coronary angioplasty, Mayo Clin. Proc. **55**:45-49, 1980.

152. Hirzel, H.O., et al.: Percutaneous transluminal coronary angioplasty: late results at 5 years following intervention, Am. Heart J. **109**:575-581, 1985.

153. Berger, E., et al.: Sustained efficacy of percutaneous transluminal coronary angioplasty, Am. Heart J. **111**:233-236, 1986.

154. Hamm, C., et al.: Factors predicting recurrent stenosis in patients with successful coronary angioplasty (abstract), J. Am. Coll. Cardiol. **5**:518, 1985.

155. Williams, D.O., et al.: Efficacy of repeat percutaneous transluminal coronary angioplasty for coronary restenosis, Am. J. Cardiol. **53**:32C-35C, 1984.

156. Levine, S., Ewels, C.J., Rosing, D.R., and Kent, K.M.: Coronary angioplasty: clinical and angiographic follow-up, Am. J. Cardiol. **55**:673-676, 1985.

157. Wijns, W., et al.: Early detection of restenosis after successful percutaneous transluminal coronary angioplasty by exercise-redistribution thallium scintigraphy, Am. J. Cardiol. **55**:357-361, 1985.

158. Leimgruber, P.P., et al.: Restenosis after successful coronary angioplasty in patient with single-vessel disease, Circulation **73**:710-717, 1986.

159. Corcos, T., et al.: Failure of diltiazem to prevent restenosis after percutaneous transluminal coronary angioplasty, Am. Heart J. **109**:926-931, 1985.

160. Abi-Mansour, P., et al.: Initial and late outcome after a third coronary angioplasty (PTCA) for recurrent native coronary restenosis (abstract), Circulation **72**(suppl. III-141):561, 1985.

161. DiSciascio, G., Cowley, M.J., Vetrovec, G.W., and Wolfgang, T.C.: Clinical recurrence rates following coronary angioplasty of single lesions, multiple (tandem) lesions, and multiple vessels (abstract), Circulation **72**(suppl. III-398):1590, 1985.

162. Whitworth, H.B., Pilcher, G.S., Roubin, G.S., and Gruentzig, A.R.: Do proximal lesions involving the origin of the left anterior descending artery (LAD) have a higher restenosis rate after coronary angioplasty (PTCA)? (abstract), Circulation **72**(suppl. III-398):1591, 1985.

163. Hoffmeister, J.M., et al.: Analysis of anatomic and procedural factors related to restenosis after double lesion coronary angioplasty (PTCA) (abstract), Circulation **72**(suppl. III-398): 1592, 1985.

164. Serruys, P.W., et al.: Incidence of restenosis 30 and 60 days after successful PTCA: a quantitative coronary angiographic study in 200 consecutive patients (abstract), Circulation **72**(suppl. III-140):559, 1985.

165. Leimgruber, P.P., et al.: Risk factors for restenosis after coronary angioplasty (PTCA) in patients with single vessel disease (SVD) (abstract), Circulation **72**(suppl. III-140):560, 1985.

166. Reeder, G.S., et al.: Is percutaneous coronary angioplasty less expensive than bypass surgery? N. Engl. J. Med. **311**:1157-1162, 1984.

167. Kelly, M.E., et al.: Comparative cost of myocardial revascularization: percutaneous transluminal angioplasty and coronary artery bypass surgery, J. Am. Coll. Cardiol. **5**:16-20, 1985.

168. Jang, G.C., et al.: Comparative cost analysis of coronary angioplasty and coronary bypass surgery: results from a national cooperative study, Circulation **66**(suppl. 2):123, 1982.

169. Kouchoukos, N.T.: Percutaneous transluminal coronary angioplasty: a surgeon's view, Circulation **72**:1144-1146, 1985.

170. Spears, J.R., et al.: In vivo coronary angioscopy, J. Am. Coll. Cardiol. **1**:1-4, 1983.

171. Abela, G.S., et al.: Angioscopy for guidance of laster recanalization in man (abstract), J. Am. Coll. Cardiol. **7**:153A, 1986.

172. Slager, C.J., et al.: Vaporization of atherosclerotic plaques for spark erosion, J. Am. Coll. Cardiol. **5**:1382-1386, 1985.

173. Lee, G., et al.: Limitations, risks and complications of laser recanalization: a cautious approach warranted, Am. J. Cardiol. **56**:181-185, 1985.

174. Lee, G., et al.: Applicability of laser to assist coronary balloon angioplasty, Am. Heart J. **110**:1233-1236, 1986.

175. Crea, F., et al.: Transluminal laser irradiation of coronary arteries in live dogs: an angiographic and morphologic study of acute effects, Am. J. Cardiol. **57**:171-174, 1986.

176. Crea, F., et al.: Laser recanalization of acutely thrombosed coronary arteries in live dogs: early results, J. Am. Coll. Cardiol. **6**:1052-1056, 1985.

177. Lai, P., et al.: Non-surgical human coronary endarterectomy: use of a mechanical rotary catheter (abstract), Circulation **72**(suppl. III-371):1482, 1985.

178. Anderson, H.V., et al.: Distal coronary artery perfusion during percutaneous transluminal coronary angioplasty, Am. Heart J. **110**:720-726, 1985.

179. Kuhl, A., et al.: A new balloon catheter and pressure generating device for R-wave–triggered coronary dilatation with diastolic

flow maintenance (abstract), J. Am. Coll. Cardiol. 7:51A, 1986.

180. McDonald, F.M., et al.: Haemodynamic and antiarrhythmic protective effects of intracoronary perfusion during percutaneous transluminal coronary angioplasty, Eur. Heart J. **6:**284-293, 1985.

181. Sibley, D.H., Whitlow, P.L., Millar, H., and Hartley, C.J.: Use of a new steerable Doppler coronary catheter to subselectively measure coronary blood flow velocity (abstract), Circulation **72**(suppl. III-20):80, 1985.

Chapter Sixteen

Thrombolytic therapy

ARA G. TILKIAN
ELAINE K. DAILY

Acute myocardial infarction is frequently precipitated by thrombotic occlusion of a coronary artery already narrowed by atherosclerotic plaque.[1,2] Thrombi also play a role in the syndrome of unstable (preinfarctional) angina.[3] Coronary arteriography or angioscopy in the setting of acute myocardial infarction, as well as unstable angina, has documented the presence of intracoronary thrombi partially or totally occluding the vessel.[4-9]

Intracoronary infusion of thrombolytic agents, first reported by Rentrop,[10] has proved effective in promoting lysis of these thrombi and reestablishing flow and myocardial perfusion. The extent of myocardial infarction may be reduced by reperfusion, depending on the promptness of coronary thrombolysis, the size of the infarct-related artery and the completeness of the occlusion, the presence of collateral vessels, the degree of reperfusion established, the myocardial oxygen demand, and probably other factors not well understood. If myocardial perfusion is reestablished within 1 to 2 hours of acute occlusion, the size of the myocardial infarction is appreciably reduced, whereas successful coronary thrombolysis 5 to 6 hours after total and continuous vessel occlusion without the presence of collaterals may not significantly alter the course of the myocardial infarction.[11-13]

Preliminary studies suggest that early successful thrombolysis reduces the short-term mortality of acute myocardial infarction.[14-17] Thrombolytic therapy was effective when used intravenously or via the coronary artery. Intravenous thrombolysis has become popular because of its simplicity and availability. The advantages and disadvantages of intracoronary therapy versus intravenous therapy are listed in Table 16-1. Many issues remain unresolved, and clinical studies are in progress.[18-25] Pending the results of such studies, thrombolytic therapy of acute myocardial infarction is still considered investigational.

In this chapter we will review the procedural and technical aspects of intracoronary and intravenous (systemic) thrombolytic treatment.

INDICATIONS

Indications for thrombolytic therapy of acute myocardial infarction are in an evolving phase. The following are guidelines:

- Acute myocardial infarction in progress (chest pain with persistent ST segment elevation despite nitroglycerin use), with substantial left ventricular myocardium at risk, where successful reperfusion may be achieved *within 3 to 4 hours* after the onset of infarction; in this setting thrombolytic treatment may be administered via either intravenous or intracoronary route (in the remainder of the indications, intracoronary infusion is the preferred method)
- Unstable angina or preinfarction state, with angiographic documentation of intracoronary thrombus
- Acute coronary artery thromboembolism during cardiac catheterization study
- Angiographic evidence of coronary artery thrombus, with or without acute occlusion, before or after elective angioplasty
- Acute graft occlusion: acute thrombosis at least 7 to 10 days after aortocoronary bypass surgery

ABSOLUTE CONTRAINDICATIONS

- Active internal bleeding
- Recent intracerebral or spinal surgery or stroke
- Recent major trauma

RELATIVE CONTRAINDICATIONS

- Conditions requiring fibrin plugs for establishment of hemostasis (surgery within the preceding 1 week, recent biopsy, trauma)
- Peptic ulcer disease (active)

Table 16-1. Comparison of intracoronary and intravenous (systemic) thrombolytic therapy of acute myocardial infarction

Comparative features	Intracoronary	Intravenous
Widespread availability	No	Yes
Delay in institution	1-2 hr frequent	None
Complexity	Yes	No
Risks of coronary catheterization	Yes	No
Risk of arterial puncture site complications	Yes	No
Risk of systemic bleeding complications	Probably less	Probably more
Cost	High	Low
Success in achieving prompt coronary thrombolysis*	75%-80%	50%-60% (75% with t-PA)
Risk of rethrombosis*	20%	20%
Time required for thrombolysis*	25-35 min	50-60 min
Doses of thrombolytic agent used*	Generally less; therefore early surgery possible	Larger—early surgery risks bleeding complications
Coronary anatomy	Known (initial and residual)	Not known or deferred to later study
Coronary angioplasty	May be first approach or may follow thrombolytic therapy	Not available
Documentation of success or failure	Yes	Not always possible

*Applies to conventional agents (streptokinase, urokinase).

- Pregnancy and postpartum period (menstruation does not seem to be a contraindication)[26]
- Recent puncture of central noncompressible vessel
- Coagulation defect
- Extensive chest wall trauma resulting from CPR
- Uncontrolled severe hypertension
- Allergy: history of anaphylactic reaction to streptokinase (urokinase or human tissue–type plasminogen activator [t-PA] may be used)
- Prior streptokinase use: within a 5-day to 6-month period (urokinase or t-PA may be used)

EQUIPMENT

If the thrombolytic agent is administered via the intracoronary route, cardiac catheterization facilities are required. For IV administration, no specialized equipment is needed. An infusion pump is desirable.

THROMBOLYTIC AGENTS[16,21-44]

Streptokinase

Streptokinase (Streptase, Kabikinase) is a nonenzymatic protein obtained from group C beta-hemolytic streptococci. It interacts with the proactivator of plasminogen and forms the active complex streptokinase-plasminogen, which catalyzes the conversion of circulating and fibrin-bound plasminogen to the fibrinolytic enzyme plasmin. Plasmin (both circulating and fibrin bound) lyses fibrin in clots. In addition, free circulating plasmin degrades fibrinogen and other coagulation fac-

tors (factors V and VIII) (Fig. 16-1). Streptokinase is available as lyophilized powder and is reconstituted in 0.9% saline or 5% dextrose solution.

Urokinase

Urokinase (Abbokinase) is an endogenous proteolytic enzyme produced in vivo by mast cell types, including endothelial cells, and secreted into the plasma in the latent form (the proenzyme prourokinase).

Commercially, urokinase is prepared from cultures of human renal cells. It acts *directly* on circulating and fibrin-bound plasminogen and activates it to the fibrinolytic enzyme plasmin, which in turn degrades fibrin, fibrinogen, and other procoagulant plasma proteins.

Urokinase is available as a lyophilized powder and is reconstituted by sterile water (without preservatives) and further diluted with 0.9% saline or 5% dextrose in water.

Tissue-type plasminogen activator

Tissue-type plasminogen activator (rt-PA) (Activase)[22,23,29-34] is a relatively fibrin-specific endogenous plasminogen activator commercially produced by using recombinant DNA techniques. rt-PA has relatively low affinity for circulating plasminogen and preferentially binds to fibrin in the thrombus, converts plasminogen to plasmin on the fibrin surface, and initiates thrombolysis, with relatively limited activation of circulating plasminogen and limited degradation of circulating fi-

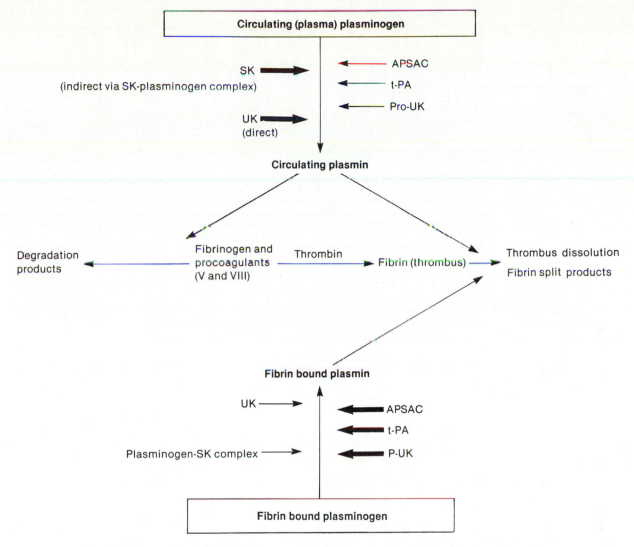

Fig. 16-1. Summary of thrombolytic cascade, indicating the site of action of the various thrombolytic (fibrinolytic) agents. (*Pro-UK,* Prourokinase; *SK,* streptokinase; *UK,* urokinase; *t-PA,* tissue type plasminogen activator; *APSAC,* anisoylated plasminogen–streptokinase activator complex; →, lesser effect [dose dependent]; →, major effect.)

brinogen. It has been shown to be an effective thrombolytic agent when given via the intracoronary or intravenous route.

Anisoylated plasminogen–streptokinase activator complex

Acylated plasminogen–streptokinase activator complex (APSAC) is another relatively fibrin-specific (clot-specific) thrombolytic agent.[40-42] It is a complex of streptokinase with acylated human plasminogen. The plasminogen selectively binds to fibrin rather than fibrinogen, causing the complex to seek out and selectively bind to thrombus. Thus most of the thrombolysis

is achieved in the thrombus, with limited systemic defibrination. Premature activation of streptokinase by plasminogen is prevented by the anisoyl group, which is hydrolyzed in vivo (permitting activation of the streptokinase), with a half-life of approximately 37 minutes.

This investigational agent has been shown to be effective via the intracoronary or intravenous route. It is subject to inactivation by circulating antistreptokinase antibodies.

Human prourokinase

Human prourokinase (Pro-UK)[36,37] is a precursor of urokinase. Its exact mechanism of action is not estab-

Table 16-2. Comparison of thrombolytic agents

Factors	Streptokinase	Urokinase	Tissue-type plasminogen activator*	Anisoylated plasminogen–streptokinase activator complex*	Prourokinase*	Fibrin antibody–streptokinase or urokinase complex*
Effective thrombolysis†	+4	+4	+4	+4	?+4	?+4
Relative clot selectivity† (fibrin specificity)	+1	+2	+4	+4	?+3±4	+4
Systemic (circulating) fibrinolysis†	+4	+2+3	+1	+1	?+1	?
Pyrogenicity	Yes	Rare	No	Yes	No	Yes ‖
Antigenicity (development of blocking antibodies after 1st use; risk of allergic reaction on retreatment)	Yes (5% of patients already have blocking antibodies)	No	Probably not	Yes	No	Yes ‖
Effective dose (IV)‡	750,000-1.5 million IU	1-2 million IU	50-80 mg	30 mg	40 mg	?
Frequently used duration of infusion‡	1 hr	1hr	1½-3 hr	2-4 min	1 hr	?
Plasma half-life	1-1½ hr§	10-20 min	6-8 min	40 min	4-5 min	?
Approximate cost	$100/million units	$500/million units	$500-1000	?	?	?
Manufacturer	Hoechst-Roussel Pharmaceuticals, Inc. (Streptase) Pharmacia Laboratories (Kabikinase)	Abbot Laboratories (Abbokinase)	Genentech, Inc., & Burroughs Wellcome Co.	Beecham Laboratories	Mochida Pharmaceutical Research Laboratory	?

*Preliminary data.

†Arbitrary scale of 0 to 4. *0*, no effect; *4*, maximal or full effect; effect is dose dependent.

‡Dose and duration used in studies reported. These are not necessarily the optimal doses or durations of infusion. For t-PA and prourokinase longer maintenance infusion may be required. For urokinase, larger doses may be appropriate because the specific activity of urokinase and rt-PA are comparable—100,000 IU/mg.

§After the effect of antibodies is overcome.

‖ For streptokinase.

lished, but in animal preparations it appears to induce more clot-selective thrombolysis than urokinase. Human trials are in a preliminary phase, and clot-selective coronary thrombolysis in patients with acute myocardial infarction has been demonstrated.[43]

Efforts are underway to develop and test fibrin-specific thrombolytic agents using human fibrin–specific antibody conjugated to streptokinase or urokinase.[38,39]

For further discussion of the various thrombolytic agents, see Table 16-2 and Fig. 16-1.

PATIENT PREPARATION

1. Continue supportive treatment of acute myocardial infarction or coronary insufficiency.

Table 16-3. Regimen for thrombolytic therapy

Agent	Bolus	Average infusion rate (range reported)*	Average total dose (range reported)*
Intracoronary infusion			
Streptokinase	10,000-30,000 units	4000 units/min (2000 to 5000 units/min)	250,000 IU in 100 ml D5W (100,000-400,000 units)
Urokinase	10,000-30,000 units	6000 units/min (2000-24,000 units/min)	500,000 units in 100 ml D5W (250,000-2,000,000 units)
Intravenous infusion			
Streptokinase	10,000-20,000 IU	10,000-20,000 IU/min (10,000-40,000 IU/min)	(750,000-1.5 million IU in 100-250 ml D5W over 30-60 min)
Urokinase	10,000-20,000 IU	10,000-20,000 IU	1-2 million IU

*Doses are not standardized. These are general guidelines, reflecting reports in the literature.

2. Obtain informed consent for systemic or intracoronary thrombolysis. Consent may include subsequent emergency angioplasty.

3. Obtain the following laboratory studies: ECG, cardiac enzymes, blood and platelet count, chemistry profile and coagulation studies, including fibrinogen, thrombin time, and partial thromboplastin time (PTT). Obtain a blood sample for typing and possible cross matching. Ensure availability of fresh frozen plasma. Thrombolytic therapy is not withheld until the completion of all these studies.

4. Prepare the patient for cardiac catheterization if the intracoronary route is chosen.

5. Give diphenhydramine (Benadryl) (50 mg intravenously) to reduce the chance of allergic reaction if streptokinase is used. (IV hydrocortisone, used in earlier studies, is no longer used in most centers.)

6. Administer heparin (5000 units intravenously) to stop further clot formation. Heparin may shorten the interval from the start of thrombolytic treatment to reperfusion.[44] Larger doses (7500-10,000 units) may induce reperfusion when given during the first hour of an acute myocardial infarction.[45]

7. Administer the thrombolytic agent as detailed below by the intracoronary or intravenous route.

TECHNIQUE
Intracoronary thrombolysis

1. Perform cardiac catheterization, using standard techniques described in Chapter 5. If delay is anticipated in starting the intracoronary infusion, a satisfactory alternative is to promptly introduce the arterial and venous sheaths in the proper vessels. This may be initiated in the emergency room or coronary care unit,

where an IV infusion of thrombolytic agent is started immediately. The patient may then be taken to the cardiac catheterization laboratory for selective angiography, continuation of the infusion through the intracoronary route, and consideration of mechanical methods of opening the occluded artery (e.g., guidewires or angioplasty).

2. Visualize what is thought to be the non-infarct-related artery, if this can be done quickly. Examine the collateral arteries and evaluate them for the presence of other critical disease. This will help plan subsequent strategy.

3. Promptly visualize the infarct-related coronary artery. Ventriculography is best deferred.

4. Inject intracoronary nitroglycerin 200 to 400 μg into the infarct-related artery.

5. If total or subtotal occlusion persists (as it will in more than 95% of cases), proceed with the intracoronary therapy, following the regimen outlined in Table 16-3.

6. Monitor the patient's ECG and systemic pressures.

7. Obtain hemodynamic measurements for the right side of the heart during the thrombolytic infusion. Do not lose valuable minutes by obtaining these pressures before initiation of intracoronary thrombolysis.

8. Have transcutaneous and transvenous pacing capability available on a standby basis.

9. Check coronary artery occlusion by contrast material injection every 5 to 10 minutes or if arrhythmias are observed.

10. Continue infusing the thrombolytic agent for 30 minutes after the establishment of reperfusion or until there is evidence of clot lysis and appearance of prompt perfusion. Frequently, reperfusion will occur 20 to 30

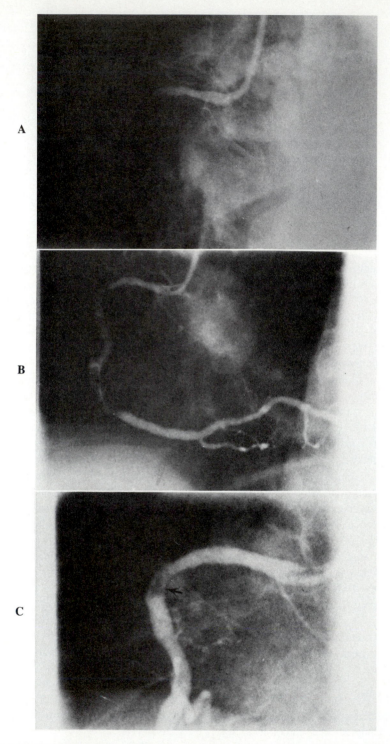

Fig. 16-2. Intracoronary thrombolysis. **A,** Injection into the right coronary artery (left anterior oblique projection) reveals a totally occluded vessel. **B,** Reperfusion is established following infusion of streptokinase. **C,** Magnified view reveals residual intracoronary thrombus within the proximal right coronary artery.

minutes after the start of intracoronary infusion (Fig. 16-2).

11. Consider mechanical measures to open the vessel if reperfusion is not achieved after approximately 30 minutes. The obstruction may be probed with a 0.016-inch (0.41 mm) flexible angioplasty guidewire. This may help promote thrombolysis by permitting more effective penetration of the agent into the thrombus. If the guidewire can be advanced distal to the obstruction and is definitely in the lumen of the obstructed artery, proceeding to coronary angioplasty (see p. 369) would be an excellent alternative to continued thrombolytic therapy.

12. After successful reperfusion, continue anticoagulation with systemic heparinization. Monitor hemoglobin, PTT, and fibrinogen levels. Start IV infusion of heparin at 600 to 700 units/hour when the PTT has returned to two to three times the control level and when fibrinogen is at least 50 to 60 mg/dl. Adjust the heparin dose every 4 hours based on PTT determination, with a view to keeping PTT two to three times the control level. Perform follow-up ECG and check creatine phosphokinase isoenzymes at 12 and 24 hours after the procedure to evaluate myocardial infarction.

13. Leave arterial and venous catheters securely in place. These are used for hemodynamic monitoring and sampling of blood. Avoid arterial or venous puncture as long as a systemic fibrinolytic state exists.

14. Residual stenosis, frequently high-grade, will be present in most patients. Individualize the follow-up therapy, which may include the use of angioplasty, revascularization surgery, or continued medical therapy with vasodilators and chronic anticoagulation.

15. Remove vascular catheters after coagulation status is competent and if urgent coronary angioplasty is not planned.

Intravenous (systemic) thrombolysis

Advantages and disadvantages of intracoronary as compared with IV thrombolytic treatment are listed in Table 16-1. The relative simplicity and general availability and the potential for earlier coronary recannalization with IV thrombolysis have made this the procedure of choice in many circumstances. The general indications, contraindications, and precautions are similar for the IV and the intracoronary techniques, as are premedication with heparin and diphenhydramine and laboratory monitoring. The following *differences* apply to the IV method.

1. Perform the procedure in the emergency department or coronary care unit with external blood pressure monitoring.

2. Insert a catheter in a large peripheral vein (medial basilic vein, brachial-cephalic vein, or femoral vein if no other large vein is available) for administrating medications and for future and frequent blood sampling without repeat venipunctures. Secure the catheter to the skin with tape and suture to prevent accidental dislodgment. Start a second IV line for the simultaneous infusion of the thrombolytic agent.

3. Start infusing the thrombolytic agent as soon as possible. The dose used is generally higher than that for intracoronary administration (see Table 16-2). The dose of streptokinase required to achieve a fibrinolytic state varies from patient to patient and is dependent on the level of antistreptokinase antibodies present in a given patient. Approximately 5% of patients may have very high titers, rendering effective therapy impossible. Such antibodies can be measured and the dose of streptokinase adjusted accordingly, but this may be time consuming. A practical alternative is to measure serum fibrinogen levels at the end of a 30-minute infusion of 750,000 units of streptokinase; if the fibrinogen level is substantially over 50 mg/dl, continue or repeat the infusion or use urokinase until a fibrinolytic state is achieved or reperfusion is observed.[46]

4. Monitor the patient's blood pressure closely during streptokinase infusion.[47] If it falls by 20 mm Hg or falls under 90 mm Hg systolic, temporarily discontinue the infusion. Be aware of the additive hypotensive effects of nitrates and morphine.

5. Watch for these signs of reperfusion: (a) relief of chest pain, (b) resolution of ECG signs of myocardial injury, and (c) reperfusion arrhythmias (accelerated idioventricular rhythm, ventricular tachycardia, bradyarrhythmia). Late-appearing clues of reperfusion are (a) early peaking of serum creatine kinase (CK)[48] and (b) a strongly positive early ^{99m}Tc-pyrophosphate image.[49]

6. Perform laboratory monitoring and use heparin as outlined in intracoronary thrombolysis.

7. Avoid intra-arterial puncture or injection of intramuscular medications.

8. Individualize coronary arteriography and follow-up treatment.

GUIDELINES[19-25,52-54]
Avoid delay

Infusion of the thrombolytic agent (intravenous or intracoronary) should commence as soon as possible. Do not waste time obtaining unnecessary laboratory or hemodynamic data or noncritical angiographic data before initiating therapy.

Prevention of myocardial damage was most successful when streptokinase was given within the first 1.5 hours after the onset of acute myocardial infarction.[17,53]

Supraselective catheter infusion

Supraselective infusion with a 3 or 4 Fr end-hole catheter, inserted through the coronary catheter via a Y adaptor, has been advocated. Mainstem coronary artery infusions appear satisfactory in most cases. Intermittent bolus infusion of the thrombolytic agent by hand may deliver more of the agent to the area of coronary artery occlusion than slow continuous drip infusion. Do not push with excessive force because this may cause reflux of the medication into the aortic sinus. Supraselective infusion may be used if it can be achieved without delay or if the mainstem coronary artery infusion does not appear to deliver the thrombolytic agent to the area of the thrombus.

Advantages of supraselective catheter infusion include simultaneous infusion and pressure monitoring and the ability to deliver a higher concentration of the thrombolytic agent to the site of occlusion, with increased chance of thrombolysis with lower overall doses.

Disadvantages include risk of coronary artery dissection and delay in instituting thrombolytic therapy.

Intra-aortic balloon pumping

Intra-aortic balloon pumping can be used before, during, or after thrombolytic therapy, depending on the patient's hemodynamic needs. Its use does not impede the passage of percutaneous femoral coronary catheters or interfere with the coronary arteriographic study.

Coronary angioplasty

Coronary angioplasty in acute myocardial infarction may be performed before or immediately after reperfusion but is probably best delayed for 1 to 2 days if adequate flow is established by thrombolytic therapy alone.[50-52] This delay will permit further lysis of thrombus, may reduce the chance of reocclusion, and will permit performance of the procedure under optimal conditions (see also Chapter 15).

Emergency coronary angioplasty without the capability to perform cardiovascular surgery if needed has been limited to attempts at opening *totally occluded vessels;* presumably, a successful result will be beneficial, and failure cannot harm the patient. In all other situations, angioplasty may be performed only if the capability to perform emergency cardiovascular surgery is available. Thus facilities where thrombolytic therapy (intravenous or intracoronary) is used but where cardiovascular surgery is not available should develop close ties and transfer arrangements with hospitals where these services are available and where such patients can be transferred after they are stable.

Bypass grafting

Although experience is limited, coronary artery bypass grafting has been performed immediately after intracoronary streptokinase infusion if total dose has been under 250,000 units and the patient's fibrinogen level has been over 100 mg/dl. Much individual variability is expected, depending on the presence or absence of antistreptokinase antibodies. Generally, surgical intervention can be carried out safely 24 hours after thrombolytic (intravenous or intracoronary) therapy, even if larger doses have been used. Intraoperative use of fresh-frozen plasma or cryoprecipitate may be needed, especially if the fibrinogen level is under 100 mg/dl. Use of rt-PA or acylated plasminogen–streptokinase complex with less systemic fibrinolytic effect and shorter half-life may permit earlier surgical intervention.

Follow-up therapy

Guidelines for follow-up therapy have not been firmly established. After successful IV thrombolytic therapy, coronary arteriography is performed to evaluate the coronary anatomy. In general, early angioplasty or revascularization surgery is considered if residual stenosis is severe, the degree of infarction is limited and especially if myocardial ischemia persists. On the other hand, with a noncritical residual stenosis, especially if the degree of myocardial infarction is substantial, such interventions are generally deferred in this acute phase of treatment. Spontaneous regression of residual stenosis may occur.[54] Decisions are guided by careful scrutiny of the postreperfusion coronary arteriogram, creatine phosphokinase assays, follow-up ECG, resting thallium myocardial perfusion study, evaluation of left ventricular function by echocardiography or radionuclide wall motion study, and most importantly the patient's clinical status.

FAILURE TO ACHIEVE REPERFUSION

Failure of thrombolytic therapy to achieve reperfusion may be secondary to:

- Use of too low a dose of a thrombolytic agent
- High titers of antistreptokinase antibodies—if streptokinase is used
- Distal thrombus, with inadequate delivery of thrombolytic agent or inadequate concentration of plasminogen at the site of the occlusion
- Presence of a platelet (versus fibrin) thrombus
- Absence of fresh thrombus in the occluded vessel: vascular obstruction resulting from raised plaque secondary to subintimal bleeding

Table 16-4. Complications of thrombolytic therapy and their prevention and treatment

Complications	Prevention and treatment
Hemorrhage (10%-20%, majority at vascular puncture sites)	For significant bleeding, stop thrombolytic agent, use fresh whole blood, packed red cells with fresh-frozen plasma, or cryoprecipitate (10 units will increase fibrinogen by 70-80 mg/dl). Consider protamine sulfate if heparin has been used.
	Secure all intravascular catheters with sutures and tape. Apply pressure as needed. Avoid/minimize venous or arterial puncture.
Gastrointestinal hemorrhage	Suppress vomiting. For prophylaxis, use antacids, ranitidine (Zantac), or cimetidine (Tagamet). Give supportive care.
Other (CNS hemorrhage, hemopericardium)	Pay close attention to contraindications and case selection. Give supportive care. Pericardiocentesis.
Reperfusion arrhythmias	Usually benign and self-limited. For sustained arrhythmias, use lidocaine or immediate cardioversion/defibrillation. IV verapamil is also effective and may be used if there is no bradyarrhythmia or left ventricular failure.
Fever (±25%), allergic reaction (±6%) (Limited to streptokinase)	Give diphenhydramine (Benadryl), hydrocortisone, or acetaminophen (Tylenol). Rarely, streptokinase infusion will have to be discontinued.
Reinfarction secondary to reocclusion (20%)	Use systemic heparin with careful monitoring. Perform coronary angioplasty or revascularization surgery or institute long-term anticoagulant therapy. Treatment must be individualized.

COMPLICATIONS

The complications of thrombolysis and their prevention and treatment are summarized in Table 16-4.

FUTURE DEVELOPMENTS

Several thrombolytic agents with clot selectivity are under investigation. These include rt-PA, anisoylated plasminogen–streptokinase activator complex, prourokinase, and fibrin-antibody conjugated to streptokinase or urokinase. These agents can cause clot lysis without inducing an extensive system lytic state. The rate of reperfusion achieved by using rt-PA intravenously approaches or exceeds that achieved by intracoronary infusion of streptokinase or urokinase. If studies in progress confirm these preliminary results and the long-term benefits of thrombolysis are demonstrated, the intracoronary infusion of thrombolytic agents will be used very infrequently and for unusual circumstances; most patients with acute myocardial infarction (and probably unstable angina) will be treated with IV fibrin-specific agents. Such IV therapy may even be initiated out of the hospital—and continued during transport of the patient to the hospital—where it may be continued.[53] The proper dosage, infusion rate, and duration of infusion of these agents are under study (Table 16-2).

The immediate benefits of safe and effective coronary thrombolysis are self-evident and may be taken for granted. Demonstration of long-term benefits must await the completion of ongoing controlled studies.

PROCEDURE CHECKLIST

- Review indications and contraindications of thrombolytic therapy.
- Inform the patient and family of therapeutic options and proposed plan of treatment and obtain informed consent.
- Notify the cardiac catheterization laboratory and prepare the patient for cardiac catheterization if the intracoronary route is to be used.
- Administer IV heparin. Administer IV diphenhydramine if streptokinase is to be used.
- Provide continuous ECG monitoring and full supportive care for the patient.
- Send a blood sample to the laboratory for analysis of enzymes, blood count, chemistry profile, coagulation studies, and blood typing and possible cross matching.
- Suture all intravascular catheters securely in place.
- Proceed to thrombolytic therapy without delay.
- After successful reperfusion, continue anticoagulation with IV heparin.
- Observe the patient for signs of gastrointestinal, genitourinary, or retroperitoneal bleeding or bleeding from puncture sites. Check PTT and adjust heparin dose every 4 hours during the early phase of therapy.
- Evaluate the patient for extent of myocardial infarction and degree of reperfusion and residual stenosis and plan follow-up therapy.

REFERENCES

1. Meade, T.W.: Thrombosis and ischaemic heart disease, Br. Heart J. **53**:473-476, 1985.
2. Davies, M.J., and Thomas, A.C.: Plaque fissuring—the cause of acute myocardial infarction, sudden ischaemic death, and crescendo angina, Br. Heart J. **53**:363-373, 1985.
3. Falk, E.: Unstable angina with fatal outcome: dynamic coronary thrombosis leading to infarction and/or sudden death. Autopsy evidence of recurrent mural thrombosis with peripheral embolization culminating in total vascular occlusion, Circulation **71**:699-708, 1985.
4. DeWood, M.A., et al.: Prevalence of total coronary occlusion during the early hours of transmural myocardial infarction, N. Engl. J. Med. **303**:897-902, 1980.
5. Holmes, D.R. Jr., et al.: Coronary artery thrombosis in patients with unstable angina, Br. Heart J. **45**:411, 1981.
6. Bresnahan, D.R., Davis, J.L., Holmes, D.R., and Smith, H.C.: Angiographic occurrence and clinical correlates of intraluminal coronary artery thrombus: role of unstable angina, J. Am. Coll. Cardiol. **6**:285-289, 1985.
7. Sherman, C.T., et al.: Fiberoptic coronary angioscopy identifies thrombus in all patients with unstable angina, Circulation **72**(suppl. III-112):446, 1985.
8. Gotoh, K., et al.: Angiographic visualization of coronary thrombus during anginal attack in unstable angina, Circulation **72**(suppl. III-112):445, 1985.
9. Haft, J.I., et al.: The coronary arteriographic lesion of acute unstable angina, Circulation **72**(suppl. III-113):451, 1985.
10. Rentrop, P., et al.: Acute myocardial infarction: intracoronary application of nitroglycerin and streptokinase in combination with transluminal recanalization, Clin. Cardiol. **5**:354, 1979.
11. Reisner, K.A., et al.: The wavefront phenomenon of ischemic cell death; myocardial infarction size vs duration of coronary occlusion in dogs, Circulation **56**:785, 1977.
12. Mathey, D.G., Sheehan, F.H., Schofer, J., and Dodge, H.T.: Time from onset of symptoms to thrombolytic therapy: a major determinant of myocardial salvage in patients with acute transmural infarction, J. Am. Coll. Cardiol. **6**:518-525, 1985.
13. Kloner, R.A., Ellis, S.G., Lange, R., and Braunwald, E.: Studies of experimental coronary artery reperfusion: effects on infarct size, myocardial function, biochemistry, ultrastructure, and microvascular damage, Circulation **68**(suppl. I):8-15, 1983.
14. Kennedy, J.W., Gensini, G.G., Timmis, G.C., and Maynard, C.: Acute myocardial infarction treated with intracoronary streptokinase: a report of the Society for Cardiac Angiography, Am. J. Cardiol. **55**:871-877, 1985.
15. Kennedy, J.W., et al.: The Western Washington randomized trial of intracoronary streptokinase in acute myocardial infarction. A 12-month follow-up report, N. Engl. J. Med. **312**:1073-1078, 1985.
16. Kambara, H., et al.: Coronary thrombolysis with urokinase infusion in acute myocardial infarction: multicenter study in Japan, Cathet. Cardiovasc. Diagn. **11**:349-360, 1985.
17. Italian Group for the Study of Streptokinase in Myocardial Infarction (GISSI): Effectiveness of intravenous thrombolytic treatment in acute myocardial infarction, Lancet **1**:344-401, 1986.
18. Stratton, J.R., et al.: Late effects of intracoronary streptokinase on regional wall motion, ventricular aneurysm and left ventricular thrombus in myocardial infarction: results from the Western Washington Randomized Trial, J. Am. Coll. Cardiol. **5**:1023-1028, 1985.
19. Jaffe, A.S., and Sobel, B.E.: Thrombolysis with tissue-type plasminogen activator in acute myocardial infarction. Potentials and pitfalls, JAMA **255**:237-239, 1986.
20. Braunwald, E.: The aggressive treatment of acute myocardial infarction, Circulation **71**:1087-1092, 1985.
21. Dunn, M.I.: Streptokinase, Arch. Intern. Med. **145**:1381-1382, 1985.
22. The TIMI Study Group: The thrombolysis in myocardial infarction (TIMI) trial: phase I findings, N. Engl. J. Med. **312**:932-936, 1985.
22a. Williams, D.O., et al.: Intravenous recombinant tissue-type plasminogen activator in patients with acute myocardial infarction: A report from the NHLBI thrombolysis in myocardial infarction trial, Circulation **73**:338-346, 1986.
23. Verstraete, M., et al.: Randomised trial of intravenous recombinant tissue-type plasminogen activator versus intravenous streptokinase in acute myocardial infarction, Lancet **1**:842-847, 1985.
24. Gersh, B.J.: Role of thrombolytic therapy in evolving myocardial infarction, Mod. Concepts Cardiovasc. Dis. **54**:13-17, 1985.
25. Health and Public Policy Committee, American College of Physicians: Thrombolysis for evolving myocardial infarction, Ann. Intern. Med. **103**:463-469, 1985.
26. de Gregorio, B., Goldstein, J., and Haft, J.I.: Administration of intracoronary streptokinase during menstruation, Am. Heart J. **109**:908-910, 1985.
27. Cowley, M.J.: Methodologic aspects of intracoronary thrombolysis. Drugs, dosage and duration, Circulation **68**(suppl. I):90-95, 1983.
28. Tennant, S.N., et al.: Intracoronary thrombolysis in patients with acute myocardial infarction: comparison of the efficacy of urokinase with streptokinase, Circulation **69**:756-760, 1984.
29. Collen, D., et al.: Coronary thrombolysis with recombinant human tissue-type plasminogen activator: a prospective, randomized, placebo-controlled trial, Circulation **70**:1012-1017, 1984.
30. Collen, D.: Human tissue–type plasminogen activator: from the laboratory to the bedside (editorial), Circulation **72**:18-20, 1985.
31. Sherry, S.: Sounding board. Tissue plasminogen activator (t-PA). Will it fulfill its promise? N. Engl. J. Med. **313**:1014-1017, 1985.
32. Collen, D., et al.: Analysis of coagulation and fibrinolysis during intravenous infusion of recombinant human tissue-type plasminogen activator in patients with acute myocardial infarction, Circulation **73**:511-517, 1986.
33. Gold, H.K., et al.: Acute coronary reocclusion after thrombolysis with recombinant human tissue-type plasminogen activator: prevention by a maintenance infusion, Circulation **73**:347-352, 1986.
34. Topol, E.J., Bell, W.R., and Weisfeldt, M.L.: Coronary thrombolysis with recombinant tissue-type plasminogen activator, Ann. Intern. Med. **103**:837-843, 1985.
35. Gurewich, V., and Pannell, R. Jr. (letter) and Wachsberg, R. (reply): Thrombolytic therapy for acute myocardial infarction, N. Engl. J. Med. **313**:825, 1985.
36. Collen, D., et al.: Coronary thrombolysis in dogs with intravenously administered human pro-urokinase, Circulation **72**:384-388, 1985.
37. Van de Werf, F., et al.: Coronary thrombolysis with intravenously administered human pro-urokinase in dogs, Circulation **72**(suppl. III-70):277, 1985.
38. Ito, R.K., et al.: Development of a thrombolytic agent using a human fibrin–specific monoclonal antibody as a conjugate-carrier of streptokinase, Circulation **72**(suppl. III-192):767, 1985.
39. Bode, C., Matsueda, G., and Haber, E.: Targeted thrombolysis

with a fibrin-specific antibody-urokinase conjugate, Circulation **72**(suppl. III-192):768, 1985.

40. Been, M., et al.: Coronary thrombolysis with intravenous anisoylated plasminogen-streptokinase complex BRL 26921, Br. Heart J. **53**:253-259, 1985.

41. Tkram, S., et al.: The use of intravenous anisoyl plasminogen streptokinase activator complex (BRL 26921) in acute myocardial infarction (abstract), J. Am. Coll. Cardiol. **7**:219A, 1986.

42. Marder, V.J., et al.: Rapid lysis of coronary artery thrombi with anisoylated plasminogen:streptokinase activator complex. Treatment by bolus intravenous injection, Ann. Intern. Med. **104**:304-310, 1986.

43. van de Werf, F., Nobuhara, M., and Collen, D.: Coronary thrombolysis with human single-chain, urokinase-type plasminogen activator (pro-urokinase) in patients with acute myocardial infarction, Ann. Intern. Med. **104**:345-348, 1986.

44. Lew, A.S., et al.: The time interval from initiation of IV streptokinase to reperfusion is directly related to the residual fibrinogen level and is shortened by pretreatment with heparin (abstract), J. Am. Coll. Cardiol. **7**:17A, 1986.

45. Berman, G.O., et al.: Heparin induces coronary reperfusion in very early myocardial infarction (abstract), J. Am. Coll. Cardiol. **7**:17A, 1986.

46. Lew, A.S., Laramee, P., and Ganz, W.: Measurement of anti-streptokinase antibodies (letter), J. Am. Coll. Cardiol. **5**:1500, 1985.

47. Lew, A.S., et al.: The hypotensive effect of intravenous streptokinase in patients with acute myocardial infarction, Circulation **72**:1321-1326, 1985.

48. Wei, J.Y., Markis, J.E., Malagold, M., and Grossman, W.: Time course of serum cardiac enzymes after intracoronary thrombolytic therapy, Arch. Intern. Med. **145**:1596-1600, 1985.

49. Wheelan, K., et al.: Early positive technetium-99m stannous pyrophosphate images as a marker of reperfusion after thrombolytic therapy for acute myocardial infarction, Am. J. Cardiol. **56**:252-256, 1985.

50. Topol, E.J., et al.: Applicability of percutaneous transluminal coronary angioplasty to patients with recombinant tissue plasminogen activator mediated thrombolysis, Cathet. Cardiovasc. Diagn. **11**:337-348, 1985.

51. Chesebro, J.H., et al.: Reocclusion and clot lysis between 90 minutes, 1 day, and 10 days after thrombolytic therapy for myocardial infarction, Circulation **72**(suppl. III-55):219, 1985.

52. Rothbard, R.L., and Fitzpatrick, P.G.: Comparison of residual coronary artery stenosis and flow immediately and 24 hours after successful thrombolysis, Circulation **72**(suppl. III-55):217, 1985.

53. Koren, G., et al.: Prevention of myocardial damage in acute myocardial ischemia by early treatment with intravenous streptokinase, N. Engl. J. Med. **313**:1384-1389, 1985.

54. Voelker, W., et al.: Spontaneous regression of residual stenosis of the infarct-related vessel after successful coronary recanalization, Cardiovasc. Rev. Reports **7**:293, 1986.

Chapter Seventeen

Transluminal catheter extraction and resolution of intracardiac catheter knots

ARA G. TILKIAN
ELAINE K. DAILY

TRANSVASCULAR EXTRACTION OF EMBOLIZED CATHETERS OR GUIDEWIRES

A catheter fragment embolism to the right atrium was first reported in 1954.[1] During the subsequent 20 years more than 200 cases of various catheter or guidewire embolization were reported while many others went unreported and even possibly unrecognized.[2-4] Almost any type of catheter, wire, or intravascular device has been reported to have embolized to the central circulation. Although improvements in catheter design and widespread practice of one-time use of catheters have reduced the risk of this potentially lethal complication, the population at risk of catheter emboli grows in number with the more frequent and more aggressive use of these devices. Earlier attempts of dealing with such complications frequently involved extensive cutdowns or major surgery including thoracotomy and cardiotomy. The first transvascular retrieval of a broken segment of a steel spring guidewire using bronchoscopy forceps was reported in 1964,[5] and numerous cases have been reported since then using various techniques.[4,6,7]

In this chapter we will review methods of preventing this iatrogenic complication and then discuss various techniques of dealing with it when it occurs.

Catheter or guidewire emboli
Types

Embolization of a catheter or guidewire fragments have been reported with most of the commonly used devices, in both the arterial and venous sides. They are listed below in order of decreasing frequency.

Polyethylene central venous catheter fragments
Guidewire fragments
Pacemaker catheter fragments
Standard diagnostic cardiac catheters
Ventriculovenous shunt catheters
Desilet-Hoffman sheath
Catheter tip occluder and wire

Complications

Embolization of these and other catheters into the central circulation or the heart is not a benign condition. The complications directly related to embolization of such devices include sepsis, endocarditis, abscess, myocardial necrosis, myocarditis, vascular or cardiac perforation, hemopericardium, thrombosis with venous or arterial occlusion, thrombosis and embolization (pulmonary or systemic), arrhythmias, and sudden death.

The morbidity directly attributed to these catheter emboli is estimated to be 50% to 70% and the mortality at 25% to 50%.[4] Thus, every precaution should be taken to prevent catheter or guidewire embolization. When emboli do occur, except for unusual circumstances, all efforts should be made to remove them, preferably using transvascular techniques.

Mechanisms

Mechanisms of catheter or guidewire emboli include the following:
- Piercing and cutting of polyethylene tubing by the sharp bevel of the needle housing the catheter
- Catheter breakage within the vessel or cardiac chamber
- Detachment of the catheter or its introducer from the hub
- Accidental severance of a catheter during dressing change

390

- Pacemaker wire fragments cut or broken during generator replacement
- Severed guidewire fragments

Understanding the mechanisms of catheter or wire emboli will help to prevent their occurrence.

Piercing and cutting of polyethylene tubing by the sharp bevel of the needle housing the catheter is a danger with the "catheter inside the needle" system. Catheter needle assemblies usually come in two configurations—"catheter over the needle" and "catheter within the needle." The "catheter over the needle" configuration consists of a combined needle and catheter unit, which is inserted into a vessel. The catheter is then passed over the needle and into the vessel; the needle is withdrawn and discarded. This is a safe method, preventing contact of the sharp needle and the catheter for any length of time. It has the disadvantage of not permitting the introduction of long catheters, as the catheter length is limited by the needle length.

With the "catheter inside the needle" system, the needle is introduced into the vascular system and a catheter is then advanced through the needle. This permits the introduction of longer catheters but leaves a sharp cutting portion of the needle in contact with the catheter. There is a risk of shearing off the catheter tip and losing it in the vessel if the catheter is withdrawn through the needle. Most polyethylene catheter emboli involve this catheter and needle system and are due to either improper handling or actual failure of the system. Various methods have been introduced by manufacturers to protect the needle tip–catheter contact area to prevent puncture or cutting of the catheter. Polyethylene catheter emboli caused by breakage of the catheter unrelated to needle puncture has not been reported.

Catheter breakage within a vessel or cardiac chamber usually occurs when catheters are used a number of times or when they are used after their expiration date and their structural integrity is compromised. Rare manufacturing defects may also be a cause.

Detachment of the catheter or its introducer from the hub occurs with multiple use of catheters, manufacturing defects, or improper and careless handling of catheters.

Accidental severance of a catheter during dressing change is a rare but embarrassing occurrence and cannot be blamed on anything except careless and hasty technique.

Guidewire fragments occur when guidewires break and embolize. Aggressive and improper use of guidewires can cause bends and kinks, and the wires can break at these points. Careless and forceful withdrawal of bent wires through a Seldinger needle or a stiff introducer can shear off a wire tip into the circulation.

Prevention

Keeping in mind the various mechanisms involved in catheter and wire embolism, the following guidelines are suggested to minimize the risk.

1. Follow the manufacturer's directions carefully. Pay special attention to the method of securing the needle-catheter interface to prevent cutting of the catheter. *Do not permit the tip of the cutting needle to be in contact with the catheter.*

2. Never forcefully pull a catheter or guidewire through a needle or introducer while the needle or introducer is still in the vessel.

3. Inspect all catheters and guidewires carefully, especially the distal tips and the catheter hub, to ensure device integrity. This is especially important in multiple-use catheters. Do not use catheters after their expiration date. Polyurethane cardiac catheters can deteriorate 3 to 5 years after manufacture and lose tensile strength, predisposing to fracture.[8]

4. A flange should be present on the hub end of the catheter to prevent accidental passage through the skin. Secure all indwelling catheters to the skin with sutures.

5. During dressing changes, use adequate light and full exposure of the catheter to avoid accidental cutting.

6. Securely suture permanent pacemaker wire fragments that cannot be removed to the subcutaneous tissue to prevent future migration.

7. Use only radiopaque catheters in the vascular system. Transvascular retrieval of nonradiopaque catheters is very difficult in case of an embolization.

8. Use catheters of known length and check the catheter integrity and length after removal.

9. When making side holes in a preshaped catheter, avoid putting the holes too close to one another, which would weaken the catheter and predispose to breakage. Make certain all hole fragments are removed before catheter insertion.

Approach to the patient

Meticulous attention to technique will reduce but not eliminate the problem of catheter or wire embolization. When such a problem does occur, two questions need to be answered.

- *Should the embolized fragment be removed?* The answer is almost always "yes." The risk of morbidity from such an event is 50% to 70% and the risk of mortality is at least 25%, whereas the risk of transvascular removal of the catheter is near zero, with a success rate of 90%.

The rare exceptions when the embolized catheter may be left in the cardiovascular system are (1) for patients with terminal illness, (2) when transvascular techniques have failed and the patient's medical condition is so poor that thoracotomy or cardiotomy is considered too great a risk, or (3) when pacemaker wires have been cut or broken during replacement of the generator and removal is very difficult or impossible and the risk of migration very small. Forced removal may risk avulsion of the tricuspid chordae tendineae and cause dysfunction of the tricuspid valve. Another exception is when the embolized catheter is discovered in the distal pulmonary artery branches many months after the event. Risk of further dislocation is small and chance of successful transvenous retrieval is small, whereas risk of surgical removal is greater than the risk of leaving the catheter fragment in the pulmonary artery.

• *Which is the best method of removing the embolized catheter?* The answer is almost always "transvascular retrieval techniques." The risk associated with transvascular wire or catheter retrieval is quite small. An aggressive approach to the problem of catheter embolization is proposed because the success rate is greater than 90%, whereas the risk is similar to that of basic cardiac catheterization (morbidity 1%, mortality <0.1%).

Contraindications

Transvascular extraction techniques are generally contraindicated when there is a large thrombus in the immediate vicinity of the foreign body or catheter to be removed, when there is perforation of a blood vessel or a cardiac chamber, and when the catheter or foreign body is known to be extravascular.

LOCATIONS OF CATHETER EMBOLI
(in decreasing frequency)

Superior vena cava
Right atrium
Superior vena cava—right atrium
Right atrium—hepatic vein
Right ventricle
Internal jugular vein
Subclavian vein
Hepatic vein
Inferior vena cava
Pulmonary artery, right and left and branches
Thoracic descending aorta

Complications

The complications of transvascular catheter fragment removal and the aftercare of the patient are similar to those of cardiac catheterization.

Failure to retrieve the fragment (10%) is usually due to fragment position (totally in a distal pulmonary artery), unrecognized extravascular position of the catheter (e.g., pleural space), permanent endocardial pacemaker catheter fragments, long duration the fragmented catheter has been in place, and lack of free end for snaring techniques alone.

Other complications that have been reported are pulmonary embolism, dislodgment and distal migration of the fragment, arrhythmias (generally benign), and vascular complications at the site of entry of the retrieval catheter.

Localization

Before any attempt can be made at transvascular retrieval of a catheter fragment, efforts should be made to localize the catheter and define its relationship to the vessel or the cardiac chamber. Of great importance are the definition of the proximal or distal tip of the catheter and the determination of whether these tips are free. These measures, to a great extent, will determine the choice of the retrieval technique used.

The locations of catheter emboli reported in a review of the literature[6] are listed in the box below. Table 17-1 lists the locations of the proximal and distal ends of embolized catheters, and Fig. 17-1 illustrates the most common of these locations.

Various imaging methods have been used to localize proximal and distal ends of embolized catheters or wire fragments. These have included multiple-view radiographs and high-quality biplane fluoroscopy as well as cineangiography.

Cineangiography is considered of great value immediately before attempted transvascular retrieval of the catheter, as it opacifies the chamber or the vessel where a catheter is lodged and shows the exact location of the catheter fragment. It also identifies its position in relationship to the vessel or chamber wall and identifies any adherent thrombus. Application of other imaging methods such as echocardiography, computerized tomographic scanning, and magnetic resonance imaging can also be valuable in localizing the catheter fragments.

Techniques of retrieval

The procedure is done in a cardiac catheterization room with standard radiographic and fluoroscopic equipment. All catheter manipulation is carried out under fluoroscopic visualization and continuous ECG

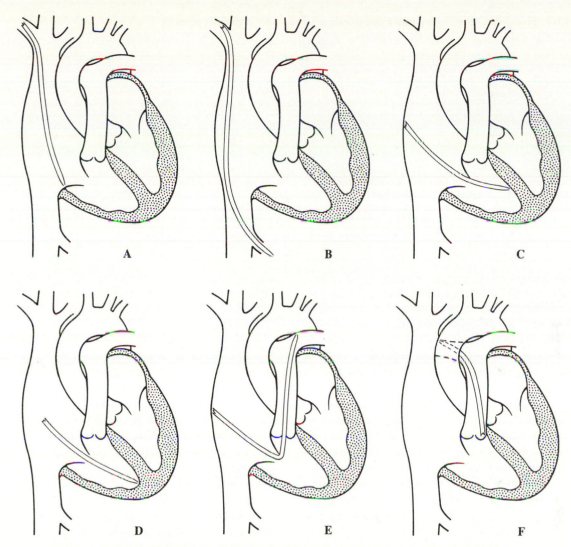

Fig. 17-1. Common lodging sites of proximal and distal ends of a broken catheter migrating from subclavian or internal jugular veins. The proximal end of the catheter is in the subclavian vein and the distal end at (**A**) the tricuspid valve/inferior vena cava junction or (**B**) the inferior vena cava/hepatic vein. **C**, The proximal end is in the right atrium and the distal end at the interventricular septum. Neither end is free. **D**, The proximal end is free in the right atrium and the distal end is in the right ventricular apex. **E**, The proximal end is in the right atrium and distal end is in the pulmonary artery. **F**, The proximal end is in the main pulmonary artery and distal end is lodged in a branch of the right pulmonary artery.

monitoring. The patient is prepared in a manner similar to that for cardiac catheterization.

Standard cardiac catheterization items are needed either for vascular cutdown or for percutaneous entry into a vessel. Choice of the vessel will depend on the location of the catheter or wire fragment and ease of access to it, a short and straight catheter course being preferable. Traditionally, the femoral vein or an antecubital vein has been used. However, the internal jugular or subclavian vein may also be used if precautions to avoid air embolism are observed.[9] The femoral artery or brachial artery may be used for arterial catheter fragments. The following special retrieval systems have been used.

Basic loop/snare technique

The basic loop/snare technique[10,11] was first described in 1967. It employs the simplest and one of the

Table 17-1. Frequency of proximal and distal lodging sites of catheter fragments*

Site	Proximal (cut) end	Distal (leading) end
Subclavian vein	11	1
Internal jugular vein	2	1
Superior vena cava	36	6
Right atrium	46	22
Right ventricle	1†	38
Pulmonary artery	33	35
Inferior vena cava	9	6
Hepatic vein	—	4
Umbilical vein	1	1

From Bloomfield, D.A.: Nonsurgical retrieval of intracardiac foreign bodies—an international survey, Cathet. Cardiovasc. Diagn. **4:**1-14, 1978.
*The proximal, most accessible end of a foreign body fragment can be expected to lie no more central in the circulation than the right atrium, unless the entire fragment passes to the pulmonary artery. The only instance of a right ventricular lodging site (†) occurred when a polyethylene catheter doubled over on itself with both ends in the ventricle and the midsection looped in the pulmonary artery.

most commonly used devices—a long guidewire folded in half and inserted through a catheter (Fig. 17-2).

This loop/snare can be made in any catheterization laboratory with a 8 Fr thin-wall catheter and a small-diameter (0.021-inch [0.53 mm]) wire. The end hole and a side hole of an angiographic catheter can also be used with this technique to provide a loop that can be rotated more easily. The advantages of this loop/snare technique include immediate availability, flexibility, changeable loop size, percutaneous use, general safety, and reasonable success rate.

This technique is not effective if the embolized fragment does not have a free end to permit snaring (Fig. 17-1, *C* and *E*). If a larger wire is used, friction in the catheter may limit flexibility or ability to change the

size of the loop. To retrieve catheter fragments from the pulmonary artery, the loop/snare is the device of choice.

Procedure

1. Insert the catheter into the vessel using the standard Seldinger technique. A vascular sheath may be used.

2. Double the guidewire over a few centimeters from its midportion and insert the loop end into the catheter. Leave only a *blunt nontraumatic loop* outside the catheter tip by withdrawing one of the free ends of the guidewire and drawing the initial tight fold of the guidewire within the catheter. The size of this loop can be altered by manipulation of the folded guidewire back and forth through the catheter (Fig. 17-3).

3. Using fluoroscopy, advance the snare with a wide loop into the vessel or chamber where the catheter fragment is lodged. Align the snare loop at approximately 90° to the estimated plane of the catheter fragment.

4. Pass varying amounts of loop repeatedly at the catheter fragment. For the loop to snare the catheter fragment, either a proximal or distal tip of the fragment must be free. Snaring will be apparent when the fragment moves with the loop (Fig 17-4, *A*).

5. Once the catheter fragment tip is snared, secure it by advancing the retrieval catheter over the wire toward the fragment (Fig. 17-4, *B*). The alternative but incorrect method of lifting the wire or pulling both ends of the guidewire to close the loop down on the object risks dislodgment of the catheter fragment.

6. Gently tighten the wire snare by withdrawing its distal end until the catheter fragment is held securely against the tip of the guiding catheter. Use a hemostat to fix the distal ends of the guidewire.

7. With continuous tension on the snare, withdraw the catheter/snare combination from the vein or the ar-

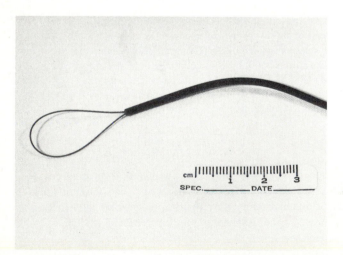

Fig. 17-2. Instrument for the loop/snare technique: a 0.021-inch (0.53 mm) guidewire folded in half and inserted through a 8 Fr catheter.

tery (Fig. 17-4, *C*), removing the fragment. Rarely a vascular cutdown is needed to remove a large catheter fragment.

Commercially available retrieval units. The Curry intravascular retrieval set uses a 100 cm long, 8 Fr radiopaque Teflon catheter with metal Cournand fitting without side ports. The snare is formed by folding over a 300 cm stainless steel guidewire, 0.021 inch (0.53 mm) in diameter. The set also contains a guidewire for the catheter, a side arm adaptor, a vessel dilator, and a plug for the flushing adaptor (Cook model CRS-1). The same catheter for pediatric use comes in 6.3 Fr, 45 cm long with a 125 cm long guidewire (0.018 inch), forming a 62.5 cm long snare (Cook model CRS-2).

The Berens atrial pacing loop wire is an alternative to the loop/snare and can be advanced through a catheter[12] (Fig. 17-5, *A* and *B*). This device is available in three sizes, small (59 mm × 45 mm), medium (72 × 55 mm), and large (85 mm × 65 mm) through USCI. The hairpin upper section of the loop makes it well suited for entrapping the catheter fragment. The use of the Berens atrial pacing loop wire for retrieval of a CVP catheter is illustrated in Fig. 17-5, *C* and *D*.

Helical basket

Initially used for retrieval of ureteral stones, the helical basket has been modified for intravascular use and

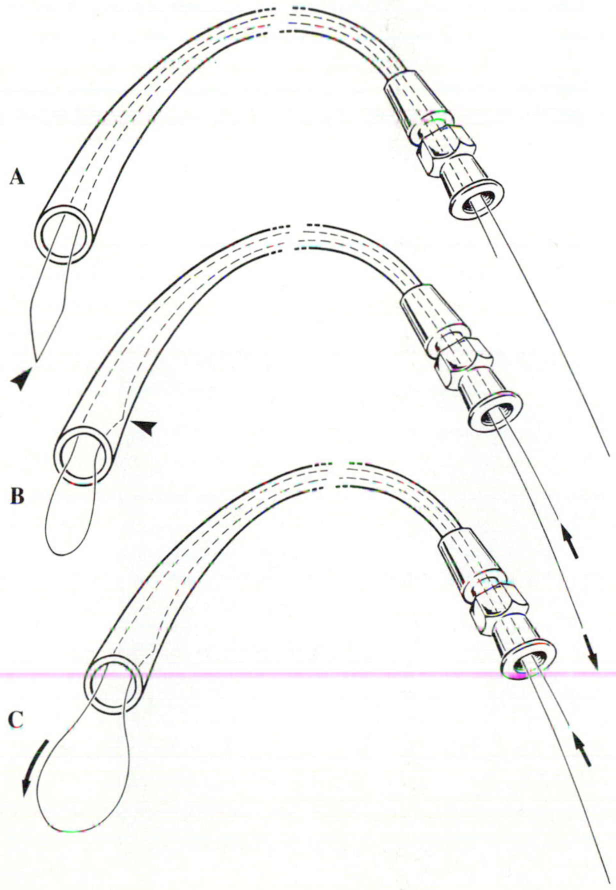

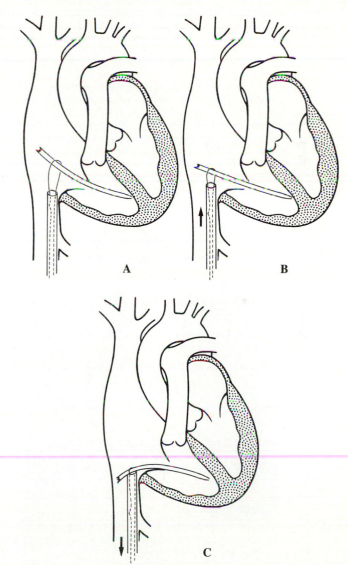

Fig. 17-3. A, Guidewire with a tight fold (arrow) beyond the catheter tip. **B,** Tight fold is withdrawn within the catheter by withdrawing one free end of the guidewire, while advancing the other end, forming a nontraumatic, blunt-tip loop/snare. **C,** The size of loop/snare is enlarged by further advancing of the guidewire end not containing the initial tight fold.

Fig. 17-4. The loop/snare technique for snaring catheter emboli. **A,** The catheter fragment is snared. **B,** The catheter is advanced, while the wire is held so that the catheter rests gently on the fragment, confirming encirclement and securing the fragment. **C,** The loop is closed down tightly and the fragment pulled out with the catheter.

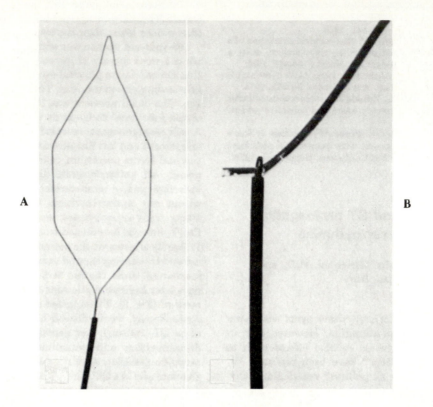

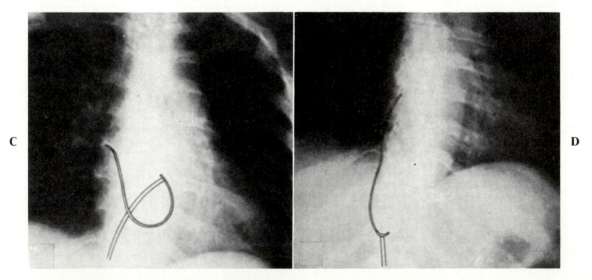

Fig. 17-5. Berens catheter **(A)** with the loop open and **(B)** with a CVP catheter trapped. **C** and **D,** Frontal plane films showing two sequential stages during CVP catheter retrieval in situ. (From Kaushik, V.S., and Ong, S.H.: Nonsurgical retrieval of intracardiac foreign body: use of Berens pacing electrode, Am. Heart J. **105:**868-870, 1983.)

A

B

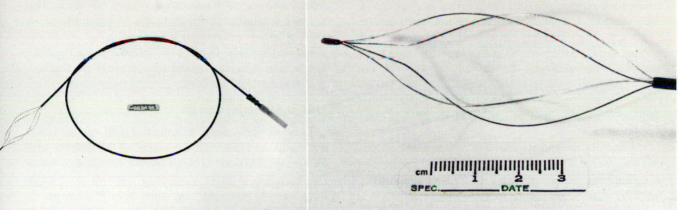

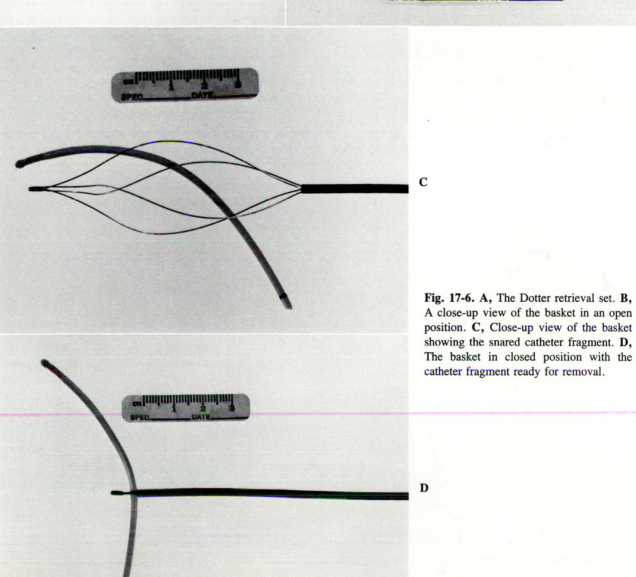

C

D

Fig. 17-6. A, The Dotter retrieval set. **B,** A close-up view of the basket in an open position. **C,** Close-up view of the basket showing the snared catheter fragment. **D,** The basket in closed position with the catheter fragment ready for removal.

is commercially available from Cook as the Dotter intravascular retrieval set (Fig. 17-6). This is a variant of the loop/snare and the techniques are similar. It can be used in the right atrium, right ventricle, superior and inferior vena cavae, and the arterial system. It is a 95 cm long 8 Fr radiopaque Teflon catheter with a Luer-Lok. There are no side ports for flushing. The set includes the helical loop basket of stainless steel wires with its long handle and an introducer sheath.

Procedure

1. Introduce the catheter through an introducer sheath using the percutaneous Seldinger technique.

2. Advance the catheter with the basket withdrawn to the level of the catheter fragment.

3. Extrude the basket past the foreign body and open it.

4. Slowly withdraw the catheter with the opened basket until the foreign body is entrapped. The spiral struts of the basket simplify fragment entrapment by providing different planes of sweep. As in the loop/snare, a free end of the catheter fragment is necessary for this device to be effective.

5. After the catheter fragment is trapped, pull the basket shut and withdraw the entire assembly from the vascular system.

6. If a Dotter retrieval set is not available, a basket-type bronchial retrieval catheter may be used. This catheter is similar in design to the Dotter retrieval set and can be passed through a 9 Fr sheath.[9]

Precaution: The Dotter helical basket has a rigid tip. Gentle manipulation is mandatory to avoid vascular/cardiac trauma.

Myocardial biopsy forceps

These devices consist of catheters with cuplike hands that open and close with movement of the catheter handle (see p. 184) and are suitable for retrieval of material from the superior vena cava, inferior vena cava, right atrium, and right ventricular apex.[13] They are 50 or 105 cm long, variably flexible, and can grasp. A free end of the fragment is not needed for these forceps to be successful (Fig. 17-7).

The design and stiffness of myocardial biopsy forceps make them unsuitable for retrieval of material from the pulmonary artery or the right ventricular outflow tract. Also, the size of the biopsy head limits its usefulness to catheter fragments of small (1 to 2 mm) diameter. Risks of vessel or myocardial perforation exist with the use of this device.

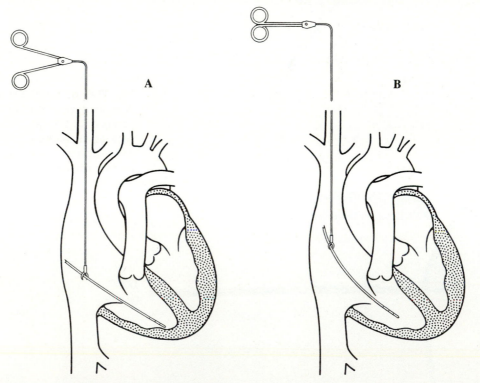

Fig. 17-7. Myocardial biopsy forceps are introduced from the right internal jugular vein to (**A**) grasp and (**B**) retrieve a lodged catheter fragment.

Grasping forceps

The grasping forceps are a variant of the myocardial biopsy forceps and are commercially available from Meditech Inc.[11] These forceps consist of four stainless steel spring wires 0.010 inch (0.25 mm) in diameter arranged like a claw and housed in a Teflon sheath with an outside diameter of 1.6 mm and a length of 120, 180, or 220 cm. The forceps open and close when the wires are advanced and withdrawn through the sheath; they measure 20 mm when fully opened. The instrument is designed for use through an 8 Fr or the Meditech steerable catheter system. This system has not received widespread use and its rate of success or risk of complication is not known. Its use inside cardiac chambers is potentially hazardous and may damage valvular structures or endomyocardium.

Procedure
1. Advance this instrument toward the catheter fragment or the foreign body with the grasping forceps closed.
2. Open the forceps by either sliding the wires forward or retracting the sheath.
3. When the prongs engage the object, advance the sheath forward to tighten the grip.
4. Withdraw the entire assembly.

We have no personal experience in the use of the grasping forceps.

Fogarty catheter

The Fogarty catheter is a balloon-tip catheter that is occasionally successful in removing a catheter fragment from a small peripheral vessel. It has no snaring or hooking ability and is not useful in central vessels. The catheter tip with its balloon is positioned beyond the foreign body, the balloon is inflated with saline solution, and the catheter is withdrawn, removing the foreign body.

Hook guidewire

The hook guidewire can be made by bending the stiff end of a steel guidewire to a tight J shape and inserting it through a catheter. An embolized catheter with no free end can be ''hooked'' using such a device. It risks vessel or cardiac perforation.

Combinations

Various combinations of angled or hooked catheters, pigtail catheters, loop wires, deflector systems, and forceps have been used at one time or another by various investigators with success.[4,6,14,15] Some of these are not commercially available and their use and modification are limited only by the imagination of the person performing the procedure.

INTRACARDIAC OR INTRAVASCULAR CATHETER KNOTTING

Intracardiac or intravascular knotting of catheters, electrodes, or wires is an infrequent but potentially serious problem. It occurs very rarely during diagnostic cardiac catheterization, where fluoroscopy is routinely used and where it is immediately recognized, and is almost always corrected by simple manipulation of the catheter, possibly with the aid of a guidewire.

The risk of catheter knotting is increased with the use of catheters with complex curves and when fluoroscopy is not used. For example, the tip of the ''headhunter'' catheter, used by neuroradiologists, has a figure-8 curve, predisposing to knot formation. The knotting risk is also increased with very soft or small catheters. Soft floatation catheters inserted into the central circulation without the aid of fluoroscopy may knot, especially if precautions are not taken. Intravascular catheter knotting is likely to become a more frequent clinical problem in parallel with an increased use of hemodynamic monitoring and use of intravascular and intracardiac catheters by physicians with limited training in cardiac catheterization techniques. In this section we review the mechanisms, prevention, and solutions of the problem of catheter knot formation.

Types of catheter knotting
Knotting of one catheter on itself

Knotting of one catheter on itself occurs most frequently with a catheter of complex distal curve design or with catheters that are soft, coil easily on themselves, and are inserted and advanced in the vascular system without fluoroscopic control. In right heart catheterization this is particularly a risk in patients with enlarged right atrium or right ventricle where the catheter can loop on itself and knot upon withdrawal.

Knotting of two different catheters in a cardiac chamber or great vessel

This may occur when multiple catheters are used in the right or left side of the heart or great vessels. It may also occur during electrophysiologic studies where three or four catheters may be inserted into the right side of the heart or when a balloon flotation catheter is inserted in a patient who has a pacing catheter in place. Using multiple catheters without fluoroscopy further increases the chance of knot formation.

Knotting of a catheter about a cardiac structure

Knotting of a catheter about a cardiac structure is a rare but potentially disastrous complication. Tricuspid valve, chordae tendineae, or right ventricular papillary muscles may be trapped in a catheter knot. This has not been reported as having occurred during cardiac catheterization but has been reported with the use of flow-directed catheters.[16,17] An extremely rare variant of this may occur during open heart surgery when a catheter may be sutured to the right atrium.

Guidelines for prevention

1. Whenever possible, use fluoroscopy to introduce and advance a catheter to the desired location in the great vessels or the heart.

2. Pay careful attention to technique when inserting a balloon-tip catheter without fluoroscopy. Partially inflate the balloon when the catheter tip reaches the subclavian vein or superior vena cava and before it reaches the right atrium.

3. Use fluoroscopy in the following circumstances:
   a. When using multiple catheters in proximity to each other
   b. During right heart catheterization in a patient with enlarged right atrium or right ventricle, especially where small and soft catheters are used (4 to 5 Fr)
   c. When catheter introduction and advancement using flotation techniques and pressure and ECG monitoring have not resulted in early success, and manipulation and repositioning are attempted
   d. When inserting catheters from the femoral vein

4. Avoid catheter kinks at all times.

5. If a catheter knot is suspected, obtain right and left anterior oblique views in addition to an anteroposterior view to ensure that a true knot is present—where the tip of the catheter is within the loop. If not, a pseudo-knot is present and is resolved by simply withdrawing the catheter.

Solutions

Once a diagnosis of knotted catheter is made there should be no further manipulation of the catheter without fluoroscopy.

Most of the methods discussed below have been used in the arterial system and involve angiographic catheters. The same techniques may also be applied with similar catheters used in the venous circulation.

The problem of the knotted catheter may be approached in several ways.

Various catheterization techniques can be used to undo the knot. These approaches have been applied mostly to arterial catheters[18,19] and should always be tried before proceeding to other techniques.

Another approach is to tighten the knot, and pull it out to a peripheral vessel, and then remove it, using a sheath technique or a surgical cutdown. This approach has been applied mostly to venous catheters.[20,21]

If these simpler measures are not successful, one may have to resort to (1) thoracotomy and surgical removal of the knotted catheter, (2) cardiotomy and surgical removal of a catheter when the knot is around cardiac structures, or (3) severing the extra portion of the catheter, suturing the proximal end in subcutaneous tissue and fascia, and leaving the knot of the catheter in the vessel or the heart (similar to the cut permanent pacing wire which cannot be removed easily).

Simple manipulation

For a knot that is loose and incomplete, gently rotate, advance, and withdraw the catheter (Fig. 17-8). This is frequently successful providing the knot is not complete, in which case such manipulation may even tighten the knot.

For a knot that is loose and complete, if there is a fairly long segment of catheter tip protruding beyond the loop of the knot (Fig. 17-9, *A*), fix the catheter tip

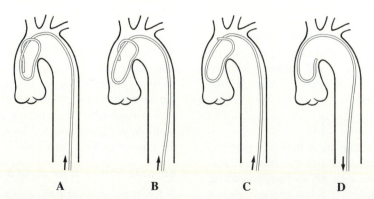

A   **B**   **C**   **D**

Fig. 17-8. A loose incomplete knot is unknotted by gently rotating and advancing (**A** to **C**) and withdrawing (**D**) the catheter.

on a vessel and advance the catheter (Fig. 17-9, *B* and *C*). This often redues the knot (Fig. 17-9, *D*).[22]

The stiff end of a standard guidewire may be inserted and advanced through the knot and close to the catheter tip to help uncoil it. The stiff guidewire tip should never extend beyond the tip of the catheter. These measures may enlarge the knot but not eliminate it. Turning the catheter clockwise and counterclockwise may untie the knot. Withdrawal of the enlarged knot (with the wire) through a smaller vessel is another method of reducing the knot. Careful observation under fluoroscopy is needed to prevent further tightening of the knot. If this is still not successful, one can try to pull the catheter over the guidewire (Fig. 17-10). If excessive force is applied the stiff distal end of the guidewire may perforate the wall of the catheter.

Manipulation with deflecting wire

When simple manipulation with or without a standard guidewire fails, a deflecting or a movable-core guidewire may be used.

1. Introduce this guidewire until its tip lies in the first turn of the knot.

2. Increase the deflection (tension) of the guidewire and "lock" the wire in this position.

3. Withdraw the catheter until the knot is reduced (Fig. 17-11, *A*).

4. Alternatively, you may advance the catheter over the fixed deflector wire, permitting progressive enlargement of the loop until its tip is released (Fig. 17-11, *B*).[23]

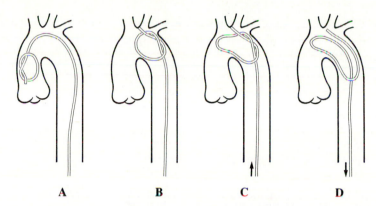

Fig. 17-9. Immobilization of the catheter tip and simple manipulation for unknotting a catheter. **A,** Knotted catheter in the ascending aorta. **B,** The protruding tip of knot is immobilized on the superior wall of the aortic arch. **C,** Advancing the catheter enlarges the loop and loosens the knot. **D,** The unknotted catheter is safely withdrawn. A guidewire advanced to the knot will facilitate this maneuver.

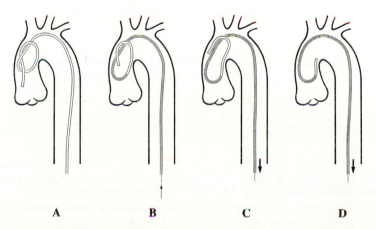

Fig. 17-10. Guidewire technique for unknotting a catheter. **A** and **B,** The stiff end of a guidewire is introduced through a catheter that is knotted in the ascending aorta. **C** and **D,** The catheter is withdrawn over the guidewire, unknotting the catheter.

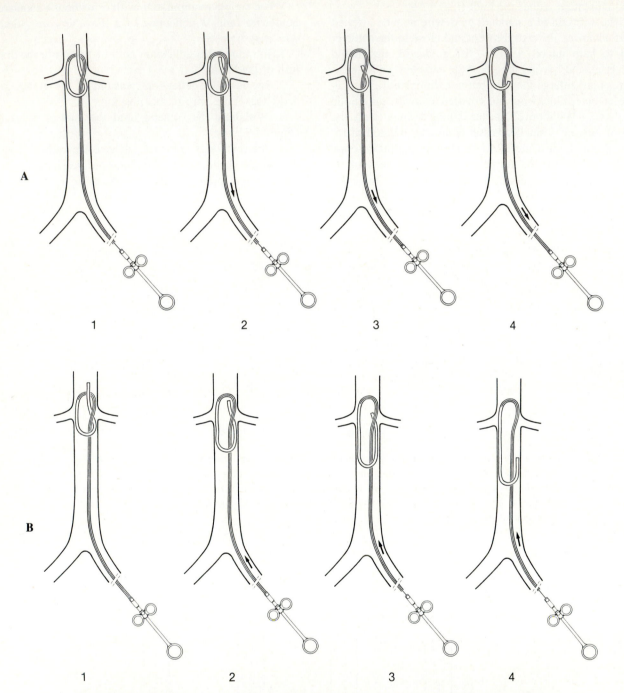

Fig. 17-11. Deflecting wire technique for unknotting a catheter. **A,** The deflecting wire is introduced until its tip lies in the first turn of the knot *(1)*. The deflecting wire is locked in position and the catheter withdrawn *(2 to 4)*. **B,** Alternatively, the catheter is advanced, enlarging the loop *(1 and 2)* until it is released *(3 and 4)*. (Adapted from Thomas, H.A., and Sievers, R.E.: Nonsurgical reduction of arterial catheter knots, A.J.R. **132:**1018-1019, © by American Roentgen Ray Society, 1979.)

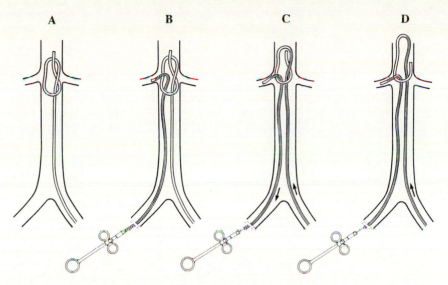

Fig. 17-12. Hook-tip catheter method. **A,** Catheter knot in abdominal aorta. **B,** Catheter with a hook is inserted and hooked over the knot loop. **C** and **D,** The knotted catheter is moved forward against the resistance exerted by the hook relieving the knot.

Untying the knot with a second catheter

Untying the knot with a second catheter may be accomplished using the deflector wire/pigtail catheter knot-reducing technique. If simple manipulation and the use of a deflecting guidewire are not successful, the knot may be reduced with the help of a second catheter. This could be a pigtail catheter with a large-caliber tip-deflecting wire forming a grasping hook in its tip.

1. Manipulate the grasping hook so that it engages the knot loop and tighten the hook so that it closes around the knotted catheter.

2. Introduce a standard guidewire through the knotted catheter to provide stiffness. Advance the knotted catheter with its guidewire within while maintaining traction on the hook catheter, reducing the knot (Fig. 17-12).[18]

Use of a snare

This technique has been used to untie a tight knot in a flow-directed balloon-tip catheter.[24] A tight knot was formed 9 cm from the tip of a Swan-Ganz catheter at the junction of the superior vena cava and right atrium. The knot was untied using a catheter tip deflector through a 7 Fr catheter introduced through the same area, hooked around the knot, and pulled while the knotted catheter was prevented from recoil by the use of a rigid Brockenbrough transseptal tip occluding wire (Fig. 17-13).

Untying the knot using a second catheter through the knot

If the knot has not been reduced with these methods, passing a second catheter through the knot will probably reduce it.

1. Withdraw the knot to the aortic bifurcation (Fig. 17-14, *A* and *B*).

2. Insert a second catheter from the opposite femoral artery and advance it through the knot and into the aortic arch (Fig. 17-14, *C*).

3. Use a to-and-fro motion of the knotted catheter to enlarge the knot. Then retract the catheter, freeing its tip (Fig. 17-14, *D* and *E*).[25] A guidewire may be in-

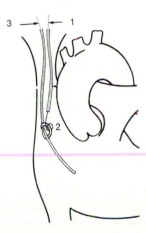

Fig. 17-13. Technique used to untie a knotted Swan-Ganz catheter. The catheter tip deflecting guidewire *(1)* is introduced through a shortened 7 Fr catheter and hooked into the loop of the knot *(2)*. A rigid transseptal tip occluding wire *(3)* is inserted into the Swan-Ganz catheter to prevent recoil of the catheter when pulling on the knot with the hook. (From Dumesnil, J.G., and Proulx, G.: A new nonsurgical technique for untying tight knots in flow-directed balloon catheters, Am. J. Cardiol. **53:**395-396, 1984.)

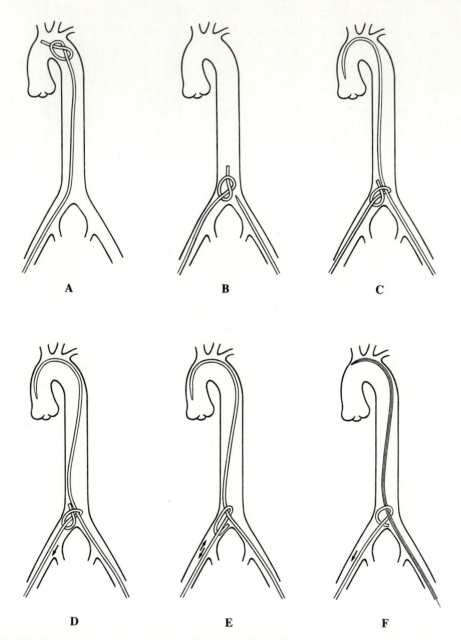

Fig. 17-14. Technique with a second catheter passed through the knot loop. **A** and **B,** Knotted catheter is withdrawn to the line of aortic bifurcation. **B** and **C,** Second catheter is introduced from contralateral side and passed through the loop. **D** and **E,** The knotted catheter is retracted with a to-and-fro motion to reduce the knot. **F,** Guidewire in the second catheter increases its anchoring force. (Adapted from Chinichian, A., et al.: Knotting of a 8 French ''head hunter'' catheter and its successful removal, Radiology **104:**282, 1972.)

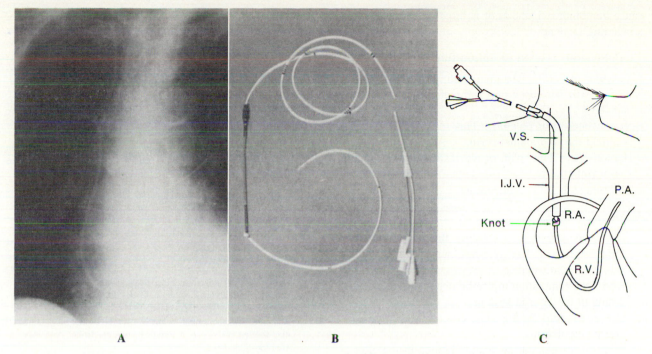

A   B   C

Fig. 17-15. A, Chest radiograph showing the tip of the Swan-Ganz catheter in the main pulmonary artery and a knot in the superior vena cava. **B,** After extraction, the tightened knot is seen against the venous sheath. **C,** Diagram showing the venous sheath *(VS)* introduced into the internal jugular vein *(IJV)* to tighten the knot in the right atrium *(RA)*. (From Kumar, S.P., et al.: Removal of a knotted flow-directed catheter by a nonsurgical method, Ann. Intern. Med. **92:**638-640, 1980.)

serted in this second (unknotted) catheter to increase its anchoring force (Fig. 17-14, *F*).

Note: This technique requires caution, because a tight knot may become tighter, especially if there is a long tip beyond its loop. Success is also determined by the type of catheter material and the size of the iliac arteries.

Methods of reducing a knot in a catheter without a lumen

Rarely, knots may form in a catheter without a lumen, such as catheters used for pacing or electrophysiologic studies. The maneuvers that have been described which do not require introduction of a guidewire into the knotted catheter may be used to reduce such knots.

Another technique involves the use of a venous introducer. Either the existing one or a new, stiffer, or longer one may be inserted over the catheter after it has been cut off from the hub. The knotted catheter is then simultaneously and slowly pulled and rotated while the introducer is held firmly in place, until the knot is reduced.[26]

The same technique may be used to tighten an irreducible knot in a soft catheter to pull out the knot without laceration of the vein. This technique has been used for a knot in a 7 Fr, balloon-tip, flow-directed catheter. The catheter was cut at its hub end and cleaned with antiseptic solution. An 8 Fr sheath was introduced over the cut end of the catheter and advanced through the superior vena cava. The knot was pulled tight against the sheath and reduced to a smaller diameter. The catheter and the sheath were then pulled out without any incident (Fig. 17-15).[20]

In a variation of this technique a 10 or 12 Fr introducer or a catheter was used and the knot pulled through it. The aim was to avoid laceration of a central, noncompressible vessel (internal jugular or subclavian vein).[21]

An alternate approach involves tightening the knot with a sheath and then pulling the knot to a peripheral vein (or snaring it to a peripheral vein using a peripherally introduced snaring catheter) and removing it directly via cutdown.

These are potentially dangerous techniques and may

cause hemothorax if the knot is large or the patient has a bleeding tendency.

Complications related to unknotting of catheters

- Vascular or cardiac chamber trauma: This may result when a stiff wire used in a soft catheter perforates the catheter
- Venous spasm or phlebitis: This may occur if a knot is pulled through a small vein
- Hemothorax: This will occur if a noncompressible vessel (internal jugular, subclavian) is lacerated
- Thromboembolic complications

Minimizing risks

1. Pay strict attention to catheter flushing during any long maneuvers. Use systemic heparinization unless it is contraindicated.
2. Resist the temptation to use branching vessels as fulcrums in the arterial system.
3. Use continuous fluoroscopic control during all catheter manipulations.
4. Perform all unknotting manipulations in the arterial system below the renal arteries if at all possible.

FUTURE DEVELOPMENTS

Continued improvement in catheter design and safety is expected. The widespread and still growing use of intravascular catheters and the increased use of interventional catheter techniques suggest that the problem of embolized catheter fragments will not disappear.

Recently introduced changes in hospital reimbursement (diagnostic-related groups [DRGs], prospective payment systems) may increase the incentive for sterilization and reuse of catheters and other medical devices. Each institution contemplating the reuse of catheters has to consider the risk of catheter fragmentation and embolism and devise quality controls to minimize this risk.

With increasing use of cardiac catheterization, hemodynamic monitoring, and a variety of catheter types, knotted catheters may become a more frequent clinical problem. Facility and ingenuity of techniques for catheter unknotting will probably develop with it!

REFERENCES

1. Turner, D.D., and Sommers, S.C.: Accidental passage of a polyethylene catheter from cubital vein to right atrium, N. Engl. J. Med. **251:**744-745, 1954.
2. Ross, A.M.: Polyethylene emboli: how many more? (editorial), Chest **57:**307-308, 1970.
3. Dotter, C.T., Rosch, J., and Bilbao, M.K.: Transluminal extraction of catheter and guide fragments from the heart and great vessels: 29 collected cases, A.J.R. **3:**467-472, 1971.
4. Fisher, R.G., and Ferreyro, R.: Evaluation of current techniques for nonsurgical removal of intravascular iatrogenic foreign bodies, A.J.R. **130:**541-548, 1978.
5. Thomas, J., Sinclair-Smith, B., Bloomfield, D., and Darachi, A.: Nonsurgical retrieval of a broken segment of steel spring guide from right atrium and inferior vena cava, Circulation 30:106-108, 1964.
6. Bloomfield, D.A.: The nonsurgical retrieval of intracardiac foreign bodies—an international survey, Cathet. Cardiovasc. Diagn. **4:**1-14, 1978.
7. Hipona, F.A., Sciammas, F.D., and Hublitz, U.F.: Nonthoracotomy retrieval of intraluminal cardiovascular foreign bodies, Radiol. Clin. North Am. **9:**583-595, 1971.
8. Schneider, R.M., et al.: Fracture of a polyurethane catheter in the aortic arch: a complication related to polymer aging, Cathet. Cardiovasc. Diagn. **9:**197-207, 1983.
9. Glatter, T.R., Scott, A., and Early, G.: Percutaneous removal of intracardiac catheter fragment: unique internal jugular venous approach, Am. Heart J. **108:**408-410, 1984.
10. Massumi, R.A., and Ross, A.M.: Atraumatic nonsurgical technique for removal of broken catheters from cardiac cavities, N. Engl. J. Med. **277:**195-196, 1967.
11. Kadir, S., and Athanasoulis, C.A.: Percutaneous retrieval of intravascular foreign bodies. In Athanasoulis, C.A., Pfister, R.C., Greene, R.E., and Roberson, G.H.: Interventional radiology, Philadelphia, 1982, W.B. Saunders Co.
12. Kaushik, V.S., and Ong, S.H.: Nonsurgical retrieval of intracardiac foreign body: use of Berens pacing electrode, Am. Heart J. **105:**868-870, 1983.
13. Bashour, T.T., Banks, T., and Cheng, T.O.: Retrieval of lost catheters by a myocardial biopsy catheter device, Chest **66:**395-396, 1974.
14. Rossi, P.: "Hook catheter" technique for transfemoral removal of foreign body from the right side of the heart, Am. J. Radiol. **109:**101, 1970.
15. Auge, J.M., Oriol, A., Serra, C., and Crexells, C.: The use of pigtail catheters for retrieval of foreign bodies from the cardiovascular system, Cathet. Cardiovasc. Diagn. **10:**625-628, 1984.
16. Meister, S.G.: Knotting of a flow directed catheter about a cardiac structure, Cathet. Cardiovasc. Diagn. **3:**171-175, 1977.
17. Schwartz, K.V., et al.: Entanglement of Swan-Ganz catheter around an intracardiac structure, J.A.M.A. **237:**1198-1199, 1977.
18. Thomas, H.A., and Sievers, R.E.: Nonsurgical reduction of arterial catheter knots, A.J.R. **132:**1018-1019, 1979.
19. Deeb, Z.L., Ahn, H.S., and Rosenbaum, A.E.: A new method for uncoiling knots in angiographic tubing, Neuroradiology **20:**197-201, 1980.
20. Kumar, S.P., et al.: Removal of a knotted flow-directed catheter by a nonsurgical method, Ann. Intern. Med. **92:**638-640, 1980.
21. Dach, J.L., Galbut, D.L., and LePage, J.R.: The knotted Swan-Ganz catheter: new solution to a vexing problem, Am. J. Radiol. **137:**1294-1295, 1981.
22. Young, D.A., et al.: Successful manipulation of a knotted intravascular catheter allowing nonsurgical removal, Radiology **94:**155-156, 1970.
23. Hawkins, I.F., et al.: Deflector method for nonsurgical removal of knotted catheters, Radiology **106:**705, 1973.
24. Dumesnil, J.G., and Proulx, G.: A new nonsurgical technique for untying tight knots in flow-directed balloon catheters, Am. J. Cardiol. **53:**395-396, 1984.
25. Chinichian, A., et al.: Knotting of a 8 French "head hunter" catheter and its successful removal, Radiology **104:**282, 1972.
26. Baldi, J., Fishenfeld, J., and Benchimol, A.: Complete knotting of a catheter and a nonsurgical method of removal, Chest **65:**93-95, 1974.

Part III

MISCELLANEOUS TOPICS

Chapter Eighteen

Cardiopulmonary resuscitation

ARA G. TILKIAN
MARY B. CONOVER

The majority of patients who have cardiac arrest have underlying coronary, myocardial, or valvular heart disease. Thus patients who undergo cardiovascular procedures are a select group likely to develop cardiac arrest. Physicians, nurses, and technologists who care for them and perform cardiovascular procedures must be experts in the response to cardiopulmonary arrest. This chapter reviews the important elements of cardiopulmonary resuscitation (CPR) and provides an up-to-date guide for effective performance of this lifesaving procedure. Formal instruction and continual training and practice are needed to acquire and maintain these skills and to ensure an appropriate response in the emergency setting of cardiac arrest.

CPR, as practiced today, has been in use for more than 25 years.[1-3] Although interest in cerebral resuscitation dates back to the beginning of this century,[4] only recently has there been active interest in this field. Because anoxic encephalopathy is an all-too-frequently observed tragedy of successful cardiac resuscitation, this recent emphasis on cerebral resuscitation is well placed.[5,6]

INDICATIONS

CPR is indicated for the treatment of cardiopulmonary arrest when there is no clear medical order stating *do not resuscitate* (DNR). Cardiopulmonary arrest is recognized by loss of consciousness, absence of carotid and femoral pulses, apnea or gasping respiratory efforts, and absence of heart sounds. If monitored, pulseless (and usually rapid) ventricular tachycardia (VT), ventricular fibrillation (VF), asystole, or electromechanical dissociation will be observed.

CONTRAINDICATIONS

Contraindications for CPR include:
• Explicit orders by the patient's physician, properly

documented in the patient's chart, stating: "In event of cardiopulmonary arrest, *do not resuscitate*" (see p. 430)
• Terminal stages of an incurable disease: CPR attempts should not be a medical "last right"
• Lack of a reasonable chance of restoring life and mentation (e.g., more than 1 hour of pulselessness in a normothermic person who has not received CPR)

RISKS AND COMPLICATIONS

Clearly, the greatest risk or complication of CPR is unsuccessful resuscitation, with the procedure ending in cardiac or brain death. Approximately 30% of survivors of CPR sustain one or more injuries directly related to the resuscitative procedure. The following list of complications is a compilation of several studies.[7,8]

Complication	Incidence
Fractured ribs/sternum	20%-47%
Permanent brain damage, vegetative state	10%-40%
Bone marrow embolization to lungs or heart	13%-27%
Pulmonary aspiration of gastric contents	10%
Liver or spleen injury	10%
Pericardial bleeding	2%-8%
Misplaced endotracheal tube	4%
Myocardial contusion	1% (30% with intracardiac injections)
Mediastinal bleeding	1%
Subcutaneous/mediastinal emphysema	1%
Gastric rupture	0.1%

Meticulous attention to CPR technique should reduce the incidence of these complications. An awareness of the possibility and nature of these complications should initiate a search for them in the successfully resuscitated patient.

EQUIPMENT

Basic CPR is performed by providing ventilatory support with mouth-to-mouth breathing and circulatory support with chest compression. Basic CPR requires no equipment, only an energetic rescuer with a pair of strong arms and healthy lungs. Ventilatory support can be provided or augmented by airway adjuncts discussed in the section on advanced cardiac life support (see p. 412).

Advanced CPR requires the following equipment:

- Defibrillator—the single most useful tool in CPR (see Chapter 12)
- Airway adjuncts:
  Oropharyngeal airway, nasopharyngeal airway, bag-valve-mask assembly, and methods of oxygen delivery (tubes, adaptors)
- Equipment for tracheal intubation:
  Laryngoscope handle with curved (MacIntosh) and straight blades
  Oral endotracheal tubes (for adults, 7 to 9 mm inner diameter) with standard 15 mm adaptor that fits bag or ventilator
  Stylets for endotracheal tube (lighted stylet may be helpful in difficult cases)
  2% Lidocaine jelly
  Topical anesthetic and applicator (2% tetracaine or 4% lidocaine)
  Magill forceps
  10 ml syringe and three-way stopcock
  Bite block and oropharyngeal airway
  Rigid pharyngeal suction tip (Yankauer) and suction apparatus
  Endotracheal suction kit with gloves, soft catheter, and water cup
  Adhesive tape, scissors, tincture of benzoin, and 4 × 4-inch gauze pads
- Other equipment:
  Hard bed board
  ECG recorder
  IV needles, catheters, IV tubing, and fluids
  Pacing capability—external transcutaneous or transvenous pacing
- Equipment for emergency cricothyrotomy:
  #11 Scalpel
  Curved Kelly clamp
  Endotracheal tube, #5 or #6
- Drugs (the following drugs are considered essential or useful during or immediately following CPR;

their role and method of use are briefly discussed on p. 420):

Oxygen	Calcium chloride
Epinephrine	Magnesium sulfate
Lidocaine	Potassium chloride
Bretylium	Verapamil
Procainamide	Propranolol
Atropine sulfate	Digitalis
Sodium bicarbonate	Phenytoin
Morphine sulfate	Dopamine
Nitroglycerin	Furosemide
Nitroprusside	

PERSONNEL AND ORGANIZATION

Out-of-hospital CPR is accomplished by the informed and motivated bystander who initiates basic cardiac life support and summons the paramedic rescue team.

In-hospital resuscitation efforts can draw on additional help and more sophisticated equipment. Each hospital should develop its own policy and procedure for dealing with patients with cardiopulmonary arrest in and out of critical care areas. Some important organizational concerns are described below.

Guidelines regarding candidates for resuscitation

The medical and nursing staff, with help from the hospital ethics committee, hospital administration, and legal counsel, should define a clear policy regarding the designation *DNR;* ambiguity in this area should be avoided.

The resuscitation team

The resuscitation team should consist of the following:

- Physician or nurse experienced in advanced life support
- Nurse experienced in CPR and familiar with cardiac drugs
- Respiratory therapist for controlling airway and ventilation
- Additional nursing and technical help for performing chest compression, monitoring ECG, performing defibrillation, obtaining arterial blood gases, and using external or transvenous pacemaker.

The minimal number of people needed is 4 to 6, depending on the difficulty of the resuscitation. One person should be responsible for keeping accurate records of the resuscitative attempt, including the time of various interventions, another for dealing with the patient's family and keeping them informed but removed from the immediate area of the resuscitation efforts. Hospital policy should deal with the problem of keeping "the crowd" out of the way and designating areas of responsibility; not everybody in the hospital who wants to help should respond to a call for resuscitation!

Within the resources and organization of each hospital the resuscitation team must be identified. Although team members may change, their roles remain for others to assume. Well-defined individual responsibilities within the team enhance the effectiveness of resuscitative efforts. An ongoing training program should be developed whereby experienced medical and nursing personnel are available to teach resuscitation skills to new members and maintain the skills of already established team members.

There should be provisions for periodic review and update of the resuscitation policies and equipment and review of actual resuscitation results in the hospital. These functions are best carried out by a multidisciplinary CPR committee with a clearly identified mandate and authority.

BASIC LIFE SUPPORT

On recognizing the onset of cardiopulmonary arrest (i.e., an unconscious person with apnea or gasping breath who shows cyanosis or pallor and who has no palpable pulses in the large arteries) the following steps must be taken in rapid sequence.

Airway

1. Establish an open airway: place the patient supine on a hard, flat surface and tilt (extend) the head backward while lifting (flexing) the back of the neck (Fig. 18-1). This maneuver should not be used in patients with suspected cervical spine injury.

2. Pull up on the angles of the jaw to displace the tongue forward (jaw lift). This will open the patient's airway and may be the only maneuver necessary. Look, listen, and feel for breathing.

3. Open the mouth and use your fingers to clear the oropharynx.

4. If airway obstruction because of food or a foreign body cannot be relieved in this way, perform the Heimlich maneuver, described and illustrated in Fig. 18-2. This maneuver does not help patients with an anatomic airway obstruction or patients with apnea.

Breathing

1. If the patient does not start breathing when you have cleared the airway, begin mouth-to-mouth ventilation. Pinch the nostrils, seal the mouth with your own, and deliver four rapid mouth-to-mouth breaths; if the oropharynx is obstructed, close the mouth and blow into the nose.

2. Check the patient's carotid pulse. If it is present, continue delivering one breath every 5 seconds. Observe for chest expansion.

Circulation

1. If the carotid pulse is absent, apply compression to the lower sternum two finger-breadths above the xiphosternal junction, displacing the sternum in the adult approximately 1½ to 2 inches.

2. A rescuer working alone delivers 15 compressions at a rate of 80-100/minute, alternating with two lung inflations.

3. If two rescuers are present, one delivers chest compressions at a rate of 80-100/minute while the other ventilates the victim during 1- to 1½-second pauses once after every fifth compression. For a discussion of new techniques in CPR, see p. 428.

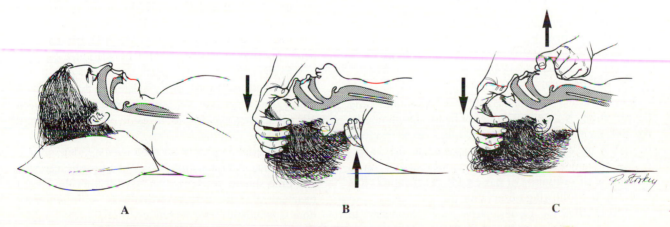

Fig. 18-1. Establish an open airway. Place the patient supine (**A**) and tilt the head backward (**B**) while lifting the neck. Pull up on the angles of the jaw to displace the tongue forward (**C**).

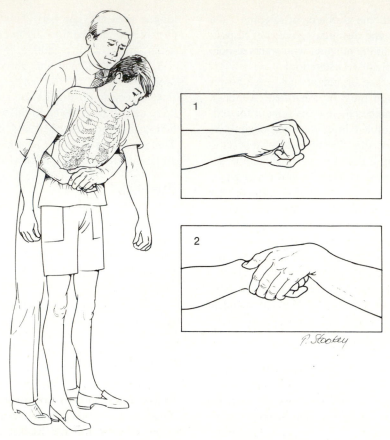

Fig. 18-2. Heimlich maneuver. Position yourself behind the victim and encircle the victim's waist with your arms. Make a fist with one hand *(1)*. The thumb should be over the index finger so that it forms a knob, which adds to the depth of the thrust. Place this knob well below the tip of the xiphoid process and slightly above the navel. Grasp the fist with the other hand *(2)* and exert a quick upward thrust into the victim's abdomen. It may be necessary to repeat the maneuver several times. Deliver the thrust with your hands only; do not exert lateral pressure on the victim's rib cage with your arms (''bear hug''). Such lateral pressure may fracture the victim's ribs.

ADVANCED CARDIAC LIFE SUPPORT

Definitive therapy of cardiac arrest may involve defibrillation, cardiac pacing, more effective ventilation and oxygenation, and the administration of drugs.

Defibrillation

The single most useful resuscitative measure is early defibrillation. If a defibrillator is at hand, this should be the first step in any witnessed cardiac arrest resulting from VT or VF and should be applied to the unwitnessed or unmonitored cardiac arrest patient as soon as possible after institution of basic CPR. This approach is based on the following observations.

• Most cases of cardiac arrest are secondary to VF.

• Basic life support may maintain organ perfusion and life but does not reverse VF.

• The earlier the defibrillation shock is delivered, the better the chance of successful defibrillation.

• Even if the rhythm appears to be asystole, it may still respond to defibrillation, indicating that the mechanism was either fine VF mimicking asystole or coarse VF mimicking asystole as a result of the null electric vector of the fibrillatory waves.[9-11]

• Resuscitation efforts for prolonged asystole or electromechanical dissociation are generally unsuccessful, and time should not be wasted establishing the precise mechanism of the cardiac arrhythmia while defibrillation is withheld. For technique of defibrillation, see Chapter 12.

ECG monitoring during CPR

During CPR, ECG monitoring via extremity leads should be initiated as soon as possible. After CPR, chest leads may be used. Defibrillating paddles have ECG electrodes (quick-look paddles) that can be used for immediate rhythm diagnosis but cannot be relied on for rhythm monitoring.

Precordial thump

Rapid hypotensive VT can sometimes be converted to a supraventricular rhythm by a forceful blow to the sternum with the fleshy part of the fist; this may be repeated once. Such a blow may deliver a low-level electric shock (approximately 5 mV) to the heart.

Disadvantages include possible conversion of VT into VF with further hemodynamic deterioration plus wasted time and effort in a situation in which seconds count. The American Heart Association recommends the precordial thump in patients with monitored VF and witnessed cardiac arrests if a defibrillator is unavailable.

Ventilation

Mouth-to-mouth breathing is applied as the first step in ventilation.[12] It is always available and delivers expired air of approximately 16% to 18% oxygen to the victim's lungs. This is capable of maintaining arterial oxygen tension of 50 mm Hg and oxygen saturation of approximately 90%, given normal lung function. Most victims of cardiac arrest cannot be adequately oxygenated for long periods of time without supplemental oxygen. Methods that improve ventilation and oxygenation are discussed below.

Measures that improve upper airway patency

The following airway adjuncts are available for improving the ventilation, oxygenation, and airway protection for the victim of cardiac arrest.[5,6,13,14]

Pharyngeal suction. The oropharynx must be suctioned thoroughly, using a rigid pharyngeal suction tip to improve upper airway patency.

Oropharyngeal airway tube. The two types of oropharyngeal airway in common use are the Berman and the Guedel tubes. The semicircular plastic or rubber airway fits over the back of the tongue and into the lower posterior pharynx, holding the tongue away from the posterior wall of the pharynx (Fig. 18-3). The airway tube is helpful in maintaining upper airway patency, facilitating suctioning, and preventing tongue biting in an *unconscious* person. In a responsive patient this tube can stimulate gagging and vomiting and should not be used.

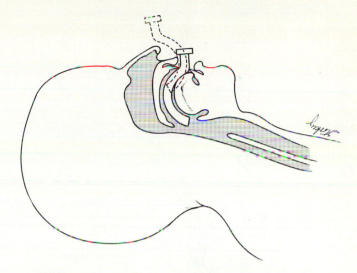

Fig. 18-3. Proper insertion and position of the Guedel oral airway.

Proper insertion and position of the oropharyngeal airway tube are important to avoid trauma or worsening of upper airway obstruction. If the jaw is somewhat relaxed, the mouth can be forced open by the crossed-finger maneuver (Fig. 18-4). However, if the jaw is tight, use the finger-behind-the-teeth maneuver. Insert the airway with a rotating motion.

Nasopharyngeal airway tube. The nasopharyngeal airway tube is a curved, soft rubber or plastic tube 15 cm long. It is inserted through the nose and into the posterior pharynx and separates the tongue from the posterior pharyngeal wall. It is better tolerated by the semiconscious patient and may be used for the patient who clenches his jaw and will not permit passage of an oral airway. It should not be forced through the nasal cavity because this may precipitate hemorrhage. Lubricants and local anesthetics help in gentle insertion.

Measures that permit delivery of supplemental oxygen

Bag/valve/mask assembly (Laerdal, Ambu). The bag/valve/mask assembly is a self-inflating bag that can deliver room air (21% oxygen) or oxygen-enriched gas via a mask that fits over the patient's nose and mouth. Tidal volumes of 500 cc can be achieved. Hyperextension of the head (unless there is cervical spinal injury) and the use of oropharyngeal or nasopharyngeal tubes are helpful in keeping the airway open. Some experience is needed to properly position the mask, apply a tight seal with one hand, and compress the bag with the other hand (Fig. 18-5).

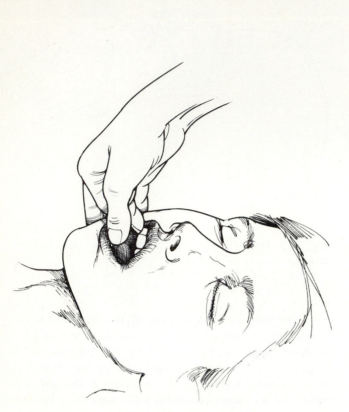

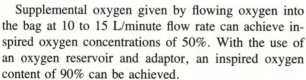

Fig. 18-4. The crossed-finger maneuver for forcing the mouth open.

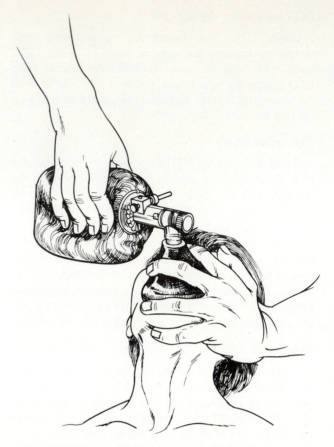

Fig. 18-5. Bag-valve-mask assembly securely held over the patient's mouth and nose with one hand, with compression of the bag with the other hand.

Supplemental oxygen given by flowing oxygen into the bag at 10 to 15 L/minute flow rate can achieve inspired oxygen concentrations of 50%. With the use of an oxygen reservoir and adaptor, an inspired oxygen content of 90% can be achieved.

Oxygen-powered manually triggered ventilation device (Elder valve). A mask is sealed over the mouth and nose and connected via the Elder valve to a compressed oxygen source. The operator squeezes a trigger to release oxygen into the mask at flow rates of 100 L/minute or more. The device is pressure limited; a relief valve opens at airway pressure of 40 mm Hg. Prolonged use frequently leads to gastric distention. This device can also be used with endotracheal tubes.

Tracheal intubation

The definitive method of airway control, ventilation, and oxygenation is tracheal intubation. It permits positive-pressure ventilation with nearly 100% oxygen and prevents progressive gastric distention and aspiration of gastric contents into the airway, a potentially serious complication of CPR.

Tracheal intubation should be performed early in CPR—as soon as a person experienced in the procedure is available, equipment is at hand, and the need for airway and ventilatory control continues. However, crucial seconds and minutes should not be lost at the initiation of CPR in clumsy attempts at tracheal intubation as the first method of ventilation, especially by inexperienced personnel. In emergency intubation the orotracheal route is faster and is preferred over the nasotracheal approach.

Key steps in tracheal intubation

1. Maintain adequate ventilation and oxygenation while preparing for intubation and between intubation attempts.

2. Choose a proper endotracheal tube—usually 8.5 to 9 mm inner diameter for men and 8 mm for women. Smaller tubes are used for children, with the size approximating the diameter of the child's little finger. Ta-

Table 18-1. Tracheal tube size for average-size persons

Age	French size	Inner diameter (mm)	Equivalent tracheotomy tube size
Children			
Premature			00
Newborn	12	2.5	00-0
6 months	16	3.5	0-1
1 year	20	4.5	1-2
2 years	22	5.0	2
4 years	24	5.5	3
6 years	26	6.0	4
8 years	28	6.5	4
10 years	30	7.0	4
12 years	32	7.5	5
14 years	34	8.0	5
Adult			
Women	34-36	7.5-8.5	5
Men	36-40	8.0-9.0	8-10

From Applebaum, E.L., and Bruce, D.L.: Tracheal intubation, Philadelphia, 1976, W.B. Saunders Co.
French size refers to external circumference of the tube.
French size divided by 3 equals external diameter in millimeters.
Internal diameter in millimeters is the preferred nomenclature.
Internal diameter is 2.4 mm less than external diameter.

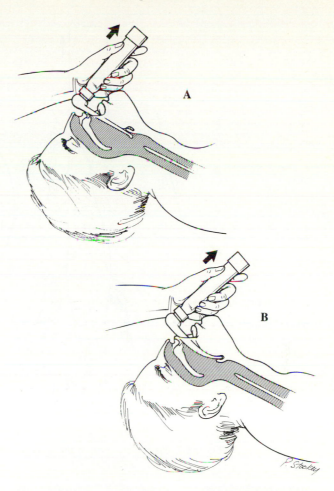

Fig. 18-6. Laryngoscopy for endotracheal intubation. Note the elevated occiput and the backward tilt of the head. **A,** Use of the straight laryngoscope blade. Note that the epiglottis is directly elevated with the tip of the blade. Do not use the teeth as a fulcrum. **B,** Use of a curved laryngoscope blade. Note that the epiglottis is indirectly elevated because the tip of the blade elevates the base of the tongue.

ble 18-1 lists the tracheal tube size for children and adults.

3. Check the cuff for leaks and then evacuate all air from the cuff (tubes less than 6 mm inner diameter frequently do not have a cuff).

4. Lubricate the tip of the endotracheal tube with a water-soluble anesthetic lubricant. If a stylet is to be used, lubricate and insert it into the endotracheal tube up to 2 cm from its tip.

5. Secure either the curved or the straight blade on the laryngoscope and check the light.

6. Remove dentures or foreign bodies from the patient's mouth and apply suction to the oropharynx.

7. You may need to sedate a combative or uncooperative patient. Diazepam (Valium), midazolam (Versed), or methohexital (Brevital) may be used (see pp. 278-279). If sedation is not adequate, you may need to use succinylcholine[13a] (Anectine) (see p. 417).

8. Remove the headboard and position the patient's head so that the mouth, pharynx, and trachea are aligned in a straight axis. Elevate the head with a small pillow and extend it by moving the chin up and back (the "sniffing position"). Apply suction to the oropharynx again.

9. Apply a topical local anesthetic to the patient's mouth, oropharynx, and hypopharynx, unless the patient is unconscious.

10. Lubricate the laryngoscope blade with sterile water.

11. Insert the blade into the widely opened mouth to the right of the midline, elevate and move the tongue to the left, maneuver the blade to the midline, and follow the contour of the pharynx toward the epiglottis. Protect the lips from trauma.

12. An assistant should apply firm backward pressure on the cricoid cartilage (Sellick's maneuver) until intubation is completed and the cuff is inflated. This will occlude the esophagus and prevent aspiration of gastric contents into the airway.

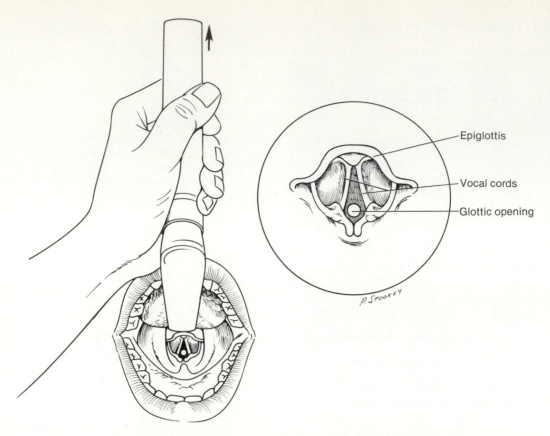

Epiglottis

Vocal cords

Glottic opening

P. STOOKEY

Fig. 18-7. Proper insertion of the laryngoscope to expose the glottic opening and landmarks.

13. If you are using a straight blade, position its tip past the epiglottis (Fig. 18-6, *A*); if you are using a curved blade, position its tip in the vallecula (Fig. 18-6, *B*).

14. Exert forceful leverage upward (in the direction of the arrow on the laryngoscope handle), using your shoulder and arm muscles. Displace the base of the tongue and the epiglottis anteriorly and expose the glottic opening (Fig. 18-7). *Caution:* Do not flex, bend, or use the wrist for this maneuver. Do not jam the blade tip in the pharynx. Do not use the upper teeth as a fulcrum. Do not use the handle with a prying motion.

15. Insert the endotracheal tube with your right hand from the right corner of the mouth, through the glottic opening, and into the trachea 5 to 6 cm beyond the vocal cords.

16. The stylet may be used to mold the tube. Lubricate it before passing it into the tube. Do not allow it to pass the tip of the endotracheal tube because it can perforate the tracheal. Use a lighted stylet in difficult cases. If successful intubation is not achieved within 30 seconds, the procedure should be interrupted and the patient's lungs should be ventilated.

17. Inflate the high-volume, low-pressure cuff to obtain an airtight seal (5 to 10 cc of air).

18. With a standard 15 mm connector, attach the proximal end of the tracheal tube to a bag-valve assembly with oxygen and manually ventilate the patient.

19. Listen for breath sounds in both right and left lungs and over the stomach to confirm correct placement of the tube.

20. After several ventilations, apply suction to the trachea if secretions are present.

21. Obtain a chest radiograph to confirm proper positioning of the tube.

22. Secure the tube in the desired position using benzoin and adhesive tape. Note the centimeter mark at the level of the mouth for reference. Trim any excess length of endotracheal tube and protect the tube from dislodgment or self-extubation.

23. If gastric distention is present, insert a nasogastric tube for decompression.

Table 18-2 compares the advantages and disadvantages of various methods of assisted ventilation.

Table 18-2. Advantages and disadvantages of various methods of ventilation

Method	Advantages	Disadvantages
Mouth-to-mouth	Immediate availability at all places Minimal training required for application Adequate ventilation and oxygenation obtained in normal lungs	Not hygienic or aesthetic Not possible to supplement oxygen Gastric distention frequent
Bag/valve/mask (Ambubag)	Available in all medical units equipped for resuscitation Permits oxygen supplementation during spontaneous and artificial ventilation Operator feels resistance to inflation—can ''control'' ventilation Permits delivery of humidified oxygen	Generally not available outside of medical facilities Difficult to use without a tracheal tube May cause gastric distention Oropharyngeal or nasopharyngeal airway frequently needed
Elder valve	Available in most medical units equipped for resuscitation Easier to use than the bag/valve/mask Permits positive-pressure ventilation with oxygen	Not available outside of medical facilities Needs compressed gas High inflation pressures can cause gastric distention and pneumothorax Cannot use humidified oxygen
Tracheal intubation	Most efficient way of ventilation and oxygenation No gastric distention or regurgitation Permits tracheal suctioning	Requires specialized training and equipment

SUCCINYLCHOLINE

Succinylcholine, a short-acting neuromuscular blocking agent, should be reserved for the difficult intubation in which sedation has not provided adequate relaxation and the patient's reflexes (coughing, gagging) and motor activity make opening of the mouth and proper positioning of the head impossible. Proceeding with such a difficult intubation without adequate muscle relaxation insures excessive upper airway trauma and frequent failure to intubate.

Preparations: Anectine (20 mg/ml) and Sucostrin (100 mg/ml)

Dose for succinylcholine: 1 to 1.5 mg/kg IV over 10 to 15 seconds

Onset of action: Less than 1 minute

Peak action: Approximately 2 minutes

Duration of action: 3 to 5 minutes and up to 10 minutes

Adverse effects: Increased intragastric pressure and vomiting with the risk of aspiration; arrhythmias—asystole (vagal stimulation) and ventricular tachycardia can occur

Precautions
- Apply backward pressure on the cricoid cartilage (Sellick's maneuver) to occlude the esophagus and prevent aspiration; this should be performed just before injection of the succinylcholine
- Monitor ECG for arrhythmias
- *Be ready for emergency cricothyrotomy*
- After succinylcholine administration, if intubation cannot be performed promptly, perform emergency cricothyrotomy
- Premedicate with diazepam if the patient is conscious and aware of his or her surroundings. This will also reduce muscular fasciculations secondary to succinylcholine.

Major contraindications
- Unfamilarity with the drug
- Cervical spine injury where orotracheal intubation is contraindicated
- Inability to control the airway following neuromuscular paralysis

Cricothyrotomy

Cricothyrotomy[14,15] is indicated in emergency situations when the patient is without an airway and standard endotracheal intubation has failed or is contraindicated or impossible (as in fixed upper airway obstruction or cervical spine injury).

Anatomy. Fig. 18-8 illustrates frontal and lateral views of the larynx. The thyroid cartilage (Adam's apple) is prominent and can easily be palpated, except in infants or obese patients. The cricothyroid membrane is between the thyroid cartilage and the cricoid cartilage, 2 to 3 cm directly below the notch of the thyroid cartilage. This membrane is approximately 20 mm wide and 10 mm high.

The cricoid cartilage is the only complete tracheal ring. Along with the posterior wall of the thyroid cartilage, the cricoid cartilage offers a "backstop" and an element of safety in the performance of cricothyrotomy.

The vocal cords are approximately 1.5 to 2 cm above the cricothyroid membrane; blood vessels traverse the membrane superiorly. The jugular and carotid vessels are lateral to the incision site and the esophagus is posterior to the incision site.

Equipment necessary for emergency cricothyrotomy
- #11 Scalpel
- Endotracheal tube (#5 or #6)
- A standard tracheotomy tray should be made available, but you should *not* wait for this

Procedure. Cricothyrotomy is a lifesaving procedure to establish an airway, using the fastest and safest possible technique and the resources instantly available. The patient is usually comatose or semicomatose, and endotracheal intubation has failed or is impossible or contraindicated. The procedure is fast and simple (except in obese patients), but it is important to be thoroughly familiar with the procedure before actually having to do it. The essence of this emergency procedure is to rapidly locate the cricoid membrane, enter the trachea through it, and ventilate the patient's lungs. The procedure is described below.

1. Elevate the larynx. A rolled towel under the shoulders will help to hyperextend the head and neck. The combative patient must be restrained by available personnel while the physician performs the procedure.

2. Identify the cricothyroid membrane. Palpably locate the thyroid cartilage and slide your finger down

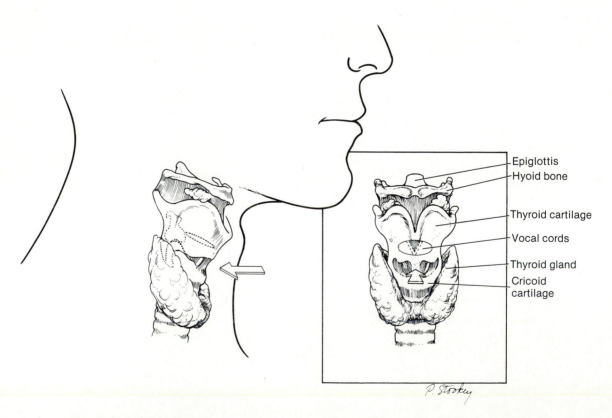

Epiglottis
Hyoid bone
Thyroid cartilage
Vocal cords
Thyroid gland
Cricoid cartilage

P. Stookey

Fig. 18-8. Frontal and lateral views of the larynx. *Arrow* points to the cricothyroid membrane, which is felt as a notch below the thyroid cartilage.

until you reach the first soft indentation—the cricothyroid membrane (Fig. 18-9). Stabilize the larynx with the nondominant hand as shown in Fig. 18-10 and make the puncture as described below.

3. Enter the trachea. Holding the scalpel so that the #11 blade is horizontal, *puncture* through the cricothyroid membrane, as illustrated in Fig. 18-10. Hold the scalpel like a pencil (between your thumb and index finger), with your hand resting on the patient so that only the tip of the blade can enter the trachea. This position will give you control even if the patient should move.

4. Slowly insert the blade until its width at the puncture site is a little less than 1 cm; this is an adequate airway. If there has been a mechanical obstruction, there will usually be a gush of air when you puncture the trachea. Do not attempt to enlarge the puncture with the blade other than to turn it vertically, creating an airway that is 1 × 1 cm. *Caution: do not remove the blade until a tube is inserted;* otherwise the airway will collapse. You now have time to get help, to apply suction if necessary, and to *slowly* and carefully insert the endotracheal tube while maintaining a place for it with the blade. Be sure to use a *puncture* wound as described; a horizontal *incision* risks severing the carotid artery or the jugular veins. Do not let the blade move deeply into the trachea because it may puncture the esophagus.

5. Insert the smallest tube with a cuff that is available. This is usually a #6 to #6½ endotracheal tube. Just barely insert the endotracheal tube through the puncture wound. Remember that the trachea is only a few centimeters away!

6. Ventilate the lungs. If there has been a mechanical obstruction, the patient will start breathing spontaneously. If there has been full respiratory arrest, inflate the balloon and energetically ventilate the patient's lungs. Once a skilled surgeon arrives, the stab wound can be dilated and a tracheostomy tube inserted.

Pacing

Emergency pacing is rarely needed *during* cardiopulmonary resuscitation. VF is treated with defibrillation and drugs. Electromechanical dissociation is difficult to reverse, frequently indicates inadequate coronary perfusion, myocardial rupture, or pericardial tamponade, and does not respond to pacing. Bradycardia and AV block can cause syncope and seizures but infrequently

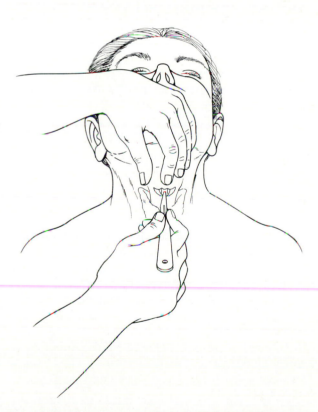

Fig. 18-10. Stabilize the larynx between the thumb and middle finger of the nondominant hand, with the index finger placed over the cricothyroid membrane. Hold the scalpel like a pencil between the thumb and index finger so that the #11 blade is horizontal and directed along the border of the nondominant index finger through the cricothyroid membrane.

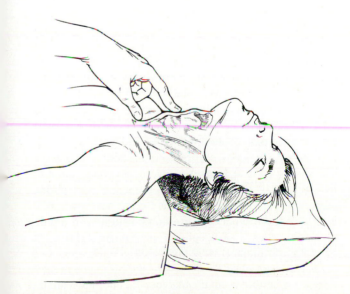

Fig. 18-9. Identifying the cricothyroid membrane. Find the thyroid cartilage and slide your finger down until you reach the first soft indentation—this is the cricothyroid membrane.

progress to full cardiac arrest with asystole. Brady-asystolic cardiac arrest is best treated by establishing an airway with effective ventilation, accompanied by chest compression and the use of drugs (such as epinephrine or atropine).

Pacing is occasionally useful for asystole. Refractory asystole usually indicates inadequate coronary perfusion. If spontaneous cardiac rhythm cannot be established, attempts at cardiac pacing are justified, although rarely successful. You may proceed to emergency external transcutaneous pacing[16,17] or emergency transvenous pacing (see Chapter 13). Transthoracic emergency pacing is generally discouraged.

DRUGS

Use of drugs for CPR has evolved over the years on an empiric basis. Recently there have been increasing attempts to study the use of these drugs in animal models of CPR or to monitor their action in CPR in humans.

Many of the traditional drugs for CPR are actually useful *after* successful resuscitation; they have little to offer during resuscitation. Oxygen and epinephrine or other sympathomimetic drugs with major alpha-adrenergic actions appear to have some value during CPR, whereas others, such as calcium, continue to be used because of tradition, even when no benefit can be demonstrated. This section is a brief review of the proper use of drugs in the setting of CPR and immediately after CPR. Table 18-3 lists the intravenous dosages of drugs used during or after CPR for adults. Table 18-4 is a list of drugs and convenient mixtures for infusion used after CPR.

Oxygen

Adequate oxygenation during CPR is critical, and supplemental oxygen should be used in all cases as soon as a bag-valve-mask system is available. High concentrations of oxygen must be used. With an endotracheal tube, nearly 100% oxygen may be used and is safe. Only after several hours (6 or more) is oxygen toxicity to the lungs a concern. Adequate oxygenation and ventilation are best followed by determination of arterial blood gases. Oxygen delivered via valveless oronasal masks, nasal canula, or Venturi mask has no role in CPR.

Epinephrine

Unless immediate defibrillation has been successful, epinephrine is used during CPR whether the rhythm is VF, asystole, or electromechanical dissociation. Epinephrine (Adrenaline) by itself is not effective treatment

Table 18-3. Intravenous dosage (adult) of drugs used during or after CPR* (see text for details)

Drug	Dosage
Atropine	0.5-1.0 mg
Bretylium (Bretylol)	400-500 mg
Calcium chloride (10%)	500 mg or 6.8 mEq of calcium (5 ml of 10% solution)
Digoxin (Lanoxin)	0.125-0.5 mg
Ephedrine	5-10 mg
Epinephrine (Adrenaline)	0.5-1.0 mg
Lidocaine (Xylocaine)	50-100 mg
Magnesium sulfate	1-2 g (5-10 ml of 20% solution)
Metaraminol (Aramine)	0.5-5.0 mg
Methoxamine (Vasoxyl)	3-5 mg
Nitroglycerin	200-400 µg
Phenylephrine (Neosynephrine)	0.2-1.0 mg
Phenytoin (Dilantin)	250-500 mg IV at 50 mg/min†
Procainamide (Pronestyl)	100 mg repeated every 5 min, or 25 mg/min to 1000 mg
Propranolol (Inderal)	1-3 mg
Sodium bicarbonate	1 mEq/kg—50-75 ml of 8.4% solution
Verapamil (Isoptin, Calan)	5-10 mg

*Usually mixed in 5 to 10 ml of 5% dextrose in water or normal saline.
†Use 0.22 to 0.45 µ filter.

for VF. During CPR, a minimum diastolic pressure of 30 to 40 mm Hg seems to be necessary for successful results. Alpha stimulation causes peripheral and splanchnic vasoconstriction without coronary or cerebral vasoconstriction, improving diastolic blood pressure and thus myocardial and cerebral blood flow during CPR and facilitating the return of spontaneous cardiac contractions. Beta stimulation (increased heart rate, myocardial contractile force, and peripheral vascular dilatation) does not improve diastolic blood pressure during CPR and has marginal or no contribution to the success of CPR. In dog experiments, epinephrine used with beta blockers remained effective, whereas it was ineffective when used in combination with alpha-blocking drugs.[18] Epinephrine and phenylephrine (a pure alpha stimulant) were compared in a dog model of cardiac arrest and CPR. There was no difference in neurologic or cardiovascular outcome.[19] Thus, pure alpha-receptor stimulants may be as effective as epinephrine in CPR. Definitive experiments to define the best adrenergic stimulant, its optimal dose, and most effective

Table 18-4. Drugs used after CPR: convenient mixtures for infusion and usual doses

Drug	Dose (per 250 ml D5W)	Concentration (per ml)	Usual dose (per minute)*
Bretylium (Bretylol)	1000 mg	4 mg	1-2 mg
Dobutamine (Dobutrex)	500 mg	2 mg	200-1000 μg
Dopamine (Intropin)	200 mg	800 μg	0.2-3 mg†
Epinephrine (Adrenaline)	1 mg	4 μg	1-8 μg
Isoproterenol (Isuprel)	2 mg	8 μg	2-20 μg
Lidocaine (Xylocaine)	1000 mg	4 mg	1-4 mg
Magnesium sulfate	4 g	16 mg	8-16 mg
Metaraminol (Aramine)	100 mg	400 μg	100-500 μg
Nitroglycerin	50 mg	200 μg	20-250 μg
Nitroprusside (Nipride, Nitropress)	50 mg	200 μg	40-800 μg
Norepinephrine (Levophed)	4 mg	16 μg	1-8 μg
Phenylephrine (Neosynephrine)	20 mg	80 μg	5-60 μg
Phenytoin (Dilantin)	500 mg	2 mg	200-300 μg
Procainamide (Pronestyl)	1000 mg	4 mg	1-4 mg
Verapamil (Isoptin, Calan)	50 mg	200 μg	100-200 μg

*Usually started at a low dose and titrated to desired action. If higher doses are used, use higher concentration ($\times 2$, $\times 4$) to limit volume of infusion.

†Low dose: 3 to 10 μg/kg/minute, high dose (predominant alpha action): 10 to 40/μg/kg/minute. For high-dose infusion, use a more concentrated solution.

route of administration are yet to be done. For other sympathomimetic amines see Table 18-5.

Dosage

The usual dosage for epinephrine is 0.5 to 1.0 mg (5 to 10 ml of a 1:10,000 solution) IV bolus, which may be repeated every 5 minutes. Epinephrine may also be given via endotracheal tube (see p. 426) but may require higher doses.[20]

Precautions

Do not mix epinephrine with sodium bicarbonate; this will cause partial inactivation of epinephrine.

Do not give epinephrine via the intracardiac route if at all possible.

Lidocaine and bretylium tosylate
Lidocaine

For more than 20 years lidocaine (Xylocaine) has been the first-line antiarrhythmic agent used during CPR. Lidocaine decreases automaticity and abolishes intraventricular reentry by depressing conduction in ischemic fibers. Clinically, it has potent antiarrhythmic (antiectopic) action and has been proved effective in reducing the frequency of premature ventricular ectopic beats and reducing the incidence of VF and VT after

Table 18-5. Sympathomimetic amines

Agent	Brand name	Receptor activity			Mode of action
		Alpha	Beta₁	Beta₂	
Dobutamine	Dobutrex		+ +	+	Direct
Dopamine	Inotropin	+ +	+ + +	+	Direct & indirect
		High dose	Low dose		
Ephedrine		+	+		Direct & indirect
Epinephrine	Adrenaline	+ +	+ + +	+ +	Direct
Isoproterenol	Isuprel		+ + +	+ + +	Direct
Methoxamine	Vasoxyl	+ + +			Direct
Metaraminol	Aramine	+ +	+		Indirect
Norepinephrine	Levophed Levarterenol	+ + +	+ + +		Direct
Phenylephrine	Neosynephrine	+ + +			Direct

CPR and in settings of acute myocardial infarction. The antifibrillatory (in contradistinction to the antiarrhythmic) action of lidocaine is probably less pronounced. In large doses, lidocaine raises the ventricular fibrillatory threshold and in combination with its antiarrhythmic action is effective in preventing recurrent VF.[21,21a]

Lidocaine has no role as a primary treatment of VF in that it does not convert VF to an organized rhythm and there is no evidence that it facilitates electric defibrillation. Animal (dog) studies show that lidocaine *increases* the energy required for defibrillation.[22]

Thus available data and 20 years of experience suggest that lidocaine is effective in the *prophylaxis* of VT or VF in patients with high risk of developing these arrhythmias (as in acute myocardial infarction and immediately following CPR). There is no evidence to support the use of lidocaine early in CPR before effective defibrillation is achieved.

Dosage. The usual dosage is 75 mg (IV bolus), which may be followed by 50 mg every 5 to 10 minutes to a maximal dose of 300 mg followed by infusion of 1 to 4 mg/minute.

Precautions. In high doses lidocaine may cause myocardial depression, mental obtundation, and seizures.

Reduce maintenance doses in elderly patients and in patients with congestive heart failure or liver disease.

Bretylium tosylate

The antifibrillatory action of bretylium (Bretylol) was described in 1966, but only during the past 5 to 10 years has it received much interest.[23] Bretylium elevates ventricular fibrillation threshold[21a] and is effective in controlling recurrent VT and VF.[24] Definitive studies comparing this function of bretylium with the prophylactic action of lidocaine are not available. In the management of out-of-hospital VF, lidocaine and bretylium were found equally effective.[25]

Current American Heart Association (AHA) guidelines recommend using bretylium during CPR only after VF has been refractory to DC shock, before and after epinephrine use. Advocates of bretylium suggest that it be used early during the initial attempt of defibrillation.[26] If the results of preliminary animal studies suggesting that bretylium reduces the defibrillatory threshold and facilitates elective defibrillation[27] are confirmed, then earlier use of this drug would seem warranted. A direct antifibrillatory action of bretylium[28] or a significant effect on defibrillation threshold[22] has been questioned in recent canine studies. VF recurring despite standard treatment (lidocaine, procainamide) has responded to bretylium in 75% of patients.[21]

Mechanism of action. Bretylium is an adrenergic neuronal blocking drug with a complex mechanism of action. Its myocardial action includes prolongation of action potential duration and the effective refractory period of Purkinje and ventricular muscle fibers.

Bretylium is not considered a potent antiarrhythmic (antiectopic) agent because it does not reduce automaticity or cardiac conduction, as does lidocaine, and is not effective in suppressing ventricular ectopic activity. On the contrary, when the blood level of bretylium is high as a result of the administration of a bolus, heart rate and ventricular ectopic beats may increase secondary to the release of norepinephrine from nerve endings. This has not led to malignant ventricular arrhythmias. Later, when the blood level is lower as a result of administration by drip infusion, bretylium inhibits this release of norepinephrine.[23]

Dosage. For treatment of VF, in conjunction with electric defibrillation, administer 500 mg of undiluted bretylium (IV bolus) followed by electroshock treatment. Repeat this dose if needed.

For prophylaxis of VF or VT, administer 5 to 10 mg/kg in 50 ml intravenously over 10 minutes.

The dose may be repeated every 1 to 2 hours. The continuous infusion rate is 1 to 2 mg/minute.

Precautions. Transient increase in heart rate, ventricular ectopic beats, and blood pressure may occur initially, followed approximately 1 hour later by hypotension, usually postural. Nausea and vomiting can occur.

Bretylium is relatively contraindicated in VT and VF secondary to digitalis toxicity.

There may be an increase in ventricular ectopy in the first 20 to 30 minutes after administration of bretylium.

Procainamide

Procainamide is an effective antiarrhythmic agent and is used in the treatment of VT and prevention of recurrent VF. It is considered a second-line antiarrhythmic agent in the setting of CPR and is generally used after lidocaine or bretylium.

Dosage

Administer as an IV bolus, 100 mg every 5 minutes (20 mg/minute) up to a dose of 1000 mg. The maintenance infusion dosage is 1 to 4 mg/minute.

Precautions

Discontinue the drug if hypotension or QRS widening of 50% or more occurs. Discontinue the drug if VT recurs in association with QT prolongation (torsade de pointes).

Atropine sulfate

Atropine increases the rate of sinus node discharge and AV conduction via its direct cardiac vagolytic action. It is used in CPR in the setting of asystole, high-grade AV block, or severe bradycardia. Full vagolytic doses should be used.

Dosage

For asystole, administer 1 mg IV bolus and repeat up to a total of 3 to 4 mg for total parasympathetic blockade.

For bradycardia, administer 0.5 mg (IV bolus). This may be repeated at 5-minute intervals a maximum of 3 times.

Precautions

Successful resuscitation of brady-asystolic cardiac arrest may be followed by tachycardia, which increases oxygen consumption and may predispose to VT and VF. Thus atropine should be used in doses necessary to reverse vagally induced asystole or AV block, but excess doses should be avoided.

Sodium bicarbonate

Hypoventilation, not perfusion failure, accounts for the acidemia observed during early CPR of victims of witnessed cardiac arrest. Thus there is no rationale for the use of sodium bicarbonate early in CPR.[9,29-31] The empirically devised and widely practiced administration of sodium bicarbonate in 1 mEq/kg doses at the onset of cardiac arrest is questioned. The following valid points have been made.

1. In the early stages of CPR (the first 1 to 5 minutes) there is no metabolic acidosis and frequently there is respiratory alkalosis. If acidosis occurs, it reflects ineffective ventilation, and sodium bicarbonate has no benefit in this setting.

2. Metabolic acidosis that appears later in CPR may not be severe and is usually not in the range in which epinephrine action or vital functions are severely compromised.

3. Sodium bicarbonate is ineffective in combating acidosis in the absence of effective ventilation. The *primary role of effective ventilation in maintaining acid-base balance during CPR* must be emphasized.

4. The dangers of excessive amounts of sodium bicarbonate in the production of metabolic alkalosis have been demonstrated. These include impaired oxygen release by hemoglobin, precipitation of VT or VF, hypernatremia, hyperosmolar states, and fluid overload. Intracellular acidosis (increased carbon dioxide produced by sodium bicarbonate diffusing intracellularly) may occur and cause myocardial depression.

5. Metabolic acidosis may be more pronounced *after* successful CPR, when circulation is restored and metabolic acids produced by anaerobic metabolism are washed into the circulation. Therefore sodium bicarbonate may be more properly used after successful CPR.

6. Benefits of sodium bicarbonate have not been proved during CPR, whereas its potential for harm has raised concern.

Recommendations for use

During CPR, make every attempt to keep the pH close to physiologic range by means of effective ventilation. Use sodium bicarbonate only if its need is documented by arterial blood gas measurements.

In prolonged CPR with effective ventilation, document arterial blood gases and administer sodium bicarbonate accordingly.

In prolonged CPR with inadequate ventilation, sodium bicarbonate has no benefit and will further increase the carbon dioxide load and aggravate intracellular acidosis.

In unwitnessed cardiac arrest in or out of the hospital, during which cardiac arrest and ventilatory arrest have existed for some time, sodium bicarbonate may be given early in CPR *after the initiation of adequate ventilation*. Follow-up doses should be guided by arterial blood gases.

Dosage

Administer 1 mEq/kg—50 to 75 ml of a 8.4% solution (1 mEq/ml) as an IV bolus.

If arterial blood gas measurements cannot be obtained, current AHA recommendations suggest repeating sodium bicarbonate in 10 to 15 minutes at one half of the initial dose. This recommendation is empiric and will probably be changed in the future.

Precautions

Use sodium bicarbonate only if its need is documented. Do not mix sodium bicarbonate with calcium or catecholamines.

Morphine sulphate

Morphine has no role during CPR. If CPR has been successful, then morphine is of value in controlling the pain of myocardial infarction or fractured ribs and relieving acute pulmonary edema. Morphine is an analgesic and its venodilating action is effective in reducing venous return and left ventricular filling pressures.

Dosage

Administer 2 to 5 mg intravenously every 5 to 15 minutes. Titrate to desired effect, with monitoring of respiratory rate and blood pressure.

Precaution

Give morphine in small IV increments to avoid respiratory depression and hypotension.

Nitroglycerin

Nitroglycerin, as a rule, is not used *during* CPR. Vasospastic coronary disease is an exception to this rule. After CPR, nitroglycerin is used to control hypertension, pulmonary edema, and myocardial ischemia with or without angina.

The vasodilating action of nitroglycerin reduces the diastolic blood pressure during CPR and is potentially harmful. However, anecdotal[32] and personal experience has shown nitroglycerin to be effective in reversing coronary artery spasm during CPR, thus permitting successful defibrillation.

Coronary artery spasm can cause total occlusion of a major coronary artery and precipitate VT, VF, AV block, or electromechanical dissociation. These arrhythmias may prove refractory to standard CPR and defibrillation or may be recurrent. It is not known how frequently coronary artery spasm is involved in the production of cardiac arrest. The role (if any) of nitroglycerin in CPR of patients with coronary artery disease has not been evaluated.

Presently nitroglycerin use during CPR can be recommended only for resuscitation of refractory VF in patients with known or suspected vasospastic coronary disease.

Dosage

Administer 200 to 400 μg (IV push); this may be repeated once after 5 minutes. If no IV route is available, give 400 μg sublingually.

For IV infusion, administer 1 to 4 μg/kg/minute, usually started at 10 to 20 μg/minute and titrated to maintenance doses.
- *Low dose:* 1 μg/kg/minute (mostly venodilating action)
- *High dose:* 4 μg/kg/minute (venous and arterial dilatation, including coronary and pulmonary arteries)

Precautions

Because of its vasodilating action, nitroglycerin can cause hypotension, especially in the presence of hypovolemia. This is potentially harmful in the setting of CPR. Therefore nitroglycerin should be used very selectively and with appropriate caution.

Sodium nitroprusside

Sodium nitroprusside (Nipride) has no role during CPR. It is used after successful resuscitation for control of hypertension, pulmonary edema, or congestive heart failure. It is a potent, rapidly acting, direct arterial and venous dilator. Its short duration of action (1 to 2 minutes) permits rapid dose titration.

Dosage

Administer 50 mg in 250 ml of 5% dextrose in water (200 μg/ml). Titrate infusion to desired clinical end point.

Precautions

During prolonged infusion, do not expose sodium nitroprusside to light. Monitor arterial blood pressure closely during administration. Thiocyanate toxicity can occur with prolonged use.

Calcium chloride

Calcium chloride has no role in the resuscitation of cardiac arrest resulting from VF or asystole unless there is documented hypocalcemia or hyperkalemia. There is no evidence for its beneficial action,[33] and it is potentially harmful because it may cause increased myocardial cellular damage and increased cerebral injury.

Infrequently (in approximately 10% of cases) cardiac arrest associated with electromechanical dissociation responds to calcium.[34,35] Calcium chloride is also effective in reversing the hypotension and AV block secondary to overdose of calcium entry–blocking agents (such as verapamil, diltiazem, nifedipine, and magnesium).

Dosage

Administer 5 ml of 10% solution of calcium chloride IV push. This dose may be repeated once in 5 to 10 minutes.

Precautions

Hypercalcemia can precipitate sinus bradycardia, sinus arrest, and digitalis toxicity. Calcium should not be mixed with sodium bicarbonate.

Magnesium

Traditionally, magnesium is not considered an essential or useful agent in CPR. All the standard sources of CPR information and AHA recommendations are silent regarding its use. Controlled studies have not been done, but the following observations suggest that there may be a role for magnesium infusion in CPR or in the stabilization of patients immediately after CPR.

Magnesium is a potent, nonselective calcium antagonist. The role of calcium entry blockers, including magnesium, in cerebral resuscitation is under intense study; early animal and human (uncontrolled) data appear encouraging.[36]

Magnesium is of proven value in treating arrhythmias caused by digitalis toxicity.[37] It is also effective in treating VT with associated hypomagnesemia.[38] Magnesium has been reported to be effective in treating VT and VF that have been refractory to other antiarrhythmic agents.[39] It is also effective in VT of the torsade de pointes variety[40] and in multifocal atrial tachycardia.[41]

Suggestions for use

Given the very limited nature of data, the following suggestions are made.

Magnesium is the treatment of choice for VT and VF secondary to documented hypomagnesemia. It is effective treatment for torsade de pointes VT, multifocal atrial tachycardia, and digitalis toxic arrhythmias.

In the treatment of VT and VF in which hypomagnesemia, digitalis toxicity, or torsade de pointes is not present, the role of magnesium therapy is not clearly defined and needs to be studied.

The use of magnesium and other calcium-blocking agents in cerebral resuscitation remains experimental.

Dosage

Administer 2 g (10 ml of 20% solution, 16 mEq) IV push over 1 to 2 minutes for treatment of VT or prophylaxis of recurrent VF. In less life-threatening situations, an infusion of 2 g over 10 minutes is safer.

For IV infusion, administer 1 to 2 g/hour for 4 to 6 hours.

Precautions

Exercise caution in using magnesium in the presence of renal failure. Life-threatening hypermagnesemia with neuromuscular paralysis and respiratory arrest can develop if renal function is compromised.

Magnesium is a vasodilator and therefore may cause hypotension when given rapidly or in large doses.

Its use should be monitored with serum levels, especially in the presence of renal dysfunction.

Potassium chloride

There is no role for administration of potassium during CPR. If hypokalemia is documented after successful resuscitation, potassium replacement should be instituted promptly.

Verapamil

The role of verapamil in CPR is limited to the control of supraventricular tachycardia (SVT), which may follow successful resuscitation. It is the treatment of choice for paroxysmal SVT that uses AV nodal conduction. It is very useful in the control of the ventricular rate in atrial fibrillation and flutter in the absence of an AV bypass tract (Wolff-Parkinson-White syndrome). In Wolff-Parkinson-White syndrome with atrial fibrillation, verapamil is contraindicated.[42] Its role, if any, in the treatment of VT and in cerebral resuscitation is under study and is currently considered experimental.

Dosage

Administer 5 mg IV push over 2 to 3 minutes, which may be repeated once in 15 minutes.

Precautions

Hypotension and high-grade AV block are extensions of the action of the drug.

If verapamil is used to treat VT (misdiagnosed as SVT) the resulting hypotension and hemodynamic deterioration may precipitate VF.

Note: The hemodynamic and antiarrhythmic action of verapamil can be reversed with calcium chloride infusion.

Propranolol

The role of propranolol (Inderal) in the treatment and prevention of VT or VF in the setting of CPR has not been studied in a controlled manner. Therefore propranolol's use in relation to lidocaine or bretylium cannot be clearly stated. Propranolol is effective therapy in VT and VF related to myocardial ischemia, excess catecholamine stimulation, and digitalis toxicity. One controlled study has shown IV propranolol to be effective in the prophylaxis of VF in the setting of acute myocardial infarction.[43] If further studies confirm this property, then the use of IV propranolol in the critical care unit may be similar to that of lidocaine.

Dosage

Administer 1 mg (IV push) every 1 to 5 minutes up to a total of 5 to 8 mg.

Precautions

Propranolol is relatively contraindicated in bronchospastic disease. It may also aggravate congestive heart failure or AV block.

Digitalis

Cardiac glycosides have no role in CPR. If, after successful resuscitation, atrial fibrillation is precipitated with a rapid ventricular rate, you may choose from verapamil, propranolol, or digitalis, or use these in combination, to control ventricular rate.

Dosage

Administer 0.125 to 0.5 mg (IV push). Full digitalization is achieved by 1 to 1.5 mg.

Precautions

Watch for subjective and ECG signs of digitalis toxicity. Sole reliance on blood levels as an indication of toxicity is not advisable.[44]

Phenytoin

Phenytoin (phenylhydantoin, Dilantin) may be used following CPR to prevent seizures and to treat arrhythmias secondary to digitalis toxicity. Phenytoin is not officially approved by the FDA for this antiarrhythmic action. Propranolol, potassium, or magnesium may be more effective for arrhythmias of digitalis toxicity.

Dosage

Administer a loading dose of 10 to 15 mg/kg (direct IV push) (mix with normal saline). Use with a 0.22 to 0.45 μ filter and do not infuse at a rate faster than 50 mg/minute. The usual maintenance dose is 300 to 500 mg/day.

Precautions

Watch for central nervous system toxicity (dizziness, ataxia, nystagmus, and dysarthria), as well as hypotension, respiratory arrest, bradycardia, and AV block.

ROUTES OF DRUG ADMINISTRATION DURING CPR
Intravenous routes

Subclavian and internal jugular veins are the intravenous routes of first choice. Ideally, a supradiaphragmatic central vein should be used if already available or if one can be accessed readily without interrupting CPR.

The antecubital vein may also be used. This is more accessible during CPR and is quite suitable.

The femoral vein is another alternative. This is most accessible during CPR but may not be the best approach. Because there are no valves in the iliac–inferior vena cava system, drugs injected in the femoral vein during CPR may not reach the central circulation because of the direction of venous blood flow during chest compression. Regional venous return to the heart and pharmacokinetics of central versus peripheral administration of drugs during CPR have not been studied in detail, and the particulars remain unknown.[45,45a]

Endotracheal routes

If a satisfactory venous route is not available, an endotracheal tube can be used to deliver epinephrine, lidocaine, atropine, naloxone, and possibly diazepam.[9,45b] Systemic absorption occurs when this route is used. Precise dosages have not been evaluated, and the *effectiveness of this route during CPR has not been demonstrated in humans*.

Epinephrine, lidocaine, and atropine should be diluted in 10 ml of 5% dextrose in water, used in twice the usual doses, and forcibly injected or delivered via a long catheter through the endotracheal tube deep into the lungs. This should be followed by four or five lung inflations with the Ambubag.

Drugs that should not be given via an endotracheal tube include sodium bicarbonate, norepinephrine, bretylium, and calcium chloride.

Intracardiac route

Intracardiac administration of drugs is discouraged because of the risk of hemopericardium, cardiac tamponade, coronary artery laceration, and intramyocardial injection. However, this route may be used in situations in which there is no alternative. The intramuscular or subcutaneous administration of drugs during CPR is probably ineffective.

INTRAVENOUS FLUIDS DURING CPR

Rapid volume expansion is critical in resuscitation efforts for hemorrhagic or hypovolemic cardiac arrest. Acute loss of 50% of blood volume will lead to cardiac arrest, usually in the form of asystole or electromechanical dissociation. In addition to efforts to control the hemorrhage and provide CPR, massive IV infusion with a plasma substitute is necessary. For acute resuscitation, hemoglobin (blood) is not necessary but will be required soon after resuscitation.

In CPR of hypovolemic cardiac arrest that is not secondary to exsanguination, volume expansion with crystalloids or colloids may be used.

If hypovolemia (relative or absolute) is not a consideration, IV fluids should be given only as vehicles for administration of drugs.

After successful CPR, measurements of central venous pressure and pulmonary artery pressure are frequently helpful in the overall management of the patient.

Alpha-receptor stimulation and a military antishock trouser (MAST) may be used to maintain perfusion pressure during and immediately after CPR.

TERMINATION OF CPR

CPR, once initiated, must continue until it is no longer required or necessary, based on the conditions described below.

- A preexisting contraindication to initiation of CPR (e.g., an order stating *do not resuscitate* or if the patient is in the terminal stages of an incurable disease)
- Cardiac death: Electric asystole (documented by a properly functioning ECG monitor) of 15 minutes or more in a normothermic patient, despite CPR efforts and drug treatment, is indicative of cardiac death

Brain death cannot be determined during CPR; thus efforts directed toward doing so are wasteful. Checking the pupillary light reflex during CPR, especially after the use of drugs such as epinephrine and atropine, is a ritual that should be abandoned. CPR that has been properly initiated on a suitable candidate may be stopped only after successful resuscitation or determination of cardiac death.

RESULTS

The outcome of CPR is determined by a combination of the patient's age, hemodynamic status before the arrest, cardiac rhythm at the time of arrest, preexisting cardiopulmonary disease, and the rescuer's speed in instituting basic and advanced life support. For example, primary VF in a young person with a stable preexisting hemodynamic status would have a favorable outcome as long as CPR was promptly instituted. Prompt resuscitation (as occurs in the cardiac catheterization laboratory) is almost universally successful. On the other hand, CPR for VF in a person with congestive heart failure or cardiogenic shock in whom there has been some delay in resuscitative effort is not as successful. CPR is rarely successful in brady-asystolic cardiac arrest.

The importance of speed in initiating resuscitative efforts is dramatically illustrated by the fact that in out-of-hospital cardiac arrest patients in whom basic life support is instituted within 4 minutes and advanced cardiac life support within 8 minutes, the survival rate approaches 50%. However, when basic cardiac life support is delayed more than 8 minutes and advanced cardiac life support more than 16 minutes, there have been no survivors.[46]

PATIENT AFTERCARE

Following successful CPR the following studies need to be obtained immediately:
- Complete reevaluation of the patient's condition
- Vital signs, including core temperature
- ECG
- Chest radiograph
- Serum electrolytes, magnesium, calcium, phosphorus, creatinine
- Arterial blood gases
- Cardiac enzymes
- Echocardiogram, if cardiac trauma is suspected or if intracardiac injection was done

Give special attention to the following:
- Control of hypotension
- Adequate ventilation and oxygenation
- Temperature control
- Control of struggling or seizures
- Prevention and treatment of sepsis and pulmonary infection
- Follow-up of renal function and electrolytes
- Precipitating causes of cardiac arrest and its prevention

CEREBRAL RESUSCITATION

Successful CPR is worthless without successful cerebral resuscitation. Currently accepted methods of cerebral resuscitation[5,6] are primarily supportive and passive. These include:
- Maintenance of adequate cerebral perfusion by transient hypertension immediately after CPR, followed by mild hypertension or normotension. Hypotension can be prevented by close monitoring and the use of vasopressors and volume expansion.
- Controlled ventilation with maintenance of PaO_2 of approximately 100 mm Hg and $PaCO_2$ of approximately 25 to 35 mm Hg.
- Use of barbiturate and/or phenytoin for seizure and restlessness. Neuromuscular blocking agents may be used for prevention of shivering and decerebrate posturing. Passive rewarming will also help alleviate shivering.
- Maintenance of the hematocrit at 30% to 35% with normal osmolality and electrolyte levels.
- Prevention of infection.

Intracranial pressure monitoring is rarely of help. Osmotic diuretics and corticosteroids have not been proved valuable. Barbiturate loading (thiopental—pharmacologic doses) is of no benefit.

If midbrain reflexes start returning 6 to 12 hours after CPR, prognosis for recovery is generally good. If a vegetative state persists for more than 2 weeks after CPR, recovery is not expected. Withholding supportive measures may be done at this time in consultation with the family and in accordance with medical, legal, and ethical constraints of the community.

Greater attention is now being given to the pathophysiology of brain damage after CPR and to active cerebral resuscitation during and after CPR.[46a] This has evolved along the paths of (1) reevaluation of CPR techniques and (2) active intervention techniques aimed at limiting cerebral injury and promoting cerebral resuscitation. Some active intervention techniques are described below.

• Hemodilution and controlled hypertension by fluid loading and the use of dextran 40, heparin, and vasopressors: Initial studies with systemic use of these agents did not improve cerebral resuscitation in humans; additional studies are underway.

• Barbiturate loading: Thiopental loading of victims of cardiac arrest was tested in the early 1980s after encouraging results in animals. When all victims of cardiac arrest were studied, it proved of no value in cerebral resuscitation. In a subgroup of patients with prolonged arrest time, some improvement in outcome was noted. Given the potential hazards of the technique and the close monitoring required, enthusiasm for this technique has faded.[46b]

• Use of calcium blockers: This is currently the most promising area of investigation. The aim of this technique is to reverse or prevent cerebral vasospasm and reduce intraneuronal calcium loading, which occurs following cerebral ischemia. Preliminary studies using verapamil, lidoflazine, nimodipine, flunarizine, and magnesium have been encouraging. Controlled study of this technique was initiated in 1984 with National Institutes of Health (NIH) support, and preliminary answers are expected by 1987.[36,47]

NEW CPR TECHNIQUES[48-53b]

CPR as practiced today is approximately 25 years old. Mouth-to-mouth-ventilation, external chest compression, and external defibrillation have been standardized and are taught in all medical, nursing, and paramedic critical care courses. To facilitate teaching and widespread application, various organizations (such as the AHA and American Red Cross) set standards of performance that were generally accepted as "ex cathedra," and seldom questioned. But some questions (and inquisitive questioners) would not go away! The major questions concerning CPR are discussed below.

1. If external chest compression produces cardiac output by compressing the heart (ventricles) between the sternum and the spine, why is the pressure equal in the iliac arteries and veins of animal models of CPR and in the aorta and the right atrium of humans? Why is external cardiac compression effective in a patient with obstructive lung disease and an emphysematous chest, in whom there is no chance of even reaching the ventricles, let alone compressing them?

2. If epinephrine is effective in CPR by stimulating myocardial contractility and increasing automaticity (beta action) why is isoproterenol not effective and why would methoxamine (Vasoxyl), a pure alpha blocker, be as effective as epinephrine?

3. Why is sodium bicarbonate given at the onset of CPR when arterial blood gas studies show that there is no metabolic acidosis? There is in fact respiratory alkalosis or respiratory acidosis, depending on the promptness, effectiveness, or lack of effectiveness of ventilation. Frequently, severe alkalosis is induced by the combination of effective ventilation (respiratory alkalosis) and "correct" administration of sodium bicarbonate.

4. Where are the data relating the benefit and harm of calcium chloride administration during CPR?

How the blood is propelled during CPR—the thoracic pump theory

Research during the past 6 years has shown that during chest compression, all intracardiac chambers have equal pressures. AV valves do not close during the "systole" of external cardiac compression, nor is there a change in left ventricular diameter. This makes the ventricular compression theory untenable.

The concept has been proposed, with much experimental evidence, that it is the increase in intrathoracic pressure (the thoracic pump) that propels blood flow during closed chest compression, and that the heart (all four chambers) acts as a passive conduit.[53a] External cardiac compression increases the intrathoracic pressure, which is then transmitted equally to all structures within the thoracic cavity. A pressure gradient is produced between the cardiac chambers (and the great vessels) within the thorax and the great vessels outside of the thorax, thus producing flow to the aortic arch and to the inferior vena cava, abdominal aorta, and superior vena cava. Because of valves in the brachiocephalic veins, this pressure is not transmitted to the cerebral veins; this creates a pressure gradient between the internal carotid artery and the jugular venous circuit and permits cerebral blood flow during the pressure gradient.

With this mechanism, the duration of chest compression becomes important. Within limits, increasing the duration of compression should increase cerebral flow.

Preliminary studies suggest that optimal duration of compression is approximately 50% of each cycle.

Because no veins guard the inferior vena caval, iliac, or femoral venous system, there is a transmission of the pressure in the arterial and venous circuits (no pressure gradient). Thus very little blood flows to organs below the diaphragm.

Arterial diastolic pressure[18,51,54,55]

The importance of maintaining arterial diastolic pressure during CPR has been rediscovered. It has been convincingly shown that the beneficial action of epinephrine is secondary to its alpha stimulation and peripheral vasoconstriction, and that beta stimulation has no beneficial action during CPR.

The two organs of immediate concern during CPR are the brain and the heart. Thus research in "new" CPR has focused on the importance of blood flow to these organs. The importance of a pressure gradient and therefore blood flow across the coronary bed and the brain have been emphasized. Coronary flow during CPR has been directly related to the "diastolic" pressure in the aorta and the atrium, or coronary sinus. Thus coronary flow during CPR is proportional to the aortic "diastolic" pressure minus the right atrial pressure. Similarly, cerebral flow is proportional to the dif-

ference between the internal carotid pressure and the jugular venous pressure. Thus measures that increase aortic diastolic pressure without increasing right atrial pressure should increase coronary blood flow. Measures that increase mean aortic pressure without increasing cerebral venous pressure should increase cerebral blood flow. Increasing blood flow to the brain and the heart should improve the outcome of cardiopulmonary cerebral resuscitative efforts. The ongoing efforts to develop a new and improved CPR are being directed at studying these functions in greater depth (Table 18-6).

The following conclusions can be drawn from the data available as of 1986.

"Old" CPR of 25 years ago remains empirically useful and effective, but far from perfect and probably can and will be improved on.

Techniques that improve (or should improve) blood flow to the heart and the brain (increased alpha stimulation, higher chest compression force, intermittent abdominal compression CPR) have the *potential* of improving the results of CPR, but their potential for damage has not been fully explored and as yet they have not been fully tested in animals or humans.

Improved techniques of CPR are gradually being incorporated into practice (see recommendations of the National Conference on Standards and Guidelines for

Table 18-6. Effects of various CPR techniques in the animal model

	Arterial pressure	Cardiac output	Cerebral perfusion	Myocardial perfusion	Survival	Comments
Epinephrine	↑	↑	↑	↑	↑	Of proven benefit in animals; other (pure alpha) stimulants being studied
Pneumatic CPR (vest and binder CPR)	↑	↑	↑	NC	NS	Animal experiments encouraging, showing improved survival
Simultaneous compression-ventilation CPR	↑	↑	↑	NC	NC	Needs intubation and mechanical ventilation; risk of lung barotrauma
Abdominal counterpulsation during conventional CPR	↑	↑	↑	NC	NC	Risk of trauma to liver and spleen; Potential of regurgitation and aspiration
Abdominal binding during conventional CPR	↑	↑ or NC		NS	NS	Animal experiments discouraging
High-impulse CPR	↑	↑	↑	↑	NS	Increased potential of trauma
Volume loading during conventional CPR	↑	↑	↓	↓	NS	Animal experiments discouraging
Military antishock trousers during CPR	↑	NS	NS	NS	NC	Requires additional equipment

Adapted and reprinted with permission from Cheng, T.O., editor: International textbook of cardiology, New York, copyright 1986, Pergamon Press.

↑, increased; ↓, decreased; *NC*, no change; *NS*, not studied.

Cardiopulmonary Resuscitation and Emergency Cardiac Care, Dallas, August 1985).* As research clarifies the benefits and risks of the techniques for increasing cerebral and coronary blood flow and cerebral and myocardial protection, these methods may be incorporated into the CPR procedure.[53b] Widespread application of these innovative and experimental techniques before adequate testing is discouraged.

COUGH CPR

Cough CPR[56] is very valuable in critical care units or cardiovascular procedure rooms. During cough there is an increase in intrathoracic and intra-abdominal pressure similar to that achieved by vigorous external chest compression with intermittent abdominal compression. Animal experiments and observations in humans have established cough CPR as an effective way to administer CPR and achieve adequate cerebral perfusion. Patients at risk of developing cardiac arrest should be instructed in the proper technique of coughing—two deep, strong coughs using chest and abdominal muscles followed by deep inspiration. At the onset of cardiopulmonary arrest, and before loss of consciousness, the resuscitation is started by cough CPR, permitting the use of drugs and defibrillation in a more orderly fashion.

OPEN-CHEST CPR

Before 1960, open-chest CPR was the only form of CPR with an overall survival rate of 28%.[57] With the widespread acceptance of closed-chest CPR and the availability of the external defibrillator, open-chest CPR was relegated to the cardiothoracic operating room. However, there is a role for open-chest CPR outside of the cardiothoracic surgical suite.

Indications for open-chest CPR are cardiac arrest with penetrating chest trauma and uncontrolled intrathoracic hemorrhage or cardiac tamponade, cardiac arrest with flail or deformed chest or following cardiac surgery when external cardiac compression may be ineffective, massive air embolism, and severe hypothermia, for which external defibrillation may not be effective.

Failed external CPR is not generally an indication for open-chest CPR. Rarely, open-chest defibrillation may be effective when external defibrillation has not been. If open-chest CPR is to be effective, it should be instituted early in the course of resuscitation and before irreversible myocardial damage has occurred. Open-chest cardiac resuscitation should not be attempted outside a fully staffed and equipped medical facility or by personnel who do not possess basic surgical skills.

---

*Montgomery, W.H.: J.A.M.A. **255**:2990-2991, 1986.

MEDICOLEGAL CONCERNS

Important medicolegal issues are involved in CPR.[58,59] A nurse or physician can be held liable for performing or not performing CPR, irrespective of the results of the resuscitative efforts. Medical, social, religious, personal, and economic issues are closely interwoven into a set of medicolegal guidelines to help patients and their physicians and nurses deal with this issue. The following recommendations are made as general guidelines.

In the absence of a written DNR order by a patient's attending physician, patients who sustain cardiopulmonary arrest should have full efforts at resuscitation. When patients reach the terminal stage of an incurable disease, the issue of resuscitation should be addressed, and such a decision documented in the patient's chart.

A DNR order is given by the physician (1) at the request or with the informed agreement of a competent patient or (2) with input from nurses, clergy, and family and with the agreement of the incompetent patient's family or guardian.

In complicated cases, such as a pregnant patient with a viable fetus, or a case in which serious disagreement exists among family members, nursing staff, or consulting physicians, then additional medical consultation should be sought. Hospital ethics committees have been helpful in such circumstances.

A DNR order should be clear, complete, and in writing. It should state "in the event of cardiac arrest, do not resuscitate." Shortcuts (such as no code, minicode, slow code, medical code only, or chemical code) should not be accepted. Such an order should be followed by clarification of the level of care and intervention to be given. Issues of intubation, mechanical ventilation, and use of defibrillator or pacemakers need to be addressed. In special situations the use of blood transfusion or fluid resuscitation may also have to be addressed. It is important to keep in mind that DNR does not mean stopping further care for the patient. The medical record should contain complete documentation as to the patient's medical condition and the circumstances of the DNR order. This record should be updated periodically.

A physician's or nurse's best protection from an unwarranted medical malpractice suit is to act in good faith, follow the standards of care of CPR formulated by the appropriate bodies, maintain the skills in basic and advanced life support, maintain necessary certification in these skills, and not deviate from these standards except for very good reasons. Document your actions in writing at the first opportunity.

FUTURE DEVELOPMENTS

Developments in cardiopulmonary cerebral resuscitation during this decade are expected in the areas described below.

Bystander defibrillation

The value of early defibrillation is universally accepted. Small portable and "user friendly" battery-operated defibrillators have been developed that distinguish between VF or asystole and deliver a defibrillating shock, based on the underlying rhythm. These units are undergoing field testing.[60,61] Such units will be placed in areas of population concentration and will be operated by minimally trained personnel. Also, patients with high risk of sudden death may go home with such units, to be operated by family members. In short, defibrillation will probably be included in basic cardiac life support.[62-65]

Techniques of basic cardiac life support

Techniques of ventilation and chest compression during basic cardiac life support will probably change after experiments in new CPR are evaluated in animal and human studies. Mechanical devices to improve chest compression (such as VEST CPR) are being tested.[66,67]

Pharmacology

Pharmacology of CPR may improve. More effective ways of maintaining or increasing arterial diastolic pressure will probably be developed.

Cerebral resuscitation

Efforts at cerebral resuscitation are in their infancy. The role (if any) of calcium-blocking agents should be clarified. The value of cerebrospinal fluid creatine phosphokinase (BB fraction) assay in the evaluation of brain injury may be tested. Interest and research in open-chest CPR may be revived.

Automatic implanted defibrillator

The automatic implanted cardioverter defibrillator (AICD) has already made an impact on survivors of CPR. More widespread use of the AICD is expected when it is further developed.

Economics

In an era of economic limits (prospective payment, cost containment measures, prepaid medical insurance plans) the use of CPR, like any other expensive medical technique, will be closely scrutinized. Utilization review will be more vigorous and decisions of whether to resuscitate a victim will be closely monitored. Medical and ethical issues may come into conflict with economic concerns.

SUGGESTED APPROACHES IN MONITORED CARDIAC ARREST

Ventricular tachycardia-fibrillation

1. Have the patient perform cough CPR if he or she is awake and able to cough.
2. Perform a precordial thump.
3. If VF is present, defibrillate the patient with 200 J; you may repeat defibrillation twice at 300 and 360 J, respectively.
4. If VF persists, initiate chest compression and positive-pressure ventilation. Start an IV infusion line.
5. Administer epinephrine 1:10,000, 5 to 10 ml (0.5 to 1 mg) intravenously or via the intratracheal route.
6. After 30 to 60 seconds of ventilation and chest compression, defibrillate the patient again with 360 J. Repeat if necessary.
7. Administer lidocaine if defibrillation is successful. Bretylium may be preferred if VF is refractory.
8. Administer sodium bicarbonate (1 mEq/kg IV push) if *metabolic acidosis* is documented by arterial blood gas studies.
9. If VF persists, try to improve ventilation and oxygenation, continue CPR, and obtain arterial blood gas measurements. Repeat sodium bicarbonate administration guided by arterial blood gases.
10. Repeat epinephrine administration (0.5 to 1 mg IV push).
11. Repeat defibrillation at 360 J.
12. Consider using other drugs (magnesium, nitroglycerin, additional bretylium).
13. Consider using methods of "new" CPR.

Asystole

1. Have the patient perform cough CPR, if applicable.
2. Attempt precordial thump pacing.
3. Institute airway control, ventilation, and external chest compression.
4. Administer epinephrine (0.5 to 1 mg) intravenously or via the intratracheal route.
5. Administer atropine (1 to 2 mg) intravenously or via the intratracheal route.
6. Continue external cardiac compression and try to improve ventilation and oxygenation.
7. Administer a DC shock of 200 to 300 J (for the possibility of VF mimicking asystole).
8. Consider using a pacemaker, either the external

transcutaneous pacer or a transvenous pacer. Transthoracic intracardiac pacing may be used if other methods are not available.

9. Try to improve CPR by applying "new" CPR techniques.

Electromechanical dissociation

In the absence of hypovolemia, cardiac tamponade, cardiac rupture, or tension pneumothorax, electromechanical dissociation usually indicates diffuse myocardial ischemia.

1. Institute basic CPR.
2. Administer epinephrine 1:10,000 (5 to 10 ml; 0.5 to 1 mg) intravenously or via the intratracheal route. This may be repeated in 5 minutes.
3. Administer calcium chloride (2.5 to 5 ml 10%) (this helps in approximately 10% of patients).
4. Try to improve ventilation and oxygenation.
5. Institute more effective CPR.
6. Administer sodium bicarbonate (1 mEq/kg) if metabolic acidosis is demonstrated.
7. Check for hypovolemia or exsanguination, ineffective CPR, cardiac tamponade (consider open-chest CPR), or tension pneumothorax.
8. Administer IV nitroglycerin if coronary spasm is a possibility.

SUGGESTED APPROACHES IN UNMONITORED CARDIAC ARREST

The approach to unmonitored cardiac arrest is similar to that for monitored cardiac arrest. The rescuer is guided by doing what can be done first.

1. Institute CPR, with control of airway, ventilation, and chest compression.
2. Defibrillate the patient as soon as possible. Do not waste precious time trying to distinguish between asystole and fine VF; defibrillation should be promptly performed. Administer a precordial thump if a defibrillator is not available.

REFERENCES

1. Kouwenhoven, W.B., Jude, J.R., and Knickerbocker, G.G.: Closed chest cardiac massage, J.A.M.A. 173:1064, 1960.
2. Kouwenhoven, W.B., Ingr, D.R., and Langworthy, O.R.: Cardiopulmonary resuscitation. An account of forty-five years of research, J.A.M.A. 226:877-881, 1973.
3. Fye, W.B.: Ventricular fibrillation and defibrillation: historical perspectives with emphasis on the contributions of John MacWilliam, Carl Wiggers, and William Kouwenhoven, Circulation 71:858-865, 1985.
4. Guthrie, C.C., Pike, F.H., and Sterrart, G.N.: The maintenance of cerebral activity in mammals by artificial circulation, Am. J. Physiol. 17:344, 1906.
5. Safar, P.: Recent advances in cardiopulmonary-cerebral resuscitation: a review, Ann. Emerg. Med. 13:856-862, 1984.
6. Safer, P.: Cardiopulmonary-cerebral resuscitation. In Shoemaker, W.C., Thompson, W.L., and Holbrook, P.R.: Textbook of critical care, Philadelphia, 1984, W.B. Saunders Co.
7. Nagel, E.L., Fine, E.G., Krischer, J.P., and Davis, J.H.: Complications of CPR, Crit. Care Med. 9:424-425, 1981.
8. Powner, D.J., et al.: Cardiopulmonary resuscitation–related injuries, Crit. Care Med. 12:54-55, 1984.
9. Ewy, G.A.: Recent advances in cardiopulmonary resuscitation and defibrillation, Curr. Probl. Cardiol. 8:5-42, 1983.
10. Ewy, G.A., Dahl, C.F., Zimmerman, M., and Otto, C.: Ventricular fibrillation masquerading as ventricular standstill, Crit. Care Med. 9:841-844, 1981.
11. Weaver, W.D., et al.: Amplitude of ventricular fibrillation waveform and outcome after cardiac arrest, Ann. Intern. Med. 102:53-55, 1985.
12. Stauffer, J.L.: Establishment and care of the airway. In Petty, T.L., editor: Intensive and rehabilitative respiratory care, Philadelphia, 1982, Lea & Febiger.
13. White, R.D., Goldberg, A.H., and Montgomery, W.H.: Adjuncts for airway control and ventilation. In McIntyre, K.M., and Lewis, A.J., editors: Advanced Cardiac Life Support, 1983, American Heart Association.
13a. Roberts, D.J., Clinton, J.E., and Ruiz, E.: Neuromuscular blockade for critical patients in the emergency department, Ann. Emerg. Med. 15:152-156, 1986.
14. Schecter, W.P., and Wilson, R.S.: Management of upper airway obstruction in the intensive care unit, Crit. Care Med. 9:577-579, 1981.
15. Kress, T.K.: Cricothyroidotomy, Ann. Emerg. Med. 11:197-201, 1982.
16. Zoll, P.M., et al.: External noninvasive temporary cardiac pacing: clinical trials, Circulation 71:937-944, 1985.
17. Dalsey, W.C., Syverud, S.A., and Hedges J.R.: Emergency department use of transcutaneous pacing for cardiac arrests, Crit. Care Med. 13:399-401, 1985.
18. Yakaitis, R.W., Otto, C.W., and Blitt, C.D.: Relative importance of alpha and beta adrenergic receptors during resuscitation, Crit. Care Med. 7:293, 1979.
19. Brillman, J.C., et al.: Comparison of epinephrine and phenylephrine for resuscitation and neurologic outcome of cardiac arrest in animals, Ann. Emerg. Med. 14:495, 1985.
20. Ralston, S.H., Showen, L., Carter, A., and Tacker, W.A.: Comparison of endotracheal and intravenous epinephrine dosage during CPR in dogs, Ann. Emerg. Med. 14:495, 1985.
21. Anderson, J.L.: Antifibrillatory versus antiectopic therapy, Am. J. Cardiol. 54:7A-13A, 1984.
21a. Chow, M.S.S., et al.: Antifibrillatory effects of lidocaine and bretylium immediately postcardiopulmonary resuscitation, Am. Heart J. 110:938, 1985.
22. Kerber, R.E., et al.: Effect of lidocaine and bretylium on energy requirements for transthoracic defibrillation: experimental studies, J. Am. Coll. Cardiol. 7:397-405, 1986.
23. Koch-Weser, J.: Bretylium, N. Engl. J. Med. 300:473-477, 1979.
24. Castle, L.: Therapy of ventricular tachycardia, Am. J. Cardiol. 54:26A-33A, 1984.
25. Haynes, R.E., Chinn, T.L., Copass, M.K., and Cobb, L.A.: Comparison of bretylium tosylate and lidocaine in management of out of hospital ventricular fibrillation: a randomized clinical trial, Am. J. Cardiol. 48:353-356, 1981.
26. Mayer, N.M.: Management of ventricular dysrhythmias in the prehospital and emergency department setting. Am. J. Cardiol. 54:34A-36A, 1984.

27. Tacker, W.A., et al.: The effect of newer antiarrhythmic drugs on defibrillation threshold, Crit. Care Med. **8:**177-180, 1980.

28. Euler, D.E., and Scanlon, P.J.: Mechanism of the effect of bretylium on the ventricular fibrillation threshold in dogs, Am. J. Cardiol. **55:**1396-1401, 1985.

29. Weil, M.H.: Iatrogenic alkalosis in CPR. In Schlunger, J.O., and Lyon, K.A., (editors): CPR and emergency cardiac care: looking to the future, New York, 1980, EM Books.

30. Nieman, J.T., and Rosborough, J.P.: Effects of acidemia and sodium bicarbonate therapy in advanced cardiac life support. II. Ann. Emerg. Med. **13:**781-784, 1984.

31. Bishop, R.L., and Weisfeldt, M.: Sodium bicarbonate administration during cardiac arrest. Effect on arterial pH, PCO_2, and osmolality, J.A.M.A. **235:**506-509, 1976.

32. Ward, W.G., and Reid, R.L.: High-dose intravenous nitroglycerin during cardiopulmonary resuscitation for refractory cardiac arrest, Am. J. Cardiol. **53:**1725, 1984.

33. Stueven, H.A., et al.: Lack of effectiveness of calcium chloride in refractory asystole, Ann. Emerg. Med. **14:**630-632, 1985.

34. Harrison, E.E., and Amey, B.D.: The use of calcium in cardiac resuscitation, Am. J. Emerg. Med. **1:**267-273, 1983.

35. Stueven, H.A., et al.: The effectiveness of calcium chloride in refractory electromechanical dissociation, Ann. Emerg. Med. **14:**626-629, 1985.

36. Schwartz, A.C.: Cerebral resuscitation in the community hospital. II. Ann. Emerg. Med. **13:**872-875, 1984.

37. French, J.H., et al.: Magnesium therapy in massive digoxin intoxication, Ann. Emerg. Med. **13:**562-563, 1984.

38. Iseri, L.T., Freed, J., and Bures, A.R.: Magnesium deficiency and cardiac disorders, Am. J. Med. **58:**837-846, 1975.

39. Iseri, L.T., Chung, P., and Tobis, J.: Magnesium therapy for intractable ventricular tachyarrhythmias in normomagnesemic patients, West. J. Med. **138:**823-828, 1983.

40. Tzivoni, D., et al.: Magnesium therapy for torsades de pointes, Am. J. Cardiol. **53:**528-530, 1984.

41. Iseri, L.T., Fairshter, R.D., Hardemann, J.L., and Brodsky, M.A.: Magnesium and potassium therapy in multifocal atrial tachycardia, Am. Heart J. **110:**789-794, 1985.

42. Jacob, A.S., Nielsen, D.H., and Gianelly, R.E.: Fatal ventricular fibrillation following verapamil in Wolff-Parkinson-White syndrome with atrial fibrillation, Ann. Emerg. Med. **14:**159-160, 1985.

43. Norris, R.M., et al.: Prevention of ventricular fibrillation during acute myocardial infarction by intravenous propranolol, Lancet **2:**883-886, 1984.

44. Selzer, A.: Role of serum digoxin assay in patient management, J. Am. Coll. Cardiol. **5:**106A-110A, 1985.

45. Doan, L.A.: Peripheral versus central venous delivery of medications during CPR, Ann. Emerg. Med. **13:**784-786, 1984.

45a. Talit, U., et al.: Pharmacokinetic differences between peripheral and central drug administration during cardiopulmonary resuscitation, J. Am. Coll. Cardiol. **6:**1073-1077, 1985.

45b. Hasegawa, E.A.J.: The endotracheal use of emergency drugs, Pharmacol. Crit. Care **15:**60-63, 1986.

46. Eisenberg, M.S., Bergner, and Hallstrom, A.P.: Cardiac resuscitation in the community: importance of rapid provision and implications of program planning, J.A.M.A. **241:**1905-1907, 1979.

46a. Bass, E.: Cardiopulmonary arrest, Ann. Intern. Med. **103:**920-927, 1985.

46b. Brain Resuscitation Clinical Trial I Study Group: Randomized clinical study of thiopental loading in comatose survivors of cardiac arrest, N. Engl. J. Med. **314:**397-403, 1986.

47. White, B.C., Winegar, C.D., Wilson, R.F., and Drause, G.S.: Calcium blockers in cerebral resuscitation, J. Trauma **23:**788-794, 1983.

48. Niemann, J.T.: Differences in cerebral and myocardial perfusion during closed-chest resuscitation. II. Ann. Emerg. Med. **13:**849-853, 1984.

49. Butler, J.: The heart is in good hands, Circulation **67:**1163-1168, 1983.

50. Rudikoff, M.T., et al.: Mechanisms of blood flow during cardiopulmonary resuscitation, Circulation **61:**345-352, 1980.

51. Joyce, S.M., Barssan, W.G., and Doan, L.A.: Use of phenylephrine in resuscitation from asphyxial arrest, Ann. Emerg. Med. **12:**418-421, 1983.

52. Kern, K.B., et al.: Twenty-four hour survival in a canine model of cardiac arrest comparing three methods of manual cardiopulmonary resuscitation, J. Am. Coll. Cardiol. **7:**859-867, 1986.

53. Criley, J.M., Niemann, J.T., and Rosborough, J.P.: Cardiopulmonary resuscitation research 1960-1984: discoveries and advances. II. Ann. Emerg. Med. **13:**756-758, 1984.

53a. Halperin, H.R., et al.: Determinants of blood flow to vital organs during cardiopulmonary resuscitation in dogs, Circulation **73:**539-550, 1986.

53b. Krause, G.S., et al.: Ischemia, resuscitation, and reperfusion: mechanisms of tissue injury and prospects for protection, Am. Heart J. **111:**768, 1986.

54. Ewy, G.A.: Current status of cardiopulmonary resuscitation, Mod. Conc. Cardiovasc. Dis. **53:**43-45, 1984.

55. Sanders, A.B., et al.: Importance of the duration of inadequate coronary perfusion pressure on resuscitation from cardiac arrest, J. Am. Coll Cardiol. **6:**113-118, 1985.

56. Criley, J.M., Blaufuss, A.H., and Kissel, G.L.: Cough-induced cardiac compression. Self-administered form of cardiopulmonary resuscitation J.A.M.A. **236:**1246-1250, 1976.

57. Stephenson, H.E. Jr.: Cardiac arrest and resuscitation, ed. 4, St. Louis, 1974, The C.V. Mosby Co.

58. Chernow, B., Seeland, A.D., and Snyder, R.: Orders not to resuscitate: the DNR patient (editorial), Crit. Care Med. **12:**922-923, 1984.

59. Lo, B., et al.: "Do Not Resuscitate" decisions: a prospective study at three teaching hospitals, Arch. Intern. Med. **145:**1115-1117, 1985.

60. Cummins, R.O., et al.: Automatic external defibrillators: clinical, training, psychological, and public health issues, Ann. Emerg. Med. **14:**755-760, 1985.

61. Cummings, R.O., Bergner, L., Eisenberg, M., and Murray, J.A.: Sensitivity, accuracy, and safety of an automatic external defibrillator, Lancet **1:**318-320, 1984.

62. Weaver, W.D., et al.: Improved neurologic recovery and survival after early defibrillation, Circulation **69:**943-948, 1984.

63. Weaver, W.D., et al.: Amplitude of ventricular fibrillation waveform and outcome after cardiac arrest, Ann. Intern. Med. **102:**53-55, 1985.

64. Stults, K.R., Brown, D.D., and Kerber, R.E.: Efficacy of an automated external defibrillator in the management of out-of-hospital cardiac arrest: validation of the diagnostic algorithm and initial clinical experience in a rural environment, Circulation **73:**701-709, 1986.

65. Weaver, W.D., et al.: Factors influencing survival after out-of-hospital cardiac arrest, J. Am. Coll. Cardiol. **7:**752-757, 1986.

66. Niemann, J.T.: Differences in cerebral and myocardial perfusion during closed-chest resuscitation, Ann. Emerg. Med. **13:**849-853, 1984.

67. Niemann, J.T., et al.: Mechanical "cough" cardiopulmonary resuscitation during cardiac arrest in dogs, Am. J. Cardiol. **55:**199-204, 1985.

ADDITIONAL SOURCES

Harwood, A.L., editor: Cardiopulmonary resuscitation, Baltimore, 1982, Williams & Wilkins Co.

Greenberg, M.I., Gernard, M.D., and Roberts, J.R., editors: Advanced techniques in resuscitation, Baltimore, 1985, Williams & Wilkins Co.

Standards and guidelines for cardiopulmonary resuscitation (CPR) and emergency cardiac care (ECC), J.A.M.A. **255:**2905, 1986.

Safar, P.: Cardiopulmonary cerebral resuscitation. A manual for physicians and paramedical instructors, Philadelphia, 1981, W.B. Saunders Co.

Chapter Nineteen

Contrast media toxicity and allergic reactions

ARA G. TILKIAN
ELAINE K. DAILY

RADIOGRAPHIC CONTRAST MEDIA TOXICITY

The first cardiac angiography was performed in dogs in 1933. In 1959 selective coronary arteriography was first performed in humans, opening the door for surgical correction of cardiovascular disease. Today the use of radiographic contrast media is widespread in diagnostic cardiology and radiology; many of the procedures described in this text require intravenous or intra-arterial injection of radiographic contrast material. These agents have a distinct toxicity and their use assumes some degree of discomfort and risk to the patient. These risks can be divided into two categories: those related to the chemical or osmolar toxicity of the agent, which will be discussed in this section, and those related to idiosyncratic reactions, which resemble anaphylactic reactions, but may not be true allergic reactions. These "allergic" reactions are discussed later in this chapter.

Conventional contrast agents

All ionic intravascular contrast media in general use until the early 1980s consisted of water-soluble salts of substituted tri-iodinated benzoic acids.[1] Three of these acids (anions) in common use are diatrizoic acid, iothalamic acid, and metrizoic acid. They are in combination with a cation, usually sodium or methylglucamine (meglumine), providing three iodine atoms per two salt molecules (Fig. 19-1). Numerous formulations of sodium or meglumine with diatrizoate, iothalamate, or metrizoate have been marketed with iodine content varying from 270 to 440 mg/ml and with a wide range of osmolality, viscosity, and sodium content.

Table 19-1 lists some of the more commonly used ionic radiocontrast media and their characteristics. These agents are marketed under a variety of names throughout the world and with a variable mixture of salts in varying concentrations and for different needs. For a detailed compilation of various trade names and concentrations see Strain.[1]

For the same iodine content (radiographic contrast capacity), sodium salt solutions have a lower viscosity than meglumine salts, permitting a higher delivery rate and better image contrast. Unfortunately, formulations with high sodium content are more toxic to the heart and brain. Thus most radiographic contrast agents used in cardiovascular medicine employ a solution of mixed sodium and meglumine salts to achieve a satisfactory combination of acceptable viscosity, toxicity, and radiocontrast. Calcium and magnesium ions are substituted for a small proportion of the sodium in some formulations (Isopaque, Triosil) to reduce toxicity while maintaining a lower viscosity.

In solution these salts dissolve into anions and cations that possess a very high osmolality of 1500 to 2000 milliosmoles (mOsm)/kg. The cationic composition of these salts, along with their increased osmolality, is primarily responsible for the clinical toxicity of radiocontrast agents. The iodinated anions are generally considered nontoxic.

Newer contrast agents

During the last decade efforts have been aimed at developing contrast media with lower osmolality and therefore reduced toxicity.[2-11a] In 1972, a high molecular weight nonionic agent, metrizamide (Amipaque), was introduced; its osmolality is one third to one quarter of other agents for a similar amount of iodine delivery. It is clearly less toxic to the central nervous system, myocardium, and arteries. Metrizamide is widely used in myelography but its cost has prohibited more general use in angiography. In addition, metrizamide is not stable in dissolved form and cannot be ster-

435

Table 19-1. Commonly used contrast media

Composition	Proprietary name (in U.S.)	Source in U.S.	Date introduced	Osmolality*
Sodium and meglumine diatrizoate	Renografin-76‡	Squibb	1953	1700
	Urografin	Schering	1953 to 1967	Variable (1400 to 2400)
	Hypaque§	Winthrop		
	Angiovist§	Berlex		
Sodium and meglumine iothalamate	Conray	Mallinckrodt		Same as above
Sodium meglumine, and calcium metrizoate	Isopaque	Winthrop		
	Triosil	Glaxo		Same as above
New low-osmolar contrast media				
Metrizamide (nonionic)	Amipaque	Winthrop	1972	580 485
Sodium and meglumine ioxaglate (ionic)¶	Hexabrix	Mallinckrodt	1976	600
Iopamidol (nonionic)	Isovue	Squibb	1979	796
Iohexol (nonionic)	Omnipaque	Winthrop-Breon	1980	844 672
Iopromide (nonionic)		Schering (Germany)	1980	670
Iotasul (nonionic)		Schering	1980	300
Iotrol (nonionic)	Iotrolan	Berlex	1983	360

*Osmolality of blood is approximately 300 mOsm/kg at 37° C (see Fig. 19-2 for more information).

†Most preparations for coronary arteriography have a sodium content of 140 to 190 mEq/L to reduce the risk of ventricular fibrillation.

‡Renografin-76, which contains 10% sodium diatrizoate, 66% meglumine diatrizoate, 0.04 mg/ml sodium EDTA, and 0.32 mg/ml sodium citrate, is used as an example. Each of these formulations come in a variety of concentrations and therefore varying iodine content, osmolality, and viscosity. For individual agent, consult appropriate product insert.

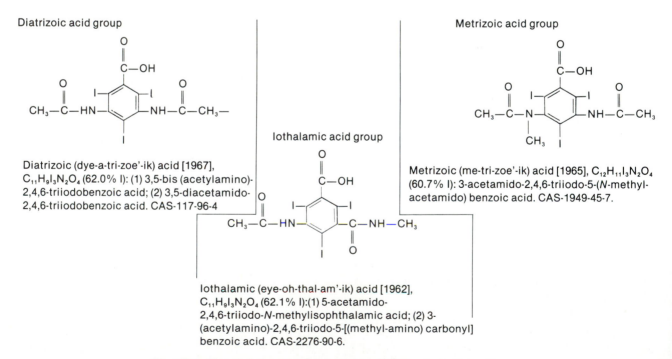

Diatrizoic acid group

Diatrizoic (dye-a-tri-zoe'-ik) acid [1967], $C_{11}H_9I_3N_2O_4$ (62.0% I): (1) 3,5-bis (acetylamino)-2,4,6-triiodobenzoic acid; (2) 3,5-diacetamido-2,4,6-triiodobenzoic acid. CAS-117-96-4

Iothalamic acid group

Iothalamic (eye-oh-thal-am'-ik) acid [1962], $C_{11}H_9I_3N_2O_4$ (62.1% I):(1) 5-acetamido-2,4,6-triiodo-N-methylisophthalamic acid; (2) 3-(acetylamino)-2,4,6-triiodo-5-[(methyl-amino) carbonyl] benzoic acid. CAS-2276-90-6.

Metrizoic acid group

Metrizoic (me-tri-zoe'-ik) acid [1965], $C_{12}H_{11}I_3N_2O_4$ (60.7% I): 3-acetamido-2,4,6-triiodo-5-(N-methyl-acetamido) benzoic acid. CAS-1949-45-7.

Fig. 19-1. Chemical formulas for diatrizoate, iothalamate, and metrizoate.

Viscosity (Centipoise at 37° C)	Iodine content (mg/ml)	pH	Sodium content† (mEq/L)	Clinical features
9	370	7-7.6	190	Reduced cardiovascular toxicity; most popular agent for cardiovascular angiography
Variable (2.5-12)	Variable (270-370)	Variable (6.5-7.5)	Variable (1-1050)	
Same as above	Same as above	Same as above	Same as above	Reduced neurotoxicity; increased cardiovascular toxicity
Same as above	Same as above	Same as above	Same as above	Slightly reduced osmolality & viscosity
16	370	7.4	0	Reduced toxicity and side effects
6.2	300			
7.5	320	6-7.6		Same as above
9.5	370‖		0	Same as above
10.4	350	6.8-7.7	0	Same as above
6.3	300			
6.2	320		0	Same as above
	400		0	Same as above
9.2	300	6-8	0	Same as above

§Hypaque-76 and Angiovist-370 have no calcium-binding sodium EDTA. Instead they contain disodium calcium EDTA and a sodium content of 140 and 150 mEq/L, respectively, and are reported to cause reduced incidence of ventricular fibrillation in animals and humans.

‖Available in lesser iodine content and proportionally less osmolality and viscosity, as illustrated for iohexol and metrizamide.

¶Ionic, but low-osmolality contrast medium, salt of the hexaiodinated acid, ioxaglate. Less toxic than conventional agents, but generally produces more side effects than nonionic agents.

ilized by heating; it therefore needs reconstitution just before use. Two other nonionic low-osmolar contrast agents, iopamidol (Isovue) and iohexol (Omnipaque), are in various stages of development and testing; they are stable in solution and can be autoclaved. Another agent approved by the FDA for clinical use is the ionic contrast medium ioxaglate (Hexabrix), which is a sodium and meglumine salt of ioxalic acid and has an iodine content that is 14% greater than meglumine iothalamate and an osmolality of only 40% of the salt (see Table 19-1). The almost ideal radiographic contrast agent may be found in iotasul, which is isoosmolar and has an iodine concentration of 400 mg/ml (Table 19-1). This agent is under investigation. Fig. 19-2 plots osmolality versus various iodine concentrations for three of the new contrast media as compared with conventional media.

It is clearly established that the newer, low-osmolar contrast media, while delivering the same amount of iodine content (same contrast effect) as conventional agents, are essentially painless and cause minimal symptoms of warmth. They cause less depression of cardiac function, less volume expansion and less injury to the endothelial lining of the vessels and organs and have reduced nephrotoxicity and neurotoxicity. The anticoagulant effect is also less pronounced. The risk of idiosyncratic anaphylactic-like reaction may also be less, but definitive data on this are not yet available.[2-11] A limiting factor in the use of these new agents is their cost. When compared with conventional agents, the cost per gram of iodine content may be 5 to 10 times greater for ioxoglate and 10 to 20 times greater for the nonionic agents, iopamidol and iohexol. Metrizamide is approximately 50 to 100 times as expensive as conventional agents per gram of iodine content.

Currently, given the limited availability of these low-osmolar agents (costly or still investigational), their use is indicated in selected cases, including infants, patients with preexisting renal disease, pulmonary hypertension, sickle cell disease, or myelomatosis, and patients with congestive heart failure, depressed left ventricular function, unstable angina, or arrhythmias. These agents

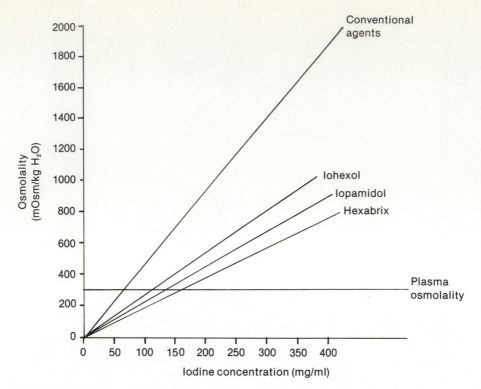

Fig. 19-2. A plot of osmolality against iodine concentration for the new and conventional contrast media. (From Dawson, P., Grainger, R.G., and Pitfield, J.: The new low-osmolar contrast media: a simple guide, Clin. Radiol. **34:**221-226, 1983.)

should also be considered for use in patients for whom arteriography is particularly painful. They may be a satisfactory alternative for patients with a past history of anaphylactic-type reaction to radiographic contrast material (see p. 444).

Types of toxicity[2,5,10,12,13]

The high osmolality of currently used radiographic contrast agents is the primary cause of their adverse reactions. The idiosyncratic anaphylactic-like reaction (see p. 442) may be an exception to this, although the early experience with the low-osmolar nonionic agent, metrizamide, suggests that even these "allergic" reactions may be avoided with the reduction of osmolality. The anions (iodinated ions) are generally considered to be nontoxic. The cations contribute to toxicity (sodium more than meglumine), especially cardiotoxicity, with increasing frequency of ventricular fibrillation during coronary arteriography if sodium content is appreciably higher or lower than 140 mEq/L. High concentrations of sodium are also neurotoxic and may cause seizures. Still, the major toxicity of the agents is the result of their hyperosmolality.

The osmolality of contrast agents ranges from 1400 to 2400 mOsm/kg, five to eight times that of plasma. When injected in large amounts (total volumes of 100 to 250 ml) or into end arteries (such as those in the brain, heart, or kidney), they can cause fluid shifts that have adverse effects on the specific organ or general adverse effects secondary to changes in equilibrium of body fluids.

Specific organ toxicities caused by contrast agents
The blood

As the hyperosmolar contrast agent is injected into the bloodstream, it raises the osmolality of the plasma, causing a shift of fluid from within the red cells to the plasma. The erythrocytes shrink and become deformed and rigid and their intracellular viscosity increases so that they cannot change their shape to fit through small capillaries. This may result in an increase in peripheral resistance to blood flow and tissue anoxia. This effect is directly proportional to the total volume of radiocontrast material and the rate at which this volume is injected into the circulation. This effect on red blood cells is particularly hazardous in patients with preexisting red blood cell abnormalities, such as sickle cell disease. It may also be a major contributing element to cardiovascular collapse and death, which may occur when a large amount of contrast agent is injected in the pulmonary vessels in a patient with severe preexisting pulmonary hypertension. These red blood cell changes may also contribute to the impairment of renal function. The low-osmolar contrast agents cause much less damage to red cells and are the agents of choice when angiography is needed for patients with sickle cell disease.

Coagulation

Radiographic contrast agents inhibit platelet aggregation and affect coagulation factors. They increase coagulation time, decrease prothombin effect, and have a slight fibrinolytic action. Clinically these effects do not seem to predispose the patient to appreciable bleeding.

Contrast media and pain

Radiographic contrast agents, when injected directly in peripheral arteries, cause pain. In clinical peripheral arteriography this pain can be severe, and occasionally studies are done with the patient under heavy sedation or even general anesthesia. The mechanism of pain is probably multifactorial. Vascular spasm or vasodilation has long been implicated. Vasodilation may be the mechanism of the warm and flushed feeling that patients experience, but it is unlikely that it is the actual cause of pain. Contrast media–induced pain is most likely secondary to biochemical processes that are activated in the capillary circulation, leading to depolarization of paravascular neuroreceptive terminals.[14] Pain is much reduced and is frequently absent when nonionic low-osmolar agents are used in peripheral arteriography.

Capillary endothelium

Damage to capillary endothelial cells and altered vascular permeability occur in direct proportion to the osmolality of the contrast agent. Most of this damage appears to be reversible. Damage to cerebral capillary endothelium may expose highly vulnerable nerve cells to the toxic anions of the contrast agents, resulting in neurotoxicity with various manifestations of central nervous system dysfunction, including seizures. Damage to venous endothelium in venography can cause phlebitis and thrombophlebitis, with their secondary complications. Vascular endothelial damage may be one mechanism producing the anaphylactic type of reaction, with activation of the coagulation, fibrinolytic, and kallikrein cascades. Nonionic or low-osmolar agents are clearly less toxic to capillary endothelium and have re-

duced neurotoxicity and cerebral edema after angiography.

Cardiovascular and hemodynamic effects and cardiotoxicity[4,5,7,8,15-24]

Local vasodilation of the peripheral vascular bed is the direct result of hyperosmolality of the radiographic contrast agent. This is perceived by the patient as a generalized sensation of warmth when a contrast agent is injected in the central circulation or as pain when it is injected in an extremity. This can cause transient reduction in peripheral vascular resistance and a drop in systemic blood pressure, which in a compromised patient (such as a patient with severe aortic stenosis or obstructive coronary artery disease) can lead to secondary complications.

Hypervolemia of the central circulation is caused by a shift of tissue fluids into the bloodstream as a result of the pull of the osmotic forces of the hyperosmolar contrast medium in the plasma. The resulting increased blood volume, especially if it occurs rapidly, can precipitate left ventricular decompensation and pulmonary edema in an already compromised heart.

Conventional hyperosmolar radiographic contrast agents, when injected into a coronary artery, cause an acute depression of left ventricular contractility, interfere with the function of the conduction system, and can cause bradycardia, AV block, and asystole. These changes generally clear within a minute. In addition to the hyperosmolality, the toxic effect of sodium directly injected into the coronary arteries is a significant factor in the production of ventricular fibrillation. If the coronary catheter wedges, preventing prompt washout of the contrast agent, the risk of ventricular fibrillation is further increased.

Recent reports from animal experiments suggest that the addition of calcium EDTA to conventional ionic contrast solution (as in Angiovist 370 or Hypaque-76) will cause less myocardial depression and reduce the incidence of ventricular fibrillation resulting from coronary arteriography. Evaluation of coronary arteriography in humans has shown a significant reduction in the incidence of ventricular fibrillation when Angiovist was used instead of Renografin (from 0.6% to 0.1%[20], and from 2.4% to 0%[21]). The newer, low-osmolar ionic contrast agent ioxaglate (Hexabrix) causes less myocardial depression and less bradyarrhythmia and may cause less ventricular fibrillation; however, experience is limited.[22-24]

Nonionic contrast agents (such as iopamidol, iohexol, and iopromide) have no negative inotropic action and may have a small positive inotropic action when injected into coronary arteries of dogs. Also, they cause fewer ECG abnormalities. The hypervolemia resulting from shifts of body fluids to the intravascular compartment and the hypotension resulting from vasodilation are clearly much reduced with these agents. Electrophysiologic (heart rate, QT interval) changes are less marked. It is anticipated that the incidence of ventricular fibrillation will also be reduced.[5,7,17,18]

Precautions. In a patient with preexisting congestive heart failure or left ventricular dysfunction, the following precautions need to be taken.

• Limit the volume and rate of radiographic contrast injections.

• Monitor left ventricular end-diastolic pressure or pulmonary artery diastolic or wedge pressure.

• Use diuretics or venodilators if a rise in left ventricular end-diastolic pressure is noted.

• Consider omitting central injection of large amounts of contrast agent (i.e., left ventricular angiogram or aortogram) and obtaining the information by other imaging means.

• Consider using digital subtraction techniques to limit the amount of contrast agent used.

• Consider using one of the low-osmolar contrast agents, especially for infants and children.

• Permit a longer time between coronary injections to allow for functional restoration.

Nephrotoxicity[25-32a]

A major problem with the use of currently available hyperosmolar radiographic contrast agents is nephrotoxicity—acute impairment of renal function following the injection of contrast material. It is estimated that 10% of all cases of acute renal failure are caused by radiographic contrast agents!

Mechanism. The mechanism of nephrotoxicity is closely related to the hyperosmolality of the agent causing reduced renal blood flow, altered red blood cell morphology and physiology, and direct tubular damage secondary to both the hypertonicity and chemical toxicity of the radiographic contrast agent.

Most of the contrast material is excreted by glomerular filtration rather than by tubular excretion. Initially, hypertonic contrast material causes vasodilation, with increased renal blood flow and increased glomerular filtration rate, followed by a reactive vasoconstriction with reduced renal blood flow and reduced glomerular filtration rate.

The ability of the red blood cells to pass through the capillary bed is compromised by red blood cell deformity and rigidity secondary to fluid shifts to the intravascular space; this further contributes to the renal tox-

Table 19-2. Patients at risk of contrast nephropathy*

Risk factor	Incidence (%)
Normal renal function	0-0.6
Nondiabetic renal insufficiency	
Serum creatinine 1.5-4.5 mg/dl	0-60
Serum creatinine >4.5 mg/dl	30-86
Diabetic nephropathy	
Serum creatinine 1.5 mg/dl	0-0.6
Serum creatinine 1.5-2 mg/dl	16
Serum creatinine 2-4.5 mg/dl	50-92
Serum creatinine > 4.5 mg/dl	76-93
Renal transplantation	36-65
Multiple myeloma	1-2

Adapted from Abraham, P., Harkonen, S., and Kjellstrand, C.: Contrast nephropathy. In Massry, S.G., and Glassock, R.J. editors: Nephrology, Baltimore, 1983, Williams & Wilkins Co.
*Contrast nephropathy is defined as a rise in serum creatinine >1 mg/dl.

icity. Compounding this is the direct toxic effect that the contrast medium has on the proximal tubular cells and some vascular endothelial damage.

Who is at risk of nephrotoxicity? Radiographic contrast agents can cause nephrotoxicity when given orally, intravenously, or intra-arterially. The risk and severity of nephrotoxicity are related to the presence and degree of preexisting renal disease and probably the dose of the contrast agent used. Particularly at risk are patients with diabetic nephropathy, renal transplantation, or multiple myeloma (Table 19-2).

The risk of nephrotoxicity is minimal and the incidence generally less than 1% in patients with normal renal function and when the total dose of contrast agent has not exceeded 5 ml/kg (or the total iodine content has not exceeded 100 g). The risks appears to increase appreciably with preexisting renal disease and may approach 50% in patients with preexisting diabetic nephropathy with serum creatinine levels greater than 2 mg/dl. This risk may approach 100% in patients with a higher creatinine level, especially when doses of the contrast agent exceed a total iodine content of 100 g.[29] A recent controlled study has suggested that these estimates of risk of contrast nephropathy may be too high, as the studies reporting these did not have a control group.[30]

The risk of nephrotoxicity increases with repeated injections of radiocontrast agent in a limited interval and with injections into the abdominal aorta or directly into the renal arteries.

Other factors that have been proposed as contributing to nephrotoxicity include hypovolemia (dehydration), congestive heart failure, hyperuricemia, and advanced age. None of these factors singly, in the absence of preexisting renal disease, seem to contribute to nephrotoxicity.

Hydration and the use of IV mannitol and lasix before, during, and after the infusion of contrast agents seem to reduce the incidence and severity of radiographic contrast nephrotoxicity in patients with preexisting renal disease (see below).

Recognition of radiographic contrast agent nephrotoxicity. Recognition of acute renal failure begins with the identification of the high-risk patient and close monitoring of urinary output, renal function, and electrolytes 24 to 48 hours after the use of radiographic contrast material. A persistent nephrogram effect is an early radiographic clue to nephrotoxicity. Another definitive clue is the rise in serum creatinine level (by at least 1 mg/dl or more). Oliguria and anuria may be present but are not consistent features of radiographic contrast agent nephrotoxicity. When present they may indicate more extensive renal dysfunction associated with irreversible or only partially reversible renal failure. Creatinine levels generally peak in 3 to 5 days, and acute renal failure is self-limited in most patients and can be managed conservatively with attention to fluids, electrolytes, and nutrition. There is no specific treatment, and diuretics and mannitol at this stage have no benefit. Occasionally, acute dialysis will be needed to control hyperkalemia or fluid overload. Rarely, acute renal failure is not reversible and proceeds to chronic renal failure.

Prevention of nephrotoxicity. The risk of radiographic contrast agent nephrotoxicity can be reduced, but not totally eliminated in most patients by following these guidelines.

1. Limit contrast agent dose in all patients to the minimal amount necessary; do not exceed 4 ml/kg of Renografin-76 or similar agent (maximum 300 ml), even in patients with normal kidneys.

2. Keep the patient well hydrated before the study.

3. Avoid use of other nephrotoxic drugs before the study.

4. Identify patients with a high risk of nephrotoxicity (prior renal dysfunction or diabetes) by history and appropriate laboratory tests; avoid the use of radiographic contrast material in these patients. Determine the absolute necessity of the study and whether the information can be obtained by other means (e.g., echocardiography or radionuclide studies).

5. If the study is necessary, attempt to reduce the risk or severity of the anticipated nephrotoxicity by following one of the three regimens listed below. If any one of these regimens is used in patients at risk of congestive heart failure, close hemodynamic monitoring of the patient is required.

REGIMEN A: One hour before the administration of contrast material, start an infusion of 500 ml of 20% mannitol plus 100 mg of furosemide for each mg/dl of the patient's serum creatinine level, infused at a rate of 20 ml/hour. Continue the infusion throughout the procedure and for 6 hours after completion of the study. Urine output is monitored and is replaced in equivalent volume with 5% dextrose in 0.45% saline with 30 mEq of potassium chloride/L intravenously. Clinical studies support the value of mannitol or loop diuretics. The rationale for their combined use is based on animal experiments.[25]

REGIMEN B: In regimen B mannitol (50 g in 180 ml of 5% dextrose solution) is given intravenously within 45 minutes of radiographic contrast agent exposure. Clinical studies have shown this regimen to be of benefit. The risk of pulmonary edema is much less than in regimen A.[31]

REGIMEN C: The third alternative relies on extracellular volume expansion, using 1500 to 2500 ml of normal saline or 5% dextrose in 0.5 normal saline IV infusion starting just before and continuing for 1 hour after completion of the study (approximately 800 ml/hr). Clinical studies have established this to be effective. *Note:* There is a risk of acute volume overload and pulmonary edema. This regimen may be used with close monitoring in patients with normal left ventricular function and no valvular abnormalities. It is contraindicated in patients at risk for congestive heart failure.[32]

The superiority of one regimen over the other is not established.[25] Regimen A seems to be the safest because it has built-in flexibility of the diuretic dose and prevents hypovolemia.

1. When the diagnostic study requires the use of a large amount of contrast agent, consider staging the study into two parts, 3 days apart, such as performing ventricular and coronary arteriography on one day, followed by peripheral or arch arteriography in 2 to 3 days or after renal function has stabilized.

2. Unless a life-threatening emergency exists, delay cardiovascular surgery requiring cardiopulmonary bypass until after renal function has returned to baseline.

3. Navigate the descending aorta with care in the presence of atherosclerotic plaques. Atherorenal emboli may mimic contrast nephropathy or may add to it.[32a]

4. Consider using one of the low-osmolar contrast agents. The cost of the contrast agent will be more than the conventional agents, but the reduced morbidity will more than compensate for the added expense.

5. Monitor urine output, renal function, and electrolytes for 24 to 48 hours after the study.

Other toxicities

Nausea is frequently encountered and may be accompanied by vomiting. This type of reaction is seen in approximately 20% of patients and more frequently with IV injections. It may reflect the hyperosmolar effect of the radiographic contrast material on the central nervous system.

General measures that will limit the toxicity of radiographic contrast agents

1. Use only the minimal amount of contrast agent necessary.

2. Space injections in end arteries or large injections in the central circulation so that the organ has "recovered" from the adverse effect of the first injection.

3. As with any drug, think of radiographic contrast agents in terms of dose per kilogram of body weight or body surface area and adjust total dose accordingly. A generally accepted maximal dose for currently used contrast agents is 4 ml/kg (Renografin-76 or similar agent) not to exceed a total dose of 300 ml. In preexisting renal disease or congestive heart failure, 150 ml may be a safer maximal dose.

ANAPHYLACTIC REACTIONS TO IODINATED RADIOGRAPHIC CONTRAST MEDIA OR LOCAL INFILTRATION ANESTHETICS

Many of the cardiovascular procedures discussed in this book involve the use of iodinated contrast media or local anesthetics. Use of these agents assumes a small but definite risk of allergic reactions, which range from a minor self-limited skin rash to potentially fatal anaphylactic reaction. It is estimated that in the United States approximately 500 deaths/year are directly attributable to such reactions. This section discusses ways to minimize this risk, recognize and treat the reactions, and manage the patient with a history of reaction to these agents. *A history of anaphylactic reaction to contrast agents or local anesthetics is not a contraindication to repeat study, but adequate patient preparation is necessary.*

Reactions to iodinated contrast media
Mechanism and mediators[33-37]

The exact mechanism of reactions to radiographic contrast agents is not known. No evidence for antibodies against the contrast agent has been convincingly shown in humans or in animals. Contaminants in the contrast agent have also been excluded as a cause, as has hypertonicity or the pH (acidity) of the agent. The most likely mechanism is a direct action of the contrast agent on mast cells and basophils, causing a release of histamine and other vasoactive agents. Whether a severe reaction will occur is not determined by previous exposure to contrast agents or even by the fact that a person had a prior reaction; first exposure may precipitate a severe reaction, repeated exposure does not lead to sensitization, and patients with prior reactions may or may not have a reaction on repeat exposure.

When the term *anaphylaxis* is used to describe such reactions, it is not meant to imply a known immunologic mechanism. This term is used because many of the signs and symptoms are identical to those of true allergic reactions (IgE-mediated antigen-antibody reaction).

Several powerful chemical mediators are involved in the production of the syndrome. Table 19-3 summarizes our current, and as yet incomplete, understanding of these mediators, histamine being the most important.[36,36a]

It is suspected that the contrast agent causes degranulation of mast cells and basophils and rapid release of histamine, which precipitates the anaphylactic reaction. In fact, some degree of direct histamine release probably occurs in most patients following injection of a radiographic contrast agent. It is postulated that a clinically significant reaction is observed in patients in whom this release is more pronounced or when there is an increased sensitivity of the host to histamine. The role of other mediators is not as clearly defined, and their contribution to the syndrome of anaphylaxis in humans is yet to be proved.

Types of reactions

All radiographic contrast media, irrespective of composition or osmolality, are capable of producing an anaphylactic type of reaction. The newer contrast agents with lower osmolality (Table 19-1) are expected to have lower nephrotoxicity and neurotoxocity and less risk of volume overload and myocardial depression. It has been suggested that they will also reduce the risk of anaphylactic reaction, and early clinical studies seem to confirm this view.[9,38]

Anaphylactic reactions to contrast agents may be classified into three categories, ranging in severity from insignificant to lethal (Table 19-4). This information has been gathered from several sources involving over 3 million patient studies.[34,35,39-41] These reactions occur with equal frequency in men and women but rarely in infants and young children. Reactions are not dose related and usually appear immediately after injections, with virtually all being manifest within 10 minutes. Late reactions are very rare. Most reported cases of mortality involve patients over the age of 50 years in

Table 19-3. Chemical mediators of anaphylaxis and their actions

Mediator	Location	Physiologic actions	Maximal action	Duration of action	Clinical manifestations	Antagonists
Histamine	Preformed in mast cells & basophils	Vasodilatation Increased vascular permeability Smooth muscle contraction Increased mucous secretion Increased gastric secretion Increased intestinal motility	1-2 min	10 min	Hypotension—shock Tissue edema, including airway & larynx Bronchoconstriction Angioedema Diarrhea, vomiting, tenesmus	H$_1$ antihistamines (diphenhydramine) H$_2$ antihistamines (cimetidine)
SRS-A	Synthesized in mast cells & other cells	Smooth muscle contraction Increased vascular permeability Increased effects of histamine	Min-hrs	Unknown	Bronchospasm Tissue edema	Diethylcarbamazine Epinephrine*
ECF-A	Preformed in mast cells	Attracts eosinophils, may inhibit action of histamine and SRS-A				?
PAF	Synthesized by cells	Platelet aggregation and serotonin release Bronchoconstriction Increased vascular permeability			Role in human clinical anaphylaxis not clear	? ?

Adapted from Saxon, A.: Immediate hypersensitivity: approach to diagnosis. In Lawlor, G.J., and Fischer, T.J., editors: Manual of allergy and immunology, Boston, 1981, Little, Brown & Co.

SRS-A, Slow-reacting substance of anaphylaxis; *ECF-A*, eosinophilic chemotactic factor of anaphylaxis; *PAF*, Platelet activating factor.
*Epinephrine will inhibit and reverse the effects of SRS-A but is not a direct antagonist.

Table 19-4. Reactions to radiocontrast media

Mild*	Moderate†	Severe‡
Nausea, vomiting	Hypotension (mild)	Hypotension (severe, with collapse)
Hot flush	Severe vomiting	Syncope
Limited urticaria	Extensive urticaria	Seizure
Mild pallor, sweating	Edema of face and glottis	Airway obstruction—laryngeal edema
Skin rash, pruritis	Bronchospasm	Severe bronchospasm
	Dyspnea	Pulmonary edema
	Chills	Major arrhythmias—bradycardia or tachycardia
	Chest pain	Myocardial infarction
	Abdominal pain	Cardiopulmonary arrest
	Headaches	
(Incidence: 5%-8%)	(Incidence: 0.1%-1%)	(Incidence: 0.01%-0.1%; Mortality: 1/40,000 to 1/50,000)

*Self-limited; diphenhydramine used for symptomatic treatment.
†Treatment required; see text.
‡Potentially fatal; intensive treatment required; see text.

whom severe cardiopulmonary complications could not be promptly reversed. Sixty to eighty percent of deaths are due to airway edema, and the remainder to irreversible vascular collapse.

Incidence of reactions to contrast material is lower with intra-arterial than with IV injections (2% versus 5% to 8%). The explanation for this is not clear.

Identification of the high-risk patient[39-42]

The risk of clinically significant idiosyncratic reaction is small. It is important to identify patients who are at increased risk and to use prophylactic measures to reduce this risk. Patient history is the best guide. Pretesting has no diagnostic value and is itself a risk. History of allergy of any type isolates a group that has increased risks of such reactions, while history of prior contrast reaction further identifies a higher risk group. Table 19-5 lists the estimate of risk to radiographic contrast agent reaction in these subgroups.

The risk of radiographic contrast material reaction is small in patients with no history of prior allergic reaction or reaction to contrast agents, and no special patient preparation is required in this group. The intermediate group with various allergies may warrant preparation, especially if the allergy has manifested life-threatening complications. Patients at greatest risk are those who have had prior reaction to contrast agents. *However, necessary diagnostic studies or procedures should not be denied to these patients based on the history of prior reaction, even if the reaction was severe and potentially life threatening*. In this group, proper patient preparation will substantially reduce but not totally eliminate the risk of reactions. The decision to proceed with or cancel the study will ultimately depend on the individual assessment of risk/benefit ratio in each case.

Preparation of the high-risk patient[36a,36b,43,45,46]

The following guidelines are recommended for patients who are to undergo contrast agent studies and have a history of acute reaction to contrast agents or who have a "highly allergic" history. Careful adherence to this regimen for these patients will reduce the risk of severe reaction to 1% or less. *However, severe anaphylactic reactions may still occur, and the angiographic team should be ready to institute immediate treatment.*

1. Review the indications for the study and ensure that the use of contrast material is clearly required.
2. Discuss the study and its risks, special precautions, and preparations with the patient. Document this in the patient's medical record. Obtain the patient's informed consent.
3. Administer the following drugs before beginning the study:

   Prednisone: three 50 mg oral doses at 6-hour intervals, with the third dose given 1 hour before the procedure. Oral prednisone is the mainstay of patient preparation.

   Diphenhydramine (Benadryl): 25 to 50 mg slow IV push just before the procedure or 50 mg orally or intramuscularly 1 hour before the procedure. The value of diphenydramine (aimed at blocking H_1 receptors) in prophylaxis remains questionable.

   Hydrocortisone sodium succinate: 500 mg IV ½ hour before the procedure. Such large doses of IV corticosteroids are generally reserved for patients with severe prior reactions, and the value of such large doses has not been rigorously tested.

Table 19-5. Identification of the high-risk patient

Patient history	Risk of developing contrast reaction without premedication*
No history of allergy	1%-2%
History of some allergy (hayfever, food allergy, asthma, hives of unknown cause, and iodine allergy)	Approx. 10%
Definite history of acute radiographic-contrast material reaction	20%-60%

*Data obtained from reports of IV use of contrast material; intra-arterial contrast has lower risk of acute reaction.

4. Secure an IV infusion line and have equipment for cardiopulmonary resuscitation and airway management in working order.
5. Have the following drugs at hand (immediately available):
   Epinephrine, 1 mg in 1/1000 and 1 mg in 1/10,000
   Diphenydramine, 100 mg for IV administration
   Aminophyllin, 500 mg for IV infusion
   Hydrocortisone, 500 mg IV
   Vasopressors (metaraminol, levarterenol, or dopamine)
6. An anesthesiologist or physician experienced in airway management should be immediately available, if needed.
7. At the completion of the study observe the patient closely for 1 hour for the rare event of a late reaction. Most acute reactions occur immediately after injection of the contrast material; virtually all reactions will manifest themselves within 10 minutes.

Alternative methods of preparation. Other methods of preparation for the high-risk patient have been proposed and are practiced, but experience with these agents is limited. These have included (1) the use of alternative contrast agents, specifically one of the low-osmolar agents (Table 19-1) or (2) additional premedications such as the following:

Cimetidine (Tagamet), 300 mg by mouth every 6 hours the day of the procedure, followed by cimetidine 300 mg IV over 5 minutes immediately before the study (with the aim of blocking H_2 receptors).

Heparin to prevent the activation of the coagulation system.

Ephedrine, 25 mg orally 1 hour before the procedure.

Aminophyllin to prevent bronchospasm.

Aspirin to suppress mast cell PGD_2 formation and platelet release reaction.

Each of these agents has theoretical benefits and may reduce the incidence and severity of acute reactions. However, side effects may occur, and the reported use of these agents has been mostly anecdotal; routine use cannot be recommended at this time. In selected high-risk patients, one or more of these agents may be added to the generally accepted regimen.

Various methods of pretesting have been used, including intradermal, subcutaneous, ocular, and intravenous injections of a test dose in an attempt to identify the patient who will have an acute reaction. *These tests are of no value.* They are useless in predicting whether a patient will have a reaction and they themselves may precipitate an acute reaction.

Recognition of acute anaphylactic reaction[47-49]

Acute anaphylactic reaction to a radiographic contrast agent may occur in a patient who has had no prior contrast studies or who has had uneventful prior studies; it rarely occurs in a patient who has had the full prophylactic preparation outlined above. This random and unpredictable occurrence mandates that personnel and facilities for treatment of anaphylactic reactions be available for every patient receiving radiographic contrast material.

Signs and symptoms of acute anaphylactic reaction are listed in Table 19-6. Three principal manifestations are airway edema, vascular collapse, and bronchospasm. Five organ systems are affected: the skin and mucous membrane, upper and lower respiratory, gastrointestinal, cardiovascular, and central nervous systems.

Rapid response is critical because death may occur within minutes. Prompt institution of treatment will almost always reverse even the most severe reaction.

1. Promptly recognize the onset of a reaction. Remember that respiratory and cardiovascular reactions can occur without cutaneous manifestations. Bronchospasm can be so severe that there may be no wheezing; the only clue could be cyanosis.

2. Differentiate the anaphylactic reaction from a vasovagal reaction (Table 19-7). For vasovagal reactions, atropine and volume expansion are sufficient treatment.

3. Appreciate the severity of the reaction (Table 19-4); institute immediate treatment based on this judgment.

Management of severe reaction[36a,36b,47-49]

1. Quickly evaluate airway patency, ventilation, and cardiorespiratory status. If there is cardiopulmonary arrest, institute CPR immediately (see Chapter 18).

2. In a severe reaction, especially if there is hypotension, immediately inject IV epinephrine (0.25 mg to 0.5

Table 19-6. Clinical aspects of anaphylaxis by target organ and mediator

Organ system	Signs and symptoms	Mediator
General (prodromal)	Malaise, weakness, sense of illness	
Dermal	Hives, erythema	Histamine
Mucosal	Periorbital edema, nasal congestion, pruritis, angioedema or flushing, pallor, cyanosis	Histamine
Respiratory	Sneezing, rhinorrhea, dyspnea	Histamine
Upper airway	Laryngeal edema, hoarseness, tongue and pharyngeal edema, stridor	Histamine
Lower airway	Dyspnea, acute emphysema, air trapping (asthma, bronchospasm, bronchorrhea), cyanosis; in severe bronchospasm, wheezing may be absent	Probably SRS-A, possible histamine, others
Gastrointestinal	Increased peristalsis, vomiting, dysphagia, nausea, abdominal cramps, diarrhea—sometimes bloody	Histamine, others—unknown
Cardiovascular	Palpitations, arrhythmias, hypotension, coronary insufficiency, coronary spasm, cardiac arrest	Histamine (H_1), others—unknown
Central nervous	Anxiety, seizures	Unknown

Adapted from Goldfrank, L., and Mayer, A.: Anaphylaxis: the IVP emergency, Hosp. Physician **14**:31, 1978.
SRA-A, Slow-reacting substance of anaphylaxis.

mg, 2.5 to 5 ml of 1/10000 solution). This may be repeated two times if needed and may be given sublingually or via endotracheal tube if an IV line is not available. In less severe reactions without cardiovascular collapse or hypotension, epinephrine may be given subcutaneously (0.3 to 0.5 mg, 0.3 to 0.5 ml of 1/1000 solution).

3. Administer diphenhydramine, 50 mg IV over 1 to 2 minutes, and cimetidine, 300 mg IV over 3 to 5 minutes.

4. Maintain airway patency; use oral airway and assisted ventilation with oxygen supplements of 10 L/minute.

5. If upper airway patency cannot be maintained, proceed to tracheal intubation via a nasotracheal or orotracheal route. In severe upper airway obstruction, emergency cricothyrotomy may be necessary (see p. 418).

6. Administer IV fluids for rapid volume expansion to maintain systolic blood pressure above 90 mm Hg. Colloid fluid is preferred, but crystalloids may be used. Acute decrease in systemic vascular resistance, coupled with increased vascular permeability, causes a decrease in venous return in early stages of anaphylaxis, and correction of hypovolemia is critical in maintaining adequate cardiac output.

7. If blood pressure cannot be maintained by epinephrine and volume expansion, vasopressors (metaraminol, levarterinol, or high-dose dopamine) may be used. See Chapter 18 for general measures of emergency resuscitation.

8. If bronchospasm persists, give aminophylline, 5 to 7 mg/kg as an IV piggyback infusion over 20 to 30 minutes, followed by a maintenance infusion of 0.5 to 1.0 mg/kg/hour.

Table 19-7. Differentiating anaphylaxis from vasovagal reaction

Conditions	Anaphylaxis	Vasovagal reaction
Pallor	+	+
Diaphoresis	+/−	+
Altered consciousness	+	+
Urticaria, angioedema	+/−	−
Dyspnea	+	+/−
Wheezing	+/−	−
Hyperinflation	+	−
Stridor	+	−
Hoarseness	+	−
Tachycardia	+	−
Hypotension	+	+
Arrhythmias	+/−	Bradycardias, sinus arrhythmia
Other ECG abnormalities	+/−	−

Adapted from Rosenblatt, H.M., et al.: Anaphylaxis. In Lawlor, G.J., and Fischer, T.J., editors: Allergy and immunology, Boston, 1981, Little, Brown & Co.
+, Usually present; +/−, may be present; −, usually absent.

9. Administer hydrocortisone sodium succinate 10 mg/kg IV and repeat 5 mg/kg every 6 hours. Discontinue in 48 hours. An equivalent dose of other corticosteroid preparations or an oral preparation may be used. Although corticosteroids are not of great value in the management of *acute* anaphylaxis, they should be used in severe reactions to prevent a prolonged course or recurrent symptoms.

LOCAL ANESTHETIC REACTIONS
Mechanism

Adverse reactions to local infiltration anesthetics are seen infrequently, and *true allergic reactions are very rare*. Most adverse reactions are due to vasovagal responses, hyperventilation, exaggerated response to the epinephrine mixed with the anesthetic, or possible toxic effects of the agent from excess doses. A carefully documented history is of some help in clarifying the type of adverse reaction. In a small group of patients the history will suggest true allergy to a local anesthetic.[50,51]

Local anesthetics

Local anesthetics can be divided into two groups based on their chemical structure (Fig. 19-3).

Group I procaine (ester prototype)	Group II lidocaine (amide prototype)
Benoxinate (dorsacaine)	Amydricaine (Alypin)
Benzocaine	Bupivacaine (Marcaine)
Butacaine (Butyn)	Cyclomethycaine (Surfacaine)
Butethamine	Dibucaine (Nupercaine)
(Monocaine)	Dimethisoquin (Quotane)
Butylaminobenzoate	Diperodon (Diothane)
(Butesin)	Dyclonine (Dyclone)
Chloroprocaine	Etidocaine (Duranest)
(Nesacaine)	Hexylcaine (Cyclaine)
Procaine	Lidocaine (Xylocaine)
(Novocain)	Mepivacaine (Carbocaine)
Tetracaine	Oxethazaine (Oxaine)
(Pontocaine)	Phenacaine (Holocaine)
	Piperocaine (Metycaine)
	Pramoxine (Tronothane)
	Prilocaine (Citanest)
	Proparacaine (Ophthaine)
	Pyrrocaine (Endocaine)

Structural formulas of procaine and lidocaine

The *ester group,* the prototype of which is procaine (Novocain), is characterized by an aromatic lipophilic group, an intermediate chain containing an ester linkage and a hydrophilic secondary or tertiary amino group.

The *amide group,* the prototype of which is lidocaine

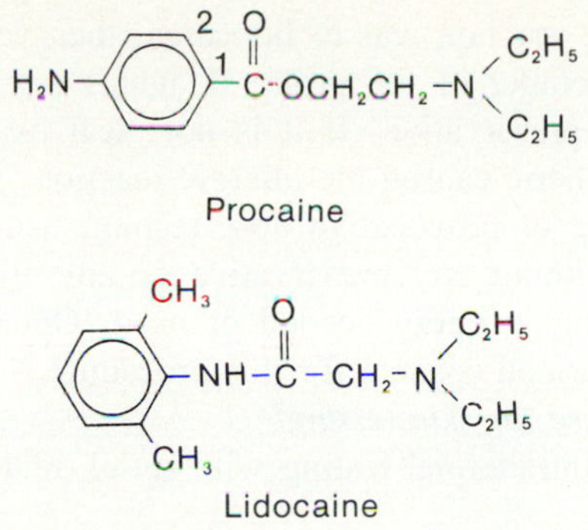

Fig. 19-3. Structural formulas of procaine and lidocaine.

(Xylocaine), consists of an aromatic lipophilic group and intermediate chain containing an amide linkage and a hydrophilic secondary or tertiary amino group.

Methylparaben or propylparaben is used as a preservative in multiple-dose containers for both group I and group II anesthetics. These preservatives can be the cause of an allergic reaction and frequently explain the apparent crossover of allergy from group I to group II agents.

True allergic reactions to local anesthetics are rare. When such reactions occur they frequently involve anesthetics in group I. Members of this group cross react with each other but do not cross react with anesthetics in group II. Nor do the various members of the group II anesthetics cross react with each other. *True allergic reaction to a pure group II anesthetic without a preservative is exceedingly rare*[52] and such a case is considered reportable.

Management of patient with history of allergy to local anesthetic[50,53,54]

For the patient who requires the use of a local anesthetic but claims to have allergy to "caine" drugs or to "local anesthetics," the following guidelines are proposed.

1. Do not cancel the procedure or perform it without anesthesia or with general anesthesia.

2. Obtain a detailed history and try to determine (1) the type of reaction (vasovagal versus toxic versus allergic), (2) the specific agent used (group I versus group II), and (3) whether the agent was pure or mixed with a preservative.

3. If a true allergic reaction is suspected and a member of group I (procaine) anesthetics was used, then a member of group II (lidocaine) anesthetics without preservatives may be used safely. Use either single vials or the 2% IV lidocaine that is used as an antiarrhythmic.

4. If the reaction was to lidocaine, then you can use another member of the group II agents (mepivacaine) without a preservative. If it is not clear exactly what local anesthetic caused the allergic reaction, proceed to skin testing or provocative dose testing, using pure lidocaine without any preservative or any epinephrine. Such testing is rarely needed or used. Obtain the patient's informed consent for this procedure.

Procedure for skin testing[54]

1. Use intradermal testing with serial dilutions of lidocaine.

2. Start with a dilution of 1/10,000 and proceed to a final dilution of 1/50 or 1/100 (the stock solution). If the tests are all negative, proceed with the use of lidocaine. False positive tests can occur.

Provocative dose testing

Provocative dose testing is the most definitive method of determining tolerance. However, this should be done in a setting where severe adverse reactions can be promptly treated.

Procedure for provocative dose testing[54]

1. Review the patient's history and ascertain if the previous reaction to local anesthetic agents was severe. If so, consider avoiding use of a local anesthetic.

2. Discuss the benefits and risks of local anesthetic use with the patient and obtain informed consent.

3. Follow the dosage and dilutional protocol below, administering the doses at 15-minute intervals:

Dose number	Route	Volume (ml)	Dilution
1	Puncture		
2	Subcutaneous	0.1	1:100
3	Subcutaneous	0.1	1:10
4	Subcutaneous	0.1	Undiluted
5	Subcutaneous	0.5	Undiluted
6	Subcutaneous	1.0	Undiluted

4. If no allergic reaction is precipitated, the drug can be used with the same risks as for persons without a history of adverse reaction.

Because a true allergy to pure lidocaine is exceedingly rare, the results of such testing will almost always be negative. Thus the procedure can be completed using lidocaine alone. In the rare event of a positive skin test to pure lidocaine, other members of the group II anesthetics may be tested. As of this writing (1986) there have been less than 10 cases of confirmed allergy to lidocaine reported in the English literature and none in which a patient was simultaneously allergic to other members of the group II local anesthetics.[51,52]

In the rare situations in which a safe local anesthetic cannot be recommended, an antihistamine such as diphenhydramine (Benadryl) may be used as a local anesthetic.

FUTURE DEVELOPMENTS

Radiographic contrast agents will remain in general use in the foreseeable future and with more experience, a clearer understanding of the mechanism of the reactions to these agents and the mediators involved may be forthcoming.

In vitro tube tests may be available that will detect the patient who is prone to develop an anaphylactic reaction to contrast material.

The ideal contrast agent has not yet been fully developed. This agent should produce adequate radiopacity without affecting the vessels or organs being studied, should have no adverse effects, and should be rapidly eliminated from the body. It should have osmolality and viscosity close to those of the blood and should be stable in solution, biologically inert and not metabolized, and able to deliver high iodine concentrations. These characteristics are approached by iotasul, which is currently in development. Further testing will determine whether or not the promise of a truly nontoxic contrast agent will be realized.[55]

Government regulatory agencies (FDA) may streamline some of the lengthy and cumbersome testing and approval processes for new contrast material, shortening the time lag from development to clinical use.

Digital subtraction techniques applied to cardiovascular and pulmonary angiography will permit reduction of the volume of contrast agent injected and therefore reduce toxicity. Combining digital subtraction techniques with low-osmolar contrast agents may further reduce this toxicity.

Future advances in imaging technology in the areas of nuclear medicine, ultrasound, computerized tomographic scanning, and magnetic resonance imaging will probably diminish the need for contrast studies in selected cases.

Magnetic resonance imaging has opened up a whole new area of imaging without the use of radiation or conventional contrast agents. A new generation of "contrast" agents, which do not rely on iodine content or radiopacity, are in development for this technique.

PROCEDURE CHECKLIST

✔ Identify the high-risk patient by history and laboratory tests. Review the procedure and its indications, risks, and complications. Is the study clearly needed? Can the information be obtained by other means?

✔ Obtain the patient's informed consent.

✔ If a patient with preexisting renal or severe cardiovascular disease needs angiographic studies, use the precautions outlined to reduce the risk of toxicity.

✔ If a patient at high risk of developing an anaphylactic type of reaction needs contrast studies, use proper premedications: prednisone, diphenhydramine, and hydrocortisone. Other possible agents (selective use) include cimetidine, heparin, ephedrine, aminophyllin, and aspirin.

✔ Secure an IV infusion line. Medications at hand should include epinephrine, diphenydramine, aminophylline, vasopressors, and a corticosteroid.

✔ Check the equipment for CPR.

✔ Observe the patient for 1 hour after the completion of the study.

✔ Document the type of preparation used and any reactions observed in the medical record.

REFERENCES

1. Strain, W.H.: The radiopaque media: nomenclature and chemical formulas. In Abrams, H.L., editor: Coronary anteriography: a practical approach, Boston, 1983, Little, Brown & Co.
2. Grainger, R.G.: Osmolality of intravascular radiological contrast media, Br. J. Radiol. **53:**739-746, 1980.
3. Grainger, R.G.: Intravascular contrast media—the past, the present and the future, Br. J. Radiol. **55:**1-18, 1982.
4. Brinker, J.A.: Advantages of non-ionic contrast in coronary angiography: a multicenter double-blind randomized trial of iopamidol (abstract), J. Am. Coll. Cardiol. **5:**432, 1985.
5. Gertz, E.W., et al.: Clinical superiority of a new nonionic contrast agent (iopamidol) for cardiac angiography, J. Am. Coll. Cardiol. **5:**250-258, 1985.
6. Levorstad, K., Simonsen, S., and Jervell, J.: Tolerability and usefulness of iohexol in cardioangiography. II. A double-blind comparison with metrizoate, Acta Radiol. (suppl. 366):101-110, 1983.
7. Bettmann, M.A., et al.: Contrast agents for cardiac angiography: effects of a nonionic agent vs. a standard ionic agent, Radiology **153:**583-587, 1984.
8. Bettmann, M.A.: Angiographic contrast agents: conventional and new media compared, A.J.R. **139:**787-794, 1982.
9. Dawson, P., Grainger, R.G., and Pitfield, J.: The new low-osmolar contrast media: a simple guide, Clin. Radiol. **34:**221-226, 1983.
10. Speck, U., Mützel, W., and Weinmann, H.J.: Chemistry, physicochemistry and pharmacology of known and new contrast media for angiography, urography and CT enhancement. In Taenzer, V., and Zeitler, E., editors: Contrast media in urography, angiography and computerized tomography, New York, 1983, Thieme-Stratton, Inc.
11. Higgins, C.B.: Mechanism of cardiovascular effects of contrast media: evidence for transient myocardial calcium ion imbalance, J. Am. Coll. Cardiol. **6:**854-855, 1985.
11a. Kawada, T.K.: Iohexol and iopamidol: second-generation nonionic radiographic contrast media, Drug Intell. Clin. Pharm. **19:**525-529, 1985.
12. Thevenin, P.: First European seminar: contrast media in radiology: evaluation and perspective—a review, neuroradiology **24:**133-137, 1983.
13. Rao, A.K., Thompson, R., Durlacher, L., and James, F.: Angiographic contrast agent–induced acute hemolysis in a patient with hemoglobin SC disease, Arch. Intern. Med. **145:**759-760, 1985.
14. Hagen, B., and Klink, G.: Contrast media and pain: hypotheses on the genesis of pain occurring on intra-arterial administration of contrast media. In Taenzer, V., and Zeitler, E., editors: Contrast media in urography, angiography and computerized tomography, New York, 1983, Thieme-Stratton, Inc.
15. Hayward, R., and Dawson, P.: Contrast agents in angiocardiography, Br. Heart J. **52:**361-368, 1984.
16. Murdock, D.K., et al.: Inotropic effects of ionic contrast media: the role of calcium binding additives, Cathet. Cardiovasc. Diagn. **10:**455-463, 1984.
17. Cumberland, D.C.: Low-osmolality contrast media in cardiac radiology, Invest. Radiol. **19**(suppl.):S301-S305, 1984.
18. Wisneski, J.A., Gertz, E.W., Neese, R.A., and Morris, D.L.: Absence of myocardial biochemical toxicity with a nonionic contrast agent (iopamidol), Am. Heart J. **110:**609-617, 1985.
19. Weikl, A., and Hubmann, M.: A survey of contrast media used in coronary angiography, Cardiovasc. Intervent. Radiol. **5:**202-210, 1982.
20. Murdock, D.K., Johnson, S.A., Loeb, H.S., and Scanlon, P.J.: Ventricular fibrillation during coronary angiography: reduced incidence in man with contrast media lacking calcium binding additives, Cathet. Cardiovasc. Diagn. **11:**153-159, 1985.
21. Zukerman, S.L., et al.: Effect of calcium-binding additives on ventricular fibrillation and repolarization changes during coronary angiography, Circulation **72**(suppl. III-401):1601, 1985.
22. Augenbraun, C.B., et al.: Effects of ioxaglate—a new low osmolality angiographic contrast agent—on coronary hemodynamics during coronary arteriography: comparison with diatriazoate, Circulation **72**(suppl. III-401):1601, 1985.
23. Wolf, G.L.: A double-blind clinical comparison of the electrophysiologic adverse effects of Hexabrix and Renografin-76, Invest. Radiol. **19:**S328-S332, 1984.
24. Tusing, T.W.: Ioxaglate, iopamidol and diatrizoate in coronary arteriography (letter), Gertz, E.W., and Wisneski, J.A. (reply), J. Am. Coll. Cardiol. **6:**956, 1985.
25. Berkseth, R.O., and Kjellstrand, C.M.: Radiologic contrast-induced nephropathy, Med. Clin. North Am. **68:**351-370, 1984.
26. Martin-Paredero, V., et al.: Risk of renal failure after major angiography, Arch. Surg. **118:**1417-1420, 1983.
27. D'Elia, J.A., et al.: Nephrotoxicity from angiographic contrast material: a prospective study, Am. J. Med. **72:**719-725, 1982.
28. Harkonen, S.: Contrast nephropathy, Am. J. Nephrol. **1:**69-77, 1981.
29. Abraham, P., Harkonen, S., and Kjellstrand, C.: Contrast nephropathy. In Massry, S.G., and Glassock, R.J., editors: Nephrology, Baltimore, 1983, Williams & Wilkins Co.
30. Cramer, B.C., et al.: Renal function following infusion of radiologic contrast material, Arch. Intern. Med. **145:**87-89, 1985.
31. Olds, C.W., et al.: Effects of mannitol in the prevention of radio contrast acute renal failure in patients with preexisting chronic renal failure, Kidney Int. **21:**158, 1982.
32. Misson, R.T., and Cutler, R.E.: Radiocontrast-induced renal failure (Medical Progress), West. J. Med. **142:**657-664, 1985.
32a. Smith, M.C., Ghose, M.K., and Henry, A.R.: The clinical spectrum of renal cholesterol embolism, Am. J. Med. **71:**174, 1981.

33. Schatz, M., et al.: The administration of radiographic contrast media to patients with a history of a previous reaction, J. Allergy Clin. Immunol. **55:**358-366, 1975.

34. Lalli, A.F.: Contrast media reactions: data analysis and hypothesis, Radiology **134:**1-12, 1980.

35. Witten, D.M.: Reactions to urographic contrast media, J.A.M.A. **231:**974-977, 1975.

36. Saxon, A.: Immediate hypersensitivity: approach to diagnosis. In Lawlor, G.J., and Fischer, T.J., editors: Manual of allergy and immunology, Boston, 1981, Little, Brown & Co.

36a. Beall, G.N., Casaburi, R., and Singer, A.: Anaphylaxis—everyone's problem, West J. Med. **144:**329-337, 1986.

36b. Bielory, L., and Kaliner, M.A.: Anaphylactoid reactions to radiocontrast materials, Int. Anesthesiol. Clin. **23:**97-118, 1985.

37. Wasserman, S.I.: Anaphylaxis. In Middleton, E.J., Read, C.E., and Ellis, E.F., editors: Allergy—principles and practice, St. Louis, 1983, The C.V. Mosby Co.

38. Rapoport, S., et al.: Experience with metrizamide in patients with previous severe anaphylactoid reactions to ionic contrast agents, Radiology **143:**321-325, 1982.

39. Ansell, G.: Adverse reactions to contrast agents: scope of problem, Invest. Radiol. **5:**374-380, 1974.

40. Witten, D.M., Hirsch, F.D., and Hartman, G.W.: Acute reactions to urographic contrast medium. Incidence, clinical characteristics and relationship to history of hypersensitivity states, A.J.R. **119:**832-840, 1973.

41. Shehadi, W.H.: Adverse reactions to intravascularly administered contrast media, A.J.R. **124:**145-152, 1975.

42. Fischer, H.W., and Doust, V.L.: An evaluation of pretesting in the problem of serious and fatal reactions to excretory urography, Radiology **103:**497-501, 1972.

43. Kelly, J.F., et al.: Radiographic contrast media studies in high-risk patients, J. Allergy Clin. Immunol. **62:**181-184, 1978.

44. Zweiman, B., Mishkin, M.M., and Hildreth, E.A.: An approach to the performance of contrast studies in contrast material-reactive persons, Ann. Intern. Med. **83:**159-162, 1975.

45. Greenberger, P.A.: Contrast media reactions, J. Allergy Clin. Immunol. **74:**600-604, 1984.

46. Mohan, J.C., Reddy, K.S., and Bhatia, M.L.: Anaphylactoid reaction to angiographic contrast media: recurrence despite pretreatment with corticosteroids, Cathet. Cardiovasc. Diagn. **10:**465-469, 1984.

47. Rosenblatt, H.M., and Lawlor, G.J.: Anaphylaxis. In Lawlor, G.J., and Fischer, T.J., editors: Manual of allergy and immunology, Boston, 1981, Little, Brown & Co.

48. Nicolas, F., Villers, D., and Blanloeil, Y.: Hemodynamic pattern in anaphylactic shock with cardiac arrest, Crit. Care Med. **12:**144-145, 1984.

49. Silverman, H.J., Van Hook, C., and Haponik, E.F.: Hemodynamic changes in human anaphylaxis, Am. J. Med. **77:**341-344, 1984.

50. deShazo, R.D., and Nelson, H.S.: An approach to the patient with a history of local anesthetic hypersensitivity: experience with 90 patients, J. Allergy Clin. Immunol. **63:**387-394, 1979.

51. Chin, T.M., and Fellner, M.J.: Allergic hypersensitivity to lidocaine hydrochloride, Int. J. Dermatol. **19:**147-148, 1980.

52. Brown, D.T., and Wildsmith, J.A.W.: Allergic reaction to an amide local anaesthetic, Br. J. Anaesth. **53:**435-437, 1981.

53. Swanson, J.G.: Assessment of allergy to local anesthetic, Ann. Emerg. Med. **12:**316-318, 1983.

54. Mellon, M.H., et al.: Drug allergy. In Lawlor, G.J., and Fischer, T.J., editors: Manual of allergy and immunology, Boston, 1981, Little, Brown & Co.

55. Grainger, R.G.: Low osmolar contrast media, Br. Med. J. **289:**144-145, 1984.

Chapter Twenty

Radiation hazards

MARY B. CONOVER

In 1895 Wilhelm Roentgen discovered the radiation he called x-rays, and within months it was used medically for the detection and treatment of a variety of diseases and injuries. X-rays were used to locate bullets and shrapnel in wounded British soldiers during World War I and were subsequently used routinely in dental work, medicine, and even shoe stores to determine shoe fit. X-rays were used not only to visualize internal body structures but also to treat acne, ringworm, asthma, whooping cough, uterine bleeding, and many other ailments, but the danger to the patient and operator was not realized. By 1902 evidence of x-ray harm began to appear; dentists and radiology technicians developed skin cancer on their fingers and hands. By 1944 it was shown that radiologists who worked regularly with x-ray apparatus were 10 times more likely to die of leukemia than other physicians, and there was an increase in thyroid cancer among adults who, as children, had received x-ray treatment for ringworm on their scalps.

At about the same time that Roentgen discovered x-rays, Becquerel discovered the radioactivity of uranium. He was working with uranium ores and chemically extracting their component metals when he noted that photographic plates were darkened by some form of radiation from these materials. Madame Curie then separated the elements formed by the radioactive decay of uranium and named two new elements, radium and polonium. Subsequently, alpha and beta particles and gamma rays were identified.

The early x-rays had to be of very high intensity because the films were slow (had a low sensitivity). Thus the image was slow to form and required a large amount of radiation. This, coupled with the fact that protective screening was minimal or nonexistent, resulted in exposure to large amounts of radiation at one time for the patient and personnel. Modern equipment has faster films (more sensitive), which reduces radiation to low levels.

In the catheterization laboratory the invisible hazard of repeated exposure to x-rays is a risk that demands just as much attention as does optimal image production and data retrieval. This chapter explains the nature and source of radiation, how it penetrates the body and causes damage, the special risk to personnel in the cardiac catheterization laboratory, and ways to minimize this health hazard for both patient and personnel.

RADIATION

Radiation is energy in motion in the form of waves or particles. It assumes many forms such as heat, microwaves, visible light, and ionizing radiations (x-rays and gamma rays, alpha particles and beta particles). Ionizing radiation has enough energy to dislodge orbital electrons from atoms (ionization), causing the disruption of molecules and subsequent biologic damage.

ATOMS

Atoms are made up of protons, electrons, and neutrons (positively and negatively charged particles and particles that are neutral). Protons repel each other and electrons are attracted by protons. The nucleus of the atom contains neutrons and protons, which are held together by a very strong attractive force. The electrons match the protons in number and are held in orbit around the nucleus of the atom by the attraction to the protons. Atoms are extremely stable but can be split into fragments if bombarded by high-energy particles.

X-RAYS

X-rays[1,2] (roentgen rays) are pulses or packets of energy (photons) released when electrons traveling at high velocities are suddenly stopped. X-rays usually have less energy than do gamma rays but are capable of striking and freeing electrons from their bond with the nucleus of the atom. The free electrons can then cause further ionization and biologic damage.

X-rays are generated from electric energy within an x-ray tube by heating a tungsten wire filament to incan-

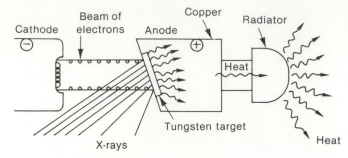

Fig. 20-1. Diagram illustrating the basic operating principles of an x-ray tube. (From Statkiewicz, M.A., and Ritenour, E.R.: Radiation protection for student radiographers, Denver, 1983, Multi-Media Publishing, Inc., p. 16.)

descence so that a cloud of electrons is formed—the hotter the filament the more electrons (Fig. 20-1). Within the same tube is a tungsten button (tungsten target) set in a heavy copper bar. A high-voltage current is applied to the terminals of the x-ray tube, which are wired to the tungsten filament and button, between which an electromagnetic field is created; the filament becomes negative (cathode) and the tungsten target positive (anode). The electrons are repelled from around the negative hot tungsten filament toward the positive tungsten button. They are traveling at high velocity (depending on the applied voltage). When suddenly arrested in their path by the tungsten target, this energy is converted into photons (x-rays) and heat. Approximately 98% of this energy is released as heat and needs to be dissipated through a cooling system, while 2% of this energy is released as x-rays. The direction that the x-rays take is influenced by the angle of the tungsten button. About half of this radiation is absorbed by the tungsten and the remainder is emitted through an arc of 180°. A small portion of this wide beam passes through the narrow opening in the housing of the x-ray tube.

X-rays travel at the speed of light; they are absorbed by and cause ionization of the matter through which they pass. The denser the matter, the greater the amount of absorption. Film protected from light is placed behind the object to be visualized. The film contains small crystals of silver bromide, which, when exposed to x-rays and developed, are reduced to grains of metallic silver. Because bones absorb more x-rays than soft tissues, their images on the film retain silver bromide. When the film is fixed the unaffected silver bromide dissolves, leaving a clear film (impression of bones), but the metallic silver remains and appears dark with variations in light depending on the density.

Tissue damage from x-rays is not only from the effect of large amounts of radiation in a short time, but also from cumulative effects of small amounts over months or years. X-rays are damaging to tissue because they can penetrate the body and cause photoelectric absorption, Compton scattering, or pair production.

If an incoming x-ray strikes an inner shell electron, it may dislodge that electron and cease to exist because it gives up all of its energy to the electron (photoelectric absorption). This is because inner shell electrons are tightly bound to their nucleus, and for dislodgment they require all of the energy possessed by the photon. In turn, the ejected electron (a photoelectron) goes on to cause more biologic damage until it uses up all of its energy. The vacancy in the inner shell is filled by the outer shell electrons until equilibrium is reached. Each time an electron moves to an inner shell, low-energy radiation is emitted. Different parts of the body can be delineated on x-ray film because photoelectric absorption differs among tissue types depending on their atomic number.

If the incoming x-ray strikes an outer shell electron, it has energy left over after the collision and continues on in a different direction (in a weakened state) to ionize other atoms (Compton scattering). It takes less energy for an x-ray photon to dislodge the loosely bound outer shell electron than an inner shell electron. The ejected electron is itself capable of ionizing atoms and finally recombines with an atom that needs another electron.

Pair production is the basis of therapeutic radiation where the object is the destruction of unwanted cells. It does not occur with diagnostic x-ray treatment because the energy involved is not high enough.

FLUOROSCOPY

Fluorescence is energy transformed into visible light. X-rays cause fluorescence of certain crystalline substances such as calcium tungstate, barium platinocyanide, or zinc sulfide. Thus a fluoroscopic screen consists of a thin coating of calcium tungstate on a piece of cardboard. When the body is placed between the x-ray tube and the fluoroscopic screen the x-rays produce visible light on the screen as they pass through the less dense structures. Thus the denser structures appear dark on the screen.

VOLTAGE AND CURRENT

Energy of the electrons inside the diagnostic x-ray tube is expressed in kilovolts at peak value (kVp). The intensity of the x-ray is determined by voltage and current (in milliamperes). The voltage determines the penetrating ability of the x-ray, and the current determines the quantity of x-ray photons in the beam. Increasing the kilovoltage increases the intensity and penetrating ability of the beam but reduces the image contrast. However, with greater penetration, there is less exposure to the patients's skin. Thus, for fluoroscopy one strives to reach a balance between adequate contrast for a particular study and protection of the patient's skin. For example, very little contrast is needed to visualize a catheter or wire within the heart, therefore the kVp can be high and the milliampere value low. One strives for the highest kVp and the lowest milliampere value for adequate contrast coupled with the shortest possible exposure time.

UNITS FOR MEASURING RADIATION AND ITS BIOLOGIC DAMAGE
The roentgen—coulomb/kilogram (SI unit)

The roentgen (R) is the traditional unit of exposure. It is a measurement of the ionization created by radiation as it travels in air. One roentgen is the ability of gamma or x-rays to produce ionization in 1 cm^3 of dry air.

The coulomb (C) is a unit of electric charge equal to 1 ampere-second. Thus in SI (système international) units the exposure is expressed as coulombs per kilogram produced by ionizing radiation in dry air. One roentgen equals 2.58×10^{-4} C/kg.

The rad—gray (SI unit)

The rad (radiation absorbed dose) is the traditional basic unit of absorbed dose of ionizing radiation. One rad is equivalent to 100 ergs (a unit of energy and work) of energy transferred to the irradiated object per gram of material. The SI unit of absorbed dose is a gray (Gy). One gray is an energy transfer of 1 J of energy/kg of irradiated object. One gray equals 100 rads.

The rem—seivert (SI unit)

The seivert is the SI unit of dose equivalent. One seivert equals 100 rem (roentgen equivalent man). A rem is the absorbed dose of any type of ionizing radiation that produces the same biologic effect as 1 rad of x-ray: 1 rem of x-ray has a different absorbed dose than 1 rem of alpha particles but has the same biologic effect.

RISKS OF EXPOSURE TO LOW-LEVEL RADIATION

In the cardiac catheterization laboratory, although the patient is briefly exposed to a relatively high level of radiation that is confined to a small area of the body, the personnel are exposed over a long period of time to relatively low levels spread over a larger area of the

Table 20-1. Common radiation exposures versus diagnostic exposure

Source of radiation	Whole body exposure (mR)
Natural environment (annual)	125
Round-trip flight, New York to California	5-10
Radiography	
Spot film of femur	10
Upper gastrointestinal studies	535
Cardiac catheterization	1400

body.[3,4] The 1980 estimations on the risks from low-level radiation by the Committee on the Biologic Effects of Ionizing Radiation (BEIR III) suggest that modern hospital radiation workers have a low lifetime risk of complications of radiation exposure (cancer [especially leukemia], cataracts, developmental abnormalities in the exposed fetus, and inherited defects in future generations).[5] To place this risk in perspective, Table 20-1 compares the radiation exposure for 1 year from natural environmental sources and a round-trip transcontinental jet flight with diagnostic radiation sustained by the patient. Note that among diagnostic procedures cardiac catheterization has the highest exposure rate, and that a spot radiograph of the femur has only twice the exposure of a transcontinental plane flight. The excessive exposure associated with cardiac catheterization is due to the length of time involved in cineradiography. The exposure sustained at high altitudes is due to cosmic radiation.

Dose responses are not the same for all tissue, thus each organ has its own degree of radiosensitivity and risk estimate.[6] The most sensitive cells are the immature blood cells and immature sperm and egg cells and in decreasing levels of sensitivity are epithelial, endothelial, and connective tissue cells; the kidney tubule; bone; and nerve, brain, and muscle cells.

Although risk values are not known, many investigators relate risk to dose, expressed by the number of expected cancers induced by a dose of 1 rad/year in a population of 1,000,000.

The risk of cataracts differs for single diagnostic radiation doses as opposed to long-term doses (200 rads in a single exposure as opposed to 500 rads over several weeks and thousands of rads of low-level occupational exposure). Thus the threshold for cataract production that would interfere with vision is a cumulative lens dose that is very high.

The thyroid gland is relatively sensitive to cancer induced by radiation, with the maximal incidence occur-

Table 20-2. Maximal dose limits for occupational exposure[13]

Area	Per year	Per 3 months
Whole body	5 rem (50 mSv)	1.25 rem (12.5 mSv)
Head & neck	5 rem	
Torso	5 rem	
Skin (including hands & forearms)	15 rem (150 mSv)	
Hands	75 rem (750 mSv)	25 rem (250 mSv)
Forearms	30 rem (300 mSv)	10 rem (100 mSv)
Other tissues & organs (e.g., thyroid)	15 rem (150 mSv)	5 rem (50 mSv)

Fetus in utero (occupational exposure of pregnant worker) 0.5 rem/gestation period (5 mSv).

Table 20-3. Planned occupational exposure under emergency conditions*

Condition	Dose
Lifesaving procedures	100 rem (1,000 mSv)
Less urgent emergencies	25 rem (250 mSv)

Data from National Council on Radiation Protection and Measurements.
*Whole body—volunteer, older than 45 years if possible.

ring at approximately 20 years after exposure. The risk appears to be 20 to 150 carcinomas/10[6] person-years/rad.

Although it is not possible to distinguish cancers resulting from radiation from those produced by other causes, it appears that the probability of developing cancer increases with radiation exposure, with the maximal incidence occurring 10 to 30 years after exposure. The risk per rad per 106 person-years for breast cancer is 30 to 200 cases, for lung cancer 20 to 100 cases, and for leukemia 10 to 60 cases.

MAXIMAL PERMISSIBLE DOSE

The upper limit of whole body radiation dose for an individual working with radiation equipment is 5 rems (0.05 seivert)/year. Tables 20-2 and 20-3 list the maximal permissible dose (MPD) limits for occupational exposure for certain portions of the body as established by the National Council on Radiation Protection (NCRP).

OPERATOR EXPOSURE DURING CORONARY ARTERIOGRAPHY AND ANGIOPLASTY

Radiation exposure to the operator and assistants during fluoroscopy and cineangiography comes from the patient in the form of scattered radiation. Because the duration of fluoroscopy is longer during coronary angioplasty, radiation exposure is twice that of routine coronary arteriography.[7,8] Of special concern is the amount of radiation exposure to the corneas, thyroid gland, and gonads of the angiographer.[9,10]

Although approximately 90% of the x-ray entering the patient's body will be absorbed, a certain amount of radiation is deflected from the patient's body into the room. Fig. 20-2 illustrates how the primary beam is backscattered circumferentially from the patient (the scattering object). The primary beam strikes the patient, and even the well-collimated beam strikes the table, bouncing off (scattering) and perhaps even hitting another object and going in yet another direction (secondary scattering). Note that the least amount of scatter radiation is received when positioned at right angles to the patient's body.[11]

Using the transbrachial technique of Sones and a rotational system, 80% of the total radiation exposure to the angiographer during an average coronary arteriogram is due to the cineangiographic study and 20% to the fluoroscopic procedure. This is because the intensity of the radiation is greater during cineangiography, causing more penetration. With more penetration, less radiation is absorbed by the patient's body and more is scattered into the room.

The use of a table-mounted lead shield decreases the radiation dosage to the eyes by 70%, the thyroid by 80%, and the legs by 90%. Table 20-4 is a comparison of measured exposures based on a study of 700 coronary arteriograms, using the brachial artery technique and a dedicated U-arm system with and without a special shield compared with the NCRP and International Commission on Radiological Protection (ICRP) guidelines.[7]

When using a rotational system, scatter radiation is at a minimum during right anterior oblique (RAO) projection for the right arm approach. Studies in the left anterior oblique (LAO) projection result in significantly higher scatter radiation exposure to the operator. Fig. 20-3 illustrates the isoexposure curves for the 50° LAO–15° cranial angulation using the Poly C Diagnost System. Each line of the isoexposure curves passes through the locations receiving the same radiation intensity. The exposure curves are shown with and without a specially designed protective shield.

In another study radiation to the hands of the physician inserting nine transvenous permanent pacemakers

Table 20-4. Comparison of measured exposures and guidelines[7]

	Probable maximal exposure (mR/examination)*		Guideline maximal exposure (mR/week)†	
	No shield	Shield	NCRP	ICRP
Eyes	8.8	3.4	100	300
Thyroid	10.0	2.7	300	600
Torso (whole body)	1.0	<0.1	100	100
Hands	9.5	4.8	1500	1500
Lower legs	46.5	2.6	300	1500

Adapted from Balter, S., Sones, F.M., and Brancato, R.: Radiation exposure to the operator performing cardiac angiography with U-arm systems, Circulation **58:**925-932, 178. Reproduced with permission. © Report of Inter-Society Commission for Heart Disease Resources, American Heart Association.

NCRP, National Council on Radiation Protection; *ICRP,* International Commission on Radiological Protection.

*There is only one chance in 40 of exceeding this exposure.
†50-week working year.

has been found to be an average of 25.5 mrems/case with an average fluoroscopy time of 12 minutes.[12]

RADIATION EXPOSURE FROM PORTABLE X-RAY UNITS

When working with portable x-ray units[2,13] the basic principles of radiation safety apply. They include collimation, the use of image intensifiers, shielding, distance from the patient, protection of nearby patients, and fluoroscopy time. Be sure to protect other patients if they are nearby.

RADIATION EXPOSURE TO CHILDREN

Because children are smaller there is increased internal scatter causing the thyroid and gonad doses to be higher than in a larger person. Children have an increased sensitivity to radiation and the dose during cinefluorography is very high, even for adults (40 to 100 R/minute). Therefore, the following additional precautions are taken when cardiac catheterization is performed in children:[14-17]

1. Use the minimal dose of cinefluorography and keep the exposure under 30 seconds.

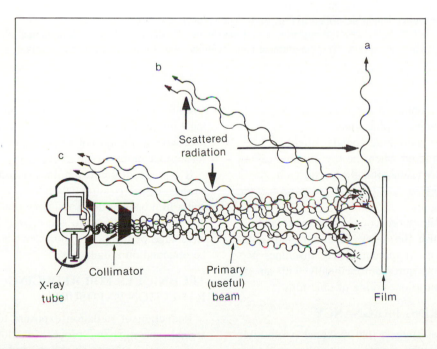

Fig. 20-2. Scatter radiation. The radiographer receives the least amount of scattered radiation by standing at right angles to the scattering object (the patient), in position *a*. The most scattered radiation is received at point *c* because of backscatter coming from the patient. (From Statkiewicz, M.A., and Ritenour, E.R.: Radiation protection for student radiographers, Denver, 1983, Multi-Media Publishing, Inc., p. 170.)

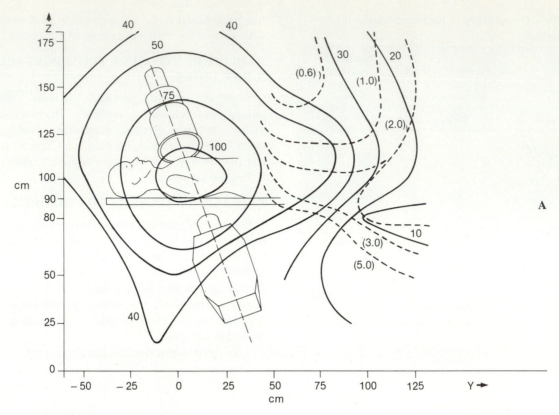

Fig. 20-3. Isoexposure curves with a rotating C-arm system with (– – –) and without (——) the protective shield described in Fig. 20-6. The vertical center of the shield is at 75 cm in both the X and Y planes with the operator behind the shield. (*Z,* Vertical plane; *Y,* longitudinal plane, *X,* horizontal plane.) **A,** The longitudinal plane with the operator at 75 cm on the Y axis.

2. Use information obtained by echocardiography to shorten cardiac angiographic time.
3. Use a large plate abdominal/gonadal shield.
4. In very small children when the thyroid area cannot be avoided when visualizing the aortic arch, use a small, malleable lead shield to selectively protect the lower nuchal region.
5. Use low-pulse-rate fluoroscopy whenever feasible.
6. If possible furnish the x-ray generator with automatic cine testing equipment. These machines perform five test exposures automatically with an exposure equivalent to one frame of cine film.

RADIATION DURING PREGNANCY

Current guidelines suggest that maximal permissible exposure to the abdomen of a pregnant radiation worker is 500 mrems (0.5 rems; 5 mSv) for the 9-month period.[18-20] Because there is some evidence that the developing embryo or fetus is especially sensitive to radiation, because we do not yet know if there is an absolutely safe low dose, and because of the explosive legal implications, some physicists maintain that a pregnant woman should not be permitted to work with fluoroscopy or mobile x-ray units at all.

If a pregnant employee does continue to work in the cardiac catheterization laboratory, a pocket dosimeter and a film badge on the abdomen (under the lead apron) are worn in addition to the regular film badges. The advantage of the pocket dosimeter is that readings can be obtained on a daily basis.

TECHNIQUES FOR REDUCING RADIATION EXPOSURE

Reduction of radiation exposure to patient and personnel encompasses proper functioning and use of equipment, adequate shielding, and monitoring of personnel. Radiation safety should be under the direction of a radiation protection officer and include education programs, equipment maintenance, and personnel monitoring.[21-26]

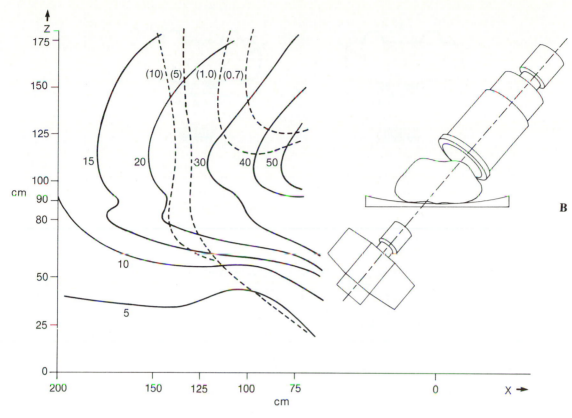

Fig. 20-3, cont'd. B, The horizontal plane with the operator at 75 cm on the *X* axis. The measurements are in milliroentgen/hour for the 50° left anterior oblique projection with 15° cranial angulation. (From Gertz, E.W., Wisneski, J.A., Gould, R.G., and Akin, J.R.: Improved radiation protection for physicians performing cardiac catheterization, Am. J. Cardiol. **50:**1283-1286, 1982.)

The most important technologic means in the reduction of radiation exposure are shielding, collimation of the beam, image intensifiers, and remote injection techniques. The single most important human variable determining radiation exposure is the duration of the procedure, which is governed by the skill and experience of the operator and difficulty of the procedure.

Patient protection

Generally speaking, reduced radiation to the patient results in reduced exposure to the operator (less scatter radiation). The patient undergoing cineangiography is exposed to high-intensity radiation over a short period of time and must be protected as much as possible. In addition to use of properly collimated and filtered beams, protection for the patient's skin can be somewhat enhanced by maintaining high kilovolt and low milliampere settings, and the exposure time can be kept to a minimum by limiting the cine filming frequency of frames per second to 30. The patient's gonads should be shielded whenever possible. For female patients a flat-contact, lead-impregnated shield should be placed over the gonads for over-table radiographic procedures and under the patient for under-table radiographic procedures. The ovaries receive about three times more exposure during any given radiographic procedure than do the testicles. However, proper shielding can reduce this by about 50%. Shaped-contact shields are available for shielding the testicles, and their use can reduce primary beam exposure for male patients by 90% to 95%.

Distance from radiation source

The further the operator and assistants stand from the radiation source, the less the radiation exposure. The inverse square law states that "the intensity of the radiation is inversely proportional to the square of the distance." This is because the area that a given amount of x-rays has to cover at a more distant spot in the room increases by the square of the distance. Thus when the distance from the x-ray target is doubled, the radiation

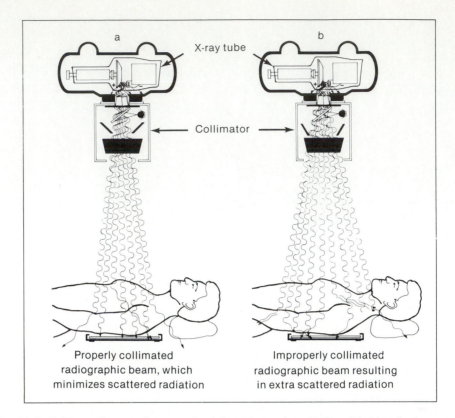

Fig. 20-4. Collimate the x-ray beam so that it is no larger than the film. Limiting the beam to the area of clinical interest decreases the dose to the patient and the scatter radiation to the operator. (From Statkiewicz, M.A., and Ritenour, E.R.: Radiation protection for student radiographers, Denver, 1983, Multi-Media Publishing, Inc., p. 132.)

is dispersed over an area that is four times larger and the intensity at the new distance is only one fourth the original.

Proper use of equipment
Collimation

Collimation of the x-ray improves image quality and is the single most important means of reducing radiation to the patient and thus scatter radiation to the operator. The collimator contains two sets of adjustable lead shutters at different levels, a light source, and a mirror. The light with the deflecting mirror permits the operator to center the x-ray over the area of interest. Collimation of the beam is then automatic to the image field size of the image intensifier. Fig. 20-4 compares the properly and improperly collimated x-ray.

Filtration

Fig. 20-5 illustrates the effect of filtration on the low-energy x-ray photons (long wavelength or "soft" x-rays). The filter decreases the amount of radiation to the

patient by allowing only the more penetrating photons to reach the patient. These photons are more likely to pass through the patient's body, whereas the low-energy ones will be scattered in the body, causing ionization and tissue damage.

Filtering devices are either built in (inherent) or added and consist of sheets of material equivalent to at least 0.5 mm of aluminum total filtration. Portable units require 2.5 mm of aluminum equivalent total filtration. If the x-ray unit produces up to 70 kilovolts (peak) (kVp), total filtration must be 1.5 mm; if it produces more than 70 kVp total filtration must be 2.5 mm.

Image intensifier

An image intensifier is a glass and metal, high-vacuum device used to convert the x-ray image pattern into a corresponding amplified, visible light pattern, reducing the amount of radiation necessary. Such a device is necessary in fluoroscopy because low current produces a poorly illuminated image. In fluoroscopy, the image intensifier is the primary protective barrier. In an auto-

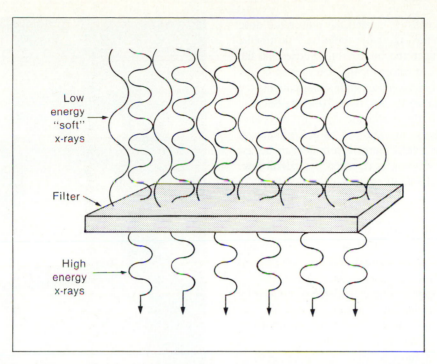

Fig. 20-5. Filtration removes low-energy photons (long-wavelength or "soft" x-rays) from the beam by absorbing them and permits higher energy photons to pass through. This reduces the patient's dose. (From Statkiewicz, M.A., and Ritenour, E.R.: Radiation protection for student radiographers, Denver 1983, Multi-Media Publishing, Inc., p. 133.)

mated system it reduces patient dose and therefore scatter radiation to the operator, saves time, and increases image brightness 7000 times, permitting fluoroscopy to be performed in a lighted room. By means of an electron vacuum tube, fluoroscopic illumination can be intensified 200 to 1000 or more times. The scanning area of the intensifier is 4 to 9 inches in diameter.

Because of the protective function of the image intensifier, the law states that if it is moved away from the x-ray tube, you should not be able to energize the fluoroscope. In fact, the two are said to be "ganged" in that the image intensifier and the x-ray tube are locked into position together. When the image intensifier is moved over the patient it clicks into place. For cinefluorography, a radiographic grid is inserted between the patient and the film to minimize the amount of scatter radiation reaching the image intensifier. The grid is made of lead strips alternated with aluminum, plastic, or wood. Such a device increases patient dose (milliampere setting must be increased); however, the improved radiographic contrast provides more diagnostic information. The maximal allowable output to the skin according to United States Federal law is 10 R/minute (5 R/minute in California).

Manual settings for fluoroscopy

The primary responsibility for current (milliampere) and voltage (kilovolt) fluoroscopic settings belongs to the physician. The hard truth is that many radiology technicians and physicians are not aware that there are different settings for spot films as opposed to fluoroscopy, resulting in fluoroscopic settings that are far too high and excessive radiation to patient and personnel.

Fluoroscopic milliampere settings should start at *the lowest possible acceptable position* (usually 1 mA) and be turned up if necessary to a maximum of 4 mA. The mA regulator may be in the control room or on the image intensifier. The setting for kilovolts is usually 80 to 100 for cardiac catheterization studies.

Uncertainty, confusion, and ignorance regarding the proper milliampere and kilovolt settings for fluoroscopy are compounded by the differences among and even within the brands of equipment and the differences between new and old equipment. In the newest models both settings are automatically adjusted to patient size. In certain older models the milliampere setting is manual and the kilovolt automatic; in others the kilovolt is manual and the milliampere automatic; in even older models both are manual. With a properly adjusted unit the panel dose rate will not exceed the prescribed dose of 5 R/minute. For the automatic units no adjustments are necessary; just push the fluoroscopy button and the voltage and current are automatically determined by the size of the patient. For example, with small patients the voltage may be reduced to as low as 70 kVp. Because of the efficiency of the automatic system, the panel dose rate usually does not exceed 1 to 3 R/minute. A timer is set so that total roentgens/minute can be assessed; a 5-minute warning is required by federal law. A physicist should check all equipment annually.

Reducing fluoroscopic and cineangiographic times

The duration of fluoroscopy should be kept at the absolute minimum. Check the fluoroscopic exposure settings (kilovolts and milliamperes) and take care not to expose your hand to the primary beam.

The fluoroscopy time can be considerably reduced by using short bursts rather than sustained viewing. Be willing to change to a different catheter or reform a catheter when manipulation time becomes prolonged. Fluoroscopy time for most routine cardiac catheterization and coronary arteriographic procedures is 2 to 5 minutes. In unusual circumstances (i.e., difficult-to-cross aortic stenosis, anomolous coronary arteries, etc.) this time may be prolonged to 30 to 40 minutes, at which time the physician must judge whether to continue with the procedure. Coronary angioplasty may also require such prolonged fluoroscopy times.

The average cineangiographic time for coronary arteriography is 30 to 35 seconds, and typical doses are 30 to 90 R/minute. The cineangiogram should run only long enough to record the necessary information, and is generally limited to 30 frames/second. Higher frame rates (hence more radiation exposure) are rarely needed, such as in patients with very rapid heart rates. It is possible to burn the skin with long exposure times. The minimal amount of radiation necessary to produce an acceptable diagnostic image is approximately 20 μR/frame. Thus a dose of 20 to 25 μR/frame represents a compromise between diagnostic image quality and minimal radiation exposure to the patient and physician.

Avoid fixed routine protocols, preplan your study, and adjust each procedure to the individual patient so that the necessary diagnostic information is obtained with minimal radiation.

Increase the distance between yourself and the source of scatter radiation (the patient's chest) during cineangiography. Use remote injection techniques and step back from the procedure table whenever feasible (e.g., aortography, ventriculography), while still maintaining catheter control. Assistants in the room should be as far as feasible from the x-ray tube.

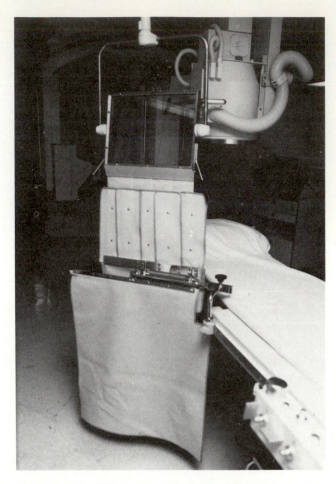

A

Fig. 20-6. A, Ceiling-mounted leaded glass and a table-mounted leaded shield (undraped).

Shielding
Multiangulated rotational equipment

Rotational C- or U-arm units pose a hazard to the operator because of the proximity of the scattered radiation, which may be as high as 3 to 5 R/hour without shielding. Make sure that the room and all personnel have proper shielding equipment and that those not directly involved in the procedure are behind a radiation barrier whenever the x-ray tube is on. This rotational equipment presents special shielding design challenges. Movable shields or drapes are available for most of the new equipment; side drapes between the patient and operator reduce scatter radiation. Reduction in exposure to the neck and face of the angiographer can be accomplished by a combination of an articulated, arm-mounted, lead-glass or lead-acrylic shield and a support-mounted lead apron (the lighter leaded acrylic is somewhat less effective).[27,28] Some companies provide

Fig. 20-6, cont'd. B, Operator adjusting the ceiling-mounted leaded glass. **C,** Same assembly, now draped and in use.

overlapping, flexible lead cloth shields that can be clamped to the patient support. This arrangement can be very effective if well thought out. Fig. 20-6 illustrates ceiling- and table-mounted shields.

Cradle for patient positioning

The patient cradle should be flush mounted with the edges of the table and flexible lead drapes hung from the cradle edges. The drapes can be made of the same material as the lead aprons. Cradles that clamp onto or mount above the table top are a source of high-level scatter radiation because of the slot created between the table top and the bottom of the cradle assembly.

Over-table x-ray tube

Scatter radiation is considerably larger when the over-table x-ray tube and under-table intensifier are used, as opposed to the under-table tube and over-table

intensifier. With the over-table tube scatter radiation is mainly from the site of entry of the beam (upper surface of the patient), whereas with the under-table tube scatter radiation comes mainly from the site of exit of the beam. One radiology department constructed a detachable rotating shielding tube out of a 0.5 mm thick sheet of lead, glued to a 6 mm thick plexiglass frame equipped with two hinged panels of different sizes. This was attached to the collimator. During the procedure the hinged panels were let down, improving the shielding in the direction of the angiographer.

A lead rubber shield may also be suspended on the compression tube of a remote control fluoroscopy apparatus by means of hooks on rods fixed to the compression tube so that it falls along the long side of the procedure table. A long, lead rubber screen may also be suspended at the head of the couch at right angles to the radiation field to protect the anesthesiologist.

Lead aprons

Lead aprons with 0.5 mm of lead shield the trunk, red bone marrow, and gonads and reduce amount of exposure by approximately 70% to 90%. Knee-length wrap-around aprons with shallow necks are best. Wrap-around and two-piece aprons are also available for persons who must turn their back to the scatter radiation. The sternum should not be exposed. Maternity lead aprons are available in which the lead content is increased to 1.0 mm decreasing the body exposure by a factor of 5 to 100 mrem, well below even background environmental exposure. However, the additional weight of these aprons makes them uncomfortable for many women.

Eye and thyroid shielding

Special glasses made of 0.5 mm lead-equivalent glass with wrap-around shields of 0.5 mm lead equivalence offer maximal protection from scatter radiation (four times more protection than regular eyeglasses for face radiation). These glasses are available with plain or prescription lenses and plain side shields. The side shields are necessary because the angiographer frequently looks at the television monitor, which is usually at an angle to source of scatter (the patient).

Separate thyroid shields, x-ray masks that protect head and neck, and aprons with built-in thyroid shields are available (see Appendix K) and should be provided for personnel directly involved in procedures. Fig. 20-7 illustrates the proper use of the lead apron, thyroid shield, and glasses.

Personnel monitoring

Personnel working with radiation should be monitored. During routine radiographic procedures, the monitoring device should be worn on the clothing on the front of the body at waist or chest level.

During fluoroscopic procedures when a lead apron is worn, the monitoring device should be worn outside the protective apron at collar level to monitor the exposure to the thyroid and eyes. A second monitoring device may be worn under the apron.

There are three types of personnel monitoring devices: film badges, pocket ionization chambers, and thermoluminescent dosimeters.

Film badge

The film badge contains metal filters and a film packet in a plastic holder. The plastic holder filters low-energy radiation, and the filters measure the approximate energy of the radiation reaching it. The film packet contains a radiation dosimetry film similar to

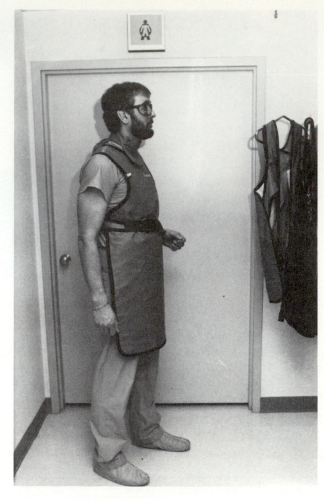

Fig. 20-7. Proper attire for the operator during cardiac catheterization. Note the leaded apron, thyroid shield, leaded glasses with the side shields, and the proper position of the film badge. Note also the specially designed rack at the entrance of the cardiac catheterization room for apron storage.

dental film and sensitive to doses as low as 10 mrem and as high as 500 rem. These badges are sent to the monitoring company for processing and exposure determination.

Pocket ionization chamber (pocket dosimeter)

This device resembles a fountain pen and contains an ionization chamber that measures radiation exposure. It is ideal for pregnant women working in the cardiac catheterization laboratory, as it provides a daily reading. The disadvantages of this device are its cost ($100/unit), the tricky read-out procedure, and the fact that it does not supply a permanent record. Also, the charge leaks out with time, giving false readings.

Thermoluminescent dosimeter

The thermoluminescent dosimeter (TLD) badge looks similar to the film badge from the outside but is far more complicated on the inside. The interior of the badge is free of light and contains a sensing material (usually the crystalline form of lithium fluoride). Ionizing radiation interacts with the sensing material much like human tissue does, thus this monitor determines dose more accurately. The electrons in the sensing material become trapped because they are excited and rearranged and absorb and store energy. When heated the trapped electrons are freed and return to their normal energy levels, releasing energy in the process in the form of visible light. The amount of light emitted is proportional to the amount of radiation sustained. An analyzer heats the sensing material and then measures the light emitted. This readout process destroys the stored information and permits the TLD to be reused.

Area monitoring devices

There are two types of gas-filled radiation survey instruments for area monitoring: the ionization chamber–type survey meter (''cutie-pie'') and the Geiger-Muller (GM) detector. These instruments detect and/or measure radiation operating on the principle that the ionizing radiation will ionize the gas (usually air) in the detector. Another gas-filled ionization chamber is the ion chamber (R-meter). This however, is not used for surveys but to calibrate x-ray equipment.

Ionization chamber–type survey meter

This is a rate meter that measures a wide range of radiation exposure within a few seconds. It is used to check scatter from x-rays using an integration mode on the meter. Its disadvantages are that it is large and of delicate construction and requires warm-up time.

Geiger-Muller detector

This unit is capable of rapid monitoring and detects individual radioactive particles or photons and can determine if an area has been contaminated by radioactive material.

Ion chamber and condenser

This is an accurate and reliable instrument for calibrating x-ray equipment. It measures radiation by recording the total exposure received during a given period.

EVALUATION OF RADIATION EXPOSURE

Measure for scatter radiation yearly. A radiation physicist makes these measurements and records them on a grid paper floor plan of the laboratory so that you can identify areas of high exposure rates. Repeat the measurements whenever new x-ray equipment is used or new components added.

Define areas to be avoided by personnel. Whenever possible, personnel should position themselves in areas of low scatter radiation.

Record total fluoroscopic and cineangiography times for all procedures on the patient record and the permanent laboratory record. The devices that turn off the x-ray after a preset time are unsatisfactory, as they may turn off at a critical time and the procedure may need to be repeated. Timers that emit alert tones are inexpensive and are required by Department of Health, Education, and Welfare regulations.

Establish limits for procedural fluoroscopic time allowed an angiographer. The physician in charge should keep strict watch over time allotments to trainees, and if no progress is being made within the allotted time, the physician in charge should complete the study.

Keep a history of each leaded apron. Mark aprons with an identification number in indelible ink and keep a fluoroscopic and radiographic record of each apron. Inspect newly purchased aprons for manufacturer defects (although the incidence is less than 5%, these defects may still be significant).[29] Do not assume that a new apron is flawless. Regulatory requirements can be satisfied with a complete fluoroscopic examination of each apron every 3 months. However, some laboratories recommend that a series of 14 × 17-inch radiographs be taken every 6 to 12 months whenever loss of integrity is suspected.

Establish a schedule for professional periodic evaluation of radiation exposure and equipment. The Joint Commission on Accreditation of Hospitals (JCAH) and some states require annual surveys by a physicist.

1. Reevaluate and remap areas of scatter following service adjustments or replacement of components.

2. Daily: Check collimators, coning devices, and the entire cineangiographic imaging chain. Do this by imaging a standard attenuator before beginning the day's work. Expose a portion of the same film to a sensitometer and take densitometric readings of the processed film. Investigate and correct any significant variance. Perform daily visual inspections of lead aprons and protective shielding devices. Some states require weekly checks of the fluoroscopic automatic exposure system.

3. Semiannually: Perform an in-depth evaluation of equipment performance, using standardized test tools secured through the Society for Cardiac Angiography to check x-ray tube housing, filter, collimation, voltage, and current calibration.

4. Every 3 months: Check aprons and protective shielding devices for radiation protection integrity. Deterioration of lead/rubber material is accelerated in the environment of the cardiac catheterization laboratory because air ionization and relay arcs cause a slight increase in atmospheric ozone.

LEGAL IMPLICATIONS OF RADIATION EXPOSURE

More years and more intensive scientific study have gone into the health effects of radiation than into any other environmental agent; still, uncertainty and controversy exist among the experts in radiation biology regarding radiation exposure. The uncertainties are compounded by the fact that no immediate effects are seen or expected from radiation exposure. Despite this lack of precision, and in the light of the emotionally charged position that radiation holds in the public eye and the general belief that radiation exposure at certain levels is associated with malignancy and genetic alterations, there is need for setting health policies and securing informed consent before exposing patients to ionizing radiation. Informed consent would include advising patients of the potential risks of radiation as compared with available options and with the risks normally accepted as a part of everyday living.[30]

FUTURE DEVELOPMENTS

Imaging techniques that do not use radiation are continually being refined and in some specific situations have replaced angiography in cardiovascular diagnosis.

Ultrasound

The use of echocardiography in cardiovascular diagnosis is commonplace. The addition of Doppler echocardiography and, more recently, flow mapping using Doppler information has advanced echocardiography to the point where valvular stenosis, degree of valvular regurgitation, and cardiac output can be estimated with increasing certainty. Cardiac tumors can be definitively diagnosed with echocardiography. Aortic, mitral, and tricuspid stenosis can be diagnosed and quantitated with Doppler echocardiography, eliminating in some cases the need for cardiac catheterization while reducing the procedure time (and the radiation exposure) in others. Further development of these ultrasound techniques is probably forthcoming.

Magnetic resonance imager

The magnetic resonance imager (MRI) is an exciting and revolutionary new instrument that offers medical science a means of visualizing the internal body structures *without any radiation whatsoever* and without the use of radiocontrast media. The technique is also called nuclear magnetic resonance (NMR).

This scanner utilizes a giant magnet to create a magnetic field that momentarily stills the body's hydrogen nuclei, which are continually in motion. A radiofrequency is then introduced into the magnetic field and the resulting behavior of the nuclei is measured by a computer, which creates a visual image. These images can be in cross section or multiple planes. Its greatest application is in imaging of the central nervous system, but the cardiovascular system can also be imaged. The clinical application of the technique is currently being developed.

PROCEDURE CHECKLIST

- On nonautomatic or semi-automatic units, check current (milliampere) and voltage (millivolt) settings yourself. Do not assume that anyone else, including radiology technician, knows the difference between cinefluoroscopy and spot film settings, which are much higher.
- Start with 1 mA and work up. Remember that if you double the milliamperage you double the dose. The kilovolt setting is usually at 80 and determines the degree of penetration into the body. The internal dose increases with kilovoltage, but damage to the skin (burning) decreases. Thus your aim is low milliampere and high kilovolt settings. If you have a totally automatic fluoroscopic unit, just press the button. But do check to see if it is truly automatic; some are only automatic for kilovoltage and not for milliamperage, and vice versa.
- Be sure that all personnel in the cardiac catheterization laboratory, including radiology technicians, are instructed by the radiation safety officer on the proper milliampere and kilovolt settings for cinefluoroscopy.
- Ensure that the equipment is inspected at determined intervals and does not deliver excessive radiation.
- Protect yourself with special equipment shields and by wearing a leaded apron, thyroid shield, and leaded glasses with side shields or x-ray mask.
- Preplan the study and make every effort to reduce the duration of fluoroscopy and cineangiography studies to the minimum necessary for definitive diagnosis.
- Increase the distance between yourself and the source of scatter radiation (the patient's chest) whenever feasible during filming.
- Collimate the x-ray and use minimal field size.

✔ Wear a film badge at your collar and keep a record of your monthly, yearly, and lifetime readings.

REFERENCES

1. Juhl, J.H.: Paul and Juhl's essentials of roentgen interpretation, ed. 4, Philadelphia, 1981, J.B. Lippincott Co., pp. 1-11.
2. Statkiewicz, M.A., and Ritenour, E.R.: Radiation protection for student radiographers, Denver, 1983, Multi-Media Publishing, Inc.
3. Hendee, W.R.: Real and perceived risks of medical radiation exposure, West. J. Med. **136:**380-386, 1983.
4. Fabrikant, J.I.: Radiation and health (editorial), West. J. Med. **138:**387-390, 1983.
5. National Research Council, Committee on the Biological Effects of Ionizing Radiation: The effects on populations of exposure to low levels of ionizing radiation. Washington, D.C., 1980, National Academy Press.
6. Martell, E.A., and Sweder, K.S.: The roles of polonium isotopes in the etiology of lung cancer in cigarette smokers and uranium miners. In Gomez, M., editor: Proceedings of the International Congress on Radiation Hazards in Mining, New York, 1982, American Institute of Mining, Metallurgical and Petroleum Engineers, pp. 383-389.
7. Balter, S., Sones, F.M., and Brancato, R.: Radiation exposure to the operator performing cardiac angiography with U-arm systems, Circulation **58:**925-932, 1978.
8. Dash, H., and Leaman, D.M.: Operator radiation exposure during percutaneous transluminal coronary angioplasty, J. Am. Coll. Cardiol. **4:**725-728, 1984.
9. Patterson, W.B., et al.: Occupational hazards to hospital personnel, Ann. Intern. Med. **102:**658-680, 1985.
10. Rueter, F.G.: Physician and patient exposure during cardiac catheterization, Circulation **58:**134-139, 1978.
11. Kan, K., Santen, B.C., Velthuyse, H.J.M., and Julius, H.W.: Exposure of radiologists to scattered radiation during radiodiagnostic examinations, Radiology **119:**455-457, 1976.
12. Antkowiak, J.G.: Scatter radiation to the hands from insertion of transvenous pacemakers, Ann. Thorac. Surg. **30:**405-406, 1980.
13. Kiviniitty, K., Lahti, R., Lahde, S., and Torniainen, P.: Radiation doses from x-ray units used outside radiology departments, Health Phys. **38:**419-421, 1980.
14. Martin, E.C., Olson, A.P., Steeg, C.N., and Casarella, W.J.: Radiation exposure to the pediatric patient during cardiac catheterization and angiocardiography: emphasis on the thyroid gland, Circulation **64:**153-158, 1981.
15. Waldman, J.D., Rummerfield, P.S., Gilpin, E.A., and Kirkpatrick, S.E.: Radiation exposure to the child during cardiac catheterization, Circulation **64:**158-163, 1981.
16. Hempelmann, L.: Risk of thyroid neoplasms after irradiation in children, Science **169:**159, 1968.
17. Leibovic, S.J., and Fellows, K.E.: Patient radiation exposure during pediatric cardiac catheterization, Cardiovasc. Intervent. Radiol. **6:**150-153, 1983.
18. Wagner, L.K., and Hayman, L.A.: Pregnancy and women radiologists, Radiology **145:**559-562, 1982.
19. Swartz, H.M., and Reichling, B.A.: Hazards of radiation exposure for pregnant women, J.A.M.A. **239:**1907-1908, 1978.
20. Review of NCRP radiation dose limit for embryo and fetus in occupationally exposed women, report no. 53, Washington, D.C., 1977, National Council on Radiation Protection and Measurements.
21. Basic radiation protection criteria, report no. 39, Washington, D.C., 1978, National Council on Radiation Protection and Measurements.
22. Medical x-ray and gamma-ray protection for energies up to 10 MeV—equipment design and use, report no. 33, Washington, D.C., 1968, National Council on Radiation Protection and Measurements.
23. Radiation protection for medical and allied health personnel, report no. 48, Washington, D.C., 1977, National Council on Radiation Protection and Measurements.
24. Laughlin, J.S.: Experience with a sustained policy of radiation exposure control and research in a medical center, Health Phys. **41:**709-726, 1981.
25. Judkins, M.P.: Guidelines for radiation protection in the cardiac catheterization laboratory, Cathet. Cardiovasc. Diagn. **10:**87-92, 1984.
26. Woodrow, T.W., King, D., Harrison, E., and Sbar, S.: Radiation exposure during cardiac catheterization (letter), Circulation **58:**1213-1214, 1978.
27. Gertz, E.W., Wisneski, J.A., Gould, R.G., and Akin, J.R.: Improved radiation protection for physicians performing cardiac catheterization, Am. J. Cardiol. **50:**1283-1286, 1982.
28. Hemmingsson, A., and Löfroth, P.O.: Radiation protection in fluoroscopy with an image intensifier, Acta Radiol. Diagn. **19:**1007-1013, 1978.
29. Glaze, S., LeBlanc, A.D., and Bushong, S.C.: Defects in new protective aprons, Radiology **152:**217-218, 1984.
30. Hendrix, T.R.: Human investigation and informed consent, A.J.R. **140:**600-601, 1983.

Chapter Twenty-one

Electrical hazards

EDWARD L. CONOVER, Jr.

In the past decade there has been an explosive growth in the use of invasive cardiac diagnostic and therapeutic procedures. The electrical shock hazard to personnel operating this equipment pales when compared with that of the "electrically sensitive patient"—one who has a direct connection from the heart to the outside world via transvenous or transthoracic catheters, needles, or wires. Because the patient's cardiac tissue is directly connected to sometimes unsuspected sources of electrical current, ventricular fibrillation caused by a level of electrical shock that would not even be perceived by another person is a frightening possibility.[1-4]

The exact number of fatal and nonfatal electric accidents involving the electrically sensitive patient will never be known. This is not solely the result of an inclination to underreport such incidents but stems also from the fact that medical personnel can actually cause an accident without being aware of their involvement.

This chapter explains the fundamental principles of electric current flow and discusses electric shock, sources of hazardous current, typically hazardous situations, and special precautions to be taken with individual cardiovascular procedures.

THE ELECTRICALLY SENSITIVE PATIENT

The primary reason for the increased shock hazard in critical care areas is the use of intracardiac and intra-arterial catheters, which provide a direct electric connection to the myocardium. Such a direct connection of the heart to the outside environment creates what is referred to as an *electrically sensitive patient*. Because the cardiac tissue is directly exposed, the patient is rendered extremely vulnerable to a level of electric current that is imperceptible to a person without a cardiac catheter.

The extreme vulnerability of an electrically sensitive patient is demonstrated by the fact that fibrillation can be induced through a cardiac catheter by a current of 200 μA, whereas attending personnel are just able to perceive a current of 1000 μA.[5]

ELECTRICAL CURRENT FLOW

Current flow is the movement of electrons around a closed loop that consists of a two-terminal voltage source and a conductive path connecting these terminals. There is a difference in potential between two points in the loop; the current then flows from the higher to the lower potential. The less the difference in potential, the less the current flow.

Conductive paths are formed by metal or ionic conductors. The flow of current through a conductive path can be likened to the flow of blood in the circulatory system. The voltage source provides a source of pressure for its closed-loop conductive path, just as the heart does for its closed-loop circulation. In the electric loop this pressure is referred to as *voltage* and is measured in volts (V). The current leaving the voltage source is referred to as the *hot* side of the electric path and corresponds to the arteries. The current returning to the voltage source is called the *neutral* side and corresponds to the veins. Just as obstructions in the arteries or veins restrict the flow of blood, so too does the nature of the electric path restrict the flow of current. This property of restricting current flow is called *resistance* and is measured in ohms. The current flow, which is analogous to the blood flow, is measured in amperes (A). The usual scaling prefixes, such as *milli* (1/1000), *micro* (1/1,000,000), *kilo* (1000), and *mega* (1,000,000), are used with these units.

In both the circulatory system and an electric system, a greater flow (current) can be achieved either by increasing the pressure (voltage) or providing a path with fewer obstructions (reduced resistance). For the electric system this relationship between applied voltage, path resistance, and the resultant current flow is known as Ohm's law. Mathematically the relationship is repre-

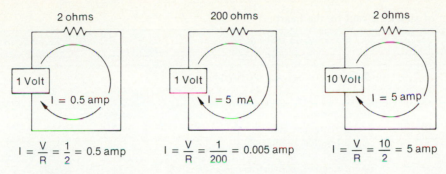

Fig. 21-1. Effect of changing resistance and voltage on current flow. (From Conover, M.B.: Understanding electrocardiography: arrhythmias and the 12 lead ECG, ed. 4, St. Louis, 1984, The C.V. Mosby Co.)

sented by the following equation:

$$\text{Current (I)} = \frac{\text{Voltage (V)}}{\text{Resistance (R)}}$$

Briefly, this expression states that the current flow increases as the applied voltage is increased and decreases as the circuit path resistance is increased. The examples in Fig. 21-1 illustrate the effect of changing resistance and voltage on curent flow.

Thus low-resistance pathways, such as catheter electrodes, allow large currents to flow in them even though the voltage source may be low. By the same token, if the resistance pathway is high, as with the V lead of the ECG, the current flow will be low, even with a high-voltage source.

ELECTRICAL SHOCK

Electrical shock repetitively stimulates the heart and can cause ventricular fibrillation. In cases of very severe shock the heart is completely stopped by sustained contraction. The shock can vary from an intensity that is almost imperceptible if the current is spread over a large area (low current density) to one that is fatal if the current is concentrated in a small area (high current density) (Table 21-1).

Macroshock

Macroshock is the result of current passing through the trunk via the intact skin. The body has two defenses against macroshock, as described below.

1. The high resistance of the skin reduces the amount of current that can flow as the result of a given impressed voltage (Ohm's law). Therefore contact with even full 120 V line voltage generally results in a painful but nonfatal shock. The intact skin exhibits a resis-

tance to the current that ranges from 1000 ohms for conditions of good contact and moist skin to 1 million ohms (1 megohm) for dry skin and low relative humidity.

2. There is a spreading effect whereby the current is distributed throughout the tissue in its path, reducing the current density. Because of this spreading, the cardiac tissue is exposed to only a small fraction of the total current passing through the body; this the operative principle in cardioversion/defibrillation. (For a full discussion on cardioversion and defibrillation, see Chapter 12.)

Microshock

Microshock is the result of current that is introduced directly into cardiac tissue. This is done therapeutically with the use of pacemakers and automatic implanted defibrillator/cardioverters. It is done unwittingly and often fatally by an attendant or because the patient himself touches the case of a piece of equipment that has leakage current.

The electrically sensitive patient may develop ventricular fibrillation as the result of current levels that are below 1 mA (Table 21-1) and that are imperceptible to medical personnel in attendance. This greatly increased vulnerability to electric shock results from the broaching of the body's two defenses, skin resistance and the spreading effect of electric current. When a catheter, needle, or wire connects the heart directly to the outside environment, any current encountered at the proximal end of the catheter, needle, or wire is concentrated in the heart at the point of contact. Because operating personnel are unable to determine when a dangerous condition exists, periodic inspection and special procedures are necessary to ensure the patient's safety.

Table 21-1. Effect of shock current on the heart

Current	Through intact skin (macroshock)	Direct contact to myocardium (microshock)
10 A ⎤ 5 A ⎦	Sustained myocardial contraction	
2 A ⎤ 1 A ⎪ 500 mA ⎬ 200 mA ⎪ 100 mA ⎦	Ventricular fibrillation (respiration continues)	
50 mA	Pain, fainting, exhaustion	
20 mA	*Let go* current (muscle contraction)	
10 mA		
5 mA	Maximum harmless current	Ventricular fibrillation (humans)
2 mA		(2.5 cm. diam. plate electrode)
1 mA	Threshold of perception	
		Ventricular fibrillation (humans)
500 µA		(0.25 cm. diam. plate electrode)
200 µA		Ventricular fibrillation in dogs
100 µA		(catheter)
50 µA		
20 µA		
10 µA		Maximum current recommended
5 µA		for electrically safe areas*

From Conover, M.B.: Understanding electrocardiography: arrhythmias and the 12-lead ECG, ed. 4, St. Louis, 1984, The C.V. Mosby Co.
*Association for Advancement of Medical Instrumentation (AAMI), type A.

SOURCES OF HAZARDOUS ELECTRICAL CURRENT
Electric power in the hospital

The basic source of all hazardous electric current in the hospital is the 120 V, 60 Hz alternating current that powers most of the instruments and equipment. This current is originally generated at an energy source (power plant) and then transmitted at very high voltage (100,000 V) to a substation, where it is transformed to lower voltage (24,000 V). Large power distribution transformers in smaller areas or at hospitals further reduce the voltage in steps until finally 120 V is made available for consumer use.

An important part of this power distribution system is the *ground*. The earth itself is a conductor of electricity, albeit a poor one. Its conductivity results from the moisture and resultant ions in the soil and, in populated areas, from an extensive network of conductive metal pipes. It is this conductive network that is referred to as ground and must be taken into consideration when planning the electrical power distribution system. The ground connection is the mainstay of patient safety. However, it is effective only to the extent that it provides an extremely low-resistance path to a true ground. Hence it is necessary that a well-designed grounding

system be used and maintained in the areas where patients are susceptible to microshock.

The three-pronged plug and line cord not only provide a safe, convenient method of connecting power to a device but also provide a low-resistance pathway to ground for potentially hazardous currents (Fig. 21-2). This plug consists of two flat blades and a longer round or U-shaped pin. One of the flat blades is the "hot" connector and conveys current to the equipment, while the other, the neutral, provides the return path. The hot wire carries a high voltage, while the neutral wire remains near zero volts. The pin is the ground wire and connects the metal case or chassis of a piece of equipment to electrical ground, providing a low-resistance pathway to dissipate leakage currents that may develop on the equipment chassis during use.

Power distribution within the hospital is illustrated in Fig. 21-3. Power is connected to the building through hot and neutral wires and is distributed to the various outlets by means of the power distribution panel. Each of the outlets is connected to ground by a direct connection and through the neutral wire. However, current can flow from the hot wire to any ground. This current flow is possible because the hot wire is at the same 120

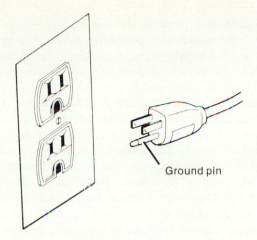

Fig. 21-2. Three-pronged grounding type of plug and receptacle. (From Conover, M.B.: Understanding electrocardiography: arrhythmias and the 12 lead ECG, ed. 4, St. Louis, 1984, The C.V. Mosby Co.)

V potential with respect to ground as it is to the neutral wire.

Leakage current
Capacitive leakage

The most probable source of current dangerous to an electrically sensitive patient is *leakage current*. Although the term suggests some sort of malfunction in a piece of electrical equipment, leakage is in fact not unusual. It is the result of a normal electrical characteristic known as *capacitive coupling,* which is the flow of current between two electric conductors that are close to each other but separated by an insulator, such as from the internal electronics of the device to its chassis. Capacitively coupled current occurs because the conductors are perfectly insulated from each other. The voltage that exists on the chassis of a piece of electric equipment will generate current that seeks the path of lowest resistance to the neutral or ground of the power line. Such a path is harmless unless an electrically sensitive patient is involved and the path that the current seeks to ground goes through the patient's heart; then it is potentially lethal!

Resistance leakage plus capacitive leakage

Resistance leakage is current that results from a deterioration of equipment insulation. The amount of leakage current increases when insulation deterioration lowers resistance, such as would result from moisture or a humid environment, dust, or corrosion. This type of leakage adds to the normal capacitive leakage so that the shock hazard may increase to a point at which even the operating personnel would be in danger of severe

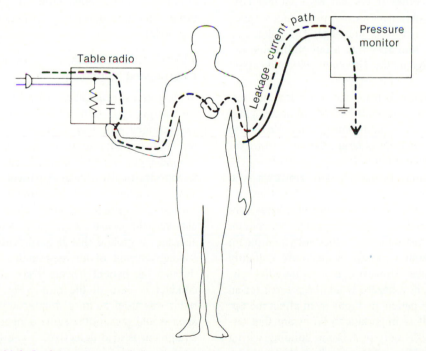

Fig. 21-3. Leakage current path for ungrounded equipment. (From Conover, M.B.: Understanding electrocardiography: arrhythmias and the 12 lead ECG, ed. 4, St. Louis, 1984, The C.V. Mosby Co.)

shock. Equipment that is normally subjected to such adverse environmental conditions (i.e., vacuum cleaners, floor waxers, electric beds, infusion pumps, intra-aortic balloon pumps, and dializers) should be rigorously inspected for leakage current.

Protection from leakage currents

To protect personnel and the patient from leakage currents, a separate wire (ground wire) is provided within the power cord that provides a very low-resistance path between exposed conducting surfaces of equipment and the power line ground. Any leakage current is then conducted harmlessly to ground. This protection is available only in a three-wire system. Two-wire systems have no such path to dissipate leakage currents and constitute a safety hazard. Certain two-wire electric devices use a technique known as *double insulation*. These devices use completely insulated cases to ensure that the leakage current is not a hazard. However, this insulation can be defeated by exposure to conductive liquids or by improper maintenance. Double-insulated devices should be treated as hazardous until approval for a specific device has been obtained from the hospital's engineering department.

Equipment faults (shorts)

A fault is a malfunction of equipment whereby an internal conductor comes in contact with another conductor or with the equipment's case, producing a shock hazard (a fault to the case, or housing). The voltage on the case can range from 120 V to a few millivolts, depending on the point in the circuit at which the fault occurs.

Protection from faults is the same as for leakage currents (i.e., ground the case with a three-pin power plug, which will conduct the fault current harmlessly to ground). If the fault current is large, the circuit breaker or fuse supplying the current will open, interrupting the current and manifesting the malfunction. However, you should be aware that circuit breakers and fuses are designed to carry 15 to 20 A without opening. Thus substantial current can flow without opening the circuit breaker or fuse. In many instances the faulty equipment will continue to operate normally or give only a slightly degraded performance. However, if the grounding circuit should be broken, a hazard would be present for an electrically sensitive patient and may even affect the operating personnel. It is important to be aware that circuit breakers and fuses only protect the building wiring from overheating and becoming a fire hazard. They provide no shock protection for either patient or operating personnel.

In addition to directing short circuit and leakage currents from equipment to power line ground, the ground wire and the building ground conductors serve another function. When several pieces of power line–operated equipment are connected to a patient, different leakage "potentials" exist on the chassis of each device. These differences in chassis potentials result in current flowing from the chassis of one device and through the patient to another device. The ground conductors of each device, in conjunction with the building power line ground, equalize the chassis potentials of all power line–operated devices. Because the potential difference between grounded devices is near zero, the resulting "leakage" current is driven to near zero, thus protecting the patient.

TYPICAL CONDUCTORS FOUND IN THE CARDIAC CATHETERIZATION LABORATORY AND ICU/CCU

Although the source of hazardous voltage is almost always the normal power used to operate equipment, conductive paths are various and at times unexpected. Any material that has mobile electrons is a conductor of electricity. This includes metals and any liquid that has free ions. Metallic conductors include pacing catheters, guidewires, electrolyte-filled angiographic catheters, metal needles, metal furniture, bed lights, and instruments. Ionic conductors include normal saline, urine, blood, and liquid refreshments (such as coffee and soda).

TYPICAL HAZARDOUS SITUATIONS
Ungrounded equipment

Ungrounded equipment can be readily identified by its two-pronged rather than three-pronged plug. The two-pronged plug has no provision for routing leakage or fault current safely to ground. Even when ungrounded equipment is in good repair, it is still a hazard to the electrically sensitive patient. For example, consider the patient who has a temporary pacing wire or a Swan-Ganz catheter in place. The pacing wire or the catheter, through its associated monitor, provides a resistance to ground that is sufficiently low to allow the leakage current of an ungrounded table radio to pass through the patient's heart if contact is made with the conductive case of the radio (Fig. 21-3). Although a radio was used as an example, any ungrounded appliance would present the same danger. If the ungrounded equipment is also defective, it can be a hazard even to the patient who is not electrically sensitive and to the operating personnel.

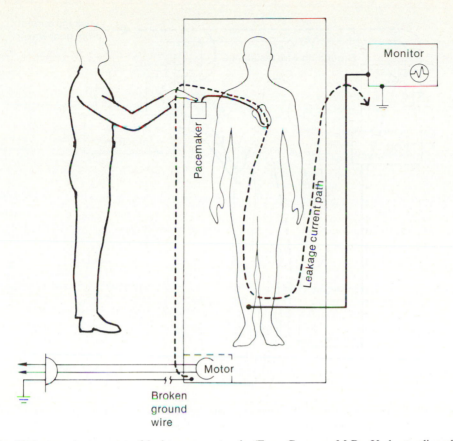

Fig. 21-4. Attendant as part of leakage current path. (From Conover, M.B.: Understanding electrocardiography: arrhythmias and the 12 lead ECG, ed. 4, St. Louis, 1984, The C.V. Mosby Co.)

Equipment with a defective ground

The hazards of a defective grounding system are the same as those of ungrounded equipment, with the added hazard that defective grounding is not as easy to spot as is ungrounded equipment (the two-pronged plug).

Fig. 21-4 illustrates a defective ground on an electric bed. If an attendant were to touch the bare pacemaker terminal while holding the bed rail, a dangerous current would flow through the patient's heart. Some authorities question the use of electric beds in an area where electrically sensitive patients are cared for.

A visual inspection of power cords is helpful, but to ensure patient safety, a resistance measurement must be made of all grounds. Fluoroscopy should be used on molded plugs and connectors.

Unequal ground potentials

The discussion so far has been concerned with one ground potential. To ensure the patient's safety, it is necessary that the various grounds associated with a given patient be at the same electrical potential. Failure to meet this requirement allows a current to pass through the patient if he is connected to two pieces of equipment that are connected to two different grounds. For example, if a patient were connected to a pressure monitor transducer that is normally grounded and to an electrocardiograph that has the usual right-leg ground, a current could flow through the patient's heart because of the difference in ground potentials between the two instruments (Fig. 21-5).

The detection of potential differences between receptacle grounds is made more difficult because the potential is usually the result of a high-leakage current flowing through the ground system. This leakage current may come from equipment that is not in the immediate area. In addition, the equipment causing the leakage current may not be in continuous operation, with the result that the difference in ground potentials will vary. To reduce the potential hazard of unequal ground potentials, separate low-resistance ground connections to a true ground should be provided in the electrically sensitive area.

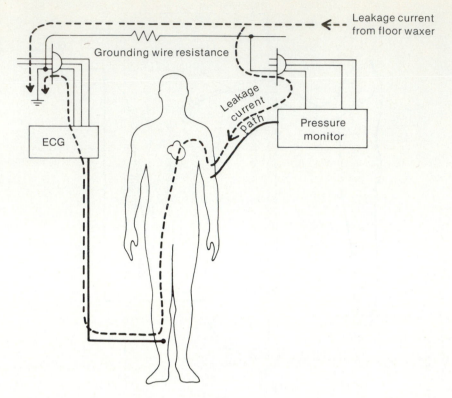

Fig. 21-5. Current flow caused by unequal ground potentials. (From Conover, M.B.: Understanding electrocardiography: arrhythmias and the 12 lead ECG, ed. 3, St. Louis, The C.V. Mosby Co.)

OPERATOR PRECAUTIONS DURING CARDIOVASCULAR PROCEDURES

Do not become part of a circuit that could allow current to flow through you and then through the patient. The following measures will help to avoid such a potentially fatal situation.

General precautions

• Have a defibrillator immediately available at all times in an electrically safe area; in spite of all precautions, accidents may occur and you must be prepared to defibrillate a patient immediately.

• Be aware that cardiac catheters, wires, and needles provide a direct electric connection to the patient's heart.

• Insulate all metal terminals, guidewires, and electrode wires by placing plastic sleeving over exposed terminals, wearing surgical gloves when handling bare electrodes, wires, or terminals.

• When recording an intracardiac ECG, be certain that the electrocardiograph is approved for intracardiac monitoring and that the intracardiac wire is connected to the V lead and not to the right-leg electrode. This lead has a high resistance in relation to power line ground. If an indifferent or ground electrode is mistakenly attached to the needle, leakage currents from other equipment contacting the patient can flow from the point of contact, through the patient's heart, and to ground via the grounded electrocardiograph or grounded personnel touching the patient.

• Be aware that intraesophageal and intratracheal devices, because of their proximity to the posterior myocardium, present a hazard almost as great as that of intracardiac catheters and should be treated with the same care.

• Make sure that all equipment being used with a single patient is plugged into adjacent receptacles.

• Be sure that every piece of electric equipment has a three-pronged plug and that two-pronged "cheater" adapters are not used.

ECG monitoring of pericardiocentesis needle tip

For a complete description of ECG monitoring of the approach of the pericardiocentesis needle tip to the heart, see p. 247. Safety rules are listed here.

• Be sure that it is the V lead that is attached to the needle and that the electrocardiograph is approved for invasive monitoring.

• Be sure that the needle and the connection to the V lead are insulated from ground; wear gloves when touching them.

Because the chest wall offers a path for the dissipation of current accidently introduced into the exploring needle, this procedure has less danger of accidental electrocution for the patient than do transvenous approaches to the heart. However, this protection is absent if the shaft of the needle is insulated by a polyethylene or Teflon sleeve (Rochester-type needle). In such a case the risks are the same as for transvenous catheters. Current carried by the needle would be concentrated at its tip and would enter the myocardium or the pericardial fluid.

Cardiac pacing

The old line-powered cardiac pacemakers have been replaced by battery-operated ones, greatly reducing the electric hazards to the patient. However, electrode catheters used for pacing offer a very low-resistance path to the heart. Even though modern pacemakers are battery powered and thus isolated from power line ground, this isolation can be negated and the patient electrocuted by attendants and electric equipment in the area.

For example, suppose a grounded attendant were to touch the pacemaker terminal of a patient being both paced and electrocardiographically monitored. The current powering the electrocardiograph would seek the low-resistance path to ground unwittingly offered by the attendant who touches the pacemaker terminal. The current would pass from the ECG chassis through the patient's heart, out of the patient's body via the low-resistance pacing electrode, and through the attendant's hand and to ground. The attendant would feel nothing and probably be unaware of having caused the accident. Likewise, as already illustrated in Fig. 21-4, leakage currents on the chassis of electric equipment can flow from the chassis, through the attendant, to the patient's heart, and to ground through the right-leg ECG grounding electrode if the pacing terminal and the electric equipment are touched simultaneously.

Cardiac catheterization and angiography

Because of the complexity and number of pieces of equipment used near the patient during cardiac catheterization and angiography, the possibility of accidental electrocution is presented.[6] The danger is particularly great when metal guidewires (without Teflon coating),

electrode catheters, and catheters carrying normal saline or radiopaque dyes are being used.

The intracardiac ECG monitoring catheter should be connected only to the V lead, which is insulated from ground, preventing significant current flow from or to the patient's heart via the V lead circuit. If the indifferent or ground electrode is used by mistake, lethal currents can flow from other equipment in use on the patient to the patient's heart and then to the mistakenly provided low-resistance ground pathway. The protective high resistance of the V lead circuit can be bypassed if grounded equipment or personnel contact the electrode terminals at their connection to the V lead. In such a case, leakage current from another piece of equipment touching the patient can flow through the heart and the grounded equipment or personnel to ground, electrocuting the patient.

Another hazard is present for the patient who is connected to two or more inadequately grounded devices and has a monitoring catheter in the heart. If the two pieces of equipment have different voltages on their chassis, current may flow from the chassis with higher voltage, through the low-resistance conductor in the patient's heart, and to the chassis with lower voltage.

Because pressure monitors are grounded, they offer a path to ground if the patient touches equipment that is not grounded and has leakage current (Fig. 21-4).

Cardioversion/defibrillation

The defibrillator generates very high voltages and discharges its storage capacitor rapidly, resulting in a pulse of several thousand volts and up to 100 A. It is not suprising that a defibrillator will generate electric transients that may affect its operation and the operation of other electronic equipment in the vicinity. One test for potential operational problems is to set the defibrillator for maximal output and discharge it thru a 25-ohm resistor.

The large currents and voltages involved in cardioversion/defibrillation require special consideration to prevent injury to the operator or patient.

Precautions

• Use adequate conductive gel with care. Gel trailing between paddles can cause the delivered energy to arc across the patient's skin, burning him and dissipating the energy meant for cardioversion or defibrillation. Gel on the operator's hands and paddle handles can result in burns and accidental shock to the operator.

• Never return or temporarily store the paddles in their case without cleaning them. A buildup of dried gel can cause accidental shock to operators.

• Nonsynchronized cardioversion could result in electric stimulation during the vulnerable period of the ECG and cause ventricular fibrillation.

• Use titrated dosage electric shock (see p. 284). Excessive amounts of electric current delivered to the heart can cause cellular damage and arrhythmias.

• Attempted cardioversion of the overdigitalized heart may result in ventricular fibrillation.

• If the resistance of the skin is not sufficiently broken down by rubbing and conductive gel, current may flow from the hot paddle to distant ground sites on the patient, such as ECG or EEG ground electrodes, causing burns.

• Be careful when touching the metal bed. If personnel are touching the metal bed and a part of the patient's body also touches it, severe shock could result.

• If other equipment attached to the patient, such as monitoring systems, has not been "defibrillation-protected," it may be damaged by the electric shock delivered to the patient's body.

• If not adequately insulated, the chassis of the charging defibrillator can carry very high leakage current because of the large AC voltage and the high DC voltage in the storage capacitor.

CONTINUED SURVEY AND CARE OF EQUIPMENT BY OPERATING PERSONNEL

• Check the chassis of all equipment by touch. If you feel a tingling sensation, investigate further. This tingling sensation is actually a mild electrical shock; it indicates that the equipment is defective and poses a definite shock hazard to the electrically sensitive patient. If the equipment is not required for life support, remove it from the area and tag it to alert others to the danger. If such equipment is required for life support, it should be repaired or preferably replaced as soon as possible.

• Keep power cords and plugs in good repair. Ask the hospital electrician to repair or replace all frayed or damaged cords. Any equipment using two-pronged plugs should not be permitted in the hospital.

• Do not allow patient-supplied appliances such as television sets, radios, or electric razors unless they are battery powered and not connected to the hospital's AC power.

• Avoid using extension cords. Two-wire extension cords defeat the grounding scheme of the equipment. If an extension cord is absolutely necessary, it must be the three-wire type and it must be inspected often for an intact ground wire. If possible, such an extension cord should be dedicated to a specific piece of equipment and inspected with that equipment.

• Investigate the cause of AC interference on an ECG tracing. The usual cause of AC interference is dried-out electrode pads or a defective patient cable. If neither of these is the case, the cause may be poorly grounded or defective electric equipment in use on the patient. By systematically disconnecting and reconnecting each piece of equipment until the interference disappears, the offending piece of equipment can be identified and should be removed from the unit and repaired.

• Ensure that the redundant green ground wires often found on electric beds, ECG monitors, and other equipment used around electrically sensitive patients are plugged into the wall ground jacks.

• Do not use equipment that has not been inspected in a reasonable amount of time or that is not intended for use around electrically sensitive patients.

• Report equipment that is operating erratically, producing a strange odor, tripping line-isolation monitors or circuit breakers, or performing in an abnormal manner.

• If ventricular fibrillation occurs in an electrically sensitive patient, assume that it has been accidentally, iatrogenically induced until all equipment and operator procedures have been checked out and proved safe.

• Do not run heavy-wheeled equipment over power cords; this may damage them.

• Do not store equipment in a manner that exposes the power cords to kinking or extremes of temperature.

A SYSTEM FOR PROFESSIONAL INSPECTION

Establish a timetable for professional inspection of medical electrical equipment.[6,7] Inspection should be performed on a regular basis and whenever new equipment has been added or there have been major repairs. This inspection must cover the entire electrically safe area and any equipment that may be brought into it. The purposes are to ensure the integrity of the grounding and the leakage current does not exceed the recommended standard.

• Check all plugs for continuity of conductors. Use an ohmmeter and fluoroscopy to evaluate molded plugs.

• Test the integrity of grounding. Inspect the electric outlets to make sure that the resistance of the ground connections does not exceed 0.15 ohms and that the polarity of the outlets is correct. Commercially available plug-in polarity testers are useful for determining that the outlet polarity is correct but are not sensitive enough to determine the integrity of the grounding system. It is necessary to remove the outlet cover plate and visually inspect the outlet for the presence and correct connection of ground wires or preferably to measure the resistance to the true ground with a milliohmmeter. All

Table 21-2. Maximum leakage current for medical equipment*

Device	Chassis leakage (µA)	Patient lead leakage (µA)
Not of a type that normally contacts a patient	500	N/A
Type likely to contact patient	100	50
All equipment with isolated inputs that are attached to patient's heart	100	10

From Conover, M.B.: Understanding electrocardiography: arrhythmias and the 12-lead ECG, ed. 4, St. Louis, 1984, The C.V. Mosby Co.
*Standards: National Fire Protection Association: NFPA 70-81, National electrical code for health care facilities, and NFPA 76B-80, Electricity in patient care areas of hospitals; Underwriters' Laboratories U1544, Standard for medical and dental equipment; Association for Advancement of Medical Instrumentation AAMI-SCL-P 10.75, Standard for safe current limits.

grounded surfaces and permanently installed equipment should meet this same resistance requirement.

• Test for leakage currents. A 1000-ohm resistor and AC voltmeter (Hewlett Packard model 400E or equivalent) should be used to determine leakage currents on the chassis of a piece of electric equipment.

The resistor simulates a patient's resistance and the voltmeter measures voltage across the resistor. The resistor is placed between the piece of equipment and the power line ground. The leakage current is determined by Ohm's law. Table 21-2 outlines the leakage current limits recommended by the National Fire Protection Association. Note that the maximal amount of leakage current that can be tolerated by the electrically sensitive patient is 10 µA.[7] This corresponds to a voltage of 10 mV across the 1000 ohm test resistor. These limits are widely accepted by both government and professional groups.

WIRING FOR THE ANGIOGRAPHIC LABORATORY

The standards of the National Electrical Code and the standards for the safe use of electricity in health care facilities are not adequate for the angiographic laboratory because the patient has multiple exposure sites.[7-9]

• All receptacles must be of the three-pin grounding type.

• The ground wire usually connected to a standard three-prong outlet is not adequate for this area. To minimize leakage current, install larger-than-normal ground wires (no. 2 wire) in the power distribution wiring. This larger wire has less resistance, thereby minimizing chassis potential differences between electrically operated devices.

• To minimize the possibility of voltages developing between equipment, the patient, and ground, isolate the chassis of all pieces of equipment completely from any electric component of the power line. In such a system there is no connection between the neutral and the ground wires.

• To maintain the grounds at a given bed at the same potential, all the ground wires from outlets serving that bed should be isolated from ground wires serving other outlets and grounded at a single true ground point.

• Connect all exposed metal items, such as water pipes, building structure, and metal furniture, to a room ground.

• If you are using equipment that grounds or is likely to ground cardiac catheters, wires, or needles, investigate the possibility of isolation transformers for the area to provide an additional margin of safety for patients in case of grounding failures.

Pitfalls of isolation transformers

Leakage current may still flow through the patient from one chassis to another if there is a voltage difference between the two chassis. This hazard exists because the two pieces of equipment have common grounds or neutral wires to the isolation transformer.

Individual isolation transformers would solve the above problem but they are extremely costly and may lose their isolation without the operator's knowledge.

EQUIPMENT SELECTION

The responsibility for the selection of new equipment and other capital improvements usually rests with hospital administrators, whose primary field of experience is business management. Thus it is usually necessary to seek advice from a consultant who is technically competent, unbiased, and aware of the necessity for a safe environment for the electrically sensitive patient.

REFERENCES

1. Burchell, H.B.: Hidden hazards of cardiac pacemakers (editorial), Circulation **24**:161, 1961.
2. Noordijk, J.A., Oey, F.T.I., and Tebra, W.: Myocardial elec-

trodes and the danger of ventricular fibrillation, Lancet **1:**975, 1961.

3. Mody, S.M., Poona, M.B., and Richings, M.: Ventricular fibrillation resulting from electrocution during cardiac catheterisation, Lancet **2:**698, 1962.

4. Pengelly, L.D., and Klassen, G.A.: Myocardial electrodes and the danger of ventricular fibrillation, Lancet **1:**1234, 1961.

5. Starmer, C.F., and Whalen, R.E.: Current density and electrically induced ventricular fibrillation, Med. Instrum. **7:**1-5, 1973.

6. Starmer, F.C., Whalen, R.E., and McIntosh, H.D.: Hazards of electric shock in cardiology, Am. J. Cardiol. **14:**537, 1964.

7. Starmer, F., McIntosh, H.D., and Whalen, R.E.: Electrical hazards and cardiovascular function, N. Engl. J. Med. **284:**181-186, 1971.

8. Starmer, F., McIntosh, H.D., and Whalen, R.E.: Determination of leakage currents in medical equipment, Am. J. Cardiol. **17:**437-438, 1966.

9. O'Dowd, W.J.: Defibrillator design and development—a review, J. Med. Engl. Technol. **7:**5-15, 1983.

Chapter Twenty-two

Medicolegal concerns

HARRY W. REIN

When diagnostic or therapeutic cardiovascular procedures are performed, physicians must be familiar with their obligations under the hospital medical staff bylaws and rules and with business, professional, and health codes of the states in which they practice. These concepts are also applied to other medical procedures.

Because there is important variation among the 50 states, only basic principles of medical law will be discussed in this chapter, with the hope that when uncertainty arises, physicians will be alerted to consult the legal advisor at their hospital or medical society or their malpractice insuror. Areas discussed include the basic elements of medical negligence suits, physician responsibility for informed consent, medical records as evidence, product liability, hospital liability, physician liability for employees, and physician responsibility under Medicare legislation.

BASIC ELEMENTS OF MEDICAL NEGLIGENCE SUITS

Most actions brought against physicians are filed as negligence complaints. Plaintiffs, to be successful, must prove all four of the following basic facts:

1. The physician assumed a duty of care to the patient.
2. The physician breached (failed) in that duty.
3. Such failure was the legal (proximate) cause of the harm that resulted to the patient.
4. The patient has sustained medical expenses, loss of earnings, pain and suffering, or other damages.

Assumption of duty of care

Assumption of duty of care is an implied agreement to provide the quality of care given by similarly trained physicians under similar patient circumstances (not necessarily the best care in the state or city). An exception may arise if a nonspecialist physician is so unwise as to represent himself or herself to the patient as a specialist.

In such a case, the duty of care assumed will be that degree of training and skill possessed by a specialist.

Assumption of duty of care requires no formal or informal verbal or written agreement; it attaches when a physician takes a medical history, examines a patient, prescribes medical treatment, performs a procedure, interprets diagnostic tests, or agrees to provide coverage for an absent attending physician.

Formerly, the assumption of a duty of care implied that the physician had training and skills possessed by similarly trained physicians in the community and would provide a quality of care accepted in that medical community. However, this concept is being eroded by national standardization of residency and fellowship programs, under the influence of national societies and their board examinations, and by effective regional and national medical education programs. The result is that a physician-defendant who argues that he or she performed coronary arteriography, for example, in a manner acceptable to similarly trained physicians in the community may be countered by an expert witness from another part of the state, whose testimony is allowed into evidence on the grounds that there is now a national standard of proficiency for performance of coronary arteriography.

Failure to perform the assumed duty

Proof that the physician breached or failed in performing the assumed duty usually requires testimony of the plaintiff's expert witness that substandard care was given. The judge makes the decision as to whether the plaintiff's witness qualifies as an expert and questions such a witness as to training, membership in medical societies, board certification, and experience. Plaintiffs frequently lose negligence suits against physicians because of difficulty in finding expert physician witnesses or witnesses whose testimony persuades juries. A "conspiracy of silence" among physicians has been often alleged, but the difficulty of plaintiffs in securing competent and credible experts sometimes reflects perceived weakness in the plaintiff's case.

When it is a matter of knowledge to a lay person (jury) that a certain untoward result does not occur in the absence of substandard care by the physician, the plaintiff is not required to have an expert physician witness show breach of duty. For example, a 38-year-old woman with uterine fibroids, who is otherwise healthy, has a hysterectomy and never regains consciousness after surgery. If the patient was under the exclusive control of the defendant physician when the harm occurred, the judge may give the jury a res ipsa loquitur (the thing speaks for itself) instruction. The persistent coma in this example is so unusual and unexpected that it is not likely to occur in the absence of physician negligence. Thus a legal inference of negligence arises, and each physician who provided care during the period that harm could have occurred has the burden of proof to show that his or her conduct did not contribute to the bad outcome. The social policy reversing the usual burden of proof in res ipsa cases is based on the notion that patients who are sedated or anesthetized would have great difficulty bearing the usual burden of proof, especially when several physicians provided care during the critical time.

Another situation in which the plaintiff is not required to have an expert physician witness testifying to substandard care is more likely to occur. In this case other competent evidence is available to show that the defendent physician failed to follow a written protocol for a diagnostic or therapeutic procedure that was in effect in the laboratory or hospital. This failure would be evidence of breach of duty, and no expert witness would be needed to say that the physician's conduct was below standard. Such protocols are readily discoverable by the plaintiff's attorney and accepted in court as the standard of care. With the use of such protocols greatly increasing in hospitals, especially in the cardiovascular field, it is important that physicians who develop them do so with the widest possible concensus of all physicians in the department or cardiovascular laboratory. Preferably, a solid majority vote should approve the protocols, and every protocol should be circulated to all physicians affected by it. Protocols should be reviewed at least annually to be certain that there is still a solid majority of support from affected physicians, that amendments are made if needed, and that the amended or reaffirmed protocols are again circulated.

Legal (proximate) cause of harm to patient

The plaintiff must prove that the defendant's care or conduct was a legally sufficient (proximate) cause of harm to the patient. If the physician's care set off a chain of events, the judge may "cut the chain" at a certain link on the grounds that the law should not hold a defendant responsible for results of sufficient remoteness from the procedure that such results could not be foreseen.

Proof of damages

The plaintiff must have means of documenting resulting medical or other care costs, evidence of the amount and likely duration of disability, actual and projected loss or diminution of earnings, loss of consortium, pain and suffering, and other lesser items that all may in the aggregate add to a very high figure. Additionally, if a physician's conduct has been sufficiently blameworthy or outrageous, punitive damages may be sought by the plaintiff and awarded by the jury. Such cases and, in many of the states, malpractice settlements or jury awards of over a stated amount are routinely investigated by a state's physician licensing board.

PHYSICIAN RESPONSIBILITY TO OBTAIN INFORMED CONSENT

The great expansion of civil and human rights that has occurred in the United States and many other countries in the past 30 years has clearly influenced the health care field. A right to privacy has been found in Justice Douglas's "Penumbra of Rights," radiating from the famous guarantees expressed in the first 10 amendments to the Constitution of the United States. Inherent in the right to privacy is the right of all competent adults to refuse or consent to medical testing, procedures, and treatment, and the right of all incompetent persons and dependent minors to have legally prescribed, substituted consent by persons who will act in such a patient's best interests. There is much variation in statutes and administrative regulations in the various states; all that can be stated here are some basic principles and the admonition that all physicians must be familiar with consent requirements in states in which they practice.

Printed consent forms used by hospitals are often signed by patients who cannot comprehend the complex phrasing. Such forms serve only as verification that the patient has received the necessary information from the physician and agrees to proceed.

The patient's right to consent to or refuse medical care implicitly carries an obligation for the recommending or performing physician, in a face-to-face exchange, to describe at least the following:

1. The procedure or treatment and the reasonably expected benefits.

2. The material complications or side effects: *Material* in this sense means those complications that the patient should know about in reaching his or her decision; even a rare complication can be material. If death, loss of limb, or stroke result only once in 1000 cardiac catheterizations, it is nevertheless a ''material'' complication and should be mentioned as one of the very remote risks.

3. Any medically reasonable alternate procedures or treatment.

4. The medically likely outcome if the patient declines the treatment or procedure that has been proposed.

Two conditions sometimes arise that will excuse a physician from disclosing less than this minimal information. The first occurs when the patient refuses to be told of the material complications; the second occurs when the physician has medical grounds for believing the patient to be so distraught that informing him of the possible complications would threaten the patient's mental stability and ability to make a reasoned decision. In both of these exceptional situations, physicians should (1) promptly document in the medical record the patient's refusal of information or the physician's reasons for withholding some information, (2) discuss the situation with the patient's closest family members, and (3) note in the patient's medical record that such a discussion occurred and what information was not transmitted to the patient. Obtaining a second opinion in these cases of less-than-complete disclosure would be additional protection for both patient and physician.

Additional methods of disclosure of information may be required by state administrative regulations. For example, in California a printed form listing alternate forms of treatment for breast cancer must be distributed to patients as part of the informed consent process.

Consent is implied, without the usual verbal exchange between physician and patient, for minor procedures without serious risks. The patient who bares and extends his or her arm to the approaching phlebotomist or turns in bed to receive a gluteal injection has implicitly consented to have blood drawn or to have an intramuscular injection.

When immediate treatment is necessary to protect a patient's life and limb, the physician may proceed after a less-than-full explanation or after no explanation; patient consent is implied provided the physician documents, at the first opportunity, the urgency of the patient's condition and the need for immediate action. In these circumstances a physician should always make an effort to provide as much information to a patient in an emergency situation as time safely permits.

When a patient is confused and unable to understand the physician's efforts to obtain informed consent, and if treatment or testing should not be deferred for sound medical reasons, the physician should provide information to the closest family members or to a guardian if one has been appointed and obtain their agreement to proceed. If there is no family or none can be contacted, it is advisable to have a second physician's concurrence in the proposed treatment or testing.

A dilemma occasionally arises when the patient's family is divided on the issue of consent or when the family refuses consent to clearly indicated and beneficial treatment. In such a case the physician should promptly consult another physician and, if the consultant concurs with the recommended care, discuss with the hospital's or insuror's legal counsel the possibility of having a guardian appointed to act for the patient.

The rules of consent for minors vary considerably among the various states, but there are some common threads. Minors who are married, who are living away from home and are self-supporting, who are close to the age of majority, or who may be pregnant or have certain communicable diseases usually may consent to treatment or testing even though they have not reached the age of majority.

MEDICAL RECORDS AS EVIDENCE

There is an ancient Chinese proverb that faded ink is more reliable than the memories of a thousand wise men; this is no less true if the wise men happen to be physicians. The primary purpose of accurate, complete, and timely recording of information in patient's charts is that a patient's health and safety depend on preservation and dissemination of that information to other physicians, nurses, and health professionals privileged to care for that person. Good recordkeeping is thus part of a physician's duty of care to his or her patient, and medical record quality is regularly monitored and enforced by hospital staffs, the Joint Commission on Accreditation of Hospitals (JCAH), and state physician licensing boards, and by Professional Review Organizations (PRO) under contract with Medicare to monitor the quality and medical necessity of care provided to Medicare patients. Quite apart from the advantages to patients of good recordkeeping by physicians, complete, accurate, and timely medical records are invaluable to the physician whose care is later questioned by medical committees or in court.

Medical records are usually a compendium of dozens or hundreds of separate entries of information entered by many persons. As written statements made outside of court, they are hearsay evidence and can only be admissible in court as evidence to support or to controvert an issue if the judge qualifies the record as an exception to rules of evidence prohibiting admission of hearsay evidence. Before a medical record may be admitted into evidence, the judge will first require live testimony or an affadavit from the hospital record administrator that the record was made contemporaneously and is complete. Any obliteration of entries or failure to record significant patient events casts substantial doubt on the accuracy of the entire record and on the credibility of the responsible physician. Furthermore, inferences of concealment may arise that could prevent the application of statutes of limitation or lead to imposition of punitive damages by juries.

The use of form reports or word-processor generated reports can be a legal pitfall for physicians, who will have an embarrassing burden of proof in court or in depositions when they try to explain disparities between the content of the form report and the actual events as shown by other competent testimony.

If a physician is in doubt as to whether to document less or more in medical records, completeness will almost always be to the physician's advantage and to the patient's benefit.

PRODUCT LIABILITY

Product liability law evolved from concepts of strict liability previously applied to food vendors for wholesomeness of food sold. Liability law is increasingly being applied in the health care field. The concepts have been refined greatly in the past 50 years by judicial decisions and by statutes as the complexity of our industrial society has greatly increased. Whereas negligence principles traditionally were applied to the delivery of services, and product liability principles to the sale of defective goods or products, the distinction blurs when a physician inserts a cardiac catheter, implants a pacemaker, or orders a transfusion of highly processed blood components or even of whole blood. A plaintiff bringing a product liability action need not show that the catheter, pacemaker, or other device was negligently designed or manufactured, but only that it had a defect that rendered it unreasonably unsafe and that damage or injury was thereby sustained.

Product liability, which was at first imposed only on manufacturers, has gradually been extended to all those in the marketing enterprise who participate in placing the product "in the stream of commerce," including wholesalers, distributors, and retailers, who should reasonably share the costs of patient injury. It is quite conceivable that a physician (retailer) who, with no knowledge of any defect, chose the particular pacemaker or device, might be a codefendant with the manufacturer

and distributor in a product liability action. If the physician used such a product without ascertaining its reliability or quality, a second, separate lawsuit for negligence could be brought against the physician.

HOSPITAL LIABILITY

Hospitals are increasingly named as codefendants in medical malpractice suits. Liability of a hospital for failure of the medical staff to perform delegated responsibilities, such as careful credentialing of medical staff applicants and effective staff monitoring of in-hospital patient care given by physicians, has resulted in large awards to plaintiffs. Hospitals are also responsible for careful selection of all nurses and other licensed professionals, for in-service training, and for periodic performance evaluations of these persons to ensure safe and effective patient care. Nurses, laboratory technicians, pharmacists, and other licensed and unlicensed hospital employees are normally "agents" of the hospital, which is responsible for any patient harm caused by its agents. An exception may arise if a physician is performing a unique or unusual procedure with the assistance of a hospital nurse or technician whose performance is continuously under physician's control. In this exception, liability for such assistant's actions may shift to the physician under the "borrowed servant" doctrine.

Physicians who bring their own employees (nurse or technician) to assist in a hospital procedure are primarily liable for acts or omissions of such employees, but the hospital may share liability if it fails to inquire into their training and qualifications, usually by evaluation before an interdisciplinary committee. By the principles of agency law, physicians are primarily liable for all acts and omissions of their employees occurring during the furtherance of employee's duties, whether in a private office or in a hospital.

Hospitals are responsible under conditions of their state license and under JCAH accreditation standards for providing safe and reliable laboratory equipment. Physicians who knowingly use unsafe or unreliable hospital equipment may share liability with the hospital for resulting patient complications or errors in diagnosis. If the physician's legitimate concerns about inadequate equipment, as expressed to medical staff committees and to hospital administration, fall on deaf ears, the physician's only ethical alternative may be to do his or her procedures in a better-equipped hospital or to obtain a "second opinion" from the state board or commission licensing hospitals.

PHYSICIAN'S RESPONSIBILITIES UNDER MEDICARE LEGISLATION

The Medicare Act of 1965 specifies that physicians have three basic responsibilities to beneficiaries:

1. The care provided must be medically indicated.
2. The care must be of sufficient quality to be acceptable to the medical community.
3. The physician must make records of sufficient quality and completeness such that peer review can determine items 1 and 2 above.

The Medicare administration contracts with nonprofit or for-profit Professional Review Organizations (PRO) to implement and monitor these basic physician obligations and to perform preadmission reviews and preprocedure reviews of nonemergency cases and reviews of interhospital transfers, certain readmissions, and cases falling outside certain length of patient stay and cost parameters.

When a physician's care of a Medicare patient is questioned by a PRO after a review of the patient's medical records by physician consultants, the physician is usually asked to meet informally with a review committee and to add any further information that could explain the questioned care. Physicians found to be providing unnecessary care or care below the accepted community standard may be subject to more intense review of their cases, or in flagrant cases, may be excluded from being compensated by Medicare for caring for Medicare beneficiaries.

Appendixes

APPENDIX A

Terminology for coronary artery anatomy. *1*, Proximal right. *2*, Mid-right. *3*, Distal right. *4*, Right posterior descending. *5*, Right posterolateral segment. *6*, First right posterior lateral. *7*, Second right posterior lateral. *8*, Third right posterior lateral. *9*, Inferior septal. *10*, Acute marginal. *11*, Left main. *12*, Proximal left anterior descending. *13*, Mid-left anterior descending. *14*, Distal left anterior descending. *15*, First diagonal. *16*, Second diagonal. *17*, First septal. *18*, Proximal circumflex. *19*, Distal circumflex. *20*, First obtuse marginal, *21*, Second obtuse marginal. *22*, Third obtuse marginal. *23*, Left atrioventricular. *24*, First left posterior lateral. *25*, Second left posterior lateral. *26*, Third left posterior lateral. *27*, Left posterior descending. (Adapted from Principal investigators of CASS and their associates: National Heart, Lung, and Blood Institute Coronary Artery Surgery Study, Circulation **63**[suppl. 1]:1-81, 1981. Used by permission of the American Heart Association, Inc.)

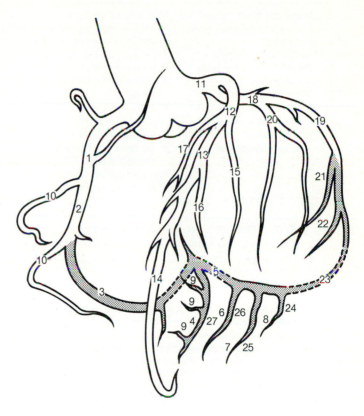

APPENDIX B

Terminology for left ventricular segments in the right anterior oblique (*RAO*) and left anterior oblique (*LAO*) projections. (*AL*, Anterolateral papillary muscle; *PM*, posteromedial papillary muscle.) (Adapted from Principal investigators of CASS and their associates: National Heart, Lung, and Blood Institute Coronary Artery Surgery Study, Circulation **63**[suppl. 1]:1-81, 1981. Used by permission of the American Heart Association, Inc.)

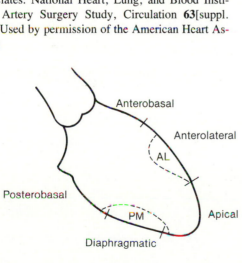

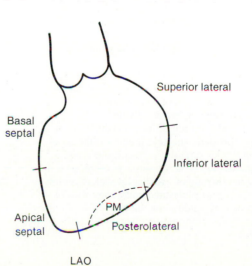

APPENDIX C—PREVENTION OF INFECTIVE ENDOCARDITIS

I. Cardiac conditions for which endocarditis prophylaxis is recommended[3]

Conditions with relatively high risk for endocarditis	Conditions with low-intermediate risk for endocarditis
Prosthetic heart valves	Mitral valve prolapse without regurgitation
Cyanotic congenital heart disease	Pure mitral stenosis
Aortic valve disease	Tricuspid valve disease
Previous infective endocarditis	Pulmonary valve disease
Mitral insufficiency	Asymmetric septal hypertrophy
Patent ductus arteriosus	Calcific aortic sclerosis
Ventricular septal defect	Alimentation or pressure monitoring catheters in the right heart or pulmonary artery
Coarctation of the aorta	Nonvalvular intracardiac prosthetic implants
Marfan's syndrome	

II. Cardiac conditions for which endocarditis prophylaxis is not considered necessary because of very low or negligible risk[3]

Atrial septal defect
Arteriosclerotic plaques
Postoperative coronary artery bypass graft surgery
Syphillitic aortitis
Cardiac pacemakers
Surgically corrected cardiac lesions (without prosthetic implants, more than 6 months after operation)

III. Procedures for which endocarditis prophylaxis is indicated

All dental procedures likely to induce gingival bleeding (not simple adjustment of orthodontic appliances or shedding of deciduous teeth)
Tonsillectomy and/or adenoidectomy
Surgical procedures or biopsy involving respiratory mucosa
Bronchoscopy, especially with a rigid bronchoscope; the risk with flexible bronchoscopy is low, and the need for prophylaxis is not well defined
Incision and drainage of infected tissue
Genitourinary and gastrointestinal procedures, such as cystoscopy, prostatic surgery, urethral catheterization, urinary tract surgery, vaginal hysterectomy, gallbladder surgery, colonic surgery, esophageal dilatation, sclerotherapy of esophageal varices, colonoscopy, upper gastrointestinal endoscopy with biopsy or proctosigmoidoscopic biopsy
Cardiac surgery including the implantation of prosthetic valves

IV. Recommended antibiotic regimens for prophylaxis of endocarditis[3]

Standard regimen

For dental procedures and oral or upper respiratory tract surgery	Penicillin V, 2.0 g orally 1 hour before procedure, then 1.0 g 6 hours later

Special regimens

Parenteral regimen for high-risk patients; also for gastrointestinal (GI) or genitourinary (GU) procedures	Ampicillin, 2.0 g intramuscularly (IM) or intravenously (IV), plus gentamicin, 1.5 mg/kg IM or IV ½ hour before
Parenteral regimen for patients allergic to penicillin	Vancomycin, 1.0 g IV slowly over 1 hour, starting 1 hour before procedure; add gentamicin, 1.5 mg/kg IM or IV, if GI or GU tract is involved
Oral regimen for patients allergic to penicillin (oral and respiratory tract only)	Erythromycin, 1.0 g orally 1 hour before procedure, then 0.5 g 6 hours later
Oral regimen for minor GI or GU tract procedures	Amoxicillin, 3.0 g orally 1 hour before procedure, then 1.5 g 6 hours later
Cardiac surgery, including implantation of prosthetic valves	Cefazolin, 2.0 g IV at induction of anesthesia, repeated 8 and 16 hours later

These recommendations are obtained from the Committee on Prevention of Rheumatic Fever and Bacterial Endocarditis of the American Heart Association,[1] consultants of the Medical Letter,[2] and expert opinion.[3] They represent the *judgment* of experts and set the standard of care in the prevention of endocarditis.[4] They are empiric suggestions; no regimen has been proven to be effective for prevention of endocarditis and prevention failures may occur with any regimen.[4,5] These regimens are not intended to cover all clinical situations. The practitioner should evaluate safety and cost/benefit issues in each individual case. One or two additional doses may be given in cases where the period of risk for bacteremia is prolonged.

Invasive procedures discussed in this book, when performed under optimal conditions, do not pose a significant risk of endocarditis. Thus, prophylactic antibiotics to prevent endocarditis are not routinely used. There are circumstances where antibiotic prophylaxis may be advisable. These include (1) patients considered to be at high risk for endocarditis (e.g., past history of endocarditis, prosthetic valves, compromised host), (2) prolonged procedure or suspected or known break in sterile technique, and (3) cardiopulmonary resuscitation with traumatic intubation. In these circumstances, one of the parenteral regimens outlined in Table IV would be advisable.

REFERENCES

1. Shulman S.T., et al.: Prevention of bacterial endocarditis: a statement for health professionals by the Committee on Rheumatic Fever and Infective Endocarditis of the Council on Cardiovascular Disease in the Young Circulation **70:**1123A-1127A, 1984.
2. The Medical Letter on Drugs and Therapeutics **23:**91-92, 1981.
3. Durack, D.T.: Current issues in prevention of infective endocarditis, Am. J. Med. **78**(suppl. 6B):149-156, 1985.
4. Kaye, D.: Prophylaxis for infective endocarditis: an update, Ann. Intern. Med. **104:**419-423, 1986.
5. Kaplan, E.L.: Bacterial endocarditis prophylaxis—tradition or necessity? Am. J. Cardiol. **57:**478-479, 1986.

APPENDIX D*

I. Normal blood oxygen saturation at various sites in cardiac chambers and great vessels

Site	Oxygen saturation (%)
IVC	80 ± 5
SVC	70 ± 5
RA	70 ± 5
RV	70 ± 5
PA	70 ± 5
LA	96 ± 2
LV	96 ± 2
AO	96 ± 2

II. Minimal percentage of oxygen saturation changes between cardiac chambers indicative of left-to-right shunts

	Minimal saturation increase (%)		
	Sets of samples		
Position	1	2	3
SVC-RA	10	7	5
RA-RV	7	5	3
RV-PA	5	3	3

III. Normal blood oxygen content at various sites in cardiac chambers and great vessels

Site	Oxygen content (vol%)
IVC	16 ± 1
SVC	14 ± 1
RA	15 ± 1
RV	15.2 ± 1
PA	15.2 ± 1
Arterial	19.1 ± 0.2

IV. Maximal normal variation in oxygen content between right heart chambers and the pulmonary artery

Site	Maximal step-up in oxygen content over proximal chamber (vol%)
PA	0.5
RV	0.9
RA	1.9

V. Typical blood oxygen contents at various sites with specific left-to-right shunts

	Oxygen content (vol%)		
Site	ASD	VSD	PDA
IVC	16	16	16
SVC	14	14	14
RA	17	14	14
RV	17	17	14
PA	17	17	17
Arterial	19	19	19

*IVC, inferior vena cava; SVC, superior vena cava; RA, right atrium; RV, right ventricle; PA, pulmonary artery; LA, left atrium; LV, left ventricle; AO, aorta.

APPENDIX E—CONVERSION FACTORS

To convert	To	Multiply by
Atmospheres	Millimeters mercury	760
Atmospheres	Pounds/square inch (psi)	14.7
Centimeters	Inches	0.3937
Centimeters water	Millimeters mercury	0.735
Feet	Meters	0.3048
French size	Millimeter diameter	0.33
Grains	Milligrams	64.799
Hybrid resistance units (HRU)	Absolute resistance units (ARU) ($dynes \cdot sec \cdot cm^{-5}$)	80 2.54
Inches	Millimeters	25.40
Kilograms	Pounds	2.205
Meters	Feet	3.281
Millimeters mercury	Centimeters water	1.36
Ounces (fl)	Milliliters	29.5735

APPENDIX F—NORMAL INTRACARDIAC AND INTRAVASCULAR PRESSURES IN ADULTS
Pressures (mm Hg)

Right atrium (RA)	Mean	0-8
	a Wave	2-10
	v Wave	2-10
Right ventricle (RV)	Systolic	15-30
	End diastolic	0-8
Pulmonary artery (PA)	Systolic	15-30
	Diastolic	5-14
	Mean	10-22
Pulmonary artery wedge (PAW)	Mean	4-12
Left atrium (LA)	Mean	4-12
	a Wave	5-15
	v Wave	5-15
Left ventricle (LV)	Systolic	90-150
	End diastolic	4-12
Aortic (AO)	Systolic	90-150
	Diastolic	60-90
	Mean	70-105

APPENDIX G—CARDIOVASCULAR FUNCTION: DERIVED DATA

Cardiovascular function tests—formulas	Units	Normal values
Oxygen (O_2) capacity = Hemoglobin (Hgb) (g/dl) × 1.39 (ml O_2/g Hgb)	vol%	17-23.5 (Hgb 12-17)
O_2 content = O_2 capacity × % saturation	vol%	19 ± 1 (arterial)
		15.2 ± 1 (mixed venous)
O_2 consumption (basal state estimate)	ml/min/m²	130 ± 10
Arteriovenous oxygen difference (avO_2 difference) = arterial O_2 content − venous O_2 content	vol%	4.1 ± 0.6
Cardiac output (Fick principle) = O_2 consumption (ml/min)/avO_2 difference (vol%) × 10	L/min	6.0 ± 2.0 (varies with body size)
O_2 delivery = Cardiac output × arterial O_2 content × 10	ml/min	1000
Cardiac index = Cardiac output/body surface area	L/min/m²	2.5-4.2
Stroke volume = End-diastolic volume − end-systolic volume or Cardiac output (ml/min)/heart rate	ml/beat	60-130
Stroke index (SI) = Cardiac index (ml/min)/heart rate	ml/beat/m²	30-65
LV stroke work index = SI × (mean arterial pressure − mean PA wedge pressure) × 0.0136	gram − m/m²	30-100
Systemic vascular resistance (SVR) = (mean arterial pressure − mean central venous pressure)/cardiac output	Hybrid resistance units (HRU) (mm Hg/L/min)	9-20
Pulmonary vascular resistance (PVR) = (Mean PA pressure − mean PAW or LA pressure)/cardiac output*	HRU	0.2-1.5
Total pulmonary resistance (TPR) = mean PA pressure/cardiac output*	HRU	1.2-3.5
$Mitral\ valve\ area = \dfrac{Mitral\ valve\ flow\ (ml/sec)}{37.7\ \sqrt{Diastolic\ gradient\ across\ the\ mitral\ valve}}$	cm²	4.0-6.0
where: Mitral valve flow = $\dfrac{Cardiac\ output\ (ml/min)}{Diastolic\ filling\ period\ (sec/min)}$		
Diastolic filling period (sec/min) = diastolic period per beat (sec/beat) × heart rate (beats/min)		
Diastolic gradient across the mitral valve (mm Hg) = left atrial mean pressure (mm Hg) − left ventricular mean diastolic pressure (mm Hg)		
37.7 = Empirical constant		
$Aortic\ valve\ area = \dfrac{Aortic\ valve\ flow\ (ml/sec)}{44.3\ \sqrt{Systolic\ pressure\ gradient\ across\ the\ aortic\ valve}}$	cm²	2.6-3.5
where: Aortic valve flow (ml/sec) = $\dfrac{Cardiac\ output\ (ml/min)}{Systolic\ ejection\ period\ (sec/min)}$		
Systolic ejection period (sec/min) = systolic ejection period per beat (sec/beat) × heart rate (beats/min)		
Systolic pressure gradient across the aortic valve (mm Hg) = left ventricular mean systolic pressure (mm Hg) − aortic mean systolic pressure (mm Hg)		
44.3 = Empirical constant		
Coronary perfusion pressure = arterial diastolic pressure − LVEDP (or mean PAW pressure)	mm Hg	60-80
Left ventricular volumes		
End systolic volume (ESV)	ml/m²	20-36
End diastolic volume (EDV)	ml/m²	50-90
Ejection fraction (ESV/EDV × 100)	%	58-75

*Assumes no intracardiac shunt, thus cardiac output = systemic blood flow = pulmonary blood flow.

APPENDIX H

Body Surface of Adults

Nomogram for determination of body surface from height and mass[1]

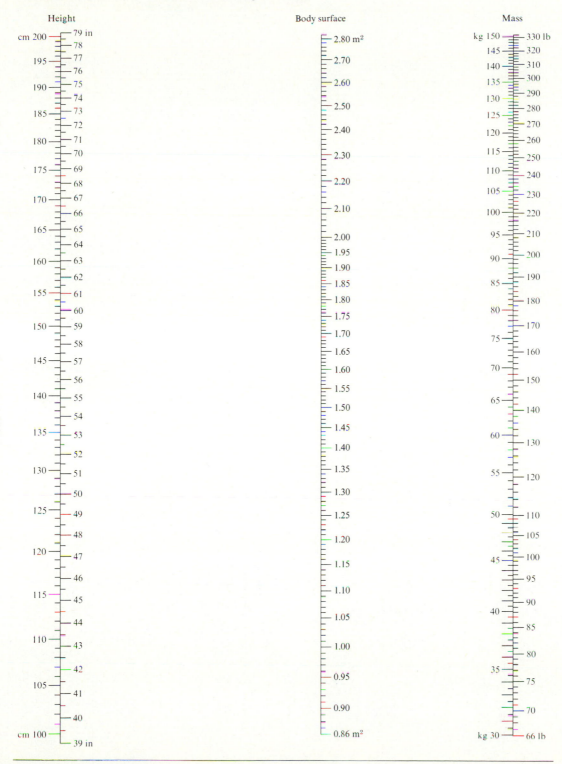

| Height | Body surface | Mass |

[1] From the formula of Du Bois and Du Bois, *Arch. intern. Med.*, **17**, 863 (1916): $S = M^{0.425} \times H^{0.725} \times 71.84$, or $\log S = \log M \times 0.425 + \log H \times 0.725 + 1.8564$ (S: body surface in cm², M: mass in kg, H: height in cm).
Reproduced with permission from Lentner, C., editor: Geigy scientific tables, ed. 8, vol. 1, Basle, Switzerland, 1981, Ciba-Geigy.

Body Surface of Children

Nomogram for determination of body surface from height and mass[1]

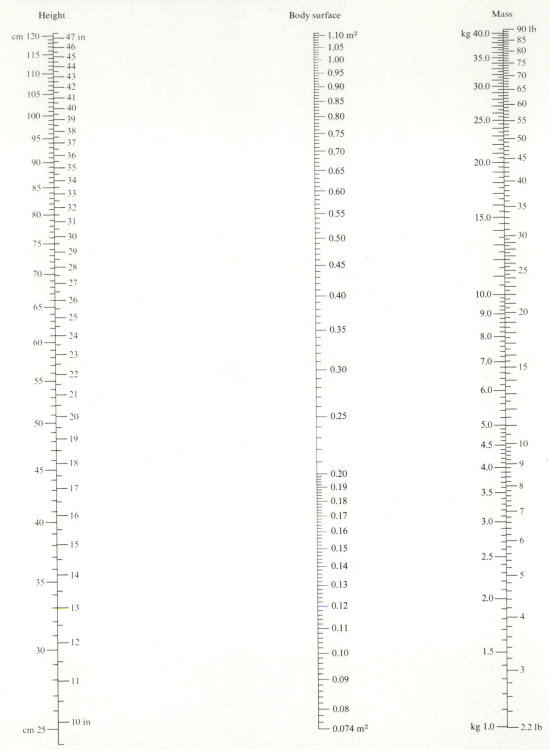

Height	Body surface	Mass

[1] From the formula of Du Bois and Du Bois, *Arch. intern. Med.,* **17**, 863 (1916): $S = M^{0.425} \times H^{0.725} \times 71.84$, or $\log S = \log M \times 0.425 + \log H \times 0.725 + 1.8564$ (S: body surface in cm², M: mass in kg, H: height in cm).
Reproduced with permission from Lentner, C., editor: Geigy scientific tables, ed. 8, vol. 1, Basle, Switzerland, 1981, Ciba-Geigy.

APPENDIX I—CENTERS EXPERIENCED IN THE EVALUATION OF ENDOMYOCARDIAL BIOPSY SPECIMENS

Europe

Arnold Forester, M.D.
Avd. for Patologi
Rikshoospitalet
Universitetet 1 Oslo
Pilestredet 32
Oslo, Norway 0027 Oslo 1

Catharina E. Essed
Dep. of Pathology I
Kijkzigt Ziekenhuis
Dr. Molenwaterplein 40
3015 GD Rotterdam
The Netherlands

Ulrik Baandrup, M.D., Ph.D.
University Institute of Pathology
Aarhus Municipal Hospital
8000 Aarhus C., Denmark

Alf Wennevold, M.D., or S.A. Mortensen, M.D.
Cardiovascular Laboratory
2014 Rigshospitalet, Blegdamsvegj
9 DK-2100 Copenhagen, Denmark

Max Eder, Prof. Dr. Med. and J. Michael Gokel,
Prof. Dr. Med.
Institute of Pathology
University of Munich
Thalkirshner Str. 36
8000 Munchen 2, West Germany

B. Kunkel, Priv. Doz. Dr.
Zentrum der Inneren Medizin
Abteilung fur Kardiologie
Theodor Stern Kai 7
6000 Frankfurt, Federal Republic of Germany

Luc A. Pierard
Institut de Medecine (Cardiologie)
Chu- Sart-Tilman
B-4000 Liege, Belgium

H. Kuhn, Prof. Dr. Med.
Staedtische Urankenanstalten
Oelmuehlenstr. 26
D-48 Bielefeld
3000 Hanover 61, Germany

Roland Hetzer, M.D.
Deutsches Herzzentrum Berlin
Histologisches Laboratorium
Augustenburger Platz 1
1000 Berlin 65

Eckhardt G.J. Olsen, M.D., F.R.C. Path., F.A.C.C.
Department of Histopathology
National Heart Hospital
Westmoreland St.
London, England, WIM 8BA

United States

William Lewis, M.D.
Division of Surgical Pathology
UCLA School of Medicine
Los Angeles, CA 90024

Cheng C. Tsai, M.D.
Immunology Laboratory
St. Louis University School of Medicine
1325 S. Grand Blvd.
St. Louis, MO 63104

Department of Pathology
Loyola University Medical Center
2160 S. First Ave.
Maywood, IL 60153

William D. Edwards, M.D.
Mayo Medical Laboratory
Mayo Clinic
Rochester, MN 55901

John J. Fenoglio, Jr., M.D.
Department of Pathology
Columbia University
630 W. 168th St.
New York, NY 10032

V.J. Ferrans, M.D.
National Institutes of Health
Bldg. 10 Rm. 10-D-48
Bethesda, MD 20205

Shi-Kaung Peng, M.D., Ph.D.
Cardiovascular Pathology
Department of Pathology
Los Angeles Co. Harbor-UCLA Medical Center
1000 W. Carson St.
Torrance, CA 90509

John T. Fallon, M.D., Ph.D.
Department of Pathology, Cardiovascular Unit
Massachusetts General Hospital
Boston, MA 02114

Frederick J. Schoen, M.S.
Cardiac Pathology Laboratory
Department of Pathology
Bringham and Women's Hospital
75 Francis St.
Boston, MA 02115

Jack L. Titus, M.D., Ph.D.
Baylor College of Medicine
6565 Fannin, M.S. 205
Houston, TX 77030

John R. Davis, M.D.
Department of Pathology
University of Arizona College of Medicine
1501 N. Campbell
Tucson, AZ 85724

Allen D. Johnson, M.D., and James Robb, M.D.
Cardiovascular Division
Scripps Clinic
1066 N. Torrey Pines Rd.
La Jolla, CA 92037

Earl F. Rose, M.D.
Department of Pathology
University of Iowa Hospital and Clinics
Iowa City, IA 52242

Ramiah Subramanian, M.D.
Department of Pathology
Middleton Memorial Veterans Administration Hospital
University of Wisconsin Medical Center
2500 Overlook Terrace
Madison, WI 53705

Thomas Colby, M.D.
Department of Pathology
University of Utah Medical Center
Salt Lake City, UT 84132

Manop Hvntrakoon, M.D.
Surgical Pathology
University of Kansas School of Medicine
39th and Rainbow
Kansas City, KS 66103

Hugh A. McAllister, M.D.
Division of Cardiovascular Pathology
St. Luke's Episcopal Hospital
6720 Bertner
Houston, TX 77030

Nelson R. Niles, M.D.
Department of Pathology
Oregon Health Sciences University
3181 S.W. Sam Jackson Park Rd.
Portland, OR 97201

Robert J. Kleinhenz, M.D.
Presbyterian Hospital
2333 Buchanan
P.O. Box 7999
San Francisco, CA 94115

Maria-Theresa Olivari, M.D.
Department of Medicine (Cardiology)
Box 508 Mayo
University of Minnesota
420 Delaware St. S.E.
Minneapolis, MN 55455

Pathology Department
Miami Heart Institute
4701 N. Meridian Ave.
Miami Beach, FL 33140

Masato Takahashi, M.D.
Director of Cardiac Catheterization
  Laboratory
Children's Hospital of Los Angeles
4650 Sunset Blvd.
Los Angeles, CA 900217

Gerald S. Spear, M.D.
Department of Pathology
University of California–Irvine Medi-
  cal Center
101 City Dr. S.
Orange, CA 92668

M.E. Billingham, M.D.
Department of Pathology
Stanford University Medical Center
Stanford, CA 94305

H. Thomas Aretz, M.D.
Department of Pathology
Lahey Clinic Medical Center
41 Mall Rd.
Burlington, MA 01805

Steven Factor, M.D.
Professor of Pathology
Albert Einstein College of Medicine
1300 Morris Parr Ave.
Bronx, NY 10461

Japan

Chuichi Kawai, M.D.
Professor of Medicine
Kyoto University
54 Kawaracho Shogoin, Sakyo-ku
Kyoto, Japan 606

Yasuo Takayama, M.D.
Sakakibara Heart Institute
2-5-4 Yoyogi, Shibuya-ku
Tokyo 151, Japan

Australia

Dr. Vincent Munro
Department of Anatomical Pathology
St. Vincent's Hospital
Victoria Street, Darlinghurst
Sydney, NSW, Australia 2010

Dr. P.J. Harris
Royal Prince Alfred Hospital
Missenden Road, Camperdown
Sydney, NSW, Australia 2050

Canada

K.M.D. Silver
Department of Pathology
Toronto General Hospital
101 College Street
Toronto, Ontario M5G 1L7

Laurel Gray, M.D.
Department of Pathology
Vancouver General Hospital
2775 Heather St.
Vancouver, British Columbia V5Z3J5

M.J. Guerard, M.D.
Department of Pathology
Montreal University
1560 Est. rue Sherhooke
Montreal, Quebec H2L 4K8

R.D.C. Forbes
Department of Pathology
Lyman Duff Bldg.
3775 University St.
Montreal, Quebec H3A 2B4

APPENDIX J—PROFESSIONAL SOCIETIES

American Association of Critical Care Nurses
1 Civic Plaza, Newport Beach, CA 92660
714-644-9310

American Association of Thoracic Surgeons
P.O. Box 1565, 13 Elm St.
Manchester, MA 01944
617-927-8330

American Cardiology Technologists Association
1 Bank St., Suite 307
Gaithersburg, MD 20760
301-258-9009

American College of Cardiology
9111 Old Georgetown Rd., Bethesda, MD 20814
301-897-5400

American College of Chest Physicians
911 Busse Hwy., Park Ridge, IL 60068
312-698-2200

American College of Emergency Physicians
P.O. Box 619911, Dallas, TX 75261
214-659-0911

American College of Radiology
1891 Preston White Dr., Reston, VA 22071
703-648-8900

American Heart Association
7320 Greenville Ave., Dallas, TX 75231
214-750-5300

American Roentgen Ray Society
428 E. Preston St., Baltimore, MD 21202

American Society of Anesthesiologists
515 Busse Hwy., Park Ridge, IL 60068
312-825-5586

American Society of Radiologic Technologists
15000 Central Ave. S.E., Albuquerque, NM 87123
505-298-4500

American Thoracic Society
1740 Broadway, New York, NY 10019
212-245-8000

Emergency Department Nurses Association
666 N. Lake Shore Dr., Chicago, IL 60611
312-649-0297

North American Society of Pacing and Electrophysiology
13 Eaton Ct., Wellesley Hills, MA 02181
617-237-1866

Radiological Society of North America
1415 W. 22nd St., Oakbrook, IL 60521
312-920-2670

Society for Cardiac Angiography
9500 Euclid Ave., Cleveland, OH 44106-4775

Society of Critical Care Medicine
223 E. Imperial Hwy., Suite 110, Fullerton, CA 92635
714-870-5243

Society of Thoracic Surgeons
111 E. Wacker Dr., Chicago, IL 60640
312-644-6610

APPENDIX K—MANUFACTURERS
Product codes

1. Catheter equipment	6. X-ray equipment, imaging equipment
2. Angioplasty equipment	7. Radiologic contrast agents
3. Hemodynamic monitoring equipment	8. Intra-aortic balloon pump
4. Pacemakers, implantable defibrillator	9. Bioptomes
5. Defibrillators (external)	10. Radiation protection supplies

Manufacturer	Product	Address	Telephone
ADAC Laboratories	6	4747 Hellyer Ave. San Jose, CA 95138	408-365-2000
Advanced Cardiovascular Systems, Inc.	1,2	1395 Charleston Rd. Mountain View, CA 94039	415-965-7360 800-227-9902
American Edwards Laboratories	1,2,3	17221 Red Hill Ave. Irvine, CA 92714	714-250-2500 800-424-3278
Angiomedics, Inc.	1,2	2905 Northwest Blvd. Minneapolis, MN 55441	612-553-8600
Angiographic Devices Corp.	6	Littleton, MA	
Angiotec	6	Burlingame, CA	
Argon Medical Corp.	1,3	214 E. Corsicana Athens, TX 75751	214-675-9321
Arrow International, Inc.	1,3	Hill & George Aves. Reading, PA 19610	215-378-0131
Bard Critical Care	1,3	129 Concord Rd. Billerica, MA 01821	617-667-8810 800-323-3419
Bloom Associates Ltd.	3	Reading, PA	
Biotronic Sales, Inc.	4	Lake Oswego, OR	
Burlington Medical Supplies, Inc.	10	14 Cedar St. P.O. Box 350 Amesbury, MA 01913	617-388-7245
Burkhart Roentgen, Inc.	10	3 River Rd. S. Cornwall Bridge, CT 06754	203-672-6695 800-243-XRAY
Camino Laboratories	1,3	7550 Trade St. San Diego, CA 92131	619-566-1750
Cardiac Control Systems Inc.	4	Palm Coast, FL	
Cardiac Pacemakers, Inc.	4	4100 N. Hamline P.O. Box 64079 St. Paul, MN 55164	612-638-4000 800-CARDIAC
Cardiac Resuscitator Corp.	4,5	12244 S.W. Garden Place Portland, OR 97223	503-620-8612
Cardiac-Pace Medical, Inc.	4	2833 N. Fairview Ave. St. Paul, MN 55113	612-483-6787
Cook, Inc.	1,3	P.O. Box 489 Bloomington, IN 47402	812-339-2235
Cook Pacemaker Corp.	4	P.O. Box 529 Leechburg, PA 15656	412-845-8621 800-245-4715
Coratomic, Inc.	4	300 Indian Springs Rd. P.O. Box 434 Indiana, PA 15701	412-349-1811
Cordis Corp.	1,3,4	P.O. Box 25700 Miami, FL 33105	800-327-7714
Critikon, Inc.	1,3	4110 George Rd Tampa FL 33614	813-887-2000

Manufacturer	Product	Address	Telephone
Daig Corp.	1	14901 Minnetonka Industrial Rd. Minnetonka, MN 55345	612-933-4700
Datascope Corp.	8	580 Winters Ave. Paramus, NJ 07652	201-265-8800
Deseret Medical, Inc.	3	9450 S. State St. Sandy, UT 84070	801-255-6851
Electro-catheter Corp.	1	2100 Felver Ct. P.O. Box 1214C Rahway, NJ 07065	201-382-5600 800-526-4243
Eigen Video	6	P.O. Box 848 Nevada City, CA 95959	916-272-3461
Elscint, Inc.	6	930 Commonwealth Ave. Boston, MA 02215	617-739-6000
F. Walter Hanel	10	P.O. Box 95-02-20 8 Munchen 95 Munich, West Germany	089-662066
General Electric Medical Systems	6	Milwaukee, WI	
Gould Inc.	3	Cleveland, OH	
G.V. Medical, Inc.	2	Minneapolis, MN	
Hewlett-Packard Co. Medical Products Division	3,5	1776 Minuteman Rd. Andover, MA 01810	617-682-1500
Honeywell Medical Electronics Division	3,5	1 Campus Dr. Pleasantville, NY 10570	914-769-6700
IMED Corp.	Infusion pump	9925 Carroll Canyon Rd. San Diego, CA 92131	619-566-9000
Intermedics, Inc.	4	240 West Second St. Freeport, TX 77541	409-233-8611 800-231-2330
International Biomedical, Inc.	5,10	P.O. Box 77 Cleburne, TX 76031	817-641-3395
IVAC Corp.	Infusion pump	10300 Campus Point Dr. San Diego, CA 92121	619-458-7000
Keymed House, Stock Road	9	Southend-on-Sea Essex SS2 5QH	0702-616333
Kimal USA, Ltd.	1	R.D. 2–Jackson Rd. Indian Mills, NJ 08088	609-268-9566
Kontron Cardio-Vascular Corp.	8	9 Plymouth St. Everett, MA 02149	617-389-6400
Linton Biomed Corp.	3	2737 77th S.E. P.O. Box 749 Mercer Island, WA 98040	206-236-0870
Mallinckrodt, Inc Science Products Division	7	675 McDonnell Blvd. P.O. Box 5840 St. Louis, MO 63134	314-895-2000 800-354-7442
Mansfield Scientific, Inc.	1,2,3	135 Forbes Blvd. Mansfield, MA 02048	617-339-4112 800-225-2732
Meadox Surgimed Inc.	1,2,3	Oakland, NJ	
Medi-Tech, Inc.	1	480 Pleasant St. P.O. Box 7407 Watertown, MA 02172	617-923-1720 800-225-3238
Medrad, Inc.	1,3	271 Kappa Dr. Pittsburgh, PA 15238	412-782-4600

Manufacturer	Product	Address	Telephone
Medtronic, Inc.	4	7000 Central Ave. N.E. Minneapolis, MN 55432	612-574-4000
Micromedical Devices, Inc.	4	12741 E. Cayley Suite 128 Englewood, CO 80111	303-790-2383
Millar Instruments, Inc.	3	6001 Gulf Freeway Houston, TX 77023	713-923-9171
Moti Enterprises International	6,10	6620 Cobb Dr. Sterling Heights, MI 48007	313-268-6900
NAMIC	2,3	Hudsonfalls, NY	
Oscor Medical Corp.	1,3	P.O. Box 459 Palm Harbor, FL 33563	813-785-0505
Oximetrix, Inc.	3	1212 Terra Bella Ave. Mountain View, CA 94043	415-961-4380
Pace Medical, Inc.	4	Waltham, MA	
Pacesetter Systems, Inc. (A Siemens Company)	4	12884 Bradley Ave. Sylmar, CA 91342	818-362-6822
Phillips Medical Systems, Inc.	6	710 Bridgeport Ave. Shelton, CT 06484	203-926-7674
Physio-Control Corp.	5	11811 Willows Rd. Redmond, WA 98052	206-881-4000
Picker International	6,10	595 Miner Rd. Highland Heights, OH 44143	216-449-3000
Schneider-Medintag A.G.	1,2,3	115 Scharenmoosstrasse CH-8052 Zurich, Switzerland	
SciMed Life Systems, Inc	1,2	13000 County Rd. 6 Minneapolis, MN 55441	612-559-9504 800-328-3320
Shiley (A Pfizer Company)	1,2	17600 Gillette Ave. Irvine, CA 92714	714-250-0500
Siemens-Elema Pacemaker Systems	4	2360 Palmer Dr. Schaumburg, IL 60195	312-397-5950
Siemens Medical Systems, Inc.	4,5	186 Wood Ave. S. Iselin, NJ 08830	201-321-4500
Scholten Surgical Instruments	9	707 Warrington Ave. Redwood City, CA 94063	415-368-5426
Squibb, Inc.	7	P.O. Box 2013 5 Georges Rd. New Brunswick, NJ 08903	201-545-1300
SMEC, Inc.	8	Route 7 Cookeville, TN 38501	615-537-6505
Sorenson Research	1,3	4455 Atherton Dr. Salt Lake City, UT 84123	801-262-2688
Survival Technology, Inc.	5	8101 Glenbrook Rd. Bethesda, MD 20814	301-656-5600
Telectronics	4	Engelwood, CO	
Thomson-CGR Medical Group	6	Columbia, MD	
Toshiba Medical Systems	6	Tustin, CA	
Transamerica Delaval Medical Products	3	Pasadena, CA	
Tremedyne, Inc.	1	1815 E. Carnegie Ave. Santa Ana, CA 92705	714-261-9041

Manufacturer	Product	Address	Telephone
UMI Corp.	1,3	P.O. Box 100 Ballston Spa, NY 12020	518-587-5095
United Shielding Technology	10	P.O. Box 542 300 Canal St. Lawrence, MA 01842	617-689-4334
USCI Division, C.R. Bard, Inc.	1,2,3	P.O. Box 566 Billerica, MA 01821	617-667-2511 800-225-0898
Vanguard Instrument Corp.	6	Melville, NY	
Vari-X, Inc.	6	17601 Fitch Ave. Irvine, CA 92714	714-754-0617
Victoreen Nuclear Associates	10	100 Voice Rd. Carle Place, NY 11514	516-714-6360
Vitatron Medical B.V.	4	P.O. Box 76 Dieren, The Netherlands	833-19010
Waters Instruments, Inc.	3	2411 N.W. Seventh St. P.O. Box 6117 Rochester, MN 55903	507-288-7777
Winthrop-Breon Laboratories	7	90 Park Ave. New York, NY 10016	212-907-2000
ZMI Corp.	4	325 Vassar St. Cambridge, MA 02139	617-576-3986 800-348-8911

Index